Winter's BASIC CLINICAL PHARMACOKINETICS

Seventh Edition

Winter's **BASIC CLINICAL PHARMACOKINETICS**

Seventh Edition

Editor

Paul M. Beringer, PharmD

Professor
Titus Family Department of Clinical Pharmacy
USC Alfred E. Mann School of Pharmacy and Pharmaceutical Sciences
University of Southern California
Los Angeles, California

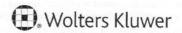

Philadelphia · Baltimore · New York · London
Buenos Aires · Hong Kong · Sydney · Tokyo

Acquisitions Editor: Matt Hauber
Development Editor: Deborah Bordeaux
Freelance Development Editor: Maria McAvey
Editorial Coordinator: Priyanka Alagar
Marketing Manager: Danielle Klahr
Production Project Manager: Justin Wright
Manager of Graphic Arts and Design: Stephen Druding
Art Director: Jennifer Clements
Manufacturing Coordinator: Margie Orzech
Prepress Vendor: S4Carlisle Publishing Services

Seventh Edition

Library of Congress Cataloging-in-Publication Data
ISBN-13: 978-1-975195-24-3
ISBN-10: 1-975195-24-8
Library of Congress Control Number: 2023910034

MPP0823

I would like to dedicate this edition to my wife, Annie Wong-Beringer, PharmD, who is a constant source of inspiration both personally and professionally.

Contributors

Timothy J. Bensman, PharmD, PhD
Clinical Pharmacologist
Division of Infectious Disease Pharmacology
U.S. Food and Drug Administration
Silver Spring, Maryland

Paul M. Beringer, PharmD
Professor
Titus Family Department of Clinical Pharmacy
USC Alfred E. Mann School of Pharmacy and Pharmaceutical Sciences
University of Southern California
Los Angeles, California

Sunita Dergalust, PharmD
Clinical Pharmacy Specialist in Neurology
Pharmacy
VA Greater Los Angeles Healthcare System
Los Angeles, California

Thomas C. Dowling, PharmD, PhD
Professor and Assistant Dean
College of Pharmacy
Ferris State University
Big Rapids, Michigan

Mary H. H. Ensom, PharmD, FASHP, FCCP, FCSHP, FCAHS
Professor Emerita, Faculty of Pharmaceutical Sciences
Emerita Distinguished University Scholar
The University of British Columbia
Vancouver, British Columbia, Canada

Reginald F. Frye, PharmD, PhD
Professor, Chair, and Associate Dean
Department of Pharmacotherapy and Translational Research
University of Florida College of Pharmacy
Gainesville, Florida

Emily Han, PharmD
Assistant Professor of Clinical Pharmacy
USC Alfred E. Mann School of Pharmacy and Pharmaceutical Sciences
University of Southern California
Los Angeles, California

James Kevin Hicks, PharmD, PhD, FCCP
Associate Member
Individualized Cancer Management
Moffitt Cancer Center
Tampa, Florida

Tony K. L. Kiang, BSc (Pharm), ACPR, PhD
Assistant Professor (Tenure-Track)
Faculty of Pharmacy and
Pharmaceutical Sciences
University of Alberta
Edmonton, Alberta, Canada

Russell E. Lewis, PharmD
Associate Professor of Infectious
Diseases
Department of Molecular Medicine
University of Padua
Padova, Italy

Emi Minejima, PharmD
Associate Professor of Clinical
Pharmacy
USC Alfred E. Mann School of
Pharmacy and Pharmaceutical
Sciences
University of Southern California
Los Angeles, California

Scott A. Mosley, PharmD
Assistant Professor of Clinical Pharmacy
USC Alfred E. Mann School of
Pharmacy and Pharmaceutical
Sciences
University of Southern California
Los Angeles, California

Viet-Huong Nguyen, PharmD, MPH, MSc
Associate Professor
Pharmacy Practice
Chapman University School of
Pharmacy
Irvine, California

Manjunath P. Pai, PharmD
Professor and Chair of Clinical
Pharmacy
University of Michigan College of
Pharmacy
Ann Arbor, Michigan

Laura F. Ruekert, PharmD
Associate Professor of Pharmacy
Practice
Pharmacy Practice
Butler University
Indianapolis, Indiana

Noha N. Salama, PhD, BSc (Pharm), RPh
Professor, Pharmaceutics,
Biopharmaceutics and
Pharmacokinetics
Department of Pharmaceutical and
Administrative Sciences
University of Health Science &
Pharmacy in St. Louis
St. Louis, Missouri

Irving Steinberg, PharmD
Associate Dean for Faculty
Affairs; Associate Professor
of Clinical Pharmacy and
Pediatrics
USC Alfred E. Mann School of
Pharmacy and Pharmaceutical
Sciences and Keck School of
Medicine
University of Southern California
Los Angeles, California

Toby Trujillo, PharmD
Associate Professor
Clinical Pharmacy
University of Colorado Skaggs School
of Pharmacy and Pharmaceutical
Sciences
Aurora, Colorado

Jeanne H. VanTyle[†]

†Deceased.

Autumn Walkerly, PharmD, BCPS, BCPP
Assistant Professor of Clinical Pharmacy
USC Alfred E. Mann School of
Pharmacy and Pharmaceutical
Sciences
University of Southern California
Los Angeles, California

Paul Wong, PharmD
Assistant Professor of Clinical
Pharmacy
USC Alfred E. Mann School of
Pharmacy and Pharmaceutical
Sciences
University of Southern California
Los Angeles, California

Preface

Since the publication of the first edition of *Basic Clinical Pharmacokinetics* more than 40 years ago, the use of serum drug concentrations as a guide for monitoring drug therapy remains a key tool to optimizing the efficacy and safety of medications for a variety of disorders. Pharmacokinetic and biopharmaceutical principles in predicting plasma drug concentrations, as well as the changes in plasma drug concentrations that occur over time, are now widely accepted as useful adjuncts in patient care. With the continued advancement of analytical technology, every healthcare institution and practitioner has access to a wide range of drug assays, and monitoring serum drug concentrations has become the standard of practice for many drugs. As we continue to gain more knowledge about both the limitations and applications of drug concentrations and their correlation with either efficacy or toxicity, concentration sampling strategies change. Appropriate use of serum drug concentrations, however, continues to be a major problem in the clinical setting. Basic pharmacokinetic principles must be applied rationally to specific patients.

Patient care continues to trend toward value-based care. This includes everything from minimizing and streamlining drug therapy and laboratory testing to the increased use of automation. The use of serum drug concentrations is not immune to the pressure of doing more with less. It is my hope that this seventh edition of *Basic Clinical Pharmacokinetics* will help the clinician in the rational application of pharmacokinetics and therapeutic drug monitoring to patient care and help to ensure that drug concentration monitoring is focused in an optimal way on the most appropriate patients.

A number of physiologic and mathematical assumptions have been made. This is a common practice in the clinical setting because of the dosing strategies and the limited number of concentrations sampled. An attempt has been made to alert the reader to these assumptions. There are a large number of texts and articles that present a much more detailed and in-depth analysis and explanation of the physiologic and pharmacokinetic principles being discussed. It is not the intent of this book to explore all of these issues. Rather, the goal of this book is to simplify pharmacokinetics so that it can be more easily understood and visualized by practitioners, and as a consequence, the use of pharmacokinetics can become part of their professional practice.

Although plasma drug concentrations are useful in evaluating drug therapy, they constitute only one source of information. They should not, therefore, be used as the sole criterion on which treatment is based. Pharmacokinetic calculations should be considered only as an adjunctive guide to the determination of dosing regimens.

If a calculated dosing regimen seems unreasonable, reevaluation is essential because sampling or assay errors, an inaccurate dosing history, or a mathematical error is always a possibility. Another problem inherent in these calculations is that the literature or assumed pharmacokinetic parameters utilized may be inappropriate for the patient under consideration. Many of the pharmacokinetic parameters available in the literature are based upon a relatively small number of patients or normal volunteers. Therefore, values obtained from these experimental data are, at best, estimates for any given patient. If the basic underlying pharmacokinetic assumptions are not applicable to the particular patient, even the most elegant calculation will be invalid.

Review articles and some texts commonly list pharmacokinetic parameters for a number of drugs and are a good initial source of pharmacokinetic information. However, the reader is encouraged to seek out the original literature to evaluate the methodology and data from which this information was derived. Some factors that should be considered in scrutinizing these studies include the number and type of subjects, type and specificity of drug assay, degree of inter- and intrasubject variability, statistical analysis of the data, and whether the drug was studied prospectively or retrospectively. The potential problems associated with using the literature data to predict disposition of a drug within a specific patient emphasize the need to obtain accurate plasma-level measurements. Clearly, the literature can serve as a guide to make initial a priori clinical decisions, but even with the best predictions, significant variance does exist. Therefore, only with a complete dosing history, appropriate drug sampling, accurate and specific assay procedures, and logical pharmacokinetic analysis can patient-specific parameters be derived that will be useful adjuncts to providing optimal patient care and improving clinical outcomes.

ORGANIZATIONAL PHILOSOPHY

The book is divided into two parts: Part I reviews basic pharmacokinetic principles and special populations, and Part II illustrates the clinical application of pharmacokinetics to specific drugs through the presentation and step-by-step solutions of common clinical problems. The reader is strongly urged to read each section in the order it appears in the book because many of the concepts discussed in the latter portions of the book are based on an understanding of those presented earlier. The appendices from previous editions—Nomograms for Calculating Body Surface Area, Common Equations Used Throughout the Text, Algorithm for Evaluating and Interpreting Plasma Concentrations, and Glossary of Terms and Abbreviations—are also included and have been updated as appropriate.

Part I

As in previous editions, Part I is divided into chapters that describe major pharmacokinetic parameters and their clinical applications. Equations that express the relationships between the various parameters and the resultant plasma concentrations are presented and discussed. Many individuals feel overwhelmed by the apparent complexity of some of the equations used to describe the pharmacokinetic behavior of drugs. Therefore, extensive explanations that emphasize major concepts accompany the more complex equations. Figures continue to be useful to help the reader visualize the concepts that are being reviewed. The principles discussed in Part I give the clinician the basis for manipulating the dosing regimens and interpreting plasma concentrations for the drugs discussed in Part II of this book.

In this seventh edition, the authors and I have attempted to maintain a simple clinical approach to the application of pharmacokinetic principles to patient care. A number of sections in Part I have been expanded, including new chapters on obesity and pregnancy.

Part II

Most of the chapters on drugs in Part II now contain cases that address pediatric considerations and pharmacogenomics information where relevant. The drugs discussed in Part II were selected because they represent the most commonly monitored drugs in the clinical setting, assays are widely available, and an understanding of their pharmacokinetic and biopharmaceutical properties can substantially aid clinicians in dosing these drugs more rationally and safely. The updates include new information on the clinical use of serum drug concentrations, and where appropriate, new cases and examples have been added to further expand and exemplify the use of pharmacokinetics in clinical practice.

Over the years, some drugs have been deleted for a variety of reasons. In some cases, the drugs have been replaced by safer, more efficacious agents that do not require drug concentration monitoring. There have been few new drugs that have gained acceptance as requiring concentration monitoring. The reasons for this vary, but, in most cases, plasma concentration monitoring is limited to those drugs that have a narrow therapeutic index and/or when toxicity or lack of efficacy is clinically unacceptable. Nonetheless, the basic pharmacokinetic principles about drug accumulation, selecting dosing intervals, and when to monitor for either efficacy or toxicity continue to be important considerations in clinical practice. In this edition, we have added a new chapter on anticoagulants and expansion of the oncology therapies in response to new data supporting pharmacogenomics of these agents.

For each of the drugs in Part II, examples of the most common pharmacokinetic manipulations, such as calculation of a loading dose and maintenance dose, are presented. An example of the process used to interpret a reported plasma concentration is also given. In addition, pathophysiologic factors and drug-drug interactions that influence the pharmacokinetics of these drugs and their significance are discussed. Examples of the most common problems encountered in clinical practice are also given to help the reader recognize when caution should be exercised in making patient care decisions based upon serum drug concentrations and pharmacokinetic principles. Ultimately, the goal is for the reader to recognize the fundamental principles that are being applied to each of the drugs. As confidence and skill in using pharmacokinetics as a clinical tool are developed, it is hoped that the reader will then be able to apply these same principles to new drugs and situations not covered in this book.

ONLINE RESOURCES

Basic Clinical Pharmacokinetics, seventh edition, includes an image bank for instructors that is available on the book's companion website at http://thePoint.lww.com/Beringer7e.

ACKNOWLEDGMENTS

The completion of the seventh edition edition of *Basic Clinical Pharmacokinetics* would not have been possible without the support of my family, friends, and colleagues. I am grateful to the highly professional coauthors who lent their expertise, knowledge, and skills to contribute new chapters and provide important updates to the individual chapters on drugs.

I would also like to recognize and thank the many students, residents, and colleagues who have provided feedback about what helps them understand and apply pharmacokinetics to their professional practice.

Most of all, I would like to thank Dr Michael Winter for introducing me to the field of clinical pharmacokinetics, serving as a role model for education in pharmacy and for providing the opportunity to contribute to this important textbook.

Contents

APPENDICES

I

BASIC PRINCIPLES

The goals and objectives in Part I, Basic Principles, should be used in concert with the goals and objectives in Part II, Drug Monographs.

GOAL

To understand and be able to apply the basic pharmacokinetic principles to the specific drugs in Part II, the learner needs to not only be able to "say the words" and write the equations that are outlined in Part I but also, just as importantly, develop an understanding of the principles and equations so that when presented in a different way, the principle can be recognized and applied. This second step is not an easy one to take. Pharmacokinetics is a language, and to truly understand the equations and become "fluent" requires patience, practice, and time. As an example, if asked "how much drug is remaining after one half-life," most can immediately answer "half." However, if asked what is the value of e^{-Kt}, where t is one half-life, most have to ponder the question for some time before arriving at the same answer.

The following set out the goals for Part I: Basic Principles:

1. Understand and appreciate the meaning of the factors that can influence drug absorption into the body.
2. Understand and be able to assign a dosing rate.
3. Appreciate the influence of plasma protein binding on the total, bound, and unbound drug concentration and the influence of altered plasma binding on the desired or target drug concentration.
4. Understand the concept of the "apparent volume of distribution" and the clinical utility of volume of distribution with regard to calculating a dose that would rapidly achieve a desired plasma concentration.
5. Understand how clearance (Cl) can be used to calculate drug loss and maintenance dosing regimens and the importance of renal and hepatic function in determining Cl.
6. Understand the first-order rate constant (K) and half-life with regard to drug elimination and accumulation and how drug concentrations will change with time. In addition, given a set of variables, the learner should be able to determine what additional pharmacokinetic parameters or information can be calculated.

1

7. Understand the relationship between $[(S)(F)(\text{Dose})]/V$, the dosing interval, the drug half-life, and the maximum and minimum plasma concentrations.

8. Given a set of pharmacokinetic parameters and a drug dosing history, be able to draw to approximate scale a plasma concentration versus time curve. Conversely, given a plasma concentration versus time curve, be able to write the equations that represent the curve.

9. Given a patient's dosing history, plasma drug concentration(s), and the literature estimates of the drug's pharmacokinetic parameters, be able to determine whether it is likely that the measured drug concentration represents steady state or non–steady state and then select the model to revise the proper pharmacokinetic parameter(s).

10. Describe the key drug Cl mechanisms in the kidney, and estimate creatinine Cl in various patient populations, including chronic kidney disease (CKD), acute kidney injury (AKI), pediatrics, obesity, and older adults.

11. Obtain an appreciation for the types of dialysis (intermittent hemo, continuous renal replacement, and peritoneal) and understand how each is likely to affect drug elimination and dosing strategies.

12. Appreciate the need for specific pediatric pharmacokinetic studies and clinical application concepts, and differences between children and adults.

13. Understand how genetic variation in drug disposition proteins affects therapeutic efficacy and toxicity.

1

PHARMACOKINETIC PROCESSES AND PARAMETERS

Paul M. Beringer

Learning Objectives

By the end of the pharmacokinetic processes and parameters chapter, the learner shall be able to:

Bioavailability (*F*)

1. Define bioavailability and list the typical conditions necessary for absorption into the systemic circulation, following oral administration (eg, stability in gastrointestinal [GI] fluids, proper lipid vs water solubility).
2. Define dosage form and salt form (*S*), and list two or more drugs that are administered as different dosage and/or salt forms.
3. Define first-pass effect with regard to hepatic metabolism and transport and what influence it can have on oral bioavailability if there is a significant first-pass effect.
4. Describe the relationship between the oral and parenteral dose of a drug that has a significant first-pass effect.

Administration Rate (R_A)

1. Define dose and dosing interval.
2. Describe the difference between a continuous infusion and an intermittent dosing regimen.
3. Explain how the units for dosing interval are usually assigned for drugs that are administered on a regular but intermittent basis.

Desired Plasma Concentration (*C*)

1. Define fraction unbound (fu).
2. Explain saturable plasma binding and at what concentrations most drugs might show saturable binding. List one drug that is known to have saturable plasma binding.

3. Describe the impact of a decrease in the plasma protein on the:
   a. Total plasma concentration
   b. Bound plasma concentration
   c. Unbound plasma concentration
4. Explain the effect on the desired plasma concentration necessary to give a normal therapeutic response when plasma binding is decreased.
5. List two or more drugs that have an fu of 0.1.
6. Know the plasma protein to which drugs that are weak acids bind most frequently.
7. Describe the effect of end-stage renal failure on the total, bound, and unbound phenytoin concentration.
8. List two reasons why assays for unbound drug concentrations would be desirable and two reasons why not.

Volume of Distribution (V)

1. Define with an equation the relationship between volume of distribution, total amount of drug in the body, and the assayed plasma concentration.
2. List two conditions or factors that would increase the apparent volume of distribution and two factors that would decrease the apparent volume of distribution.
3. Demonstrate with an equation how to calculate an initial loading dose necessary to achieve a desired plasma concentration.
4. Demonstrate with an equation how to determine the loading dose if the patient has an initial plasma concentration.
5. Explain the significance of two-compartment modeling when the end organ for response (receptors) behaves as though they are in the first compartment. Consider the rapid onset and the initial rapid decline in pharmacologic effect relative to administration of the loading dose. List at least two drugs that behave this way.
6. Explain the significance of two-compartment modeling when the end organ for response (receptors) behaves as though they are in slower equilibrating tissue compartment. List at least two drugs that behave this way.
7. Why do almost all drugs display two-compartment modeling when given intravenously (IV), but not when given orally? Name two drugs that are an exception and the distribution phase can be seen following oral administration.
8. Explain for a drug with a large volume of distribution, that is, the majority of drug is in the tissue, the impact of a decrease in plasma binding on the loading dose of a drug.

Clearance (Cl)

1. Use an equation to "define" Cl relative to a dosing regimen $[(S)(F)(\text{Dose}/\tau)]$ and the $C_{ss\ ave}$.

2. Select the proper units (volume/time) for Cl, given a dosing regimen and $C_{ss\,ave}$.
3. Calculate the third if any two of the three (dosing regimen, $C_{ss\,ave}$, and Cl) are given.
4. Approximate a patient's body surface area if weight is given.
5. Explain why, when plasma protein binding is decreased, the $C_{ss\,ave}$ of the unbound drug almost always remain unchanged. The learner shall also be able to give at least one example.
6. Calculate Cl and dosing rate adjustment factors that can be used to calculate a dose for a patient with compromised renal or hepatic function, given the renal Cl and metabolic Cl (or fractions eliminated renally and metabolically).
7. List at least four factors that can influence or alter Cl.

Elimination Rate Constant (K) and Half-life ($t_{1/2}$)

1. Define K with regard to Cl and V and be able to identify which of the variables (K, Cl, or V) are dependent and which are independent.
2. Perform a unit analysis and select units that are consistent for K, Cl, and V.
3. Calculate the expected drug concentration (C_2) after a given time interval (t), given an initial drug concentration (C_1) and K value.
4. Calculate the K value, given two drug concentrations (C_1 and C_2) and the time interval between the two.
5. Explain why the time interval between C_1 and C_2 should be a minimum of one half-life in order to make a reasonable estimate of K or $t_{1/2}$.
6. Know the number of half-lives necessary to achieve 90% of steady state, and explain why, in clinical practice, many use four or five half-lives as the time necessary to ensure steady state has been attained.
7. Calculate a non–steady-state drug concentration (C_1) t_1 hours after initiating a constant infusion and the drug concentration (C_2) t_2 hours after ending the infusion.

Maximum and Minimum Plasma Concentrations

1. Write the equations representing the maximum or minimum concentration, assuming instantaneous absorption and an intermittent, fixed dosing interval.
2. Draw a graph of the steady-state plasma concentrations that is approximately to scale, given a dosing interval and drug half-life. For example, if the dosing interval is equal to the half-life, the peak should be 2 times the trough and the line connecting the peak and trough should be slightly convexly curved.
3. Explain why, if the dosing interval is much less than the drug half-life, the C_{ss} trough can be used as $C_{ss\,ave}$ to calculate Cl.

Bioavailability (*F*)

DEFINITION

Bioavailability is the percentage or fraction of the administered dose that reaches the systemic circulation of the patient. Examples of factors that can alter bioavailability include the inherent dissolution and absorption characteristics of the administered chemical form (eg, salt, ester), the dosage form (eg, tablet, capsule), the route of administration, the stability of the active ingredient in the gastrointestinal (GI) tract, and the extent of drug metabolism and transport before reaching the systemic circulation. Drugs can be metabolized by GI bacteria, the GI mucosa, and the liver before reaching the systemic circulation.

To calculate the amount of drug absorbed, the administered dose should be multiplied by a bioavailability factor, which is usually represented by the letter *F*. For example, the bioavailability of digoxin is estimated to be 0.7 for orally administered tablets.[1-3] This means that if 250 µg (0.25 mg) of digoxin is given orally, the effective or absorbed dose can be calculated by multiplying the administered dose by *F*:

$$\text{Amount of drug absorbed or reaching the systemic circulation} = (F)(\text{Dose}) \qquad \textbf{(Eq. 1.1)}$$

$$
\begin{aligned}
\text{For the previous example, amount of drug absorbed or reaching the systemic circulation} &= (F)(\text{Dose}) \\
&= (0.7)(250\ \mu g) \\
&= 175\ \mu g
\end{aligned}
$$

It should be emphasized that this factor does not take into consideration the rate of drug absorption; it only estimates the extent of absorption. Although the rate of absorption can be important when rapid onset of pharmacologic effects is required, it is not usually important when a drug is administered chronically. The rate of absorption is important only when it is so slow that it limits the absolute bioavailability of the drug, or when it is so rapid that too much drug is too quickly absorbed. "Dose dumping" can occur under certain conditions with some sustained-release preparations.[4,5] In addition, incomplete absorption of sustained-release dosage forms should be considered in patients who have a short GI transit time. GI transit times of 24 to 48 hours are probably average, but patients with bowel disease may have transit times of only a few hours. A lower-than-average bioavailability should be considered in these patients, especially when the duration of absorption is extended.

DOSAGE FORM

As noted previously, bioavailability can vary among different formulations and dosage forms of a drug. For example, digoxin elixir has a bioavailability of approximately 80% (*F* = 0.8), whereas the soft gelatin capsules have a bioavailability of 100% (*F* = 1.0). This is in contrast to the tablets, which have a bioavailability of 70% (*F* = 0.7).[2,6,7]

When drugs are administered parenterally, the bioavailability is usually considered to be 100% ($F = 1.0$). Equation 1.1 can be rearranged to calculate equivalent doses of a drug when a patient is to receive a different dosage form of the same drug.

$$\frac{\text{Dose of new}}{\text{dosage form}} = \frac{\substack{\text{Amount of drug absorbed} \\ \text{from current dosage form}}}{F \text{ of new dosage form}} \qquad \text{(Eq. 1.2)}$$

For example, if a patient who has been receiving digoxin 250 µg (0.25 mg) in the tablet dosage form, with a bioavailability of 0.7, needs to receive digoxin elixir, an equivalent dose of the elixir would be calculated as follows:

$$\text{Dose of elixir} = \frac{(0.7)(250\,\mu g)}{0.8}$$

$$= \frac{175\,\mu g}{0.8}$$

$$= 219\,\mu g$$

If the soft gelatin capsules of digoxin were to be administered, the bioavailability or F of the new dosage form would have been 1.0, and the equivalent dose would have been 175 µg.

The bioavailability of parenterally administered drugs is usually assumed to be 1.0. Drugs that are administered as inactive precursors that must then be converted to an active product are an exception to this rule. If some of the inactive precursor is eliminated from the body (renally excreted or metabolized to an inactive compound) before it can be converted to the active compound, the bioavailability will be less than 1.0. For example, parenteral chloramphenicol is given as the succinate ester, and this chloramphenicol ester must be hydrolyzed to the active compound. The bioavailability of the parenterally administered chloramphenicol succinate ranges from 55% to 95% because 5% to 45% of the chloramphenicol ester is eliminated renally before it can be converted to the active compound.[8-10] Generally, for those drugs with nearly complete absorption ($F > 0.8$), bioavailability is usually consistent. For those drugs with a low oral bioavailability ($F < 0.5$), there is often a large variation in the extent of absorption. This is not a hard-and-fast rule because any drug under the right conditions can have an altered bioavailability.

CHEMICAL FORM (S)

The chemical form of a drug must also be considered when evaluating bioavailability. For example, when a salt or an ester of a drug is administered, the bioavailability factor (F) should be multiplied by the fraction of the total molecular weight that the active drug represents. If S represents the fraction of the administered dose that is the active drug, then the amount of drug absorbed from a salt or an ester form can be calculated as follows:

$$\text{Amount of drug absorbed or reaching the systemic circulation} = (S)(F)(\text{Dose}) \qquad \text{(Eq. 1.3)}$$

The S factor should be included in all bioavailability equations as a constant reminder of its importance in assessing bioavailability of the active drug form. When a drug is administered in its parent or active form, the S for that drug is 1.0.

Equation 1.2 can now be expanded to consider the salt factor and the bioavailability when calculating the dose of a new dosage form:

$$\text{Dose of new dosage form} = \frac{\text{Amount of drug absorbed from current dosage form}}{(S)(F) \text{ of new dosage form}} \qquad \text{(Eq. 1.4)}$$

Aminophylline and phenytoin are examples of this principle (Figure 1.1). Aminophylline is the ethylenediamine salt of the pharmacologically active moiety, theophylline. For this salt, 80% to 85% (by weight) is theophylline so that the S for aminophylline is approximately 0.8. Uncoated aminophylline tablets are considered to be completely (100%) bioavailable; the bioavailability factor (F) for this dosage form is, therefore, 1.0. It is important to consider the salt form in determining the amount of theophylline absorbed from an aminophylline tablet. When Equation 1.3 is applied to this situation, it can be demonstrated that 160 mg of theophylline is absorbed from a 200-mg aminophylline tablet.

$$\text{Amount of drug absorbed or reaching the systemic circulation} = (S)(F)(\text{Dose})$$
$$= (0.8)(1)(200 \text{ mg aminophylline})$$
$$= 160 \text{ mg theophylline}$$

Similarly, 300 mg of phenytoin sodium with an S of 0.92 represents only 276 mg of phenytoin reaching the systemic circulation, assuming complete absorption ($F = 1$).

$$\text{Amount of drug absorbed or reaching the systemic circulation} = (S)(F)(\text{Dose})$$
$$= (0.92)(1)(300 \text{ mg phenytoin sodium})$$
$$= 276 \text{ mg phenytoin}$$

In some cases, the labeled amount of drug has already taken into account the amount of active drug. Valproate sodium, the sodium salt of valproic acid, is manufactured and labeled with the amount of valproic acid; therefore, a value of 1 would be appropriate for S. Fosphenytoin sodium is the sodium salt of the phosphate ester of phenytoin. Although fosphenytoin sodium is only 61% phenytoin, the manufacturers have labeled the drug as phenytoin sodium equivalents or P.E. Therefore, to calculate

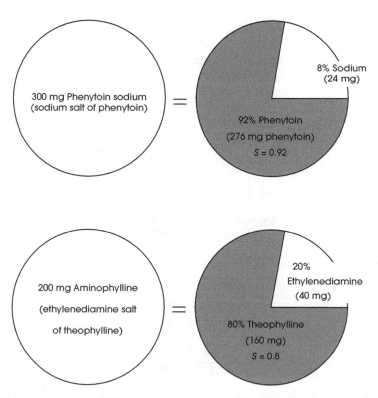

FIGURE 1.1 The effect of the chemical drug form on bioavailability. The previous examples emphasize the importance of considering the chemical form when calculating the amount of active drug actually administered. The amount of active drug administered may represent only a fraction (S) of the salt, ester, or other chemical form of the drug contained in the formulation. The bioavailability (F) of the dosage form itself must also be considered when drugs are administered by the oral route.

the amount of phenytoin in 100 mg of fosphenytoin P.E., an S value of 0.92 would be used.

The important concept is to understand and be able to calculate the amount of the labeled drug that will be available to the patient as active drug. To do this, both the fraction of the dose that is active drug (S) and the bioavailability or fraction of administered dose that will reach the systemic circulation (F) need to be considered when calculating doses and dosing regimens.

FIRST-PASS EFFECT

Because orally administered drugs are absorbed from the GI tract into the portal circulation, some drugs may be extensively metabolized by the liver or undergo intestinal efflux via transporters before reaching the systemic circulation. The term "first pass" refers to metabolism by the liver because the drug passes through the liver via the portal vein following absorption. This "first-pass effect" can substantially decrease the amount of active drug reaching the systemic circulation and thus its bioavailability (Figure 1.2).

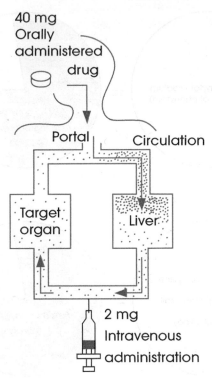

40 mg
Orally
administered
drug

Portal   Circulation

Target organ

Liver

2 mg
Intravenous
administration

FIGURE 1.2 First-pass effect. When drugs with a high "first-pass effect" are administered orally, a large amount of the absorbed drug is metabolized or undergoes intestinal efflux before it reaches the systemic circulation. If the drug is administered intravenously, the liver is bypassed and the fraction of the administered dose that reaches the circulation is increased. Parenteral doses of drugs with a high "first pass" are much smaller than oral doses necessary to produce equivalent pharmacologic effects.

Propranolol is an example of a drug that has a significant portion of an orally administered dose that does not reach the systemic circulation because it is metabolized as it passes through the liver following absorption from the GI tract. Because of this "first-pass effect," oral bioavailability is low, and orally administered doses are much larger than doses administered intravenously (IV). However, the propranolol issue is further complicated by the fact that one of the metabolites, 4-hydroxy-propranolol, is pharmacologically active.[11] Lidocaine is an example of a drug with a first-pass effect that is so great that oral administration is not practical as a route of administration if systemic effects are desired.[12] In addition, some drugs are extensively metabolized by cytochrome enzymes, primarily CYP3A4, that are located in the gut wall. As an example, the low and variable bioavailability ($F \approx 0.3$) of cyclosporine is in part because of metabolism by CYP3A4 and efflux via P-glycoprotein in the gut wall.[13]

Administration Rate (R_A)

The administration rate is the average rate at which absorbed drug reaches the systemic circulation. This is usually calculated by dividing the amount of drug absorbed (see Equation 1.3) by the time over which the drug was administered (dosing interval). The dosing interval is usually represented by the symbol τ.

$$\text{Administration rate } R_A = \frac{(S)(F)(\text{Dose})}{\tau} \qquad \text{(Eq. 1.5)}$$

When drugs are administered as a continuous infusion, the dosing interval can be expressed in any convenient time unit. For example, the theophylline administration rate resulting from aminophylline infused at a rate of 40 mg/hr is calculated using Equation 1.5 as follows:

$$\begin{aligned} \text{Administration rate } R_A &= \frac{(S)(F)(\text{Dose})}{\tau} \\ &= \frac{(0.8)(1)(40 \text{ mg})}{1 \text{ hr}} \\ &= 32 \text{ mg/hr} \end{aligned}$$

or

$$\begin{aligned} \text{Administration rate } R_A &= \frac{(S)(F)(\text{Dose})}{\tau} \\ &= \frac{(0.8)(1)(40 \text{ mg})}{60 \text{ min}} \\ &= 0.53 \text{ mg/min} \end{aligned}$$

When drugs are administered at fixed dosing intervals, the calculated administration rate would be an average value. For example, the average administration rate of digoxin resulting from an oral dose of 250 µg of digoxin given orally as tablets every day would be calculated using Equation 1.5 as follows:

$$\begin{aligned} \text{Administration rate } R_A &= \frac{(S)(F)(\text{Dose})}{\tau} \\ &= \frac{(1)(0.7)(250 \text{ mg})}{1 \text{ d}} \\ &= 175 \text{ µg/d} \end{aligned}$$

or

$$\begin{aligned} \text{Administration rate } R_A &= \frac{(S)(F)(\text{Dose})}{\tau} \\ &= \frac{(1)(0.7)(250 \text{ mg})}{24 \text{ hr}} \\ &= 7.29 \text{ µg/hr} \end{aligned}$$

Although each digoxin tablet is actually absorbed over 1 to 2 hours, the average "administration rate" is calculated over the entire dosing interval. Although the administration rate of 7.29 µg/hr and 175 µg/d are equivalent, most clinicians think of the dosing rate that is consistent with how the drug is administered. In this case, the usual interval would be 1 day because digoxin is most commonly administered once each day. In the section on clearance (Cl), we consider how the drug administration rate, drug Cl, and the usually reported units for drug concentration all need to be consistent for the purposes of performing pharmacokinetic calculations.

Desired Plasma Concentration (C)

PROTEIN BINDING

Most clinical laboratory reports of drug concentrations in plasma (C) represent drug that is bound to plasma protein plus drug that is unbound or free. It is the free or unbound drug that is in equilibrium with the receptor site and is, therefore, the pharmacologically active moiety. Thus, in the case of a drug with significant plasma binding, the reported plasma drug concentration indirectly reflects the concentration of free or active drug (Figure 1.3).

Some disease states are associated with decreased plasma proteins or with decreased binding of drugs to plasma proteins.[14-17] In these situations, drugs that are usually highly protein bound have a larger percentage of free or unbound drug present in plasma. Therefore, a greater pharmacologic effect can be expected for any given drug concentration in plasma (C). Clinicians must always consider altered protein binding

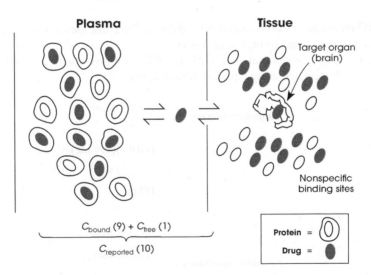

FIGURE 1.3 Plasma concentration of a highly protein-bound drug: normal plasma protein concentration. The plasma drug concentration reported by the laboratory represents a total of both "bound" and "free" drugs. It is the "free" drug that is in equilibrium with the target organs and is the pharmacologically active moiety. In this illustration, fu (or the fraction of free drug to total drug concentration) is 0.1.

and whether the fraction of free drug concentration or fraction unbound (fu) is altered when interpreting or establishing the desired plasma drug concentrations.

$$fu = \frac{Free\,drug\,concentration}{Total\,drug\,concentration}$$

$$fu = \frac{C_{free}}{C_{bound} + C_{free}} \qquad \text{(Eq. 1.6)}$$

The fraction of drug that is unbound (fu) does not vary with the drug concentration for most drugs that are bound primarily to albumin. This is because the number of protein-binding sites far exceeds the number of drug molecules available for binding. When the plasma concentrations for drugs bound to albumin exceed 25 to 50 mg/L, however, albumin-binding sites can start to become saturated. As a result, fu, or the fraction of drug that is free, will change with the plasma drug concentration. For example, valproic acid can saturate plasma protein-binding sites when plasma concentrations exceed 25 to 50 mg/L.[18] For those drugs that do not reach serum concentrations capable of saturating protein-binding sites, the plasma protein concentration (in many cases, this is albumin) and the binding affinity of the drug for the plasma protein are the two major factors that control the fu.

LOW PLASMA PROTEIN CONCENTRATIONS

Low plasma protein concentrations decrease the plasma concentration of bound drug (C_{bound}); however, the concentration of free drug (C_{free}) generally is unaffected. Therefore, the fraction of drug that is free (fu) increases as plasma protein concentrations decrease. Free or unbound drug concentrations are not significantly increased because the free drug that is released into plasma secondary to low plasma protein concentrations equilibrates with the tissue compartment (compare Figure 1.4 with Figure 1.3). Therefore, if the volume of distribution (V) is relatively large (eg, phenytoin 0.65 L/kg), only a minor increase in C_{free} will result (also see Volume of Distribution [V]).

The relationship between the plasma drug concentration and the plasma protein concentration can be expressed as follows:

$$\frac{C'}{C_{normal\,binding}} = (1 - fu)\left[\frac{P'}{P_{NL}}\right] + fu \qquad \text{(Eq. 1.7)}$$

This equation can be used to estimate the degree to which an altered plasma protein concentration will affect the desired therapeutic drug concentration. C' represents the patient's plasma drug concentration, and P' represents the patient's plasma protein concentration. $C_{normal\,binding}$ is the plasma drug concentration that would be expected if the patient's plasma protein concentration were normal (P_{NL}). Note that fu is the free fraction associated with "normal plasma protein binding." The $C_{normal\,binding}$ for any given drug can be calculated by rearranging Equation 1.7 as follows:

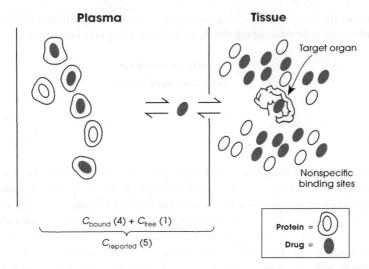

Plasma   **Tissue**

Target organ

Nonspecific
binding sites

C_{bound} (4) + C_{free} (1)

$C_{reported}$ (5)

Protein =

Drug =

FIGURE 1.4 Effect of decreased plasma protein concentration on plasma drug concentration. Compare this figure with Figure 1.3. The decreased protein concentration decreases the plasma drug concentration reported by the laboratory. In this situation, the concentration of free, or active, drug remains the same because free drug that is released as a result of the lowered plasma protein concentration is taken up by nonspecific tissue-binding sites and/or cleared from the body. For this reason, the pharmacologic effect, which can be expected from the reported C of 5, will be the same as that produced by the reported C of 10 in Figure 1.3. In this illustration, fu (or the fraction of free drug to total drug concentration) is increased to 0.2 because of the decrease in the bound concentration.

$$C_{normal\,binding} = \frac{C'}{(1-fu)\left[\dfrac{P'}{P_{NL}}\right]+fu} \qquad \text{(Eq. 1.8)}$$

For example, a patient with a low serum albumin of 2.2 g/dL (normal albumin, 4.4 g/dL) and an apparently low plasma phenytoin concentration of 5.5 mg/L still has a therapeutically acceptable plasma drug concentration when it is adjusted for the low serum albumin. When the normal free fraction (fu) for phenytoin of 0.1 is substituted into Equation 1.8, an adjusted phenytoin plasma concentration of 10 mg/L is calculated.

$$C_{normal\,binding} = \frac{C'}{(1-fu)\left[\dfrac{P'}{P_{NL}}\right]+fu}$$

$$= \frac{5.5\ mg/L}{(1-0.1)\left[\dfrac{2.2\ g/dL}{4.4\ g/dL}\right]+0.1}$$

$$= \frac{5.5\ mg/L}{(0.9)(0.5)+0.1}$$

$$= 10\ mg/L$$

The phenytoin concentration that would have been reported from the laboratory if the patient's albumin concentration was "normal" would be approximately 10 mg/L. This calculation is based on the assumption that phenytoin is primarily bound to albumin and that an average normal albumin concentration is 4.4 g/dL (range: 3.5-5.5 g/dL). Although Equation 1.8 could be used to adjust for any drug significantly bound to albumin, the degree to which the drug concentration will be adjusted or "normalized" for the alteration in serum albumin between 3.5 and 5.5 g/dL will be minimal and is generally unwarranted.

Many other drugs are bound primarily to globulin rather than albumin. Adjustments of plasma drug concentrations for these drugs based on serum albumin concentrations would, therefore, be inappropriate. Unfortunately, adjustments for changes in globulin binding are difficult, because drugs usually bind to a specific globulin that is only a small fraction of total globulin concentration. In general, acidic drugs (eg, phenytoin, most of the antiepileptic drugs, and some neutral compounds) bind primarily to albumin; basic drugs (eg, lidocaine and quinidine) bind more extensively to globulins.[15,19-22]

ELEVATED PLASMA PROTEIN CONCENTRATIONS

The fu value (fraction of total drug concentration that is free or unbound) for selected drugs is provided in Table 1.1. Because increases in serum albumin are uncommon in the clinical setting, the use of Equation 1.8 for high serum albumin would be rare. Many basic drugs, however, are bound to the acute phase reactive protein,[26,27] α_1-acid glycoprotein (AAG). This plasma protein has been known to be significantly decreased and increased under certain clinical conditions. For example, increases in plasma quinidine concentrations have been observed following surgery or trauma.[19,28] The change in the quinidine concentration is the result of increased concentrations of the plasma-binding proteins (AAGs) and increased bound concentrations of quinidine. There appears to be little or no change in the free quinidine level because reequilibration with the larger tissue stores occurs. In this situation, there would be a decrease in fu, and the therapeutic levels of free or unbound drug should correlate with higher-than-usual drug concentration ($C_{bound} + C_{free}$). Other basic compounds with significant binding to AAGs would be expected to be similarly affected. Unfortunately, AAG concentrations are seldom assayed in the clinical setting, thereby making it difficult to evaluate the relationship between the total drug concentration and the fu. For this reason, evaluation of plasma levels for basic drugs that are significantly protein bound is often difficult. A careful evaluation of the patient's clinical response to a measured drug level, as well as an evaluation of any concurrent medical problems (such as surgery, trauma, or inflammatory disease) that could influence plasma protein concentrations and drug binding, is required.

Patients with cirrhosis vary considerably in their plasma protein–binding characteristics. Some patients have significantly elevated binding capabilities, whereas others have significantly decreased binding capabilities. This variation probably reflects the fact that some cirrhotic patients have a strong stimulus for the production of AAGs, whereas others with more serious hepatic disease are unable to manufacture these binding proteins.[26,28,29]

TABLE 1.1   Drugs and fu Values for Plasma Protein Binding

DRUG	fu VALUE
Amitriptyline	0.04[a]
Carbamazepine	0.2
Chlordiazepoxide	0.05
Chlorpromazine	0.04[a]
Cyclosporine	<0.1[b]
Diazepam	0.01
Digoxin	0.70
Digitoxin	0.10
Ethosuximide	1.0
Gabapentin	0.97
Gentamicin	0.9
Imipramine	0.04[a]
Lidocaine	0.30[a]
Lithium	1.0
Methadone	0.13[a]
Methotrexate	0.5
Nafcillin	0.10
Nelfinavir	0.02
Phenobarbital	0.5
Phenytoin	0.10
Propranolol	0.06[a]
Quinidine	0.20[a]
Salicylic acid	0.16[c]
Valproic acid	0.15[c]
Vancomycin	0.9
Warfarin	0.03

fu, unbound fraction.
[a]Basic drugs that are bound significantly to plasma proteins other than albumin.[14,19,20,23]
[b]Bound to lipoproteins and other blood elements.[24,25]
[c]Concentration-dependent plasma protein binding (eg, valproic acid).

BINDING AFFINITY

The binding affinity of plasma protein for a drug can also alter the fraction of drug that is free (fu) (compare Figure 1.5 with Figure 1.3). For example, the plasma proteins in patients with uremia (severe end-stage renal failure) have less affinity for phenytoin than that in individuals without uremia.

As a result, the fu for phenytoin in patients with uremia is estimated to be in the range of 0.2 to 0.3 in contrast to the normal value of 0.1.[22,30] The "effective" or free drug concentration can be calculated by rearranging Equation 1.6 as follows:

$$\text{fu} = \frac{C_{\text{free}}}{C_{\text{bound}} + C_{\text{free}}}$$

$$= \frac{C_{\text{free}}}{C_{\text{total}}}$$

$$C_{\text{free}} = (\text{fu})(C_{\text{total}}) \qquad \textbf{(Eq. 1.9)}$$

According to Equation 1.9, the concentration of free phenytoin in patients with uremia is comparable to that in patients without uremia—despite lower phenytoin plasma concentrations (C_{total}). In the patient with uremia, the fu is increased because

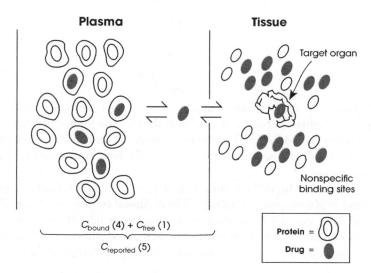

FIGURE 1.5 Effect of decreased binding affinity on plasma drug concentration. Compare this figure with Figure 1.3. Although the protein concentration is normal, the decreased binding affinity of the drug for protein has decreased the reported drug concentration. The concentration of free, or active, drug remains the same because drug that is released from the plasma-binding sites as a result of this decreased affinity is taken up by nonspecific binding sites in the tissue and/or cleared from the body. Thus, the pharmacologic effect that can be expected from the reported C of 5 will be the same as that produced by the reported C of 10 in Figure 1.3. In this illustration, fu (or the fraction of free drug to total drug concentration) is increased to 0.2 because of a decrease in the bound concentration.

the bound concentration is decreased, and as a result, the C_{total} is decreased. The important point is that the unbound concentration is not increased. The patient with uremia with an fu of 0.2 and a reported phenytoin concentration of 5 mg/L would have the same free drug concentration (and same pharmacologic effect) as a patient with normal renal function who has a reported phenytoin concentration of 10 mg/L (using Equation 1.9):

$$C_{free} = (fu)(C_{total})$$

$$C_{free} \text{ (in a patient with uremia)} = (0.2)(5 \text{ mg/L})$$

$$= 1 \text{ mg/L}$$

$$C_{free} \text{ (in a patient with normal renal function)} = (0.1)(10 \text{ mg/L})$$

$$= 1 \text{ mg/L}$$

In summary, any factor that alters protein binding becomes clinically important when a drug is highly protein bound (ie, if fu is <0.1 or 10% unbound). For example, if fu is increased from 0.1 (10% free) to 0.2 (20% free), the concentration of free or active drug *for any given value of C* (bound + free) would be double the usual values, that is:

$$C_{free} = (fu)(C_{total})$$

$$= (0.1)(10 \text{ mg/L})$$

$$= 1 \text{ mg/L}$$

versus

$$= (0.2)(10 \text{ mg/L})$$

$$= 2 \text{ mg/L}$$

Although, in the previous example, it is true that the patient with altered binding had a higher unbound concentration, the increase in the unbound concentration was not caused by the decrease in binding. The unbound concentration of 2 mg/L is the result of a larger amount of drug in the body from either a loading or maintenance dose.

If, on the other hand, the fu for a drug is 0.5 or higher (50% free), it is unlikely that changes in plasma protein binding will be of clinical consequence. As an illustration, if the fu for a drug is increased from a normal value 0.5 (50% free) to 0.6 (60% free) because of decreased protein concentrations, the concentration of free active drug (assuming the same total concentration) would actually be increased by only 20%.

$$C_{free} = (fu)(C_{total})$$

$$= (0.5)(10 \text{ mg/L})$$

$$= 5 \text{ mg/L}$$

versus

$$= (0.6)(10 \text{ mg/L})$$

$$= 6 \text{ mg/L}$$

As a general rule, if fu is increased in any given situation, the clinician should reduce the desired C by the same proportion.[14] That is, if fu is increased 2-fold, the desired C or "therapeutic range" should be reduced to one-half the usual value.

What is often misunderstood is that for drugs with significant plasma protein binding, changes in plasma binding will have a profound effect on the plasma drug concentration because the bound concentration has been altered but generally the unbound concentration is unchanged. As a consequence, the fu of drug in plasma is altered. Again, the unbound drug concentration is, in most cases, relatively unaffected.[31] When considering changes in binding, it should be kept in mind that the fu is the ratio of unbound drug concentration to total drug concentration, as outlined in Equation 1.6.

$$\text{fu} = \frac{C_{free}}{C_{bound} + C_{free}}$$

As depicted in Equation 1.6, fu is dependent on the binding characteristics and is not the "cause" of the free or unbound drug concentration as might be suggested in Equation 1.9.

$$C_{free} = (\text{fu})(C_{total})$$

As an example, let us consider four patients, the first two with phenytoin concentrations of 10 and 20 mg/L, respectively. If both these patients had normal plasma binding (fu = 0.1), their respective C_{free} phenytoin concentrations would be 1 and 2 mg/L. The increased potential effect of the C_{total} phenytoin concentration of 20 mg/L with a C_{free} of 2 mg/L seems intuitively obvious. The fact that the drug concentration (C_{bound} and C_{free}) is higher in the second patient is probably the result of either higher-than-average doses or decreased elimination.

Now let us consider two other patients each with a phenytoin concentration of 10 mg/L. However, in this case, the first patient has normal plasma binding and an fu of 0.1. The second patient has decreased plasma binding and, as a result, an fu of 0.2. In this situation, the first patient with a normal binding fu of 0.1 and C_{total} of 10 mg/L would have a C_{free} of 1 mg/L. The second patient with an altered binding fu of 0.2 and a C_{total} of 10 mg/L would have a C_{free} of 2 mg/L. It is important to recognize that although both patients have a phenytoin concentration of 10 mg/L, the second patient would be expected to have an increased drug effect because of the higher C_{free} or unbound drug concentration. The reason that the second patient has an increased C_{free} is not because of altered binding, but probably because the patient has been given higher-than-average doses or their metabolism is less than average.

MONITORING FREE OR UNBOUND PLASMA CONCENTRATIONS

Although many clinicians believe that monitoring free or unbound plasma concentrations is desirable, it is not common in general clinical practice. The reasons are several and include the fact that assay procedures for free or unbound drug are not commercially available for many compounds. Furthermore, the assay procedures available for free drug concentrations are more expensive and increase the cost of providing patient care. In addition, most patients exhibit reasonably normal binding characteristics; therefore, monitoring unbound drug concentrations would not add significantly to the evaluation of their clinical status. Whereas, in theory, monitoring unbound drug concentrations should be clinically superior, there is little evidence demonstrating that monitoring unbound drug levels improves the correlation between the plasma concentration and the pharmacologic effect or therapeutic outcome.

If unbound drug concentrations are to be used in clinical practice, the clinician must be aware of factors that can alter the relationship between in vitro and in vivo plasma-binding characteristics. For example, the method used to determine the free drug level (equilibrium dialysis, ultrafiltration, saliva sampling) and the conditions under which the sample is obtained can alter the in vitro assay results. This, in turn, can result in an inaccurate estimate of the in vivo binding characteristics.[17,32-35] For these reasons, the use of unbound or free plasma level monitoring is not the standard of practice and is used in only a limited number of clinical settings. If unbound serum drug concentrations are used infrequently, the results should be carefully evaluated and compared to both the expected free drug level and the clinical response of the patient.

Volume of Distribution (V)

The volume of distribution for a drug or the "apparent volume of distribution" does not necessarily refer to any physiologic compartment in the body.[1,36] It is simply the size of a compartment necessary to account for the total amount of drug in the body if it was present throughout the body at the same concentration found in the plasma (Figure 1.6A). The equation for the volume of distribution is expressed as follows:

$$V = \frac{Ab}{C} \qquad \text{(Eq. 1.10)}$$

where V is the apparent volume of distribution, Ab the total amount of drug in the body, and C the plasma concentration of drug.

The plasma volume of the average adult is approximately 3 L. Therefore, apparent volumes of distribution that are larger than the plasma compartment (>3 L) only indicate that the drug is also present in tissues or fluids outside the plasma compartment. The actual sites of distribution cannot be determined from the V value. For example, a drug with a volume of distribution similar to total body water (0.65 L/kg) does not indicate that the drug is equilibrated equally throughout the total body water. The drug may or may not be bound in or excluded from certain tissues. However, the average binding results in an apparent volume of distribution that is approximately equal to that of total body water. Without additional specific information, the actual sites of a drug's distribution are only speculative.

The apparent volume of distribution is a function of the lipid versus water solubilities and of the plasma and tissue protein-binding properties of the drug. Factors that tend to keep the drug in the plasma or increase C (such as high water solubility,

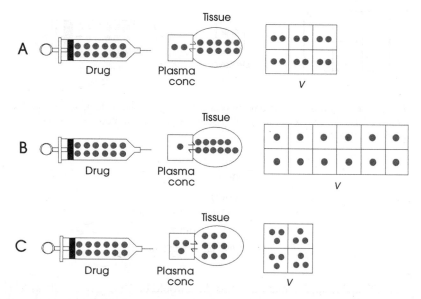

FIGURE 1.6 Volume of distribution. **A.** The administration of a drug into the body produces a specific plasma concentration. The apparent volume of distribution (V) is the volume that accounts for the total dose administration based on the observed plasma concentration. **B.** Any factor that decreases the drug plasma concentration (eg, decreased plasma protein binding) will increase the apparent volume of distribution. **C.** Conversely, any factor that increases the plasma concentration (eg, decreased tissue binding) will decrease the apparent volume of distribution.

increased plasma protein binding, or decreased tissue binding) tend to reduce the apparent volume of distribution. It follows then that factors that decrease C in plasma (such as decreased plasma protein binding, increased tissue binding, and increased lipid solubility) tend to increase the apparent volume of distribution.

LOADING DOSE

Because the volume of distribution is the factor that accounts for all of the drug in the body, it is an important variable in estimating the loading dose necessary to rapidly achieve a desired plasma concentration:

$$\text{Loading dose} = \frac{(V)(C)}{(S)(F)} \qquad \textbf{(Eq. 1.11)}$$

where V is the volume of distribution, C the desired plasma level, and $(S)(F)$ the fraction of the dose administered that will reach the systemic circulation (Figure 1.7).

For example, if one wishes to calculate an oral loading dose of digoxin (ie, using digoxin tablets) for a 70-kg man that produces a plasma concentration of 1.5 µg/L, Equation 1.10 can be used. If S is assumed to be 1.0, F to be 0.7, and V to be 7.3 L/kg,[1,3,37] the loading dose will be 1,095 µg or 1.095 mg based on the following calculation:

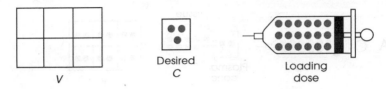

FIGURE 1.7 Loading dose. The volume of distribution is the major determinant of the loading dose. If the V for a drug is known, the loading dose that produces a specific concentration can be calculated (see Equation 1.11).

$$\text{Loading dose} = \frac{(V)(C)}{(S)(F)}$$

$$= \frac{(7.3 \text{ L/kg})(70 \text{ kg})(1.5 \text{ µg/L})}{(1)(0.7)}$$

$$= 1,095 \text{ µg or } 1.095 \text{ mg}$$

A reasonable approximation of this dose would be 1 mg given orally as tablets. The usual clinical approach is to give the loading dose in divided doses (0.25 mg per dose every 6 hours). The patient is observed and evaluated for therapeutic response, and digoxin toxicity before each successive dose is administered. In addition, some clinicians use a bioavailability factor of greater than 0.7 (eg, 0.75 or 0.8), which would further decrease the chance of exceeding the desired drug concentration.

Equation 1.11 can also be used to estimate the loading dose that will be required to achieve a higher plasma concentration than the present concentration (Figure 1.8). This new formula is derived by replacing the C in Equation 1.10 with an expression that represents the increment in plasma concentration that is desired.

$$\text{Incremental loading dose} = \frac{(V)(C_{\text{desired}} - C_{\text{initial}})}{(S)(F)} \qquad \textbf{(Eq. 1.12)}$$

For example, if the previous patient had a digoxin level of 0.5 µg/L and the desired concentration was 1.5 µg/L, the loading dose would have been:

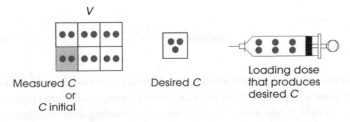

FIGURE 1.8 Loading dose to produce an increment in plasma level. If the V and initial plasma concentration for a drug are known, the incremental loading dose that produces a higher desired plasma concentration can be calculated (see Equation 1.12).

$$\text{Incremental loading dose} = \frac{(V)(C_{\text{desired}} - C_{\text{initial}})}{(S)(F)}$$

$$= \frac{(7.3 \text{ L/kg})(70 \text{ kg})(1.5 \text{ μg/L} - 0.5 \text{ μg/L})}{(1)(0.7)}$$

$$= 730 \text{ μg or } 0.73 \text{ mg}$$

A reasonable incremental loading dose in this case would be about 0.75 mg.

FACTORS THAT ALTER VOLUME OF DISTRIBUTION (V) AND LOADING DOSE

In analyzing Equation 1.11, it becomes clear that any factor that alters the volume of distribution will theoretically influence the loading dose.

Decreased tissue binding of drugs in patients with uremia is a common cause of a reduced apparent volume of distribution for several agents (Figure 1.6C).[38,39] Decreased tissue binding will increase the C by allowing more of the drug to remain in the plasma (Figure 1.6C). Therefore, if the desired plasma level remains unchanged, a smaller loading dose will be required. Digoxin is an example of a drug whose loading dose should be altered in patients with uremia.

Decreased plasma protein binding, on the other hand, tends to increase the apparent volume of distribution because more drug that would normally be in plasma is available to equilibrate with the tissue and the tissue-binding sites (Figure 1.6B). Decreased plasma protein binding, however, also increases the fraction of free or active drug so that the desired C that produces a given therapeutic response decreases. To summarize, diminished plasma protein binding increases V and decreases C in Equation 1.11, resulting in no net effect on the loading dose.

$$\frac{\leftrightarrow}{\text{Loading dose}} = \frac{(\uparrow V)(C \downarrow)}{(S)(F)}$$

This is based on the assumption that the majority of drug in the body is actually outside the plasma compartment and that the amount of drug bound to plasma protein comprises only a small percentage of the total amount in the body.

This principle is illustrated by the pharmacokinetic behavior of phenytoin in patients with uremia. Plasma phenytoin concentrations in patients with uremia are frequently one-half of those observed in normal patients given the same dose. The lower plasma levels, however, produce the same free or pharmacologically active phenytoin concentration as levels twice as high in normal patients because the fu is increased from 0.1 to 0.2 in these individuals, indicating that the target plasma concentrations (bound + free) in patients with uremia should be about half of the usual target concentration. Furthermore, a loading dose of phenytoin that produces a normal therapeutic effect is the same for patients with and without uremia, because the volume of distribution increases by approximately 2-fold (0.65-1.44 L/kg) in individuals with uremia.[27] Equation 1.11 indicates that there would be no change in the loading dose if the volume of distribution is increased by a factor of 2 and the desired drug concentration is decreased by a factor of ½.

$$\overset{\leftrightarrow}{\text{Loading dose}} = \frac{(2 \times V)\left(\frac{1}{2} \times C\right)}{(S)(F)}$$

TWO-COMPARTMENT MODELS

Pharmacokinetic Parameters

If one thinks of the body as a single compartment, pharmacokinetic calculations are relatively simple. However, there are some situations in which it is more appropriate to conceptualize the body as two, and occasionally, more than two compartments when thinking about drug distribution, elimination, and pharmacologic effect. The first compartment can be thought of as a smaller, rapidly equilibrating volume, usually made up of plasma or blood and those organs or tissues that have high blood flow and are in rapid equilibrium with the blood or plasma drug concentration. This first compartment has a volume referred to as V_i or initial volume of distribution. The second compartment equilibrates with the drug over a somewhat longer period. This volume is referred to as V_t or tissue volume of distribution.[36,40] The half-life for the distribution phase is referred to as the α half-life, and the half-life for drug elimination from the body is referred to as the β half-life. The sum of V_i and V_t is the apparent volume of distribution (V). Drugs are assumed to enter into and be eliminated from V_i. That is, any drug that distributes into the tissue compartment (V_t) must reequilibrate into V_i before it can be eliminated (Figure 1.9).

Effects of a Two-Compartment Model on the Loading Dose and Plasma Concentration (C)

Because some time is required for a drug to distribute into V_t, a rapidly administered loading dose calculated on the basis of V ($V_i + V_t$) would result in an initial C that is higher than predicted, because the initial volume of distribution (V_i) is always smaller than V. The consequences of a higher-than-expected C depend on whether the target organ for the clinical response behaves as though it were located in V_i or V_t.

Drugs such as lidocaine, phenobarbital, and theophylline exert therapeutic and toxic effects on target organs that behave as though they are located in V_i. In these instances, when loading doses are calculated based on the total volume of distribution, the concentration of drug delivered to the target organs could be much higher than expected and produce toxicity if the loading dose is not administered appropriately. This problem can be circumvented by first calculating the loading dose based on the total volume of distribution (V) and then administering the loading dose at a rate slow enough to allow for drug distribution into V_t. This approach is common in clinical practice, and the guidelines for rates of drug administration are often based on the principle of two-compartment modeling, with the receptors for clinical response (toxic or therapeutic) responding as though they were located in V_i. A second approach is to administer the loading dose in sufficiently small individual bolus doses such that the C in V_i does not exceed some predetermined critical concentration.[41,42]

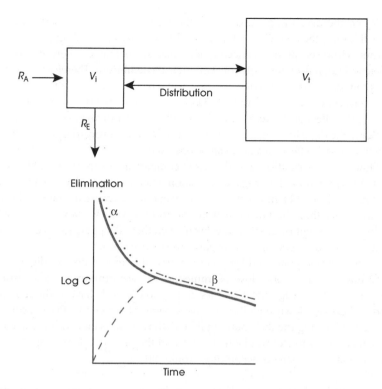

FIGURE 1.9 Two-compartment model: volumes of distribution. V_i is the initial volume of distribution. Drug administration (R_A) and elimination (R_E) are assumed to occur in V_i. The lower graph shows that, following rapid administration of drug into V_u, the plasma concentration (*solid line*) follows a biphasic decay pattern. The initial decay half-life ($\alpha t_{1/2}$) is usually primarily because of drug distribution into V_t. The second decay half-life ($\beta t_{1/2}$) is usually because of drug elimination from the body. The dotted line represents the drug effect when the end organ for effect is located in V_i. Note that drug effect parallels the plasma concentration at all times. The dashed line represents the drug effect when the end organ for effect is located in V_t. Note that initially when all of the drug is in V_i, there is no drug effect. However, as distribution takes place, the drug effect increases and begins to parallel the plasma concentration only in the elimination phase after distribution is complete.

Although not commonly discussed in pharmacokinetic terms, potassium is a good example of a drug that follows this principle of two-compartment modeling with the end organ being located in V_i. Potassium is primarily an intracellular electrolyte, but its cardiac effects parallel the plasma concentration. In addition, there is a slow equilibrium between plasma and tissue potassium concentrations. When potassium is given IV, the rate of administration must be carefully controlled as serious cardiac toxicity and death can occur if the patient experiences excessive potassium concentrations in the plasma (V_i).

This concept of two-compartment modeling is also important in evaluating the offset of drug effect. For drugs with the end organ for clinical response located in V_i, rapid achievement of a therapeutic response followed quickly by a loss of the therapeutic response may be the result of drug being distributed into a larger volume of distribution rather than drug being eliminated from the body.

When the drug's target organ is in the second or tissue compartment, V_t (eg, digoxin, lithium), the high C, which may be observed before distribution occurs, is not dangerous. However, plasma concentrations that are obtained before distribution is complete will not reflect the tissue concentration at equilibrium. Therefore, these plasma samples cannot be used to predict the therapeutic or toxic potential of these drugs.[43,44] For example, clinicians usually wait 1 to 3 hours after an IV bolus dose of digoxin before evaluating the effect and 4 to 6 hours before obtaining a digoxin concentration. This delay allows the digoxin to distribute to the site of action (myocardium) so that the full therapeutic or toxic effects of a dose can be observed.

Slow drug distribution into the tissue compartment can pose problems in the accurate interpretation of a drug concentration when a drug is given by the IV route. It is not generally a problem when a drug is given orally because the rate of absorption is usually slower than the rate of distribution from V_i into V_t. Nevertheless, digoxin and lithium are exceptions to this rule. Even when these drugs are given orally, several hours are required for complete absorption and distribution.

Plasma samples obtained less than 6 hours after an oral dose of digoxin or less than 12 hours after an oral dose of immediate-release lithium are of questionable value. For these two drugs, the receptors in the end organs behave as though they are located in the more slowly equilibrating tissue compartment or V_t. Plasma concentrations obtained during the distribution phase (before equilibrium with the deep tissue compartment is complete) will be increased, and the pharmacologic response will be much less than the plasma concentration would indicate.

As a general rule, sampling of drug concentrations during the absorption/distribution phase should be avoided because these concentrations are changing very rapidly and are difficult to interpret.

Drugs With Significant and Nonsignificant Two-Compartment Modeling

As illustrated in Figure 1.9, the α phase for most drugs represents distribution of drug from V_i into V_t, and relatively little drug is eliminated during the distribution phase. Drugs that behave in this way are generally referred to as "nonsignificant" two-compartmental drugs. The term "nonsignificant" means that if the patient is not harmed by the initially elevated drug concentration in the α phase and no drug samples are taken in the α phase, then the drug can be successfully modeled as a one-compartment drug (ie, only the elimination or β phase is considered). It is important to recognize that for some drugs, increased drug plasma concentrations during the α phase can be clinically significant because the patient may experience serious toxicity if the end organ behaves as though it lies within the initial volume of distribution (V_i). These drugs are considered to exhibit "nonsignificant" two-compartmental modeling only after the α phase or distribution has been completed. That is, plasma samples are obtained for pharmacokinetic modeling only during the β or elimination phase.

Drugs with "significant" two-compartment modeling are those that are eliminated to a significant extent during the initial α phase. For these drugs (eg, methotrexate), the α phase cannot be thought of simply as distribution because significant elimination occurs as well. Two drugs that border on having significant two-compartment modeling are lithium and lidocaine. When a one-compartment model is used for drugs that exhibit significant drug elimination in the α phase, the actual trough concentrations will be lower than those predicted by the one-compartment model.

Some clinicians have suggested that these drugs could be more successfully monitored by using two-compartmental model pharmacokinetics. The complexity of these models, however, as well as the number of plasma samples required for patient-specific dose adjustments, usually limits the use of two-compartmental modeling techniques.

Two-compartment computer models are available for therapeutic drug monitoring. Usually, the value of these two-compartment computer models is that they can compensate or adjust for drug samples that have been obtained in the distribution phase. If care is taken to avoid obtaining samples in the distribution phase, very similar pharmacokinetic interpretations are usually arrived at using the simpler one-compartment model.

Clearance (Cl)

Cl can be thought of as the intrinsic ability of the body or its organs of elimination (usually the kidneys and the liver) to remove drug from the blood or plasma. Cl is expressed as a volume per unit of time. It is important to emphasize that Cl is not an indicator of how much drug is being removed; it only represents the theoretical volume of blood or plasma that is completely cleared of drug in a given period. The amount of drug removed depends on the plasma concentration of drug and the Cl (Figure 1.10).

STEADY STATE

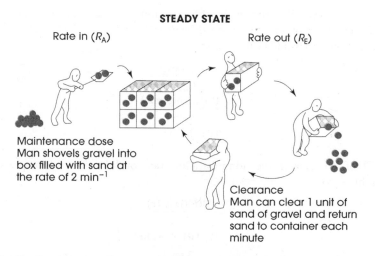

Rate in (R_A) Rate out (R_E)

Maintenance dose
Man shovels gravel into
box filled with sand at
the rate of 2 min^{-1}

Clearance
Man can clear 1 unit of
sand of gravel and return
sand to container each
minute

FIGURE 1.10 Steady state, maintenance dose, clearance, and elimination rate constant. At steady state, the rate of drug administration (R_A) is equal to the rate of drug elimination (R_E), and the concentration of drug remains constant. In this example, the man on the left is able to shovel gravel or "drug" into a container of sand at the rate of 2 min^{-1}. The man on the right is able to remove 1 unit of sand containing gravel or "drug" from the container, dump the gravel, and return the sand to the container each minute. The amount of gravel or "drug" removed per unit of time (rate of elimination) will be determined by the concentration of gravel per unit of sand as well as the clearance (volume of sand cleared of gravel). The elimination rate constant (K) can be thought of as the fraction of the total volume cleared per unit of time. In this case, K would be equal to $\frac{1}{6}$ or 0.17 min^{-1}.

At steady state, the rate of drug administration (R_A) and rate of drug elimination (R_E) must be equal (also see Elimination Rate Constant [K] and Half-life [$t_{1/2}$]: Elimination Rate Constant [K]).

$$R_A = R_E \qquad \text{(Eq. 1.13)}$$

Cl can best be thought of as the proportionality constant that makes the average steady-state plasma drug level equal to the rate of drug administration (R_A):

$$R_A = (Cl)(C_{ss\ ave}) \qquad \text{(Eq. 1.14)}$$

where R_A is $(S)(F)(\text{Dose})/\tau$ (see Equation 1.5), and $C_{ss\ ave}$ is the average steady-state drug concentration.

If an average steady-state plasma concentration and the rate of drug administration are known, the Cl can be calculated by rearranging Equation 1.14 as follows:

$$Cl = \frac{(S)(F)(\text{Dose}/\tau)}{C_{ss\ ave}} \qquad \text{(Eq. 1.15)}$$

For example, if IV lidocaine is infused continuously at a rate of 2 mg/min and if the concentration of lidocaine at steady state is 3 mg/L, the calculated lidocaine Cl using Equation 1.15 would be 0.667 L/min

$$Cl = \frac{(S)(F)(\text{Dose}/\tau)}{C_{ss\ ave}}$$
$$= \frac{(1)(1)(2\ \text{mg}/\text{min})}{3\ \text{mg/L}}$$
$$= 0.667\ \text{L}/\text{min}$$

or a Cl of 40 L/hr if the administration rate of lidocaine was expressed as 120 mg/hr.

$$Cl = \frac{(S)(F)(\text{Dose}/\tau)}{C_{ss\ ave}}$$
$$= \frac{(1)(1)(120\ \text{mg/hr})}{3\ \text{mg/L}}$$
$$= 40\ \text{L/hr}$$

F is considered to be 1.0 because the drug is being administered IV. S is also assumed to be 1.0 because the hydrochloride salt represents only a small fraction of the total molecular weight for lidocaine and because correction for the salt form is unnecessary.

MAINTENANCE DOSE

If an estimate for Cl is obtained from the literature, the Cl formula (Equation 1.15) can be rearranged and used to calculate the rate of administration or maintenance dose that produces a desired average plasma concentration at steady state:

$$\text{Maintenance dose} = \frac{(Cl)(C_{ss\,ave})(\tau)}{(S)(F)}$$

(Eq. 1.16)

For example, using the literature estimate for theophylline Cl of 2.8 L/hr, the rate of IV administration for theophylline that produces a steady-state plasma theophylline concentration of 10 mg/L is given in the following equation:

$$\text{Maintenance dose} = \frac{(Cl)(C_{ss\,ave})(\tau)}{(S)(F)}$$

$$= \frac{(2.8\ \text{L/hr})(10\ \text{mg/L})(1\ \text{hr})}{(1)(1)}$$

$$= 28\ \text{mg given qh}$$

Because τ is 1 hour, the rate of administration is 28 mg/hr. If the theophylline was to be given every 12 hours, the dose would be 336 mg or 12 times the hourly administration rate to maintain the same average steady-state concentration.

$$\text{Maintenance dose} = \frac{(Cl)(C_{ss\,ave})(\tau)}{(S)(F)}$$

$$= \frac{(2.8\ \text{L/hr})(10\ \text{mg/L})(12\ \text{hr})}{(1)(1)}$$

$$= 336\ \text{mg to be given q12h}$$

The units for volume and time in Cl are somewhat arbitrary but must be consistent with the units for the drug administration rate and drug concentration.

Administration rate	Mass/time
Drug concentration	Mass/volume
Clearance	Volume/time

As an example, if the drug administration rate is in mg/hr and concentration is in mg/L, then Cl would be in L/hr. Conversely, if the administration rate was mg/d and concentration in mg/L, then Cl be in L/d. Again, the units are somewhat arbitrary, but clinicians usually use values that are consistent with how the drug is used in clinical practice.

In some cases, conversions need to be made. Digoxin is usually prescribed as milligrams (eg, 0.25 mg) given once daily. The plasma concentration is usually reported as µg/L (ng/mL). Therefore, the units of Cl would be either L/d or L/hr depending on whether the dosing interval is thought of as daily or every 24 hours. Another example is methotrexate that is usually administered as grams or milligrams, but methotrexate concentrations are reported as µg/L (ng/mL) (see Chapter "Precision Oncology: Pharmacokinetics and Genomics to Guide Cancer Therapy"). Care should be taken to ensure that the appropriate units and conversions are used when performing pharmacokinetic calculations.

FACTORS THAT ALTER CLEARANCE (Cl)

Body Surface Area

Most literature values for Cl are expressed as volume/kg/time or as volume/70 kg/time. There is some evidence, however, that drug Cl is best adjusted on the basis of body surface area (BSA) rather than weight.[45-50] BSA can be calculated using Equation 1.16, or it can be obtained from various charts and nomograms[51-53] (see Appendix II).

$$\text{BSA in m}^2 = \left(\frac{\text{Patient's weight in kg}}{70 \text{ kg}} \right)^{0.7} (1.73 \text{ m}^2) \qquad \textbf{(Eq. 1.17)}$$

The value of a patient's weight divided by 70 taken to the 0.7 power is an attempt to scale or size a patient as a fraction of the average 1.73 m² or 70-kg individual. Weight divided by 70 taken to the 0.7 power has no units and should be thought of as the fraction of the average-sized person.

As an example, a 7-kg patient has a weight ratio relative to 70 kg of 0.1 and, therefore, may be thought of as having a size and thus a metabolic and renal capacity that is one-tenth of the average 70-kg person.

$$\left(\frac{7 \text{ kg}}{70 \text{ kg}} \right) = 0.1$$

If the same weight individual was compared to the 70-kg standard using weight to the 0.7 power, the ratio becomes 0.2 or 20% the size and Cl capacity of the standard 70-kg or 1.73-m² individual.

$$\left(\frac{7 \text{ kg}}{70 \text{ kg}} \right)^{0.7} = 0.2$$

In the previous example, the difference between 0.1 and 0.2 is large. However, when patients do not differ significantly from 70 kg, the difference between using weight versus weight to the power 0.7 or BSA becomes less significant.

It is also important to remember that 0.2 has no units and represents the fraction of the average-sized (1.73 m² or 70 kg) individual. Occasionally, the value of 0.2 is mistaken for the surface area or size of the patient in square meters. This is not correct and can lead to dosing errors.

The following formulas can be used to adjust the Cl values reported in the literature for specific patients. There are other equations one can use depending on units used in the literature for Cl.

$$\text{Patient's Cl} = (\text{Literature Cl/m}^2)(\text{Patient's BSA}) \qquad \textbf{(Eq. 1.18)}$$

$$\text{Patient's Cl} = (\text{Literature Cl}/70\,\text{kg})\left(\frac{\text{Patient's BSA}}{1.73\,\text{m}^2}\right) \qquad \textbf{(Eq. 1.19)}$$

$$\text{Patient's Cl} = (\text{Literature Cl}/70\,\text{kg})\left(\frac{\text{Patient's weight in kg}}{70\,\text{kg}}\right) \qquad \textbf{(Eq. 1.20)}$$

$$\text{Patient's Cl} = (\text{Literature Cl}/\text{kg})\,(\text{Patient's weight in kg}) \qquad \textbf{(Eq. 1.21)}$$

Equations 1.20 and 1.21 adjust Cl in proportion to weight, whereas Equations 1.18 and 1.19 adjust Cl in proportion to BSA.

The underlying assumption in using weight or surface area to adjust Cl is that the patient's liver and kidney size (and hopefully function) vary in proportion to these physical measurements. This may not always be the case; therefore, Cl values derived from the patient populations having a similar age and size should be used whenever possible. If the patient's weight is reasonably close to 70 kg (BSA = 1.73 m²), the patient's calculated Cl will be similar whether weight or BSA is used to calculate Cl. If, however, the patient's weight differs significantly from 70 kg, then the use of weight or surface area is likely to generate substantially different estimates of the patient's Cl. When a patient's size is substantially greater or less than the standard 70 kg, or 1.73 m², a careful assessment should be made to determine whether the patient's body stature is normal, obese, or emaciated. In patients who are obese and emaciated, neither weight nor surface area is likely to be helpful in predicting Cl, because the patient's body size will not reflect the size or function of the liver and kidney (Table 1.2).

Plasma Protein Binding

For highly protein-bound drugs, diminished plasma protein binding is associated with a decrease in reported steady-state plasma drug concentrations (total of unbound and free drug) for any given dose that is administered (see Figures 1.4 and 1.5 and Desired Plasma Concentration [C], this part). According to Equation 1.15, a decrease in the denominator, $C_{ss\ ave}$, increases the calculated Cl.

$$\text{Cl} = \frac{(S)(F)(\text{Dose}/\tau)}{C_{ss\ ave}}$$

It would be misleading, however, to assume that because the calculated Cl is increased, the amount eliminated per unit of time has increased. Equation 1.15 assumes that when $C_{ss\ ave}$ (total of bound and free drug) changes, the free drug concentration, which is available for metabolism and renal elimination, changes proportionately. In actuality, the free or unbound fraction of drug in the plasma generally increases (even though $C_{ss\ ave}$ decreases) with diminished plasma protein binding.[15,54] As a result, the amount of free drug eliminated per unit of time remains unchanged.[28] This should be apparent if one considers that at steady state, the amount of drug administered per unit of time (R_A) must equal the amount eliminated per unit of time (R_E). If R_A has not changed, R_E must remain the same.

TABLE 1.2   Factors that Alter Clearance

Body weight
Body surface area
Cardiac output
Drug-drug interactions
Extraction ratio
Genetics
Hepatic function
Plasma protein binding
Renal function

In summary, when the same daily dose of a drug is given in the presence of diminished protein binding, an amount equal to that dose will be eliminated from the body each day at steady state despite a diminished steady-state plasma concentration and an increase in the calculated Cl. This lower plasma concentration ($C_{bound} + C_{free}$) is associated with a decreased C_{bound}, no change in C_{free}, and as a result, there is an increase in the fraction of unbound drug (fu).

$$\uparrow fu = \frac{C_{free}}{\downarrow C_{bound} + C_{free}} \qquad \text{(Eq. 1.22)}$$

Therefore, the pharmacologic effect achieved will be similar to that produced by the higher serum concentration observed under normal protein-binding conditions. This example reemphasizes the principle that Cl alone is not a good indicator of the amount of drug eliminated per unit of time (R_E) (Figures 1.11 and 1.12).

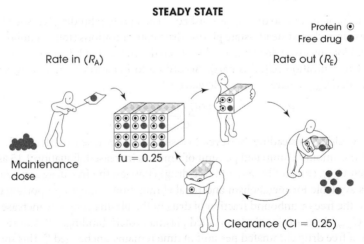

STEADY STATE

Protein ◉
Free drug ●

Rate in (R_A)   Rate out (R_E)

Maintenance dose

fu = 0.25

Clearance (Cl = 0.25)

FIGURE 1.11 Clearance (Cl) of a highly protein-bound drug with a low extraction ratio. The free or unbound drug is available for Cl. Protein-bound drug is returned to the container so that the actual volume cleared of drug is one-fourth of the total volume removed by the man and presented to the clearing organ (eg, kidney or liver). (Compare with Figure 1.10.)

STEADY STATE

Rate in (R_A)   Rate out (R_E)

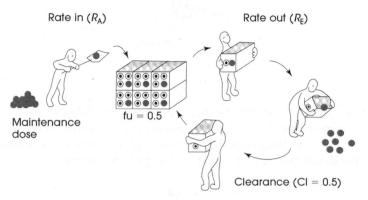

Maintenance
dose

fu = 0.5

Clearance (Cl = 0.5)

FIGURE 1.12 Effect of diminished protein binding on clearance (Cl) of a highly protein-bound drug that has a low extraction ratio. Compare this figure with Figure 1.11. The plasma concentration of drug has decreased, but the free concentration remains the same (fu is increased) (see Figure 1.4). The volume cleared of drug has increased (½) compared to that cleared in Figure 1.11, even though the unbound concentration and amount of drug cleared per unit of time remained unchanged. This illustrates the principle that the amount of a highly protein-bound drug cleared per unit of time or rate of elimination (R_E) remains the same if the increase in Cl is owing to a decrease in plasma binding and the intrinsic metabolism or renal elimination remains unchanged.

This principle is illustrated by comparing phenytoin in a patient with or without uremia at steady state. As noted previously in the discussion of desired plasma concentration, the steady-state unbound plasma phenytoin concentration (C_{free}) will be the same in individuals with or without uremia receiving the same daily dose and having the same metabolic capability. However, owing to decreased protein binding, C_{bound} and, therefore, C_{total} will be lower in patients with uremia than those without.

As an example, consider two patients with the same metabolic capability receiving phenytoin 300 mg/d. The first patient is nonuremic with a phenytoin concentration of 10 mg/L and normal plasma binding (fu = 0.1). The second patient is uremic with a phenytoin concentration of 5 mg/L and decreased plasma binding (fu = 0.2). If these two patients were to have their Cl calculated using Equation 1.15, it would appear as though the patient with uremia has a higher Cl.

$$Cl = \frac{(S)(F)(Dose/\tau)}{C_{ss\,ave}}$$

Nonuremic:

$$Cl = \frac{(S)(F)(Dose/\tau)}{C_{ss\,ave}}$$
$$= \frac{(1)(1)(300\ mg/d)}{10\ mg/L}$$
$$= 30\ L/d$$

Uremic:

$$Cl = \frac{(S)(F)(Dose/\tau)}{C_{ss\,ave}}$$

$$= \frac{(1)(1)\left(300\,mg/d\right)}{5\,mg/L}$$

$$= 60\,L/d$$

Although the calculated Cl for the patient with uremia is higher than that for the patient without uremia (60 vs 30 L/d), the amount of drug cleared per day (300 mg) is the same because, at steady state, the rate of drug administration (R_A) is equal to the rate of drug elimination (R_E) for patients with and without uremia.

$$R_A = R_E$$
$$300\ mg/d = 300\ mg/d$$

When protein binding is decreased, the increase in calculated Cl is generally proportional to the change in fu. Although the calculated Cl may be used to estimate a maintenance dose, careful selection of the plasma level that will produce the desired unbound or free plasma level and pharmacologic effect is critical to the determination of a therapeutically correct maintenance dose.

Extraction Ratio

The direct proportionality between calculated Cl and fu does not apply to drugs that are so efficiently metabolized or excreted that some (perhaps all) of the drug bound to plasma protein is removed as it passes through the eliminating organ.[28,47,55] In this situation, the plasma protein acts as a "transport system" for the drug, carrying it to the eliminating organs, and Cl becomes dependent on the blood or plasma flow to the eliminating organ. To determine whether the Cl for a drug with significant plasma binding will be influenced primarily by blood flow or plasma protein binding, its extraction ratio is estimated and compared to its fu value.

The extraction ratio is the fraction of the drug presented to the eliminating organ that is cleared after a single pass through that organ. It can be estimated by dividing the blood or plasma Cl of a drug by the blood or plasma flow to the eliminating organ. If the extraction ratio exceeds the fu, then the plasma proteins are acting as a transport system and Cl will not change in proportion to fu. If, however, the extraction ratio is less than fu, Cl is likely to increase by the same proportion that fu changes. This approach does not take into account other factors that may affect Cl, such as red blood cell binding, elimination from red blood cells, or changes in metabolic function.

Renal and Hepatic Function

Drugs can be eliminated or cleared as unchanged drug through the kidney (renal Cl) and by metabolism in the liver (metabolic Cl). These two routes of Cl are assumed to be independent of one another and additive.[36,40]

$$Cl_t = Cl_m + Cl_r \qquad \text{(Eq. 1.23)}$$

where Cl_t is total clearance, Cl_m the metabolic clearance or the fraction cleared by metabolism, and Cl_r the renal clearance or the fraction cleared by the renal route. Because the kidneys and liver function independently, it is assumed that a change in one does not affect the other.

Most pharmacokinetic adjustments for drug elimination are based on renal function (see Chapter "Drug Dosing in Kidney Disease and Dialysis") because hepatic function is usually more difficult to quantitate. Elevated liver enzymes do reflect liver damage but are not a good measure of function. Hepatic function is often evaluated using the prothrombin time, serum albumin concentration, and serum bilirubin concentration. Unfortunately, each of these laboratory tests is affected by variables other than altered hepatic function. For example, the serum albumin may be low owing to decreased protein intake or increased renal or GI loss, as well as decreased hepatic function. Although liver function tests do not provide quantitative data, pharmacokinetic adjustments must still take into consideration liver function because this route of elimination is important for a significant number of drugs.

Cardiac Output

Cardiac output also affects drug metabolism. Hepatic or metabolic Cl for some drugs can be decreased by 25% to 50% in patients with congestive heart failure. For example, the metabolic Cls of theophylline[56] and digoxin[45] are reduced by approximately one-half in patients with congestive heart failure. Because the metabolic Cl for both of these drugs is much lower than the hepatic blood or plasma flow (low extraction ratio), it would not have been predicted that their Cls would have been influenced by cardiac output or hepatic blood flow to this extent. The decreased cardiac output and resultant hepatic congestion must, in some way, decrease the intrinsic metabolic capacity of the liver. The effect of diminished Cl on plasma drug concentrations is illustrated in Figure 1.13 (compare with Figure 1.10).

Elimination Rate Constant (K) and Half-life ($t_{1/2}$)

It is often desirable to predict how drug plasma levels will change with time. For drugs that are eliminated by first-order pharmacokinetics, these predictions are based on the elimination rate constant (K). The key characteristic of first-order elimination is that both Cl and volume of distribution do not vary with dose or concentration.

FIRST-ORDER PHARMACOKINETICS

First-order elimination pharmacokinetics refers to a process in which the amount or concentration of drug in the body diminishes logarithmically over time (Figure 1.14).

NON–STEADY-STATE

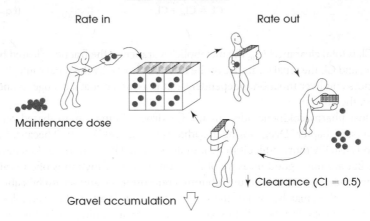

NEW STEADY STATE

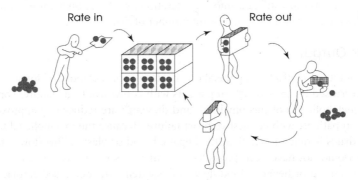

FIGURE 1.13 Effect of changes in clearance (Cl) on steady-state serum concentrations. Compare this figure with Figure 1.10. In this illustration, the maintenance dose or amount of gravel added to the container per unit of time remains the same; however, the volume of sand cleared of gravel (Cl) has been halved. Initially, the amount of gravel or "drug" cleared per unit of time is less than the maintenance dose; the concentration of gravel in the container increases until a new steady state is reached. At this point, the rate at which gravel is added to the container again equals the rate at which gravels is eliminated from the container. If Cl had increased, the concentration of gravel would have decreased until the amount removed per unit of time (R_E) again equaled the rate of administration (R_A).

The rate of elimination (R_E) is proportional to the drug concentration; therefore, the amount of drug removed per unit of time (R_E) will vary in direct proportion to drug concentration. The fraction or percentage of the total amount of drug present in the body (Ab) that is removed at any instant in time, however, will remain constant and independent of dose or concentration. That fraction or percentage is expressed by the elimination rate constant, K. The equations that describe first-order elimination of a drug from the body are as follows:

$$Ab = (Ab_0)(e^{-Kt})$$

(Eq. 1.24)

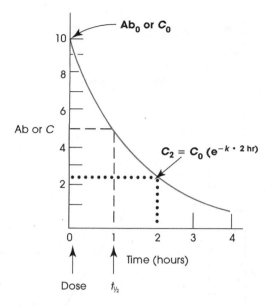

FIGURE 1.14   First-order elimination C versus time. The initial amount (Ab_0) or concentration (C_0) diminishes logarithmically over time. The half-life ($t_{1/2}$) is the time required to eliminate one-half of the drug. The concentration at the end of a given time interval (in this example, 2 hours) is equal to the initial concentration times the fraction of drug remaining at the end of that time interval ($e^{-K \cdot 2 \, hr}$). The amount or concentration of drug lost in each 1-hour interval diminishes over time (5, 2.5, and 1.25); however, the fraction of drug that is lost in each unit of time remains constant (0.5). For example, over the first hour (0-1 hour), of the total amount of drug in the body (10), one-half was lost (5). In the next time interval (1-2 hours), of the amount of drug that remained (5), one-half was lost (2.5).

or

$$C = (C_0)(e^{-Kt})$$ (Eq. 1.25)

where in Equation 1.24, Ab_0 and Ab represent the total amount of drug in the body at the beginning and end of the time interval, t, respectively; and e^{-Kt} is the fraction remaining at time t. In Equation 1.25, C_0 and C are the plasma concentrations at the beginning and end of the time interval, respectively. Because the drug concentration diminishes logarithmically, a graphic plot of the logarithm of the plasma level versus time yields a straight line (Figure 1.15).

This type of graphic analysis of declining plasma drug concentrations is often used to determine whether a drug is eliminated by a first-order process. The key element is that the drug concentration decay curve when plotted as C versus time is a concave curve (see Figure 1.14) and when plotted as log C versus time is a straight line (see Figure 1.15). One important assumption in this analysis is that there is no additional drug being absorbed or placed into the body during the decay process.

Because first-order drugs have a volume of distribution and Cl that are constant (assuming no change in a patient's clinical status), many but not all the

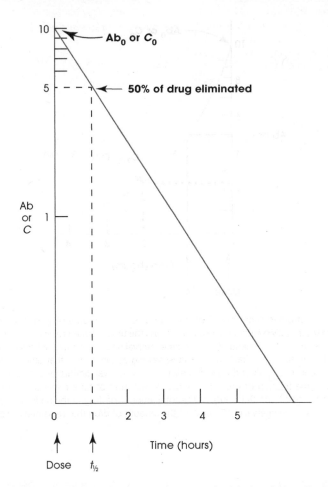

FIGURE 1.15   First-order elimination log C versus time. A graph of the log of Ab or C versus time yields a straight line. The half-life is the time required for Ab or C to decline to one-half the original value.

dose-to-concentration relationships are proportional. As an example, the average steady-state concentration will be proportional to the dosing rate. Therefore, the steady-state concentration can be adjusted by altering the drug dosage rate in proportion to the desired change in concentration (Figure 1.16).

Equation 1.25 can also be thought of as any initial drug concentration C_1 that is decayed over some time interval t_1 to calculate the subsequent drug concentration C_2.

$$C_2 = (C_1)(e^{-Kt}) \qquad \textbf{(Eq. 1.26)}$$

ELIMINATION RATE CONSTANT (K)

The elimination rate constant, K, is the fraction or percentage of the total amount of drug in the body removed per unit of time and is a function of Cl and volume of distribution.

NON-STEADY-STATE

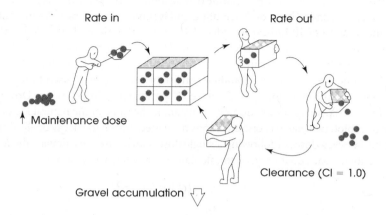

NEW STEADY STATE

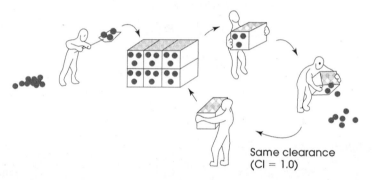

FIGURE 1.16 Effect of changes in maintenance dose on steady-state plasma concentrations. Compare this figure with Figure 1.10. In this illustration, the clearance or volume of sand cleared of gravel remains the same; however, the maintenance dose or the amount of gravel added to the container per unit of time has been increased from 2 to 3 min^{-1}. Therefore, the concentration of gravel or "drug" increases until a new steady state is reached. At this point, the rate at which gravel is added to the container again equals the rate at which gravel is eliminated from the container. If the maintenance dose decreased, the concentration of gravel would have gradually decreased until a new steady state had been achieved.

$$K = \frac{Cl}{V} \qquad \text{(Eq. 1.27)}$$

As Equation 1.27 shows, K can also be thought of as the fraction of the volume of distribution that will be cleared of drug per unit of time (see Figure 1.10). For example, a drug with a Cl of 10 L/d and a V of 100 L would have an elimination rate constant of 0.1 d^{-1}.

$$K = \frac{10 \text{ L/d}}{100 \text{ L}}$$
$$= 0.1 \text{ day}^{-1}$$

The elimination rate constant of 0.1 d^{-1} indicates that in 1 day, the volume cleared is 1/10 or 10% of the total volume of distribution. The value of K is based on the units used for Cl and volume of distribution and is somewhat arbitrary. As an example, using the same Cl of 10 L/d expressed as 0.417 L/hr (10 L/d divided by 24 hr/d) and the V of 100 L, the corresponding K value would be 0.00417 hr^{-1} or 0.417% of the total volume of distribution cleared in 1 hour. As previously discussed, the units chosen for Cl and volume of distribution should be consistent with the units used to report the dose, concentration, and dosing interval (see Clearance [Cl]: Maintenance Dose).

Because the drug elimination rate constant is the slope of the natural log or ln C versus time plot, two plasma concentrations measured during the decay or elimination phase (ie, between doses or following a single dose) can be used to calculate the K for a specific patient. The equation used to calculate K is a rearrangement of Equation 1.26:

$$C_2 = (C_1)(e^{-Kt})$$

$$\frac{C_2}{C_1} = e^{-Kt}$$

$$\ln\left(\frac{C_2}{C_1}\right) = -Kt$$

$$\ln\left(\frac{C_1}{C_2}\right) = Kt$$

$$\frac{\ln\left(\frac{C_1}{C_2}\right)}{t} = K$$

or

$$K = \frac{\ln\left(\frac{C_1}{C_2}\right)}{t} \qquad \text{(Eq. 1.28)}$$

where C_1 is the first or higher plasma concentration, C_2 is the second or lower plasma concentration, and t is the time interval between the plasma samples. For example, if C_1 is 5 mg/L and C_2 is 2 mg/L, and the time interval between the samples is 8 hours, the elimination rate constant (K) will be 0.115 hr^{-1}.

$$K = \frac{\ln\left(\frac{C_1}{C_2}\right)}{t}$$

$$= \frac{\ln\left(\frac{5\,\text{mg/L}}{2\,\text{mg/L}}\right)}{8\,\text{hr}}$$

$$= 0.115\,\text{hr}^{-1}$$

One of the key issues in using Equation 1.28 is that to estimate K accurately, the time between C_1 and C_2 should be at least one half-life (see Elimination Rate Constant [K] and Half-life [$t_{1/2}$]: Half-life [$t_{1/2}$]). In other words, C_2 should be equal to or less than half of C_1. This time interval of one half-life is a minimum, and an interval of longer than a half-life is desirable. Whereas K can be calculated from any two drug concentrations during a decay phase, when the interval is less than one half-life, assay error alone results in highly variable and inaccurate estimates of K.

HALF-LIFE ($t_{1/2}$)

The elimination rate constant is often expressed in terms of a drug's half-life, a value that is more conveniently applied to the clinical setting. The half-life ($t_{1/2}$) of a drug is the time required for the total amount of drug in the body or the plasma drug concentration to decrease by one-half (see Figure 1.15). It is sometimes referred to as the $\beta t_{1/2}$ to distinguish it from the half-life for distribution ($\alpha t_{1/2}$) in a two-compartment model, and it is a function of the elimination rate constant, K.

$$t_{1/2} = \frac{0.693}{K} \qquad \text{(Eq. 1.29)}$$

If the K used in Equation 1.29 is derived from plasma concentrations obtained during the decay phase, then the time interval in which the samples are drawn should span at least one half-life as previously mentioned (see discussion of Equation 1.28).

Because the dosing interval is frequently equal to or shorter than the usual half-life for many drugs, it is often impractical to obtain peak and trough levels within a dosing interval to determine the half-life (eg, theophylline, digoxin, and phenobarbital).

If the volume of distribution and Cl for a drug are known, the half-life can be estimated using Equation 1.30. The half-life, like K, is dependent on and determined by Cl and V. This relationship is illustrated in Equation 1.30, which was obtained by substituting Equation 1.27 into Equation 1.29:

$$t_{1/2} = \frac{0.693(V)}{\text{Cl}} \qquad \text{(Eq. 1.30)}$$

The dependence of $t_{1/2}$ or K on V and Cl is emphasized because the volume of distribution and Cl for a drug can change independently of one another and thus affect the half-life or elimination constant in the same or opposite directions. Another caution is appropriate at this point. It is a common misconception that because Equation 1.27 can be rearranged to

$$\text{Cl} = (K)(V) \qquad \text{(Eq. 1.31)}$$

that Cl is determined by K (or $t_{1/2}$) and V; however, this is incorrect considering the physiologic model that is used in the application of pharmacokinetics to the clinical setting. Instead, K and $t_{1/2}$ depend on Cl and the volume of distribution. Therefore, caution should be used when making any assumptions about the volume of distribution or Cl of a drug based solely on knowledge of its half-life. For example, if the half-life of a drug is prolonged, the Cl may be increased, decreased, or unchanged depending on corresponding changes in the volume of distribution. As a general principle, however, when the half-life is longer than the usual value for that drug, it is more likely owing to a decrease in Cl than an increase in volume of distribution. This is because the variability in both renal and hepatic function (ie, Cl) is more likely to be altered than is the plasma and tissue distribution characteristics (volume of distribution) of a drug. However, there are situations when the volume of distribution is significantly altered and should be considered when using pharmacokinetics in the clinical setting (eg, aminoglycosides and digoxin).

CLINICAL APPLICATION OF ELIMINATION RATE CONSTANT (K) AND HALF-LIFE ($t_{1/2}$)

Time to Reach Steady State

Half-life is an important variable to consider when answering questions concerning time such as "How long will it take a drug concentration to reach steady state on a constant dosage regimen?" or "How long will it take for the drug concentration to reach steady state if the dosage regimen is changed?" (For clinical application of half-life, see Table 1.3.)

When drugs are given chronically, they accumulate in the body until the amount administered in a given period (maintenance dose) is equal to the amount eliminated in that same period, that is, rate in equals rate out. When this occurs, drug concentrations in the plasma will plateau and will have reached "steady state" (see Figures 1.10 and 1.16). The time required for a drug concentration to reach steady state is determined by the drug's half-life. It takes 1 half-life to reach 50%, 2 half-lives to reach 75%, 3 half-lives to reach 87.5%, 3.3 half-lives to reach 90%, and 4 half-lives to reach 93.75% of steady state. With each additional half-life, the residual fraction from steady state diminishes, and at some point (usually ≤10%), this residual is considered negligible, and steady state is assumed to have been achieved. In most clinical situations, the attainment of steady state can be assumed after three to five half-lives (Figure 1.17).

TABLE 1.3 Clinical Application of the Elimination Rate Constant (K) and Half-life ($t_{1/2}$)

1. Estimating the time to reach steady-state plasma concentrations after initiation or change in the maintenance dose
2. Estimating the time required to eliminate all or a portion of the drug from the body once it is discontinued
3. Predicting non–steady-state plasma levels following the initiation of an infusion
4. Predicting a steady-state plasma level from a non–steady-state plasma level obtained at a specific time following the initiation of an infusion
5. Given the degree of fluctuation in plasma concentration desired within a dosing interval, determine that interval; given the interval, determine the fluctuation in the plasma concentration

---

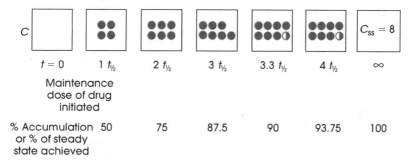

FIGURE 1.17 First-order accumulation. When a maintenance dose is initiated, it takes 3 to 5 half-lives to reach steady-state plasma levels; 3.3 half-lives represent 90% of steady state. This example assumes that the maintenance dose administered will produce an average steady-state level ($C_{ss\ ave}$ or C_{ss}) of 8.

Time for Drug Elimination

The half-life can also be used to determine how long it will take to effectively eliminate all of the drug from the body after the drug has been discontinued. It takes 1 half-life to eliminate 50%, 2 half-lives to eliminate 75%, 3 half-lives to eliminate 87.5%, 3.3 half-lives to eliminate 90%, and 4 half-lives to eliminate 93.75% of the total amount of drug in the body. Again, in most clinical situations, it can be assumed that all of the drug has been effectively eliminated after three to five half-lives (Figure 1.18).

Prediction of Plasma Levels Following Initiation of an Infusion

Often, when drugs are given by constant infusion, it is useful to predict the plasma concentrations that will be achieved at a specific period (Figure 1.19). The rate at which a drug approaches steady state is also governed by the elimination rate constant;

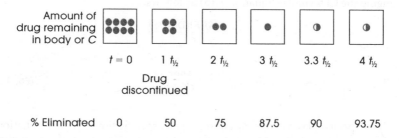

FIGURE 1.18 First-order elimination: amount of drug remaining in the body after one to four half-lives have passed. The amount of drug eliminated per unit of time diminishes over time, but the fraction eliminated in each time interval (in this case, 0.5 as the interval is $1t_{1/2}$) remains the same; $3.3t_{1/2}$ represents 90% eliminated or only 10% remaining.

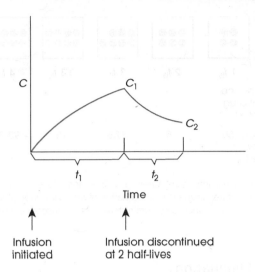

FIGURE 1.19   Graphic representation of an infusion that is discontinued before steady state. C_1 is a concentration that is achieved any time (t_1) after the infusion is initiated, and C_2 is a concentration that results any interval of time (t_2) after the infusion has been discontinued.

therefore, this parameter can be used to calculate the fraction of steady state that is achieved at any time after initiation of the infusion (t_1):

$$C_1 = \frac{(S)(F)(\text{Dose}/\tau)}{\text{Cl}}\left(1 - e^{-Kt_1}\right)$$

$$C_2 = \frac{(S)(F)(\text{Dose}/\tau)}{\text{Cl}}\left(1 - e^{-Kt_1}\right)\left(e^{-Kt_2}\right)$$

$$\begin{array}{l}\text{Fraction of steady state} \\ \text{achieved at time } t_1\end{array} = 1 - e^{-Kt_1} \qquad \textbf{(Eq. 1.32)}$$

The average plasma concentration at steady state ($C_{\text{ss ave}}$) can be calculated by rearranging the Cl formula (Equation 1.15) as follows:

$$\text{Cl} = \frac{(S)(F)(\text{Dose}/\tau)}{C_{\text{ss ave}}}$$

$$C_{\text{ss ave}} = \frac{(S)(F)(\text{Dose}/\tau)}{\text{Cl}} \qquad \textbf{(Eq. 1.33)}$$

The expected plasma concentration (C_1) at a specific time (t_1) after initiation of the infusion can be calculated by multiplying the average steady-state concentration ($C_{\text{ss ave}}$) by the fraction of steady state achieved at t_1.

$$C_1 = (C_{\text{ss ave}})\left(\begin{array}{l}\text{Fraction of steady state} \\ \text{achieved at } t_1\end{array}\right) \qquad \textbf{(Eq. 1.34)}$$

By substituting the appropriate parts of Equations 1.32 and 1.33 into Equation 1.34, a new equation for plasma concentration C_1 at t_1 is derived:

$$C_1 = \frac{(S)(F)(\text{Dose}/\tau)}{\text{Cl}}\left(1 - e^{-Kt_1}\right) \qquad \text{(Eq. 1.35)}$$

All the units in Equation 1.35 must be consistent (eg, time in τ, Cl, and t_1; volume in Cl, V, and C; mass in dose and C). According to Equation 1.35, as the duration of the infusion (t_1) approaches three to five half-lives, the fraction of steady state achieved approaches 1, and, for all practical purposes, the patient is at steady state. Conversely, if a drug plasma concentration (C_1) was obtained before steady-state concentration was attained, the approximate steady-state concentration that should eventually be achieved can be estimated through rearrangement of Equation 1.35 and substituting $C_{\text{ss ave}}$ for $[(S)(F)(\text{Dose}/\tau)]/\text{Cl}$:

$$C_{\text{ss ave}} = \frac{C_1}{1 - e^{-Kt_1}} \qquad \text{(Eq. 1.36)}$$

If the predicted steady-state concentration is unacceptably high, side effects or toxicities might be avoided by reducing the maintenance infusion before the achievement of steady state.

Prediction of Plasma Levels Following Discontinuation of an Infusion

The plasma concentration any time after an infusion is discontinued (C_2) can be estimated by multiplying the measured or predicted plasma concentration (C_1) at the time the infusion is discontinued by the fraction of drug remaining at t_2 hours from the end of the infusion (Figure 1.19).

$$\text{Fraction of drug remaining at } t_2 = e^{-Kt_2} \qquad \text{(Eq. 1.37)}$$

$$C_2 = \left(C_1\right)\left(e^{-Kt_2}\right) \qquad \text{(Eq. 1.38)}$$

If the right side of Equation 1.35

$$C_1 = \frac{(S)(F)(\text{Dose}/\tau)}{\text{Cl}}\left(1 - e^{-Kt_1}\right)$$

is substituted for C_1 in Equation 1.38, the plasma concentration (C_2) at any time (t_2) after an infusion is discontinued is given as follows (see Fig. 1.19):

$$C_2 = \frac{(S)(F)(\text{Dose}/\tau)}{\text{Cl}}\left(1 - e^{-Kt_1}\right)\left(e^{-Kt_2}\right) \qquad \text{(Eq. 1.39)}$$

Although Equation 1.39 may look complicated, it is really a series of simpler equations linked together to model the continuous infusion that was discontinued before steady state (Equation 1.35) followed by a first-order decay (Equation 1.37).

Calculation of a theophylline concentration, which will be expected 8 hours after a theophylline infusion of 80 mg/hr is discontinued, can be used to illustrate this principle. Assume that theophylline has been administered for 16 hours to a patient with a theophylline Cl of 2.8 L/hr and a half-life of 8 hours (K of 0.087 hr^{-1}). The calculations can be accomplished step by step as follows:

1. The expected steady-state theophylline concentration resulting from a theophylline infusion of 80 mg/hr to a patient with a theophylline Cl of 2.8 L/hr and an assumed S and F of 1 can be calculated using Equation 1.33:

$$C_{ss\,ave} = \frac{(S)(F)(Dose/\tau)}{Cl}$$

$$= \frac{(1)(1)\left(80\,mg/hr\right)}{2.8\,L/hr}$$

$$= 28.6\,mg/L$$

2. The expected concentration after 16 hours of infusion (t_1) can be calculated using Equation 1.35:

$$C_1 = \frac{(S)(F)(Dose/\tau)}{Cl}\left(1 - e^{-Kt_1}\right)$$

$$C_1 = 28.6\ mg/L\left(1 - e^{-\left(0.087\,hr^{-1}\right)\left(16\,hr\right)}\right)$$

$$= 28.6\ mg/L\left(1 - e^{-1.392}\right)$$

$$= 28.6\ mg/L\left(1 - 0.25\right)$$

$$= 21.49\ mg/L$$

3. The expected concentration 8 hours after the end of the infusion can be calculated using Equation 1.38:

$$C_2 = \left(C_1\right)\left(e^{-Kt_2}\right)$$

$$C_2 = 21.49\ mg/L\left(e^{-\left(0.087\,hr^{-1}\right)\left(8\,hr\right)}\right)$$

$$= 21.49\ mg/L\left(e^{-0.696}\right)$$

$$= 21.49\ mg/L\left(0.5\right)$$

$$= 10.7\ mg/L$$

Of course, these three steps could have been combined by using Equation 1.39, where t_1 would be 16 hours and t_2 would be 8 hours.

$$C_2 = \frac{(S)(F)(Dose/\tau)}{Cl}\left(1 - e^{-Kt_1}\right)\left(e^{-Kt_2}\right)$$

Whether the stepwise or single combined equation is used depends on how the sequence of events is visualized and, therefore, how the problem or equation is expressed (see Figure 1.19).

Dosing Interval (τ)

The half-life can also be used to estimate the appropriate dosing interval or τ for maintenance therapy when a drug is administered intermittently and the absorption or input into the body is relatively rapid. For example, if the goal of therapy is to minimize plasma fluctuations to no more than 50% between doses, the dosing interval τ should be less than or equal to the half-life. The maintenance dose can be calculated using Equation 1.16:

$$\text{Maintenance dose} = \frac{(Cl)(C_{ss\,ave})(\tau)}{(S)(F)}$$

If τ is less than or equal to the half-life of a drug, the calculated maintenance dose will produce plasma concentrations that will fluctuate by 50% or less during that dosing interval. The plasma levels will be above the average steady-state plasma level for the first half of the dosing interval and below the average steady-state plasma level during the second half of the dosing interval (Figure 1.20).

$$C_{ss\,ave} = \frac{(S)(F)(\text{Dose}/\tau)}{Cl}$$

$$C_{ss\,max} = \frac{\dfrac{(S)(F)(\text{Dose})}{V}}{1 - e^{-K\tau}}$$

$$C_{ss\,min} = \frac{\dfrac{(S)(F)(\text{Dose})}{V}}{1 - e^{-K\tau}} e^{-K\tau}$$

$$C_{ss_1} = \frac{\dfrac{(S)(F)(\text{Dose})}{V}}{1 - e^{-K\tau}} e^{-Kt_1}$$

If the approximate half-life and dosing interval are known, the degree of change in plasma drug concentration that will occur over a dosing interval can be determined. Once the degree of fluctuation is known, one can then determine whether the primary determinant of plasma levels between dosing intervals is the volume of distribution or the Cl or, in some cases, both volume and Cl.

In certain situations, the dosing interval is much longer than the half-life and, for practical purposes, all of the drug is eliminated before the next dose. Therefore, each new dose is essentially a new loading dose. In this situation, each new peak concentration will be determined primarily by the volume of distribution because almost no drug remains from the previous dose.

Antibiotics are commonly dosed in this manner. The therapeutic index for antibiotics is usually so large that wide fluctuations in plasma levels are acceptable and perhaps even desirable.[57,58] Furthermore, the therapeutic effect may require a plasma level that is above the minimal bactericidal or inhibitory concentration for only a brief period relative to the dosing interval.[59]

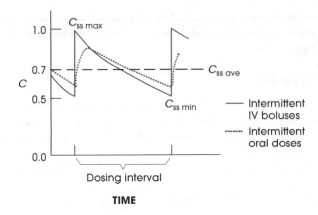

FIGURE 1.20   Plasma level-time curve for intermittent dosing at steady state. When the dosing interval is equal to the half-life, plasma concentrations are above the average steady-state plasma concentration ($C_{ss\ ave}$) ~50% of the time. Oral administration dampens the curve, and the maximum concentration at steady state ($C_{ss\ max}$) occurs later and is lower than that produced by IV bolus. The minimum concentration at steady state ($C_{ss\ min}$) is greater than that produced by IV bolus doses because of the effect of absorption. In the previous equations, τ is the interval between doses and t_1 is the time from the theoretical peak concentration following a dose to the time of sampling. IV, intravenous.

When the dosing interval is much shorter than the half-life, the plasma concentration fluctuates very little throughout the dosing interval. In this case, the plasma concentration will be primarily determined by Cl. Digoxin and phenobarbital given orally and any drug administered by a constant infusion or as a sustained-release dosage form that releases the drug over the entire dosing interval are good examples of such a situation (also see Maximum and Minimum Plasma Concentrations, this part).

Determining the parameter that primarily affects plasma concentration for any given dosage regimen (when τ is longer or shorter than $t_{1/2}$) is important because one then knows which parameters can be calculated reliably from the reported steady-state plasma concentrations. For example, if a patient who has been taking a dose of 0.375 mg of digoxin daily has a reported steady-state trough plasma concentration of 3.8 µg/L, one can reliably calculate the digoxin Cl for this patient using Equation 1.15.

$$Cl = \frac{(S)(F)(Dose/\tau)}{C_{ss\ ave}}$$

Because the dosing interval is much shorter than the half-life, the trough concentration is a good approximation of the $C_{ss\ ave}$, and, therefore, Cl is the major determinant of the patient's plasma concentration. One cannot reliably use the reported plasma concentration to calculate a patient-specific V because the average steady-state concentration is only a function of Cl (see Maximum and Minimum Plasma Concentrations, page 49).

With a new revised Cl value, one can estimate a new maintenance dose. Loading doses are based on the volume of distribution and would require a literature estimate, because no patient-specific information about V can be determined from this drug level. In addition, using the value of V from the literature and our revised Cl, a new estimate of K (Equation 1.27) or $t_{\frac{1}{2}}$ (Equation 1.30) can be obtained:

$$K = \frac{Cl_{revised}}{V_{assumed}}$$

$$t_{\frac{1}{2}} = \frac{0.693\left(V_{assumed}\right)}{Cl_{revised}}$$

Of course, the confidence in this new K or $t_{\frac{1}{2}}$ would depend on the confidence in the assumed value of V derived from the literature.

Maximum and Minimum Plasma Concentrations

It is often important to estimate the maximum ($C_{ss\,max}$ or peak) and minimum ($C_{ss\,min}$ or trough) plasma drug concentrations produced by a given dose of drug within the dosing interval at steady state (see Figure 1.20). For example, whereas it is critical in gentamicin therapy to achieve an acceptable peak concentration for efficacy, it is also important that the trough level be below a specified concentration to minimize concentration-related toxicity.

For drugs with a narrow therapeutic index (eg, theophylline), it is useful to determine the degree of fluctuation in plasma drug concentration that will occur between doses. This can be particularly important if the dosing interval is longer than the half-life (ie, fluctuations will be large) and $C_{ss\,min}$ levels are being used to monitor therapy.

Most frequently, plasma samples for drug assays are drawn as a trough or just before a dose because $C_{ss\,min}$ levels are the most reproducible. The reported plasma drug concentrations for these samples are often considered to be average steady-state concentrations ($C_{ss\,ave}$). However, when the dosing interval approaches or exceeds the drug's half-life, a patient's pharmacokinetic parameters can be more accurately estimated using an equation that describes $C_{ss\,min}$ rather than $C_{ss\,ave}$ (see Maximum and Minimum Plasma Concentrations: Minimum Plasma Drug Concentration [$C_{ss\,min}$]).

MAXIMUM PLASMA DRUG CONCENTRATION ($C_{ss\,max}$)

The maximum plasma drug concentration can be calculated from Equation 1.41 if the dose, salt form (S), bioavailability (F), volume of distribution (V), and elimination rate constant (K) are known:

$$C_{ss\,max} = \frac{\Delta C}{\text{Fraction of drug lost in}\,\tau} \qquad \text{(Eq. 1.40)}$$

or

$$C_{ss\,max} = \frac{\dfrac{(S)(F)(\text{Dose})}{V}}{1 - e^{-K\tau}} \qquad \text{(Eq. 1.41)}$$

where ΔC and $(S)(F)(\text{Dose})/V$ represent the change in drug concentration that occurs over the dosing interval, and $(1 - e^{-K\tau})$ represents the fraction of drug that is eliminated in the dosing interval.

Some pharmacokineticists have chosen to describe the fraction lost in a dosing interval $(1 - e^{-K\tau})$ as the "accumulation factor" and express it as

$$\frac{1}{1 - e^{-K\tau}}$$

and the $C_{ss\,max}$ equation as

$$C_{ss\,max} = \left(\frac{(S)(F)(\text{Dose})}{V}\right)\left(\frac{1}{1 - e^{-K\tau}}\right)$$

This equation is the same as Equation 1.41 expressed in a slightly different format.

Equation 1.41 assumes that drug absorption and distribution rates are rapid in relation to the drug elimination half-life and the dosing interval. This assumption is valid as long as drug concentrations are not sampled during the absorption and distribution phases. Following IV injection, the absorption and distribution phases are relatively short compared to the dosing interval and half-life for most drugs. When drugs are administered orally, the primary concern is with the absorption phase because the distribution component associated with two-compartment modeling is usually negligible. Digoxin and lithium are two notable exceptions in that a distribution phase continues for several hours after oral administration.

For digoxin, the observed peak concentration following oral administration will be greater than that predicted by Equation 1.41 for $C_{ss\,max}$ because drug distribution into tissue requires a minimum of 6 hours. When theophylline is dosed every 6 to 8 hours as an immediate-release product, the observed peak concentration will be slightly lower than that predicted by Equation 1.41 because absorption is relatively slow compared to the dosing interval and the half-life of the drug. This tends to blunt or dampen the peak- and trough-level fluctuations of theophylline because elimination begins before the entire drug enters the body. For most drugs, following oral administration as an immediate-release product, the time required to reach peak concentrations after oral administration is between 1 and 2 hours.

MINIMUM PLASMA DRUG CONCENTRATION ($C_{ss\,min}$)

The minimum plasma drug concentration can be estimated by subtracting ΔC or the change in plasma concentration in one dosing interval from the maximum plasma concentration:

$$C_{ss\,min} = C_{ss\,max} - \Delta C \qquad \text{(Eq. 1.42)}$$

or

$$C_{ss\,min} = C_{ss\,max} - \left(\frac{(S)(F)(\text{Dose})}{V}\right) \qquad \text{(Eq. 1.43)}$$

Alternatively, $C_{ss\,min}$ can be calculated by multiplying $C_{ss\,max}$ by the fraction of drug that remains at the end of the dosing interval ($e^{-K\tau}$).

$$C_{ss\,min} = C_{ss\,max}\,(e^{-K\tau}) \qquad \text{(Eq. 1.44)}$$

Substituting Equation 1.41 for $C_{ss\,max}$ into Equation 1.44 enables one to calculate $C_{ss\,min}$ if the dose, elimination rate constant (K), volume of distribution (V), salt form (S), and bioavailability (F) are known.

$$C_{ss\,min} = \frac{\dfrac{(S)(F)(\text{Dose})}{V}}{1 - e^{-K\tau}}\,e^{-K\tau} \qquad \text{(Eq. 1.45)}$$

If a steady-state sample is obtained at some time other than the peak or trough, the concentration can be calculated as follows:

$$C_{ss_1} = \frac{\dfrac{(S)(F)(\text{Dose})}{V}}{1 - e^{-K\tau}}\,e^{-Kt_1} \qquad \text{(Eq. 1.46)}$$

where t_1 is the number of hours since the last dose, and C_{ss_1} is the steady-state plasma concentration "t_1" hours after the last dose or $C_{ss\,max}$, which is "assumed" to occur at the time of dose administration (ie, absorption or drug input is assumed to be instantaneous). Note that although steady state has been achieved, not all plasma concentrations within the dosing interval represent the average concentration or $C_{ss\,ave}$. If the dosing interval (τ) is short compared to the half-life, the plasma concentration changes very little within the dosing interval and all concentrations are a close approximation of $C_{ss\,ave}$ (see Figures 1.20 and 2.11).

Note that when a slow absorption rate significantly dampens the plasma drug concentration versus time curve (eg, sustained-release dosage forms), the $C_{ss\,min}$ can usually be assumed to be a close approximation of the average steady-state concentration ($C_{ss\,ave}$) and Equation 1.15,

$$\text{Cl} = \frac{(S)(F)(\text{Dose}/\tau)}{C_{ss\,ave}}$$

is used to calculate the patient's pharmacokinetic parameter (ie, Cl) (see Figures 1.20 and 2.11). This assumption is also applicable when the dosing interval is short relative to the half-life. Although it would not be incorrect to use Equation 1.46,

$$C_{ss_1} = \frac{\dfrac{(S)(F)(\text{Dose})}{V}}{1 - e^{-K\tau}}\,e^{-Kt_1}$$

when the dosing interval is much shorter than the drug half-life, the complexity of the equation tends to obscure the fact that all drug concentrations within the dosing interval are essentially an approximation of $C_{ss\,ave}$. In addition, if pharmacokinetic revisions are made by manipulating K and/or V in Equation 1.46, it should be kept in mind that it is the product of K times V or Cl that has the most value or accuracy from the revision process. Again, when the dosing interval is much shorter than the half-life, peak and trough plasma levels are about equal to the average concentration and are, therefore, primarily determined by Cl. Although the product of the V and K obtained by manipulating Equation 1.46 may closely approximate Cl, there is less confidence in the V and K values.

REFERENCES

1. Huffman DH, Manion CV, Azarnoff DL. Absorption of digoxin from different oral preparations in normal subjects during steady state. *Clin Pharmacol Ther.* 1974;16(2):310-317.

2. Iisalo E. Clinical pharmacokinetics of digoxin. *Clin Pharmacokinet.* 1977;2(1):1-16.

3. Mooradian AD. Digitalis. An update of clinical pharmacokinetics, therapeutic monitoring techniques and treatment recommendations. *Clin Pharmacokinet.* 1988;15(3):165-179.

4. Weinberger M, Hendeles L, Bighley L. The relation of product formulation to absorption of oral theophylline. *N Engl J Med.* 1978;299(16):852-857.

5. Hendeles L, Weinberger M, Milavetz G, Hill M, Vaughan L. Food-induced "dose-dumping" from a once-a-day theophylline product as a cause of theophylline toxicity. *Chest.* 1985;87(6):758-765.

6. Mallis GI, Schmidt DH, Lindenbaum J. Superior bioavailability of digoxin solution in capsules. *Clin Pharmacol Ther.* 1975;18(6):761-768.

7. Marcus FI, Dickerson J, Pippin S, Stafford M, Bressler R. Digoxin bioavailability: formulations and rates of infusions. *Clin Pharmacol Ther.* 1976;20(3):253-259.

8. Nahata MC, Powell DA. Bioavailability and clearance of chloramphenicol after intravenous chloramphenicol succinate. *Clin Pharmacol Ther.* 1981;30(3):368-372.

9. Burke JT, Wargin WA, Sherertz RJ, Sanders KL, Blum MR, Sarubbi FA. Pharmacokinetics of intravenous chloramphenicol sodium succinate in adult patients with normal renal and hepatic function. *J Pharmacokinet Biopharm.* 1982;10(6):601-614.

10. Kramer WG, Rensimer ER, Ericsson CD, Pickering LK. Comparative bioavailability of intravenous and oral chloramphenicol in adults. *J Clin Pharmacol.* 1984;24(4):181-186.

11. Nies AS, Shand DG. Clinical pharmacology of propranolol. *Circulation.* 1975;52(1):6-15.

12. Boyes RN, Scott DB, Jebson PJ, Godman MJ, Julian DG. Pharmacokinetics of lidocaine in man. *Clin Pharmacol Ther.* 1971;12(1):105-116.

13. Fahr A. Cyclosporin clinical pharmacokinetics. *Clin Pharmacokinet.* 1993;24(6):472-495.

14. Koch-Weser J, Sellers EM. Binding of drugs to serum albumin (first of two parts). *N Engl J Med.* 1976;294(6):311-316.

15. Levy RH, Shand D, eds. Clinical implications of drug-protein binding. Proceedings of a symposium sponsored by Syva Company. Washington DC, 5th and 6th August, 1983. *Clin Pharmacokinet.* 1984;(9 suppl 1):1-104.

16. Levine M, Chang T. Therapeutic drug monitoring of phenytoin. Rationale and current status. *Clin Pharmacokinet.* 1990;19(5):341-358.

17. Barre J, Didey F, Delion F, Tillement JP. Problems in therapeutic drug monitoring: free drug level monitoring. *Ther Drug Monit.* 1988;10(2):133-143.

18. Perucca E. Pharmacological and therapeutic properties of valproate: a summary after 35 years of clinical experience. *CNS Drugs.* 2002;16(10):695-714.

19. Fremstad D, Bergerud K, Haffner JF, Lunde PK. Increased plasma binding of quinidine after surgery: a preliminary report. *Eur J Clin Pharmacol.* 1976;10(6):441-444.

20. Tucker GT, Boyes RN, Bridenbaugh PO, Moore DC. Binding of anilide-type local anaesthetics in human plasma. I. Relationships between binding, physicochemical properties, and anesthetic activity. *Anesthesiology.* 1970;33(3):287-303.

21. Borgå O, Piafsky KM, Nilsen OG. Plasma protein binding of basic drugs. I. Selective displacement from alpha 1-acid glycoprotein by tris(2-butoxyethyl) phosphate. *Clin Pharmacol Ther.* 1977; 22(5 Pt 1):539-544.

22. Adler DS, Martin E, Gambertoglio JG, Tozer TN, Spire JP. Hemodialysis of phenytoin in a uremic patient. *Clin Pharmacol Ther.* 1975;18(1):65-69.

23. Thummel KE, Shen DD. Appendix II: design and optimization of dosage regimens: pharmacokinetic data. In: Hardman JG, ed. *Goodman and Gilman's the Pharmacologic Basis of Therapeutics.* 10th ed. McGraw-Hill; 2001:1917-2023.

24. Lemaire M, Tillement JP. Role of lipoproteins and erythrocytes in the in vitro binding and distribution of cyclosporin A in the blood. *J Pharm Pharmacol.* 1982;34(11):715-718.

25. Niederberger W, LeMaire M, Maure G, et al. Distribution and binding of cyclosporine in blood and tissue. *Transplant Proc.* 1983;15:2419-2421.

26. Piafsky KM. Disease-induced changes in the plasma binding of basic drugs. *Clin Pharmacokinet.* 1980;5(3):246-262.

27. Pike E, Skuterud B, Kierulf P, Fremstad D, Abdel Sayed SM, Lunde PK. Binding and displacement of basic, acidic and neutral drugs in normal and orosomucoid-deficient plasma. *Clin Pharmacokinet.* 1981;6(5):367-374.

28. Edwards DJ, Lalka D, Cerra F, Slaughter RL. Alpha-1-acid glycoprotein concentration and protein binding in trauma. *Clin Pharmacol Ther.* 1982;31(1):62-67.

29. Routledge PA, Shand DG, Barchowsky A, Wagner G, Stargel WW. Relationship between alpha-1-acid glycoprotein and lidocaine disposition in myocardial infarction. *Clin Pharmacol Ther.* 1981;30(2):154-157.

30. Odar-Cederlöf I, Borgå O. Kinetics of diphenylhydantoin in uraemic patients: consequences of decreased plasma protein binding. *Eur J Clin Pharmacol.* 1974;7(1):31-37.

31. Benet LZ, Hoener BA. Changes in plasma protein binding have little clinical relevance. *Clin Pharmacol Ther.* 2002;71(3):115-121.

32. Svensson CK, Woodruff MN, Baxter JG, Lalka D. Free drug concentration monitoring in clinical practice. Rationale and current status. *Clin Pharmacokinet.* 1986;11(6):450-469.

33. Booker HE, Darcey B. Serum concentrations of free diphenylhydantoin and their relationship to clinical intoxication. *Epilepsia.* 1973;14(2):177-184.

34. Cornford EM, Pardridge WM, Braun LD, Oldendorf WH. Increased blood-brain barrier transport of protein-bound anticonvulsant drugs in the newborn. *J Cereb Blood Flow Metab.* 1983;3(3):280-286.

35. Tozer TN, Gambertoglio JG, Furst DE, Avery DS, Holford NH. Volume shifts and protein binding estimates using equilibrium dialysis: application to prednisolone binding in humans. *J Pharm Sci.* 1983;72(12):1442-1446.

36. Rowland M. Drug administration and regimens. In: Melmon K, Morelli H, eds. *Clinical Pharmacology and Therapeutics.* 2nd ed. Macmillan; 1978:25-29.

37. Reuning RH, Sams RA, Notari RE. Role of pharmacokinetics in drug dosage adjustment: I. Pharmacologic effect kinetics and apparent volume of distribution of digoxin. *J Clin Pharmacol New Drugs.* 1973;13(4):127-141.

38. Gibaldi M, Perrier D. Drug distribution and renal failure. *J Clin Pharmacol New Drugs.* 1972;12(5):201-204.

39. Kappel J, Calissi P. Nephrology: 3. Safe drug prescribing for patients with renal insufficiency. *CMAJ.* 2002;166(4):473-477.

40. Rowland M, Tozer TN. *Clinical Pharmacokinetics: Concepts and Applications.* 2nd ed. Lea & Febiger; 1989.

41. Benowitz NL. Clinical applications of the pharmacokinetics of lidocaine. *Cardiovasc Clin.* 1974;6(2):77-101.

42. Mitenko PA, Ogilvie RI. Rapidly achieved plasma concentration plateaus, with observations on theophylline kinetics. *Clin Pharmacol Ther.* 1972;13(3):329-335.

43. Walsh FM, Sode J. Significance of non-steady-state serum digoxin concentrations. *Am J Clin Pathol.* 1975;63(3):446-450.

44. Shapiro W, Narahara K, Taubert K. Relationship of plasma digitoxin and digoxin to cardiac response following intravenous digitalization in man. *Circulation*. 1970;42(6):1065-1072.

45. Sheiner LB, Rosenberg B, Marathe VV. Estimation of population characteristics of pharmacokinetic parameters from routine clinical data. *J Pharmacokinet Biopharm*. 1977;5(5):445-479.

46. Barot MH, Grant RH, Maheendran KK, Mawer GE, Woodcock BG. Individual variation in daily dosage requirements for phenytoin sodium in patients with epilepsy. *Br J Clin Pharmacol*. 1978;6(3):267-271.

47. Vogelstein B, Kowarski A, Lietman PS. The pharmacokinetics of amikacin in children. *J Pediatr*. 1977;91(2):333-339.

48. I.V. dosage guidelines for theophylline products. *FDA Drug Bull*. 1980;10(1):4-6.

49. Lack JA, Stuart-Taylor ME. Calculation of drug dosage and body surface area of children. *Br J Anaesth*. 1997;78(5):601-605.

50. Sawyer M, Ratain MJ. Body surface area as a determinant of pharmacokinetics and drug dosing. *Invest New Drugs*. 2001;19(2):171-177.

51. Diem K, Lentner C, eds. *Documenta Geigy: Scientific Tables*. 7th ed. Ciba-Geigy; 1972.

52. Gunn VL, Nechyba C, eds. *The Harriet Lane Handbook: A Manual for Pediatric House Officers*. 16th ed. Mosby; 2003.

53. Taketomo CK, ed. *Pediatric Dosage Handbook*. 9th ed. Lexi-Comp; 2002.

54. Ohnhaus EE, Spring P, Dettli L. Protein binding of digoxin in human serum. *Eur J Clin Pharmacol*. 1972;5(1):34-36.

55. Pang KS, Rowland M. Hepatic clearance of drugs. I. Theoretical considerations of a "well-stirred" model and a "parallel tube" model. Influence of hepatic blood flow, plasma and blood cell binding, and the hepatocellular enzymatic activity on hepatic drug clearance. *J Pharmacokinet Biopharm*. 1977;5(6):625-653.

56. Powell JR, Vozeh S, Hopewell P, Costello J, Sheiner LB, Riegelman S. Theophylline disposition in acutely ill hospitalized patients. The effect of smoking, heart failure, severe airway obstruction, and pneumonia. *Am Rev Respir Dis*. 1978;118(2):229-238.

57. ter Braak EW, de Vries PJ, Bouter KP, et al. Once-daily dosing regimen for aminoglycoside plus β-lactam combination therapy for serious bacterial infection: comparative trial with netilmicin plus ceftriaxone. *Am J Med*. 1990;89(1):58-66.

58. Nicolau DP, Freeman CD, Belliveau PP, Nightingale CH, Ross JW, Quintiliani R. Experience with a once-daily aminoglycoside program administered to 2,184 adult patients. *Antimicrob Agents Chemother*. 1995;39(3):650-655.

59. Craig WA, Vogelman B. The postantibiotic effect. *Ann Intern Med*. 1987;106(6):900-902.

2

SELECTING THE APPROPRIATE EQUATION AND INTERPRETATION OF MEASURED DRUG CONCENTRATIONS

Paul M. Beringer

Learning Objectives

By the end of the selecting the appropriate equation and interpretation of measured drug concentrations chapter, the learner shall be able to:

Selecting the Appropriate Equation
1. Draw to approximate scale of a plasma concentration versus time curve, given a set of pharmacokinetic parameters and a drug dosing history. Write the equations that represent the curve, given a plasma concentration versus time curve.

Loading Dose or Bolus Dose
1. Calculate the initial drug concentration and subsequent drug concentration at any time t_1 following the loading dose, given the salt form, bioavailability, elimination rate constant, volume of distribution, and a loading dose.

Continuous Infusion to Steady State
1. Calculate the steady-state drug concentration and the drug concentration at any time t_1 following the discontinuation of the infusion, given the salt form, bioavailability, clearance, elimination rate constant, and an infusion or input rate.

Initiation and Discontinuation of Infusion Before Steady State
1. Calculate the drug concentration as it accumulates toward steady state at t_1 or t_{in} hours after initiating the infusion and the drug concentration at

any time t_2 following the discontinuation of the infusion, given the salt form, bioavailability, clearance, elimination rate constant, and an infusion or input rate.

2. Explain when the instantaneous input or bolus versus short infusion model can be used and, given a set of pharmacokinetic parameters and the duration of drug input, select the simplest model that will approximate the drug concentrations with 10% error.

3. Describe the different pharmacokinetic functions of t_{in} in $[(S)(F)(Dose)]/t_{in}$ versus $1 - e^{-Kt_{in}}$ for the short infusion model, that is, which one is used to determine "rate" and which to determine "duration" of the infusion.

Loading Dose Followed by Infusion

1. Calculate the expected concentration C_1 at any time t_1 following a loading dose and immediate initiation of a continuous infusion, given the pharmacokinetic parameters S, F, dose, volume of distribution, clearance, and K.

Intermittent Administration at Regular Intervals to Steady State

1. Predict steady-state peak and trough concentrations and the drug concentration at any time t_1 following the steady-state peak concentration, given the pharmacokinetic parameters S, F, dose, volume of distribution, and K.

Series of Individual Doses

1. Predict a drug concentration at any time after the administration of a series of individual doses given at irregular intervals by summing the concentration remaining for each of the individual doses, given the pharmacokinetic parameters S, F, dose, volume of distribution, clearance, and K.

2. Predict a drug concentration at any time after the administration of a series of individual doses (N doses) given at regular intervals, given the pharmacokinetic parameters S, F, dose, volume of distribution, clearance, and K.

Sustained-Release Dosage Forms

1. Define the conditions that allow the use of a continuous uninterrupted infusion model for sustained-release oral dosage forms (ie, $\tau - t_{in}$ vs drug $t_{1/2}$), assuming zero-order input, and recognize when the continuous uninterrupted infusion model would not be appropriate, given a set of pharmacokinetic parameters.

Algorithm for Choosing the Appropriate Equation

1. Determine whether steady state has or has not been achieved, given a set of pharmacokinetic parameters and a dosing history.

2. Determine whether steady state has been achieved:
   a. If a continuous or intermittent input model is required to predict plasma concentrations.

   b. If an intermittent input model is required to determine whether it is the bolus model or short infusion model that would be most appropriate to predict plasma concentrations.
3. Determine whether steady state has not been achieved:
   a. Whether a series of individual bolus or short infusion models would be required to predict the drug concentrations if dose and τ are not consistent.
   b. Whether a non–steady-state continuous infusion, non–steady-state bolus, or non–steady-state short infusion model would be required to predict the plasma concentrations if dose and τ are consistent.

Interpretation of Plasma Drug Concentrations
1. Determine whether it is likely that the measured drug concentration represents steady state or non–steady state and then select the model to revise the proper pharmacokinetic parameter(s), given a patient's dosing history, plasma drug concentration(s), and the literature estimates of the drug's pharmacokinetic parameters.

Plasma Sampling Time
1. Explain why, in most cases, trough drug samples are preferred to peak drug samples.
2. Recognize whether or not the drug sample is likely to have been obtained in the absorption/distribution phase when given a dosing history and drug sampling time(s).

Revising Pharmacokinetic Parameters
1. Define the conditions with regard to drug input (absorption and distribution) and the time interval (absorption and decay) that must be met in order to be able to revise the volume of distribution.
2. Explain why the average steady-state concentration is determined by clearance.
3. Explain when a steady-state trough concentration can be substituted for steady-state average concentration to revise clearance.
4. Recognize when the change in the literature or predicted versus revised pharmacokinetic parameter is much different than the change in predicted versus measured drug concentration when performing pharmacokinetic revisions.
5. Identify and explain why volume, clearance, or neither volume nor clearance can be revised, given a patient's dosing history, drug sampling times, and the literature estimates of the drug's pharmacokinetic parameters.

Choosing a Model to Revise or Estimate a Patient's Clearance at Steady State
1. Determine, by comparing $[(S)(F)(\text{Dose})]/V$ versus $C_{ss\ min}$, the approximate relationship between τ and the drug $t_{1/2}$.

2. Choose the simplest equation necessary to revise clearance using a single C_{ss} trough concentration when:
   a. $\tau \leq \frac{1}{3}t_{\frac{1}{2}}$
   b. $\tau \leq t_{\frac{1}{2}}$
   c. $\tau > t_{\frac{1}{2}}$
3. Know the conditions required for (2) and, given a patient dosing history and time of drug sampling, recognize when one or more of the conditions have not been met.
4. Explain why confidence in the revised clearance increases when $\tau \leq t_{\frac{1}{2}}$ and decreases as τ increases beyond $t_{\frac{1}{2}}$.

Non–Steady-State Revision of Clearance (Iterative Search)
1. Recognize which equations can be rearranged to solve directly for clearance and which cannot.
2. Explain why it is important, when performing non–steady-state revisions, for the change in the predicted relative to the revised clearance to approximate the change in the predicted relative to the measured drug concentration. That is, sensitivity analysis.
3. Recognize when the percentage change in the literature or predicted versus revised clearance is very much different from the percentage change in the predicted versus measured drug concentration.

Non–Steady-State Revision of Clearance (Mass Balance)
1. Use the mass balance approach to calculate a revised clearance, given two non–steady-state drug concentrations, a literature estimate of volume of distribution, and the drug dosing history between the two concentrations.
2. Know the conditions required for using the mass balance approach, time interval in $t_{\frac{1}{2}}$s between the two concentrations, the allowable change from the first to the second concentration, and consistency of the dosing rate.
3. Recognize when one or more of the abovementioned conditions have not been met, for example, compare the interval between the two concentrations to the revised $t_{\frac{1}{2}}$ as calculated from the predicted volume of distribution and the mass balance revised clearance.

Single-Point Determination of Clearance
1. Demonstrate graphically the impact on the drug concentration decay from a single bolus dose when clearance is held constant and volume of distribution is increased or decreased.
2. Explain why, although in principle, the single-point determination of clearance is appealing, but its clinical use is limited.

Bayesian Analysis
1. Explain the basic concepts of Bayesian analysis and why this type of approach will help to avoid "making too much out of too little" when performing pharmacokinetic revisions.

2. Give at least one example of where Bayesian analysis would help to avoid making an inappropriate revision of a pharmacokinetic parameter.

Assay Specificity
1. List at least two factors that may make a reported drug concentration inaccurate.
2. Recognize that drug assay procedures are often changed so that knowledge of the specific assay used is the only way to know for sure whether there are likely to be conditions that alter the utility of the reported drug concentration.
3. List at least two drugs that have active metabolites.

Selecting the Appropriate Equation

It is often difficult to determine which of the many equations should be used to solve specific clinical problems. A technique used by this author to avoid the use of inappropriate equations is to draw a graphic representation of the plasma drug concentration versus time curve that would be expected on the basis of the dosage regimen the patient is receiving. Once the graph is drawn and the plasma concentration visualized, mathematical equations that describe the drug's pharmacokinetic behavior are selected. To facilitate this process, a series of typical plasma level-time curves and their corresponding formulas is presented in Figures 2.1 to 2.7.

LOADING DOSE OR BOLUS DOSE

When a loading dose or a bolus of drug has been administered (Figure 2.1), the initial plasma concentration (C) can be determined by rearranging the "loading dose" equation (see Equation 1.11):

$$C = \frac{(S)(F)(\text{Loading dose})}{V} \qquad \text{(Eq. 2.1)}$$

A subsequent plasma level (C_1) at any time (t_1) after the dose has been administered can be calculated by using a variation of Equation 1.26 that describes first-order elimination:

$$C_2 = (C_1)(e^{-Kt_1})$$

where C_1 is replaced by $C = \dfrac{(S)(F)(\text{Loading dose})}{V}$ and C_2 by C_1.

$$C_1 = \frac{(S)(F)(\text{Loading dose})}{V}(e^{-Kt_1}) \qquad \text{(Eq. 2.2)}$$

C_1 now represents the concentration remaining t_1 hours after the loading dose.

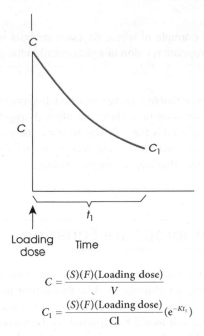

$$C = \frac{(S)(F)(\text{Loading dose})}{V}$$

$$C_1 = \frac{(S)(F)(\text{Loading dose})}{Cl}(e^{-Kt_1})$$

FIGURE 2.1 Graphic representation of the change in plasma level that occurs over time following a loading dose. C represents the initial concentration immediately following the administration of a loading dose, and C_1 represents the concentration at any interval of time (t_1) after the dose has been administered. Assume a one-compartment model and rapid absorption if the drug is given orally.

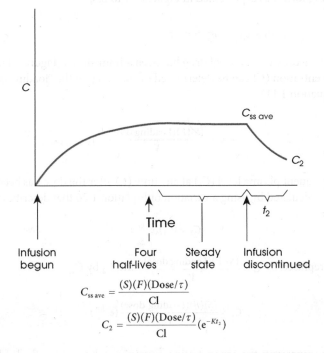

$$C_{\text{ss ave}} = \frac{(S)(F)(\text{Dose}/\tau)}{Cl}$$

$$C_2 = \frac{(S)(F)(\text{Dose}/\tau)}{Cl}(e^{-Kt_2})$$

FIGURE 2.2 Graphic representation of the plasma concentration versus time curve that results when an infusion is continued until steady state is reached and then discontinued. $C_{\text{ss ave}}$ is the steady-state concentration, and C_2 is the concentration at any interval of time (t_2) after the infusion has been discontinued.

CONTINUOUS INFUSION TO STEADY STATE

The plasma concentration versus time curve produced by a continuous infusion, which has been administered until steady state has been achieved, is represented by Figure 2.2. The average steady-state concentration ($C_{ss\,ave}$) that will be produced by the infusion can be calculated using Equation 1.33.

$$C_{ss\,ave} = \frac{(S)(F)(Dose/\tau)}{Cl}$$

DISCONTINUATION OF INFUSION AFTER STEADY STATE

The curve representing a change in plasma concentration after the infusion has been discontinued is also represented in Figure 2.2. The concentration (C_2) produced at any time (t_2) after the infusion has been discontinued can be calculated using a variation of the first-order elimination equation (Equation 1.26):

$$C_2 = (C_1)(e^{-Kt_1})$$

where C_1 is replaced by $C_{ss\,ave}$ and t_1 by t_2:

$$C_2 = (C_{ss\,ave})(e^{-Kt_2}) \qquad\qquad \text{(Eq. 2.3)}$$

or substituting for $C_{ss\,ave}$ gives:

$$C_2 = \frac{(S)(F)(Dose/\tau)}{Cl}(e^{-Kt_2}) \qquad\qquad \text{(Eq. 2.4)}$$

INITIATION AND DISCONTINUATION OF INFUSION BEFORE STEADY STATE

When an infusion is initiated and discontinued before steady state is achieved (<3 to $5t_{1/2}$), the plasma concentration versus time curve can be described, as depicted in Figure 1.19. In this situation, the concentration (C_1) that occurs at any time (t_1) after the infusion has been initiated and the concentration (C_2) that occurs at any time (t_2) after the infusion was discontinued can be approximated by Equation 1.35:

$$C_1 = \frac{(S)(F)(Dose/\tau)}{Cl}(1 - e^{-Kt_1})$$

and Equation 1.39:

$$C_2 = \frac{(S)(F)(Dose/\tau)}{Cl}(1 - e^{-Kt_1})(e^{-Kt_2})$$

The input model for Equations 1.35 and 1.39 is an infusion model. Whether a bolus or an infusion model is used to represent the input or absorption of drug into the body depends on the relationship between the duration of drug input relative to the drug's half-life. For example, if a drug is administered rapidly as an intravenous (IV) bolus or if an orally administered drug is absorbed rapidly relative to the drug's half-life, very little drug will be cleared or eliminated during the administration or absorption process. Therefore, absorption can be thought of as instantaneous, and the bolus model can be used. If, however, a drug is absorbed over a long time relative to its half-life, a significant amount of drug will be eliminated during the input or absorption period, and the plasma-level concentrations resulting from oral adminis-tration would resemble those resulting from an infusion model. As a general rule, if the drug input time (t_{in}) is less than one-tenth its half-life, then it can be successfully modeled as a bolus dose; however, if the drug input time is greater than one-half its half-life, it is more appropriate to use an infusion model. When the duration of drug input falls between one-tenth and one-half of its half-life, an arbitrary choice can be made between a bolus dose and an infusion model.

As a clinical guideline, the author uses one-sixth of a drug's half-life as an ar-bitrary break point. That is, for those drugs that are absorbed over a period equal to one-sixth of a half-life or less, the bolus model is used; for those drugs absorbed over a period that is greater than one-sixth of the half-life, the short infusion model is used. Whereas the one-sixth of a half-life "rule" is arbitrary, it was selected because the dif-ference in the calculated plasma concentrations when using the bolus or short infusion model is less than 10% (see Figure 2.4).

If there is any uncertainty about which model is more appropriate, the short infusion model should be used because it more closely approximates the actual ab-sorption and plasma concentration curve during drug absorption and elimination. Figure 2.3 represents the plasma concentration obtained at the end of a short infusion, as calculated by Equation 2.5.

$$C_{t_{in}} = \frac{(S)(F)(\text{Dose}/t_{in})}{Cl}(1 - e^{-Kt_{in}}) \hspace{2cm} \textbf{(Eq. 2.5)}$$

Note, in this equation, that t_{in} represents the duration of drug input and $1 - e^{-Kt_{in}}$ represents the fraction of steady state that would be achieved during the infusion time. This concentration $(C_{t_{in}})$, therefore, represents the peak level at the end of the infusion.

Conceptually, it is useful to compare Equation 2.5 with Equation 1.35.

$$C_1 = \frac{(S)(F)(\text{Dose}/\tau)}{Cl}(1 - e^{-Kt_1})$$

Both equations represent the process of multiplying a steady-state average con-centration by the fraction of steady state achieved. The dosing interval (τ) and duration of infusion (t_1) in Equation 1.35 are replaced in Equation 2.5 with the duration of drug input (t_{in}). Although both equations represent the same basic process, Equation 1.35

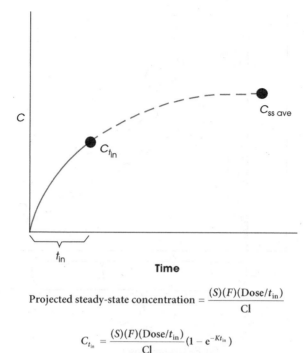

$$\text{Projected steady-state concentration} = \frac{(S)(F)(\text{Dose}/t_{\text{in}})}{Cl}$$

$$C_{t_{\text{in}}} = \frac{(S)(F)(\text{Dose}/t_{\text{in}})}{Cl}(1 - e^{-Kt_{\text{in}}})$$

FIGURE 2.3 Graphic representation of a short infusion. The plasma concentration at the end of a short infusion $(1 - e^{-Kt_{\text{in}}})$ can be calculated by multiplying the "projected steady-state concentration" (dotted line) by the fraction of steady state achieved $(1 - e^{-Kt_{\text{in}}})$ during the infusion period (t_{in}).

is most commonly used when a continuous infusion (eg, theophylline, lidocaine) is discontinued or sampled before steady state is achieved, and Equation 2.5 is used when a dose is to be administered over a relatively short period (eg, aminoglycoside antibi-otics). Note, in Equation 2.5, that the "function" of t_{in} in $(S)(F)(\text{Dose}/t_{\text{in}})$ is to convert the dose into a rate of drug input, and the t_{in} in $(1 - e^{-Kt_{\text{in}}})$ is the duration over which the drug input occurs. Although the value of t_{in} is usually the same in Equation 2.5, for example, 0.5 hour as one generally thinks of the dose being infused over 0.5 hour, the pharmacokinetic function of the two t_{in}s is different.

Once the infusion has been concluded, any subsequent drug concentration (C_2) can be calculated by multiplying the concentration at the end of the infusion $(C_{t_{\text{in}}})$ by the fraction remaining at any time interval since the end of the infusion (t_2).

$$C_2 = \frac{(S)(F)(\text{Dose}/t_{\text{in}})}{Cl}(1 - e^{-Kt_{\text{in}}})(e^{-Kt_2}) \qquad \text{(Eq. 2.6)}$$

The relationship between plasma concentrations predicted by the bolus dose equation (Equations 2.1 and 2.2) and the short infusion equation (Equations 2.5 and 2.6)

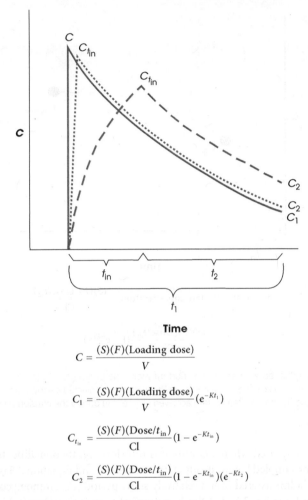

$$C = \frac{(S)(F)(\text{Loading dose})}{V}$$

$$C_1 = \frac{(S)(F)(\text{Loading dose})}{V}(e^{-Kt_1})$$

$$C_{t_{in}} = \frac{(S)(F)(\text{Dose}/t_{in})}{Cl}(1 - e^{-Kt_{in}})$$

$$C_2 = \frac{(S)(F)(\text{Dose}/t_{in})}{Cl}(1 - e^{-Kt_{in}})(e^{-Kt_2})$$

FIGURE 2.4 Graphic representation of a drug administered as a bolus (solid line) or as a short infusion (dashed line and dotted line). The bolus dose model assumes that drug input or absorption is instantaneous. The decay interval, t_1 (ie, $t_{in} + t_2$), is, therefore, assumed to begin at the start of the infusion. In contrast, the infusion model assumes that the decay interval (t_2) begins at the conclusion of the infusion period (t_{in}). When t_{in} is $\leq \frac{1}{6}t_{\frac{1}{2}}$ (dotted line), the concentrations are approximately the same for the short infusion and bolus dose model. When t_{in} is considerably $> \frac{1}{6}t_{\frac{1}{2}}$ (dashed line), the concentrations calculated by the short infusion and bolus dose model are substantially different.

is depicted in Figure 2.4. Note that the bolus dose is assumed to be instantaneously absorbed at the beginning of the infusion; therefore, the initial peak concentration is higher than would be predicted by the short infusion model.

However, plasma concentrations corresponding to the conclusion of the short infusion model (t_{in} hours after starting the infusion) and all subsequent plasma levels are lower for the bolus dose model than for the infusion model. If the infusion time t_{in} is less than one-sixth of a drug's half-life, then the difference between the plasma concentrations predicted by the bolus dose and the short infusion model will be minimal. Although either equation can be used, the bolus dose model is much simpler.

LOADING DOSE FOLLOWED BY INFUSION

When a patient is given a loading dose followed by an infusion, the plasma concentration (C_1) at any time (t_1) can be calculated by summing the equations that describe the concentration produced by the loading dose at t_1 (Equation 2.2) and the concentration produced by the infusion at t_1 (Equation 1.35) (refer to C_1 in Figure 2.1 and C_1 in Figure 1.19).

$$C_1 = \begin{matrix} \text{Concentration} \\ \text{produced by the} \\ \text{loading dose at } t_1 \end{matrix} + \begin{matrix} \text{Concentration} \\ \text{produced by the} \\ \text{infusion at } t_1 \end{matrix}$$

$$C_1 = \left[\frac{(S)(F)(\text{Loading dose})}{V}(e^{-Kt_1}) \right] + \left[\frac{(S)(F)(\text{Dose}/\tau)}{\text{Cl}}(1 - e^{-Kt_1}) \right]$$

Note that $(S)(F)(\text{Dose}/\tau)$ in the second portion of the equation represents the infusion rate. It is important to recall in this situation that the loading dose is eliminated according to first-order pharmacokinetics, as described in Figure 2.1, even when a maintenance infusion is initiated. This must be taken into account when predicting a plasma concentration. In other words, the maintenance infusion is accumulating, whereas the concentration resulting from the loading dose is diminishing (Figure 2.5).

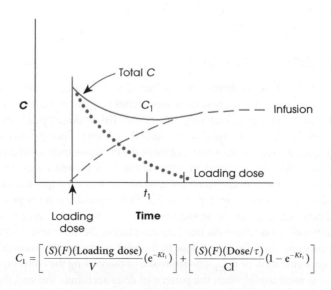

$$C_1 = \left[\frac{(S)(F)(\text{Loading dose})}{V}(e^{-Kt_1}) \right] + \left[\frac{(S)(F)(\text{Dose}/\tau)}{\text{Cl}}(1 - e^{-Kt_1}) \right]$$

FIGURE 2.5   Graphic representation of the plasma level-time curve that results from a loading dose followed by a maintenance infusion. The curve (solid line) represents a summation of a loading dose curve (dotted line) and an infusion curve (dashed line). C_1 is the concentration at any time (t_1) after the loading dose has been administered and after the maintenance infusion has been initiated.

INTERMITTENT ADMINISTRATION AT REGULAR INTERVALS TO STEADY STATE

When a drug is administered intermittently at regular dosing intervals until steady state is achieved (at least three to five half-lives), the average steady-state concentration can be calculated using Equation 1.33.

$$C_{ss\ ave} = \frac{(S)(F)(Dose/\tau)}{Cl}$$

Assuming absorption is rapid relative to $t_{1/2}$, the steady-state maximum and minimum concentrations can be approximated using Equations 1.41 and 1.45, respectively.

$$C_{ss\ max} = \frac{\dfrac{(S)(F)(Dose)}{V}}{1 - e^{-K\tau}}$$

$$C_{ss\ min} = \frac{\dfrac{(S)(F)(Dose)}{V}}{1 - e^{-K\tau}} e^{-K\tau}$$

Prediction of a plasma concentration at any time (t_1) following the peak can be accomplished using Equation 1.46. Figure 2.6 depicts the plasma concentration versus time curve that occurs with this type of dosing regimen "Maximum and Minimum Plasma Concentrations" section in Chapter "Pharmacokinetic Processes and Parameters").

$$C_{ss_1} = \frac{\dfrac{(S)(F)(Dose)}{V}}{1 - e^{-K\tau}} e^{-Kt_1}$$

SERIES OF INDIVIDUAL DOSES

When a series of individual doses is administered and a concentration before steady state must be calculated, there are several approaches that can be taken. One approach is to sum the contributions of each individual dose. This is done by decaying the peak concentration of each dose to the time at which the plasma concentration needs to be predicted. Figure 2.7 represents a series of three doses whose individual contributions were calculated and then summed to estimate the total plasma concentration existing at some time point after the third dose. Note that this is simply the sum of three individual doses, as modeled by Equation 2.2. This approach is most practical when the interval between doses or the amount of drug administered with each dose varies. Note that depending on where the brackets are placed, the summation equation may predict the concentration from one dose to the next or the contribution of each dose to the final concentration or C_{sum}. The approach of calculating the concentration from dose to dose is most useful when the pattern of drug accumulation and the potential of drug effect at each point in time are of interest. However, if the intent is to see how much each of the individual doses contribute or if an iterative solution for revision of

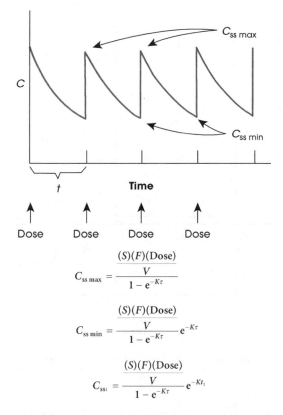

$$C_{ss\,max} = \dfrac{\dfrac{(S)(F)(Dose)}{V}}{1 - e^{-K\tau}}$$

$$C_{ss\,min} = \dfrac{\dfrac{(S)(F)(Dose)}{V}}{1 - e^{-K\tau}}\,e^{-K\tau}$$

$$C_{ss1} = \dfrac{\dfrac{(S)(F)(Dose)}{V}}{1 - e^{-K\tau}}\,e^{-Kt_1}$$

FIGURE 2.6   Graphic representation of the steady-state plasma concentration versus time curve that occurs when drugs are given intermittently at regular dosing intervals. Any maximum concentration ($C_{ss\,max}$) is interchangeable with any other maximum concentration, and any minimum concentration ($C_{ss\,min}$) is interchangeable with any other minimum concentration. In addition, any concentration (C_{ss1}) at time t_1 within a dosing interval is interchangeable with a corresponding concentration at the same t_1 within any other interval.

a pharmacokinetic parameter is to be performed, then the approach that allows one to see how much each dose is contributing to the final solution is preferred.

If each dose and the intervals between doses are the same, it may be simpler to multiply $C_{ss\,max}$ or the peak concentration that would be achieved at steady state (Equation 1.41)

$$C_{ss\,max} = \dfrac{\dfrac{(S)(F)(Dose)}{V}}{1 - e^{-K\tau}}$$

by the fraction of steady state achieved after N doses.

Fraction of steady state achieved after (N) doses $= 1 - e^{-K(N)\tau}$ **(Eq. 2.7)**

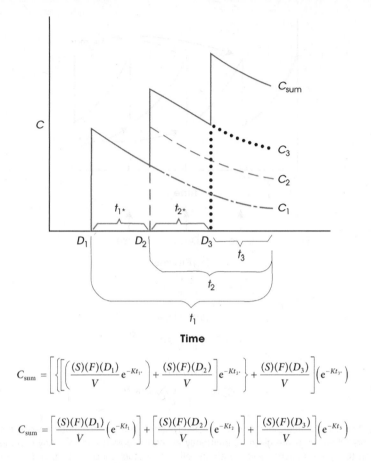

$$C_{\text{sum}} = \left[\left\{ \left[\left(\frac{(S)(F)(D_1)}{V} e^{-Kt_1\cdot} \right) + \frac{(S)(F)(D_2)}{V} \right] e^{-Kt_2\cdot} \right\} + \frac{(S)(F)(D_3)}{V} \right] \left(e^{-Kt_3\cdot} \right)$$

$$C_{\text{sum}} = \left[\frac{(S)(F)(D_1)}{V} \left(e^{-Kt_1} \right) \right] + \left[\frac{(S)(F)(D_2)}{V} \left(e^{-Kt_2} \right) \right] + \left[\frac{(S)(F)(D_3)}{V} \right] \left(e^{-Kt_3} \right)$$

FIGURE 2.7 · Graphic representation of non–steady-state summation of individual doses. The solid line represents the top summation equation and a plasma concentration because each dose is administered (D_1, D_2, D_3) as they accumulate. $t_1\cdot$ is the time from D_1 to D_2, $t_2\cdot$ is the time from D_2 to D_3, and t_3 is the time from D_3 to the time at which the plasma concentration (C_{sum}) is to be calculated. The dashed and dotted lines represent the bottom summation equation and the contribution of each of the individual doses to the total concentration or C_{sum}. The t_1, t_2, and t_3 represent the time from each administered dose to the time at which the plasma concentration (C_{sum}) is to be calculated.

In Equation 2.7, τ is the interval between each dose, and N represents the number of doses that have been administered. The peak concentration following N doses can be calculated by combining Equations 1.41 and 2.7. Any concentration (C_2) following the Nth dose can be calculated by multiplying the peak concentration following N doses by e^{-Kt_2}, where t_2 is the number of hours since the last dose.

$$C_{ss_2} = \frac{\dfrac{(S)(F)(\text{Dose})}{V}}{1 - e^{-K\tau}} \left(1 - e^{-K(N)\tau} \right) \left(e^{-Kt_2} \right) \qquad \text{(Eq. 2.8)}$$

Note that if the doses and dosing intervals were the same in Figure 2.7, the concentration (C_{sum}) could be calculated using Equation 2.8, where N would be 3 and t_2 would be the number of hours after the third dose. Equation 2.8 is most useful when a number of doses have been administered with a consistent τ, but steady state has not yet been achieved. Equation 2.8 represents the concentration of drug produced by a series of consistently administered bolus doses that have not yet achieved steady state. This equation can be further expanded to represent a series of doses that are absorbed over a significant fraction of the drug's half-life (ie, $t_{in} > {}^1\!/_6 t_{\frac{1}{2}}$).

$$C_{ss_2} = \frac{\dfrac{(S)(F)(\text{Dose}/t_{in})}{Cl}}{1 - e^{-K\tau}}\left(1 - e^{-K(N)\tau}\right)\left(e^{-Kt_2}\right) \qquad \textbf{(Eq. 2.9)}$$

Equation 2.9 is similar to Equation 2.8, except that the bolus dose input model is now replaced with the short infusion input model. Equation 2.9 is seldom used in clinical practice. This is because the half-life of the drug, which requires the use of a short infusion input model, is likely to be sufficiently brief such that steady state will be achieved after two to three doses have been administered.

SUSTAINED-RELEASE DOSAGE FORMS

Most sustained-release dosage forms are designed to produce concentrations that fluctuate little within the dosage interval. Therefore, in most cases, concentrations produced by sustained-release products can be estimated by use of the equation that describes the average steady-state concentration (Equation 1.33):

$$C_{ss\ ave} = \frac{(S)(F)(\text{Dose}/\tau)}{Cl}$$

As illustrated in the following equation, the use of the $C_{ss\ ave}$ formula for sustained-release products is based on the assumption that the time required for absorption (t_{in}) is approximately equal to the dosing interval (τ).

$$C_{ss_2} = \frac{\dfrac{(S)(F)(\text{Dose}/t_{in})}{Cl}\left(1 - e^{-Kt_{in}}\right)}{1 - e^{-K\tau}}\left(e^{-Kt_2}\right) \qquad \textbf{(Eq. 2.10)}$$

$$C_{ss_2} = \frac{\dfrac{(S)(F)(\text{Dose}/\tau)}{Cl}\left(1 - e^{-K\tau}\right)}{1 - e^{-K\tau}}\left(e^{-Kt_2}\right)$$

In this equation, the $1 - e^{-K\tau}$ in the numerator and denominator cancel, and assuming t_2 is 0, we have Equation 1.33.

$$C_{ss\ ave} = \frac{(S)(F)(Dose/\tau)}{Cl}$$

If the t_{in} is exactly equal to τ, the input from one dose stops at the same time the next dose begins its infusion process. As a result, an average steady-state concentration with no rise or fall within the dosing interval is achieved. This would be exactly the same as changing an IV bag for a constant infusion without interrupting the infusion process. In practice, absorption times are not exactly equal to the dosing interval, but for most sustained-release drug products, they are reasonably close, and therefore, plasma concentrations can be considered an average steady-state value. It should be emphasized, however, that the use of Equation 1.33 is not universal and depends on not only the absorption of the drug product but also the dosing interval selected and half-life of the drug in the specific patient. As a general rule, absorption times that exceed the dosing interval are not a problem. However, if the duration of absorption (t_{in}) is substantially less than the dosing interval, then there will be some fluctuation in the plasma concentrations. A useful approach is to consider the duration over which the plasma concentrations will decay following the end of absorption. This can be approximated by subtracting the absorption time from the dosing interval.

$$\tau - t_{in} = \begin{array}{l}\text{Time within the dosing}\\\text{interval with no drug absorption}\end{array} \qquad \textbf{(Eq. 2.11)}$$

If this time within the dosing interval when there is no drug input is short compared to the drug's half-life, it suggests that there will be little fluctuation of the plasma concentration within the dosing interval. As a clinical guideline, if $\tau - t_{in}$ is $\leq \frac{1}{3}t_{1/2}$, the average steady-state equation (Equation 1.33) can be used. Note that this guideline is very similar to the guidelines used for substituting the average steady-state equation (Equation 1.33) for the intermittent bolus dose equation (Equation 1.46) (see Figure 2.11 and Interpretation of Plasma Drug Concentrations: Choosing a Model to Revise or Estimate a Patient's Clearance at Steady State). Note, however, in Figure 2.11, that the time of decay is considered to be the entire dosing interval, because the absorption is assumed to be instantaneous and t_{in} is 0.

ALGORITHM FOR CHOOSING THE APPROPRIATE EQUATION

Selecting the appropriate equation to use in a specific clinical situation can be a complex process. The algorithm in Figure 2.8 offers a stepwise approach to this process. The rules follow those outlined in the text. First, one must consider whether steady state has been achieved; then, the appropriate model is chosen to predict or calculate drug concentrations.

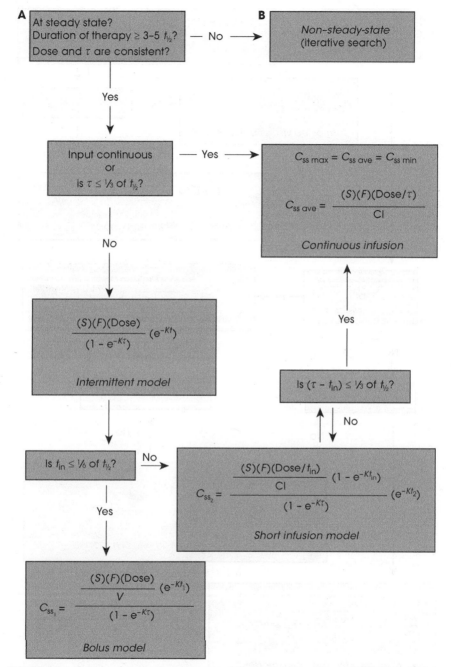

FIGURE 2.8 Algorithm for choosing the appropriate pharmacokinetic model. **(A)** At steady state and **(B)** non–steady state.

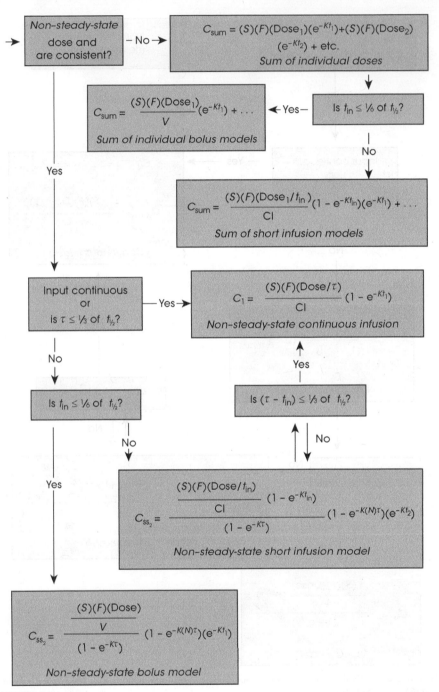

FIGURE 2.8 (continued)

Interpretation of Plasma Drug Concentrations

Plasma drug concentrations are measured in the clinical setting to determine whether a potentially therapeutic or toxic concentration has been produced by a given dosage regimen. This process is based on the assumption that plasma drug concentrations reflect drug concentrations at the receptor and, therefore, can be correlated with pharmacologic response. This assumption is not always valid. When plasma samples are obtained at inappropriate times or when other factors (such as delayed absorption or altered plasma binding) confound the usual pharmacokinetic behavior of a drug, the interpretation of serum drug concentrations can lead to erroneous pharmacokinetic and pharmacodynamic conclusions and ultimately inappropriate patient care decisions. These factors are discussed in the subsequent sections.

PLASMA SAMPLING TIME

To properly interpret a plasma concentration, it is essential to know when a plasma sample was obtained in relation to the last dose administered and when the drug regimen was initiated. If a plasma sample is obtained before distribution of the drug into tissue is complete (eg, digoxin), the plasma concentration will be higher than predicted based on the dose and response. Peak ($C_{ss\,max}$) plasma levels are helpful in evaluating the dose of antibiotics used to treat severe, life-threatening infections. Although serum concentrations for many drugs peak 1 to 2 hours after an oral dose is administered, factors such as slow or delayed absorption can significantly delay the time at which peak serum concentrations are attained. Large errors in the estimation of $C_{ss\,max}$ can occur if the plasma sample is obtained at the wrong time (Figure 2.9). Therefore, with few exceptions, plasma samples should be drawn as trough or just before the next dose

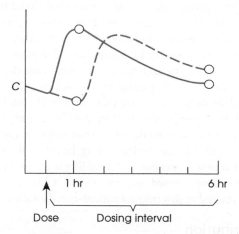

FIGURE 2.9 Schematic representation of the effect of delayed absorption (dashed line) on plasma-level measurements (solid line). Note the magnitude of error at 1 hour (theoretical time to reach $C_{ss\,max}$) as compared to 6 hours ($C_{ss\,min}$).

($C_{ss\,min}$) when determining routine drug concentrations in plasma. These trough levels are less likely to be influenced by absorption and distribution problems.

When the full therapeutic response of a given drug dosage regimen is to be assessed, plasma samples should not be obtained until steady-state concentrations of the drug have been achieved. If drug doses are increased or decreased based on the drug concentrations that have been measured while the drug is still accumulating, disastrous consequences can occur. Nevertheless, in some clinical situations, it is appropriate to measure drug levels before steady state has been achieved. For example, pharmacokinetic parameters for a drug administered to a patient who is severely ill may change so rapidly that extrapolations from a reported plasma concentration may not be valid from one day to the next. Similarly, if there is reason to suspect that the pharmacokinetic parameters in a given patient are likely to differ substantially from those reported in the literature (eg, lidocaine in a patient with congestive heart failure),[1] or the accumulation process is prolonged because of a long $t_{1/2}$ (eg, phenobarbital),[2,3] it may be reasonable to obtain plasma samples before steady state to avoid excessive accumulation or unnecessarily prolonged subtherapeutic concentrations from the current dose. If possible, plasma samples should be drawn after a minimum of two half-lives because clearance (Cl) values calculated from drug levels obtained less than one half-life after a regimen has been initiated are very sensitive to small differences in the volume of distribution and minor assay errors (Figure 2.10).

REVISING PHARMACOKINETIC PARAMETERS

The process of using a patient's plasma drug concentrations and dosing history to determine patient-specific pharmacokinetic parameters can be complex and difficult. If the relationship between pharmacokinetic equations, the specific parameters, and the resultant plasma levels is understood, however, this process can be simplified. A single plasma sample obtained at the appropriate time can yield information to revise only one parameter, either the volume of distribution or Cl, but not both. Drug concentrations measured from poorly timed samples may prove to be useless in estimating a patient's V or Cl values. Thus, the goal is to obtain plasma samples at times that are likely to yield data that can be used with confidence to estimate pharmacokinetic parameters. In addition, it is important to evaluate available plasma concentration data to determine whether they can be used to estimate, with some degree of confidence, V and/or Cl. Which pharmacokinetic parameter is revised has much to do with the timing of the sample and the drug's pharmacokinetic profile. The goal in pharmacokinetic revisions is not only to recognize which pharmacokinetic parameter can be revised but also to find the accuracy or confidence one has in the revised or patient-specific pharmacokinetic parameter. In the clinical setting, based on the way drugs are dosed and the recommended time to sample, bioavailability is almost never revised, volume of distribution is sometimes revised, and, most often, Cl is the pharmacokinetic parameter that can be revised to determine a patient-specific value.

Volume of Distribution

A plasma concentration that has been obtained soon after the administration of an initial bolus is primarily determined by the dose administered and the volume of

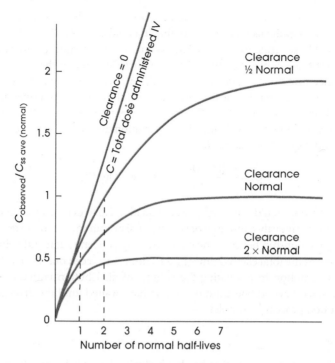

FIGURE 2.10 Relationship between observed plasma concentrations ($C_{observed}$) and the normal steady-state concentration ($C_{ss\ ave(normal)}$) following initiation of a maintenance regimen at various clearance values. At steady state, the plasma concentrations are inversely proportional to clearance. Plasma concentrations obtained at or before one normal half-life are all very similar, regardless of clearance. After two half-lives, alterations in a patient's clearance and ultimately steady-state concentrations can be detected by unexpectedly high or low plasma drug concentrations. After three half-lives, more confident predictions of steady-state concentrations can be made. IV, intravenous.

distribution. This assumes that both the absorption and distribution phases have been avoided. This is illustrated by Equation 2.2 (also see Figures 2.1 and 2.12):

$$C_1 = \frac{(S)(F)(\text{Loading dose})}{V}(e^{-Kt_1})$$

When e^{-Kt_1} approaches 1 (ie, when t_1 is much less than $t_{1/2}$), the plasma concentration (C_1) is primarily a function of the administered dose and the apparent volume of distribution. At this point, very little drug has been eliminated from the body. As a clinical guideline, a patient's volume of distribution can usually be estimated if the absorption and distribution phases are avoided and t_1, or the interval between the administration and sampling time, is less than or equal to one-third of the drug's half-life. Because t_1 exceeds one-third of a half-life, the measured concentration is increasingly influenced by Cl. Because more of the drug is eliminated (ie, t_1 increases), it is difficult to estimate the patient's V with any certainty. The specific application of this clinical guideline depends on the confidence with which one knows Cl. If Cl is extremely variable and uncertain, a time interval of less than one-third of a half-life would be necessary to revise the volume of distribution. On the other hand, if a patient-specific value for Cl has already been determined, then t_1 could exceed one-third of a half-life, and a reasonably accurate estimate of the volume of distribution could be obtained. It is important to recognize that the pharmacokinetic parameter that most influences the drug concentration is not determined by the model chosen to represent the drug level. For example, even if the dose is modeled as a short infusion (Equation 2.6), the volume of distribution can still be the important parameter controlling the plasma concentration. V is not clearly defined in the equation; nevertheless, it is incorporated into the elimination rate constant (K).

$$C_2 = \frac{(S)(F)(\text{Dose}/t_{in})}{\text{Cl}}(1 - e^{-Kt_{in}})(e^{-Kt_2})$$

Although one would not usually select Equation 2.6 to demonstrate that the drug concentration is primarily a function of volume of distribution, it is important to recognize that the relationship between the observed drug concentration and volume is not altered as long as the total elapsed time ($t_{in} + t_2$) does not exceed one-third of a half-life.

Our assumption in evaluating the volume of distribution is that although we have not sampled beyond one-third of a $t_{\frac{1}{2}}$, we have waited until the drug absorption and distribution process is complete.

Clearance

A plasma drug concentration that has been obtained at steady state from a patient who is receiving a constant drug infusion is determined by Cl. This is illustrated by Equation 1.33:

$$C_{ss\,ave} = \frac{(S)(F)(\text{Dose}/\tau)}{\text{Cl}}$$

Note that the average steady-state plasma concentration is not influenced by the volume of distribution. Therefore, plasma concentrations that represent the average steady-state level can be used to estimate a patient's Cl value, but they cannot be used to estimate a patient's volume of distribution. As illustrated in Figure 2.11, all steady-state plasma concentrations within a dosing interval that is short relative to a drug's half-life ($\tau \leq \frac{1}{3}t_{\frac{1}{2}}$) approximate the average concentration. Therefore, these concentrations are also primarily a function of Cl and only minimally influenced by V. If the average drug concentration is assumed to occur approximately in the middle of the dosing interval, the trough concentration will have decayed from the average for only half of the dosing interval or by one-sixth of a drug's half-life (assuming the dosing interval is one-third of a half-life or less). Under these conditions, the trough concentration is approximately 90% of the average drug level, an error that is usually acceptable in clinical practice. Thus, in this circumstance, the equation for $C_{ss\,ave}$ (Equation 1.33) or the equation that represents a steady-state plasma concentration sampled at any time within the dosing interval (Equation 1.46) can be used to estimate a patient-specific Cl.

$$C_{ss_1} = \frac{\dfrac{(S)(F)(\text{Dose})}{V}}{1 - e^{-K\tau}}e^{-Kt_1}$$

If Equation 1.46 is used, the expected volume of distribution should be retained, and the elimination rate constant should be adjusted such that C_{ss1} at t_1 equals the observed drug plasma concentration. Cl could then be calculated using Equation 1.31:

$$Cl = (K)(V)$$

Sensitivity Analysis

Whether a measured drug concentration is a function of Cl or volume of distribution is not always apparent. When this is difficult to ascertain, one can examine the sensitivity or responsiveness of the predicted plasma concentration to a parameter by changing one parameter while holding the other constant. For example, Equation 1.35 represents a plasma concentration (C_1) at some time interval (t_1) after a maintenance infusion has been started.

$$C_1 = \frac{(S)(F)(\text{Dose}/\tau)}{Cl}(1 - e^{-Kt_1})$$

When the fraction of steady state that has been reached $(1 - e^{-Kt_1})$ is small, large changes in Cl are frequently required to adjust a predicted plasma concentration to the appropriate value. If a large percentage change in the Cl value results in a disproportionately small change in the predicted drug level, then something other than Cl is controlling (responsible for) the drug concentration. In this case, the volume of distribution and the amount of drug administered are the primary determinants of the observed concentration. In addition, in cases where the drug concentration is very low, it might be assay error or sensitivity that is the predominant factor in determining the drug concentration, thereby making the ability to revise for any pharmacokinetic parameter limited if not impossible. This concept is illustrated graphically in Figure 2.10. Note that plasma concentrations within the first two half-lives are all very similar, whereas the steady-state concentrations are quite different. Within the first two half-lives of initiating a maintenance regimen, very large changes in Cl are required to account for small changes in plasma levels.

This type of sensitivity analysis is useful to reinforce the concept that the most reliable revisions in pharmacokinetic parameters are made when the predicted drug concentration changes by approximately the same percentage as the pharmacokinetic parameter undergoing revision. To illustrate this principle, let us examine the relationship between a theophylline drug concentration obtained 6.93 hours after starting a theophylline infusion of 30 mg/hr in a patient with the following expected parameters for theophylline: Cl 3 L/hr, V 30 L, K 0.1 hr^{-1}, $t_{1/2}$ 6.93 hours. Because the drug being administered is theophylline, S and F are assumed to be 1.0. Using Equation 1.35, the expected plasma concentration (C_1) is calculated to be 5 mg/L.

$$C_1 = \frac{(S)(F)(\text{Dose}/\tau)}{Cl}(1 - e^{-Kt_1})$$

$$= \frac{(1)(1)(30 \text{ mg/hr})}{3 \text{ L/hr}}(1 - e^{-(0.1 \text{ hr}^{-1})(6.93 \text{ hr})})$$

$$= 10 \text{ mg/L} (1 - 0.5)$$

$$= 5 \text{ mg/L}$$

As can be seen from the calculations, the expected steady-state concentration is 10 mg/L, and the fraction of steady state achieved $(1 - e^{-Kt1})$ is 0.5 because the time of sampling is at one drug half-life and 50% of the steady-state plasma concentration has been achieved. If the observed plasma concentration was 6 mg/L, only slightly higher than the calculated or expected value of 5 mg/L, one might expect the patient's Cl on revision to be only slightly less than the expected 3 L/hr. This relationship, however, is deceiving because, in order to calculate a plasma concentration of 6 mg/L at 6.93 hours with a volume of 30 L, a Cl of approximately 1.32 L/hr with a corresponding K and $t_{\frac{1}{2}}$ of 0.044 hr^{-1} and 15.7 hours, respectively, is required.

$$C_1 = \frac{(S)(F)(\text{Dose}/\tau)}{Cl}(1 - e^{-Kt_1})$$

$$= \frac{(1)(1)\ (30 \text{ mg/hr})}{1.32 \text{ L/hr}}(1 - e^{-(0.044 \text{ hr}^{-1})(6.93 \text{ hr})})$$

$$= 22.7 \text{ mg/L} (1 - 0.737)$$

$$= 22.7 \text{ mg/L} (0.263)$$

$$= 5.97 \text{ mg/L}$$

As can be seen from this illustration, the Cl value of 3 L/hr had to be reduced by more than one-half (ie, from 3 to 1.32 L/hr) to increase the predicted drug concentration by approximately 20%. This poor response of the calculated drug concentration to a change in Cl suggests that Cl is not the primary pharmacokinetic parameter responsible for the drug concentration. Therefore, any estimates of Cl and future dosing regimen based on these calculations would be tenuous at best. Although knowing that the patient's theophylline concentration is 6 mg/L may be a useful clinical information, it is important to recognize that very little additional pharmacokinetic information can be obtained from this drug level. Therefore, while it may be that the patient's theophylline Cl is approximately as predicted, it is also possible that it is quite different, and additional drug levels later in the accumulation process would be necessary to determine what the final steady-state theophylline concentration would be (see Figure 2.10).

When a predicted drug concentration changes in direct proportion or inverse proportion to an alteration in only one of the pharmacokinetic parameters, it is likely that a measured drug concentration can be used to estimate that patient-specific parameter. When both Cl and volume of distribution have a significant influence on the prediction of a measured drug concentration, revision of a patient's pharmacokinetic parameters will be less certain because there is an infinite number of combinations for Cl and volume of distribution values that could be used to predict the observed drug concentration. When this occurs, the patient-specific pharmacokinetic characteristics can be estimated by adjusting one or both of the pharmacokinetic parameters. Nevertheless, in most cases such as this, additional plasma-level sampling will be needed to accurately predict the patient's Cl or volume of distribution so that subsequent dosing regimens can be adjusted.

If a plasma drug concentration calculated from a specific equation is similar to the reported value, the pharmacokinetic parameters used in that equation may not necessarily be the most important determinants of the drug concentration. Equation 1.46 and Figure 2.11 can be used to demonstrate this principle.

$$C_{ss_1} = \frac{\dfrac{(S)(F)(\text{Dose})}{V}}{1 - e^{-K\tau}} e^{-Kt_1}$$

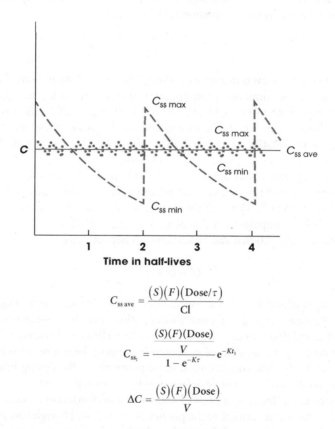

$$C_{ss\,ave} = \frac{(S)(F)(\text{Dose}/\tau)}{\text{Cl}}$$

$$C_{ss_1} = \frac{\dfrac{(S)(F)(\text{Dose})}{V}}{1 - e^{-K\tau}} e^{-Kt_1}$$

$$\Delta C = \frac{(S)(F)(\text{Dose})}{V}$$

FIGURE 2.11 Plasma concentrations relative to $C_{ss\,ave}$ (solid line) when τ is much less than (dotted line) and greater than (dashed line) the half-life. When τ is much less than $t_{1/2}$ (dotted line), all plasma concentrations approximate the average concentration ($C_{ss\,ave}$) and are, therefore, primarily a function of clearance. When τ is much greater than $t_{1/2}$ (dashed line), the plasma concentrations fluctuate significantly. The degree to which plasma concentrations are determined by clearance and/or volume of distribution is a function of when the plasma level is obtained within the dosing interval. Also, note that with the bolus model, the difference between $C_{ss\,max}$ and $C_{ss\,min}$ (ΔC) is a function of the dose and volume of distribution.

When the dosing interval is much shorter than the drug's half-life, the changes in concentration within a dosing interval are relatively small, and any drug concentration obtained within a dosing interval can be used as an approximation of the average steady-state concentration. Even though Equations 1.41 and 1.45

$$C_{ss\ max} = \frac{\frac{(S)(F)(\text{Dose})}{V}}{1 - e^{-K\tau}}$$

$$C_{ss\ min} = \frac{\frac{(S)(F)(\text{Dose})}{V}}{1 - e^{-K\tau}} e^{-K\tau}$$

could be used to predict peak and trough concentrations, a reasonable approximation could also be achieved by using Equation 1.33 for $C_{ss\ ave}$:

$$C_{ss\ ave} = \frac{(S)(F)(\text{Dose}/\tau)}{Cl}$$

This suggests that even though Equations 1.41 and 1.45 do not contain the parameter Cl per se, the elimination rate constant functions in such a way that the Cl derived from Equations 1.41 or 1.45 and 1.33 would all essentially be the same.

In the situation in which the dosing interval is greater than one-third of a half-life, the use of Equations 1.41 and 1.45 is appropriate, because not all drug concentrations within the dosing interval can be considered as the $C_{ss\ ave}$. However, as long as the dosing interval has not been extended beyond one half-life, Cl is still the primary pharmacokinetic parameter that is responsible for the drug concentrations within the dosing interval. Although the elimination rate constant and volume of distribution might be manipulated in Equations 1.41 and 1.45, it is only the product of those two numbers (ie, Cl) that can be known with any certainty:

$$Cl = (K)(V)$$

If a drug is administered at a dosing interval that is much longer than the apparent half-life (see Figure 2.11), peak concentrations may be primarily a function of volume of distribution. Because most of the dose is eliminated within a dosing interval, each dose can be thought of as something approaching a new loading dose. Of course, for steady-state conditions, at some point within the dosing interval, the plasma concentration ($C_{ss\ ave}$) will be determined by Cl. Trough plasma concentrations in this situation are a function of both Cl and volume of distribution. Because Cl and volume of distribution are critical to the prediction of peak and trough concentrations when the dosing interval is much longer than the drug $t_{1/2}$, a minimum of two plasma concentrations is needed to accurately establish patient-specific pharmacokinetic parameters and a dosing regimen that will achieve the desired peak and trough concentrations. Aminoglycoside antibiotics are examples of drugs that are administered at dosing intervals that greatly exceed their apparent half-life; therefore, if it is important to achieve targeted peak and trough concentrations, at least two plasma concentrations would be needed (see Chapter "Aminoglycoside Antibiotics").

When an observed drug concentration correlates with the level that was pre-dicted based on pharmacokinetic parameters from the literature, the particular pharmacokinetic parameter that is the primary determinant of the observed drug concentration should be determined before making future predictions. For example, successful prediction of an appropriate loading dose to achieve a specific plasma level does not guarantee that the maintenance dose is correct. Therefore, critical evaluation of the parameters affecting a patient's measured drug concentration will minimize in-correct assumptions about the applicability of literature-based pharmacokinetic pa-rameters to a specific patient's situation or about the predictability of future plasma concentrations.

CHOOSING A MODEL TO REVISE OR ESTIMATE A PATIENT'S CLEARANCE AT STEADY STATE

As previously discussed, a drug's half-life often determines the pharmacokinetic equation that should be used to make a revised or patient-specific estimate of a phar-macokinetic parameter. A common problem encountered clinically, however, is that the half-life observed in the patient often differs from the expected value. Because a change in either Cl or volume of distribution or both may account for this unexpected value, the pharmacokinetic model is often unclear. One way to approach this dilemma is to first calculate the expected change in plasma drug concentration associated with each dose:

$$\Delta C = \frac{(S)(F)(\text{Dose})}{V} \qquad \text{(Eq. 2.12)}$$

where ΔC is the change in concentration following the administration of each dose $[(S)(F)(\text{Dose})]$ into the patient's volume of distribution (V). This change in concentra-tion can then be compared to the steady-state trough concentration measured in the patient.

$$\frac{(S)(F)(\text{Dose})}{V} \text{ versus } C_{ss\,min}$$

or

$$\Delta C \text{ versus } C_{ss\,min}$$

Note, in Figure 2.11, that when the dosing interval (τ) is much less than the drug's half-life, ΔC will be small when compared to $C_{ss\,min}$. As the dosing interval increases relative to τ, ΔC will increase relative to $C_{ss\,min}$. Therefore, a comparison of ΔC or $(S)(F)(\text{Dose})/V$ to $C_{ss\,min}$ can serve as a guide to estimating the drug $t_{1/2}$ and the most appropriate pharmacokinetic model or technique to use for revision. With few exceptions, drugs that have plasma-level monitoring are most often dosed at intervals less than or equal to their half-lives. Therefore, Cl is the pharmacokinetic parameter most often revised or calculated for the patient in question. The following guidelines can be used to select the pharmacokinetic model that is the least complex and, therefore, the most appropriate to estimate a patient-specific pharmacokinetic parameter.

Condition 1

When

$$\frac{(S)(F)(Dose)}{V} \leq \frac{1}{4} C_{ss\,min}$$

then

$$\tau \leq \frac{1}{3} t_{\frac{1}{2}}$$

Under these conditions,

$$C_{ss\,min} \approx C_{ss\,ave}$$

and Cl can be estimated by Equation 1.15:

$$Cl = \frac{(S)(F)(Dose/\tau)}{C_{ss\,ave}}$$

Rules/Conditions: must be at steady state.

Condition 2

When

$$\frac{(S)(F)(Dose)}{V} \leq C_{ss\,min}$$

then

$$\tau \leq t_{\frac{1}{2}}$$

Under these conditions,

$$C_{ss\,min} + \left(\frac{1}{2}\right)\frac{(S)(F)(Dose)}{V} \approx C_{ss\,ave} \qquad \text{(Eq. 2.13)}$$

and Cl can be estimated by Equation 1.15:

$$Cl = \frac{(S)(F)(Dose/\tau)}{C_{ss\,ave}}$$

Rules/Conditions: must be at steady state C is $C_{ss\,min}$.
    Bolus model for absorption is acceptable.
    That is, dosage form is not sustained release.
    Short infusion model is not required, that is, $t_{in} \leq \frac{1}{6}t_{\frac{1}{2}}$.

Condition 3

When

$$\frac{(S)(F)(Dose)}{V} > C_{ss\,min}$$

then

$$\tau \leq t_{\frac{1}{2}}$$

Under these conditions,

$$C_{ss\,min} + \frac{(S)(F)(Dose)}{V} \approx C_{ss\,max} \qquad \text{(Eq. 2.14)}$$

where V is an assumed value from the literature.

K is revised ($K_{revised}$):

$$K_{revised} = \frac{\ln\left(\dfrac{C_{ss\,min} + \dfrac{(S)(F)(Dose)}{V}}{C_{ss\,min}}\right)}{\tau} = \frac{\ln\left(\dfrac{C_{ss\,max}}{C_{ss\,min}}\right)}{\tau} \qquad \text{(Eq. 2.15)}$$

Cl is revised ($Cl_{revised}$) using $K_{revised}$ in Equation 1.31: $Cl_{revised} = (K_{revised})(V)$
Rules/Conditions: must be at steady state C is $C_{ss\,min}$.
  Bolus model for absorption is acceptable.
  That is, dosage form is not sustained release.
  Short infusion model is not required, that is, $t_{in} \leq \frac{1}{6}t_{\frac{1}{2}}$

Note that the approaches used become more complex as the dosing interval increases relative to the drug's half-life. If a drug is administered at a dosing interval less than or equal to one-third of its half-life and the technique in Condition 3 is used to revise Cl, the revised Cl would be correct. The calculation is not wrong, just unnecessarily complex. However, if a drug is administered at a dosing interval that exceeds one half-life and the technique in Condition 1 is used to revise Cl, the revised Cl value would be inaccurate because $C_{ss\,min}$ cannot be assumed to be approximately equal to $C_{ss\,ave}$. Although it could be argued that the technique used in Condition 3 would suffice for all the previous conditions, it is more cumbersome and tends to focus on the intermediate parameters, K and V, rather than Cl. One should also be aware that as the dosing interval increases relative to the drug's half-life, the confidence in a revised Cl diminishes because the volume of distribution, which is an assumed value from the literature, begins to influence the revised Cl to a greater degree. As a general rule, the confidence in Cl is usually good when the dosing interval is less than $t_{\frac{1}{2}}$, steady state has been achieved, and drug concentrations are obtained properly.

NON–STEADY-STATE REVISION OF CLEARANCE (ITERATIVE SEARCH)

The techniques described in the previous section allow one to calculate a revised Cl directly. However, there are a number of situations in which revision of the Cl value is possible, but there are no explicit solutions. These situations require an iterative search technique. The first situation is when the parameter being revised appears in both the exponential and nonexponential portions of the equations, as illustrated by Equation 1.35.

$$C_1 = \frac{(S)(F)(\text{Dose}/\tau)}{\text{Cl}}(1 - e^{-Kt_1})$$

Although it may not be obvious that Cl appears in both the exponential and nonexponential portions of the equation, the elimination rate constant consists of both Cl and V.

$$C_1 = \frac{(S)(F)(\text{Dose}/\tau)}{\text{Cl}}(1 - e^{-\left(\frac{\text{Cl}}{V}\right)t_1})$$

Therefore, if V is held constant, the revision process would be associated with a changing Cl (and the corresponding elimination rate constant) to match the observed plasma concentration (C_1). The Cl that "fits" or calculates a value for C_1 that is the same as the assayed concentration would be the revised Cl. As stated earlier, there is no direct solution, and the Cl value (which when placed in Equation 1.35 calculates the specific C_1) can only be found by trial and error. The second situation that requires an iterative search is any time there are multiple exponential terms (e^{-Kt}) where t differs. This might occur when there are multiple bolus doses being administered and the plasma concentration is the sum of the residual of each of these doses (see Figure 2.7). Another example is the short infusion model at steady state or Equation 2.10.

$$C_{ss_2} = \frac{\dfrac{(S)(F)(\text{Dose}/\tau)}{\text{Cl}}\left(1 - e^{-K\tau}\right)}{1 - e^{-K\tau}}\left(e^{-Kt_2}\right)$$

In Equation 2.10, Cl is expressed in both the exponential (ie, $K = \text{Cl}/V$) and nonexponential portions. In addition, each of the exponential terms has a different value for t, which, in itself, is a condition that would require an iterative search to find a unique solution for Cl.

Although an iterative search process can be cumbersome, in most cases, approximate values for the revised Cl can be arrived at within one to three attempts. One technique is to adjust the Cl by the ratio that the predicted C_1 and the assayed drug concentration are different. If, for example, the predicted drug concentration is 10 mg/L and the assayed drug concentration is 12 mg/L, the Cl in Equation 2.10 would be decreased by about 20% in the hope that a 20% decrease in Cl would increase the calculated C_1 by 20%. However, this may not be the case because, in Equation 2.10, the relationship between Cl and C_1 is not proportional. If the required change in Cl is significantly out of proportion to the ratio of C_1 to the assayed drug concentration, it is a strong indication that Cl is not the only pharmacokinetic parameter responsible for C_1. Therefore, any estimates of Cl under conditions where a large change in Cl is required to make small changes in C_1 would be tenuous at best. Many pharmacokineticists use programmed calculators or computers to facilitate these repetitive trial and error calculations. Although the use of computers is to be encouraged as a labor-saving device, the user must understand the fundamental process and the limits of the method (see Interpretation of Plasma Drug Concentrations: Revising Pharmacokinetic Parameters: Sensitivity Analysis: Interpretation of Plasma Drug Concentrations: Bayesian Analysis).

NON–STEADY-STATE REVISION OF CLEARANCE (MASS BALANCE)

The mass balance technique has been suggested as a more direct alternative to the iterative approach.[4,5] The mass balance technique is relatively simple and can be best visualized by examining the relationship between the rate of drug administration and the rate of drug elimination. At steady state, the rate of drug elimination (R_E) is equal to the rate of administration (R_A) and the change in the amount of the drug in the body with time is 0.

$$R_A - R_E = \text{Change in the amount of drug in the body with time} = 0$$

Under non–steady-state conditions, however, there will be a change in the amount of drug in the body with time. This change can be estimated by multiplying the difference in the plasma concentration (ΔC) by the volume of distribution and dividing by the time interval between the two drug concentrations.

$$R_A - R_E = \frac{(\Delta C)(V)}{t} \qquad \text{(Eq. 2.16)}$$

By substituting the appropriate values in this equation, an estimate of Cl can be derived as follows:

$$R_A - R_E = \frac{(\Delta C)(V)}{t}$$

$$(S)(F)(\text{Dose} / \tau) - R_E = \frac{(C_2 - C_1)(V)}{t}$$

$$(S)(F)(\text{Dose}/\tau) - \frac{(C_2 - C_1)(V)}{t} = R_E$$

$$(S)(F)(\text{Dose}/\tau) - \frac{(C_2 - C_1)(V)}{t} = (\text{Cl})(C_{ave})$$

$$(S)(F)(\text{Dose}/\tau) = \frac{\dfrac{(C_2 - C_1)(V)}{t}}{C_{ave}} = \text{Cl} \qquad \text{(Eq. 2.17)}$$

Note that the average plasma concentration (C_{ave}) is generally assumed to be the average of C_1 and C_2.

$$C_{ave} = \frac{C_1 + C_2}{2} \qquad \text{(Eq. 2.18)}$$

Although this C_{ave} is not the steady-state average, it is assumed to be the average concentration that results in the elimination of drug as the concentration proceeds toward steady state. Equation 2.17 is an accurate method for estimating Cl if the following conditions are met:

1. t, or time interval between C_1 and C_2, should be equal to at least one but no longer than two of the revised drug half-lives. This rule helps to ensure that the time interval is not so short as to be unable to detect any change in concentration and yet not so long that the second concentration (C_2) is at steady state.
2. The plasma concentration values should be reasonably close to one another. If the drug concentrations are increasing, C_2 should be less than 2 times C_1; if the plasma concentrations are declining, C_2 should be more than one-half of C_1 (ie, $0.5 < C_2/C_1 < 2.0$). This rule limits the change in concentration so that the assumed value for V will not be a major determinant for the value of Cl calculated from Equation 2.17.
3. The rate of drug administration $[(S)(F)(\text{Dose}/\tau)]$ should be regular and consistent. This rule helps to ensure a reasonably smooth progression from C_1 to C_2 such that the value of C_{ave} $[(C_1 + C_2)/2]$ is approximately equal to the true average drug concentration between C_1 and C_2.

The mass balance approach is a useful technique if the abovementioned conditions are met. It is relatively simple and allows for the calculation of Cl under non–steady-state conditions by a direct solution process. There are certain situations in which these conditions are not met but the mass balance technique still works relatively well. For example, if the time interval between C_1 and C_2 is substantially greater than two half-lives but the value of C_2 is very close to C_1, then Equation 2.17 approximates Equation 1.15 because the average plasma concentration approximates the average steady-state value.

$$\frac{(S)(F)(\text{Dose}/\tau) - \dfrac{(C_2 - C_1)(V)}{t}}{C_{ave}} = Cl$$

$$\frac{(S)(F)(\text{Dose}/\tau) - (\approx 0)}{C_{ave}} = Cl$$

$$\frac{(S)(F)(\text{Dose}/\tau)}{C_{ave}} = Cl$$

The mass balance approach is most commonly applicable for drugs that are given as a continuous IV infusion, as a sustained-release product, or at a dosing interval that is much less than the half-life.

As an example, let us look at a patient who has a phenobarbital level of 10 mg/L on day 1 and is given 100 mg daily for 10 days. At the end of day 10, the phenobarbital level is reported to be 18 mg/L. Given that the usual $t_{1/2}$ of phenobarbital is approximately 4 or 5 days, it seems unlikely that the phenobarbital level of 18 mg/L represents steady state (ie, <3 to $5t_{1/2}$s on this regimen). One of several approaches could be taken to resolve this problem. One approach would be to write an equation that was the sum of the initial concentration decayed to the time of the second sample plus each of the 10 doses decayed individually to the time of the second sample. To solve the equation, values of S, F, and V would have to be assumed and then, in an iterative manner, values of K would be substituted until the equation equaled the observed phenobarbital level of 18 mg/L.

$$C_{sum} = C\left(e^{-Kt}\right) + \left[\frac{(S)(F)(D_1)}{V}\left(e^{-Kt_1}\right)\right] + \left[\frac{(S)(F)(D_2)}{V}\left(e^{-Kt_2}\right)\right] + \cdots$$

The K value could then be used in combination with the assumed V in Equation 1.31 to calculate a Cl value.

$$Cl = (K)(V)$$

A second approach might be to again start with the initial concentration decayed to the time of the second sample and add to that concentration the contribution of a continuous infusion model that was accumulating toward steady state. The continuous infusion model could be used because the interval of 1 day between the phenobarbital doses is sufficiently short compared to the $t_{1/2}$ so that the accumulation is a relatively smooth process.

$$C_1 = \left[C\left(e^{-Kt_1}\right)\right] + \left[\frac{(S)(F)(Dose / \tau)}{Cl}\left(1 - e^{-Kt_1}\right)\right]$$

In this equation, Cl/V would be substituted for K or $(K)(V)$ for Cl, so there is only one unknown to be resolved in the equation.

Lastly, the mass balance approach could be used.

$$\frac{(S)(F)(Dose/\tau) - \dfrac{(C_2 - C_1)(V)}{t}}{C_{ave}} = Cl$$

where t would be the 10-day interval between the initial phenobarbital level and the second level. This last approach using mass balance is a direct solution and does not require an iterative search. The solution for Cl should be reasonably good as long as the three rules previously mentioned are met. If there are concerns that the value of Cl is incorrect, this value of Cl could be used in one of the previous equations to see whether the more complex equation will predict the observed second phenobarbital concentration. A word of caution: If the Cl value predicts the phenobarbital concentration well (the calculated value is close to the observed value), it does not necessarily mean the Cl is correct—only that regardless of which equation is used, you will calculate the same answer.

SINGLE-POINT DETERMINATION OF CLEARANCE

A drug concentration obtained approximately 1.44 half-lives after a single bolus dose is primarily a function of Cl and is also referred to as the mean residence time. This concept is represented in Figure 2.12. The ability to predict Cl using this principle is based on a complex relationship between the volume of distribution, Cl, and half-life. As can be seen from Equation 2.1 for C and Equation 1.30 for $t_{1/2}$:

$$C = \frac{(S)(F)(Loading\ dose)}{V} \qquad t_{1/2} = \frac{(0.693)(V)}{Cl}$$

if Cl is held constant, and the volume of distribution is decreased, the initial plasma levels will be higher and the elimination half-life will be decreased. However, if the

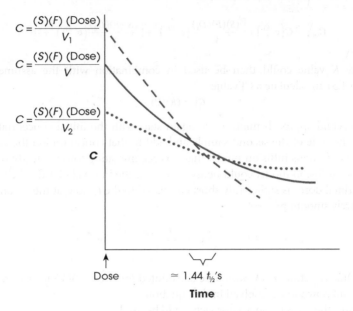

FIGURE 2.12   Single-point determination of clearance. The plasma concentrations following a single bolus dose when clearance is held constant and volume of distribution is altered tend to pivot around a single point that occurs at ~1.44 half-lives after the dose. When the volume of distribution is smaller (dashed line V_1), the concentrations before 1.44 half-life points are elevated, relative to the concentrations found in patients with larger volumes of distribution (dotted line V_2). The opposite is true after the 1.44 half-life point.

volume of distribution is increased, the initial plasma concentrations will be lower and the elimination half-life will be longer.

By examining Figure 2.12, it can be seen that over a range of volume of distribution values, there is a locus or point about which the decaying plasma concentration versus time curves appear to pivot. This pivot point is at 1.44 half-lives. For this reason, a single plasma concentration obtained at 1.44 half-lives following an initial bolus dose can be used to estimate a Cl.[6-8] This approach is essentially a rearrangement of Equation 1.28:

$$K = \frac{\ln\left(\dfrac{C_1}{C_2}\right)}{t}$$

where $(S)(F)(Dose)/V$ is substituted for C_1, and C_2 is the measured plasma concentration at time t after the loading dose.

$$K = \frac{\ln\left(\dfrac{(S)(F)(\text{Loading dose})/V}{C_2}\right)}{t} \qquad \textbf{(Eq. 2.19)}$$

Equation 1.31 can then be used with the assumed value for V to calculate the patient's Cl.

$$\text{Cl} = (K)(V)$$

It is important to recognize that if the patient's Cl or volume of distribution values differ substantially from those assumed, a sampling time based on a literature-derived half-life may not represent 1.44 half-lives for the patient. In this instance, accurate patient-specific Cl would not be derived from this method outlined using Equations 2.19 and 1.31. For example, if a patient has a very low Cl and a longer-than-expected elimination half-life, plasma samples obtained at 1.44 times the drug's reported half-life will represent a sampling time that is sooner than 1.44 times the patient's actual half-life. Plasma samples obtained at this time are primarily a function of volume of distribution and would be influenced much less by Cl. Conversely, if the patient's Cl is much greater than the literature value, a sample obtained at 1.44 of the usual $t_{1/2}$ may represent several of the patient's true half-lives. Under these conditions, the observed plasma concentration is influenced to a large degree by both the volume of distribution and Cl. As a result, the ability to extract (with any level of confidence) revised values for Cl or volume of distribution is extremely limited. As can be seen from the previous discussion, the single-point determination of Cl only works when patient's $t_{1/2}$ is approximately as predicted. When the patient is much different from predicted, Cl cannot be accurately determined from a single sample.

It is often difficult to accurately plan a sampling time that can be used for the single-point method. However, if sensitivity testing reveals that Cl is the primary determinant of a concentration obtained approximately 1.44 half-lives after a bolus dose, this concentration may be used to ascertain a patient-specific Cl.

BAYESIAN ANALYSIS

As previously discussed, the usual approach when using pharmacokinetics in the clinical setting is to solve our kinetic problem by using simple manipulations of an equation and then solving the equation by revising or changing one or sometimes two variables, usually volume of distribution and/or Cl. This technique works well if the clinician has a good understanding of pharmacokinetics and good clinical judgment. One of the potential dangers is that a clinical decision might be made using pharmacokinetic data that have a very low level of reliability. To help guard against this type of error, many pharmacokinetic computer programs use Bayesian analysis.

The mathematics in this approach is complicated and requires significant computational capacity. However, the concept is relatively simple. The basic approach used in this analysis technique is to adjust each element in the equation to the degree that it helps solve the equation and to the degree that it is likely that the initial estimates are wrong. Depending on the way the program is designed, everything from adherence to bioavailability, concentration measurement variability, and our usual parameters of Cl and volume of distribution can be considered in the revision process. There are three key issues with the Bayesian approach. One is that the average population value is a good and reasonable estimate for the patient. Second is that the uncertainty or variability in the individual parameters is known. Third is that the pharmacokinetic model is appropriate.

As an example, we can consider Equation 2.2:

$$C_1 = \frac{(S)(F)(\text{Loading dose})}{V}(e^{-Kt_1})$$

If we take a situation in which we obtain two drug samples relatively soon after a loading dose of 100 mg is administered, both of the drug concentrations would have information about V but very little information about Cl. In this problem, we start by assuming that S and F are 1, V is 10 L, Cl is 1 L/hr, $K = 0.1$ hr^{-1} ($t_{1/2} = 6.93$ hours), and the two sampling times are at 0.5 and 1 hour after the dose.

$$C_1 = \frac{(S)(F)(\text{Loading dose})}{V}(e^{-(K)(t_1)})$$

$$= \frac{(1)(1)(100 \text{ mg})}{10 \text{ L}}(e^{-(0.1 \text{ hr}^{-1})(0.5 \text{ hr})})$$

$$= 10 \text{ mg/L} \ (0.951)$$

$$= 9.51 \text{ mg/L}$$

And the second concentration would be:

$$= \frac{(1)(1)(100 \text{ mg})}{10 \text{ L}}(e^{-(0.1 \text{ hr}^{-1})(1 \text{ hr})})$$

$$= 10 \text{ mg/L} \ (0.905)$$

$$= 9.05 \text{ mg/L}$$

If the laboratory reported the drug concentration at 0.5 and 1 hour to be 9.8 and 8.7 mg/L, respectively, we would, from a clinical point of view, simply look at the expected values of 9.51 and 9.05 and consider the predictions to be excellent. We would assume that the less than 10% differences in the predicted and observed drug concentrations were owing to assay error. Knowing that the two drug levels were obtained very soon after the initial loading dose suggests that our volume of distribution is approximately correct. However, very little information about Cl is "contained" in the two drug samples. This would mean that our maintenance dosing regimen should be based on our original estimate of 1 L/hr for Cl. We would use the expected Cl value not because we know it is correct, but rather because we do not have any additional information that would suggest changing our original expectation.

There are computer programs (and clinicians with calculators) that would use what is commonly thought of as an "exact fit" method of analysis. This method tries to make everything fit the drug concentrations as closely as possible. In our example, S, F, t_1, and C_1 would be assumed to be exact values, and any differences between the observed values in C and the expected value are because of differences in our expected V and Cl. Following this line of reasoning, Equation 1.28 and the two drug concentrations can be used to calculate a new elimination rate constant of 0.238 hr^{-1}.

$$K = \frac{\ln\left(\dfrac{C_1}{C_2}\right)}{t}$$

where C_1 is 9.8 mg/L, C_2 8.7 mg/L, and t the 0.5-hour time interval between the first and second sample. (Note that these two samples were obtained $<1t_{1/2}$ apart, indicating that the calculated K will be suspect.)

$$K = \frac{\ln\left(\dfrac{9.8 \text{ mg/L}}{8.7 \text{ mg/L}}\right)}{0.5 \text{ hr}}$$

$$= 0.238 \text{ hr}^{-1}$$

Now using Equation 1.26 and rearranging to solve for C_1, just after the bolus dose or 0.5 hour before the first sample, we calculate a drug level of 11.04 mg/L.

$$C_2 = C_1(e^{-(K)(t)})$$

$$9.8 \text{ mg/L} = C_1(e^{-(0.238 \text{ hr}^{-1})(0.5 \text{ hr})})$$

$$9.8 \text{ mg/L} = C_1(0.888)$$

$$\frac{9.8 \text{ mg/L}}{(0.888)} = C_1$$

$$11.04 \text{ mg/L} = C_1$$

Now using this concentration of 11.04 mg/L that would correspond to the C in Equation 2.1, we can calculate a revised volume of distribution of 9.1 L.

$$C = \frac{(S)(F)(\text{Loading dose})}{V}$$

$$11.04 \text{ mg/L} = \frac{(1)(1)(100 \text{ mg})}{V}$$

$$V = \frac{(1)(1)(100 \text{ mg})}{11.04 \text{ mg/L}}$$

$$V = 9.1 \text{ L}$$

Note that the revised V of 9.1 L is reasonably close to the initial estimate of 10 L. This is because we would expect considering that the timing of the samples is close to the loading dose.

However, if we use the revised K of 0.238 hr^{-1} and V of 9.1 L in Equation 1.31 to calculate a revised value for Cl, we would obtain 2.17 L/hr.

$$\text{Cl} = (K)(V)$$

$$\text{Cl} = (0.238 \text{ hr}^{-1})(9.1 \text{ L})$$

$$\text{Cl} = (2.17 \text{ L/hr})$$

This revised Cl is more than twice our initial estimate of 1 L/hr and would have a major impact on the maintenance regimen.

This revision is an example of making too much out of too little information. A Bayesian pharmacokinetics program would try to balance the change in the calculated drug concentrations as a result of a change in Cl and attempt to come up with a reasonable estimate or compromise considering that there is an expected assay error as well as some error in V and Cl. The end result would probably be a slightly higher Cl, a slightly smaller volume of distribution, and some slight differences in the observed and predicted drug concentrations. This approach would help avoid the huge change in Cl that occurred using the "exact fit" type of analysis. The Bayesian analysis would be similar to our initial conclusion that the observed and predicted drug concentrations are a close fit and confirm V but do not contain much information on Cl.

When drug levels are obtained at an "optimal" time, and the appropriate pharmacokinetic parameter is being analyzed, both the "exact fit" and Bayesian approaches usually give essentially the same answer. It should also be pointed out that although the Bayesian approach will help prevent the error of making too much of too little, it cannot correct or account for large real errors. Bayesian computer programs cannot adjust for gross errors. For example, errors in dose (200 mg administered vs 100 mg recorded as given), sample labeling (sample labeled with incorrect patient name or peak labeled as a trough), model (linear vs nonlinear elimination), and so on cannot be successfully corrected by Bayesian or any other type of computer program. Another potential problem with Bayesian programs occurs when the patient is truly different from the expected patient population. In this situation, the computer will tend to place less emphasis on the drug concentrations of the patient and try to revise toward parameters that are more like the average patient. This problem should be taken in the context that in most clinical situations, data that are very unusual are often the result of an error. Regardless of what type of approach is taken, it is important for the clinician to evaluate the drug concentration in the context of the patient and use rational judgment as to how pharmacokinetics is used in designing drug regimens.

ASSAY SPECIFICITY

The accuracy and specificity of assays used by the clinical laboratory to measure serum drug concentrations are critical. Historically, laboratories developed their assay procedures using a variety of analytical methods ranging from radioimmunoassays to high-performance liquid chromatography assay procedures. Currently, however, the vast majority of drug assays performed in the clinical setting are some variant of commercially available immunobinding assay procedures. The most commonly used procedures are variants of the fluorescence polarization immunoassay and enzyme immunoassay (enzyme-multiplied immunoassay technique and enzyme-linked immunosorbent assay).[9,10]

These assays are generally specific; however, in isolated instances, metabolites or other drug-like substances are also recognized by the antibody.[11-15] Most assay

TABLE 2.1   Examples of Drugs With Active Metabolites[2,22]

Amitriptyline
Carbamazepine
Chlordiazepoxide
Chlorpromazine
Chlorpropamide
Diazepam
Lidocaine
Meperidine
Metronidazole
Primidone
Propranolol
Warfarin

interferences are the result of cross-reactivity with the drug's metabolites, but, in some cases, endogenous compounds or drugs with similar structures can cross-react, resulting in either a falsely elevated or a decreased assayed drug concentration.[14-19]

Pharmacokinetic parameters derived from nonspecific assays or plasma concentrations that are in error may influence clinicians to make decisions that are not optimal for patient care.[16-19] Whereas the current literature is usually associated with relatively specific drug assays, caution should always be exercised when using serum drug concentrations as part of the clinical decision-making process.[20,21] This is especially true when the older literature is used because pharmacokinetic parameters that have been derived from assays with differing specificities are not interchangeable. The usual therapeutic range will also be altered when more specific assays are used.

For assays that measure the parent compound only, it is important to determine the pharmacologic activity and pharmacokinetic behavior of the metabolites. Many drugs have active metabolites that may affect a patient's pharmacologic response (Table 2.1); the pharmacokinetic behavior of these metabolites cannot be predicted by assaying only the parent compound.[22]

Whenever possible, one should evaluate the patient's clinical response directly. If drug levels and clinical response do not correlate as predicted, it may be owing to a laboratory error. Similarly, factors unique to the patient, such as concurrent disease states or antagonist drug therapy, may alter one's interpretation of the plasma drug concentration. For example, it is a common clinical observation that higher-than-usual plasma concentrations of digoxin are required to achieve a clinical response in patients with atrial fibrillation. Furthermore, for drugs that have high plasma protein binding, the same therapeutic effect will be achieved with a lower plasma concentration when plasma protein binding is decreased. This is because, for most clinical assays, the total plasma concentration (bound + free) is reported. As discussed earlier, decreased binding lowers the bound concentration, but not the free, pharmacologically active concentration. The formation of aberrant metabolites and tachyphylaxis are other reasons why plasma drug concentrations fail to correlate with an expected therapeutic response.

REFERENCES

1. Zeisler JA, Skovseth JR, Anderson JR, Meister FL. Lidocaine therapy: time for re-evaluation. *Clin Pharm.* 1993;12:527-528.

2. Thummel KE, Shen DD. Appendix II: design and optimization of dosage regimens: pharmacokinetic data. In: Hardman JG, ed. *Goodman and Gilman's the Pharmacologic Basis of Therapeutics.* 10th ed. McGraw-Hill; 2001:1917-2023.

3. Wilensky AJ, Friel PN, Levy RH, Comfort CP, Kaluzny SP. Kinetics of phenobarbital in normal subjects and epileptic patients. *Eur J Clin Pharmacol.* 1982;23(1):87-92.

4. Chiou WL, Gadalla MA, Peng GW. Method for the rapid estimation of the total body drug clearance and adjustment of dosage regimens in patients during a constant-rate intravenous infusion. *J Pharmacokinet Biopharm.* 1978;6(2):135-151.

5. Vozeh S, Kewitz G, Wenk M, Follath F. Rapid prediction of steady-state serum theophylline concentration in patients treated with intravenous aminophylline. *Eur J Clin Pharmacol.* 1980;18(6):473-477.

6. Slattery JT, Gibaldi M, Koup JR. Prediction of maintenance dose required to attain a desired drug concentration at steady-state from a single determination of concentration after an initial dose. *Clin Pharmacokinet.* 1980;5(4):377-385.

7. Koup JR. Single-point prediction methods: a critical review. *Drug Intell Clin Pharm.* 1982; 16(11):855-862.

8. Unadkat JD, Rowland M. Further considerations of the "single-point single-dose" method to estimate individual maintenance dosage requirements. *Ther Drug Monit.* 1982;4(2):201-208.

9. Glazko AJ. Phenytoin: chemistry and methods of determination. In: Levy RH, Mattson RH, Meldrum BS, et al, eds. *Antiepileptic Drugs.* 3rd ed. Raven Press; 1989:159-176.

10. Steijns LS, Bouw J, van der Weide J. Evaluation of fluorescence polarization assays for measuring valproic acid, phenytoin, carbamazepine and phenobarbital in serum. *Ther Drug Monit.* 2002;24(3):432-435.

11. Patel JA, Clayton LT, LeBel CP, McClatchey KD. Abnormal theophylline levels in plasma by fluorescence polarization immunoassay in patients with renal disease. *Ther Drug Monit.* 1984;6(4):458-460.

12. Hicks JM, Brett EM. Falsely increased digoxin concentrations in samples from neonates and infants. *Ther Drug Monit.* 1984;6(4):461-464.

13. Flachs H, Rasmussen JM. Renal disease may increase apparent phenytoin in serum as measured by enzyme-multiplied immunoassay [letter]. *Clin Chem.* 1980;26(2):361.

14. Frank EL, Schwarz EL, Juenke J, Annesley TM, Roberts WL. Performance characteristics of four immunoassays for antiepileptic drugs on the IMMULITE 2000 automated analyzer. *Am J Clin Pathol.* 2002;118(1):124-131.

15. Dasgupta A. Digoxin-like immunoreactive substances in elderly people. Impact on therapeutic drug monitoring of digoxin and digitoxin concentrations. *Am J Clin Pathol.* 2002;118(4):600-604.

16. Steimer W, Müller C, Eber B. Digoxin assays: frequent, substantial, and potentially dangerous interference by spironolactone, canrenone, and other steroids. *Clin Chem.* 2002;48(3):507-516.

17. Somerville AL, Wright DH, Rotschafer JC. Implications of vancomycin degradation products on therapeutic drug monitoring in patients with end-stage renal disease. *Pharmacotherapy.* 1999;19(6):702-707.

18. Sym D, Smith C, Meenan G, Lehrer M. Fluorescence polarization immunoassay: can it result in an overestimation of vancomycin in patients not suffering from renal failure? *Ther Drug Monit.* 2001;23(4):441-444.

19. Kingery JR, Sowinski KM, Kraus MA, Klaunig JE, Mueller BA. Vancomycin assay performance in patients with end-stage renal disease receiving hemodialysis. *Pharmacotherapy.* 2000;20(6):653-656.

20. Rainey PM, Rogers KE, Roberts WL. Metabolite and matrix interference in phenytoin immunoassays. *Clin Chem.* 1996;42(10):1645-1653.

21. Roberts WL, Annesley TM, De BK, Moulton L, Juenke JM, Moyer TP. Performance characteristics of four free phenytoin immunoassays. *Ther Drug Monit.* 2001;23(2):148-154.

22. Drayer DE. Pharmacologically active drug metabolites: therapeutic and toxic activities, plasma and urine data in man, accumulation in renal failure. *Clin Pharmacokinet.* 1976;1(6):426-443.

3

DRUG DOSING IN KIDNEY DISEASE AND DIALYSIS

Noha N. Salama and Thomas C. Dowling

By the end of the drug dosing in kidney disease and dialysis chapter, the learner shall be able to:

Renal Drug Clearance and Creatinine Clearance (Cl_{Cr})

1. Describe the key drug clearance mechanisms in the kidney and estimate Cl_{Cr} in various patient populations including chronic kidney disease (CKD), acute kidney disease, pediatrics, obesity, and older adults.
2. Describe the role of passive and active drug transport on renal drug elimination and mechanisms of renal drug-drug interactions.
3. Describe the production of creatinine and the inverse relationship between serum creatinine and Cl_{Cr}.
4. Know the usual Cl_{Cr} and glomerular filtration rate (GFR) for a young adult with normal renal function.
5. Calculate, using the Cockcroft and Gault equation, a patient's estimated Cl_{Cr}.
6. Compare the creatinine production (mg/kg/d) with the expected production of creatinine for the patient, and if the two values differ significantly, list the possible reasons.
7. Compare the estimated Cl_{Cr} as calculated by the Cockcroft and Gault equation with the value calculated from a 24-hour collection, and if the two values differ significantly, list the possible reasons.
8. Estimate lean body weight and recognize/identify when a patient is considered "obese," using body mass index (BMI) as an indicator.
9. Estimate Cl_{Cr} for children in mL/min/1.73 m^2.
10. Convert Cl_{Cr} in mL/min/1.73 m^2 to Cl_{Cr} in mL/min for a child using either body surface area or weight per 70 kg raised to the power 0.7.
11. Estimate Cl_{Cr} from two non–steady-state serum creatinine values.

12. Identify at least one reason why a rising serum creatinine makes estimates of renal function difficult.
13. Calculate a patient's Cl_{Cr} using a 24-hour urine collection.
14. Compare and contrast equations that estimate GFR (estimated glomerular filtration rate [eGFR], Modification of Diet in Renal Disease [MDRD], Chronic Kidney Disease Epidemiology Collaboration [CKD-EPI]) and the Cockcroft and Gault equation regarding appropriate use, units of measure, and patient size.
15. Give examples of situations where eGFR equations should NOT be used to estimate kidney function for the purpose of adjusting doses of drugs that are cleared by kidney mechanisms.

Dialysis of Drugs

1. Obtain an appreciation for the types of dialysis (intermittent, continuous, and peritoneal) and know how each is likely to affect drug elimination and dosing strategies.
2. Choose the appropriate model for postdialysis replacement dosing, given the patient's residual drug clearance and the estimated dialysis clearance.
3. Calculate the expected predialysis and postdialysis drug concentrations, given a patient's steady-state peak drug concentration.
4. Explain why, in most cases, immediate postdialysis sampling of drugs is not recommended.
5. Explain the impact of unbound volume of distribution on the extent of drug removed by dialysis.
6. Know the usual limit for drug clearance by hemodialysis and the typical residual patient clearance above which it is unlikely that hemodialysis will remove significant additional drug.
7. Know the molecular weight (molecular mass) cutoff for low- and high-flux hemodialysis above which it is unlikely that dialysis will be able to remove a significant amount of drug.
8. Describe the difference in molecular weight cutoff between low- and high-flux hemodialysis.
9. Give examples of drugs significantly removed by high-flux hemodialysis, but not by low-flux hemodialysis.
10. Describe the typical total continuous renal replacement therapy (CRRT) flow rate (ultrafiltration and dialysis) and the relationship of the flow to the fraction unbound (fu) and CRRT clearance.
11. Given a target drug concentration and the CRRT flow rate and given a patient's residual drug clearance, volume of distribution, and fu:
    a. Determine whether a continuous input and the average steady-state concentration ($C_{ss\ ave}$) model or an intermittent bolus model can be used to calculate a dosing regimen.
    b. Calculate a maintenance dose, using the appropriate model.
12. Describe the typical peritoneal volume exchange and duration or dwell time.
13. Calculate the expected continuous ambulatory peritoneal dialysis clearance (Cl_{CAPD}), given a drug's fu and the peritoneal dialysate exchange rate.

Because many drugs are partially or totally eliminated by the kidney, it is important to understand the impact of altered kidney function on drug pharmacokinetics. Drugs can be eliminated or cleared as unchanged drug through the kidney (renal clearance) and liver (including biliary secretion and metabolic biotransformation). These two routes of clearance are assumed to be independent of one another and additive.[1,2]

$$Cl_t = Cl_m + Cl_r$$

where Cl_t is total clearance, Cl_m the metabolic clearance or the fraction cleared by metabolism, and Cl_r the renal clearance or the fraction cleared by the renal route.

The primary mechanisms within the kidney that contribute to drug clearance are glomerular filtration, tubular secretion, and tubular reabsorption (Table 3.1). In patients with chronic kidney disease (CKD), the capacity of these renal mechanisms to eliminate drugs is reduced, leading to an overall reduction in total drug clearance. Because the volume of distribution for most drugs remains largely unchanged until severe renal impairment (CKD stage 5), the reduced elimination rate constant leads to a proportional increase in half-life ($t_{1/2}$). If dose adjustments are not made, then excessive accumulation may occur, leading to toxicity and unwanted pharmacologic side effects.

Although there are several endogenous markers of glomerular filtration, creatinine clearance (Cl_{Cr}) remains the primary clinical biomarker of glomerular filtration rate (GFR) and overall kidney function.[3-5]

Estimating Cl_{Cr} is typically the first step in personalized drug dosing for drugs that rely primarily on the kidney for elimination.

Creatinine Clearance (Cl_{Cr})

Estimating kidney function is an important component in the application of pharmacokinetics to designing drug therapy regimens. Cl_{Cr} as determined by a urine

TABLE 3.1   Factors Affecting the Three Renal Drug Elimination Mechanisms

Glomerular filtration
Molecular weight
Plasma protein binding
Glomerular capillary pressure

Tubular secretion
Membrane transporters (organic anion transporter [OAT], P-glycoprotein [PgP], multidrug-resistant protein [MRP])
Drug-transporter interactions
Renal blood flow

Tubular reabsorption
Drug pK_a
Urine pH
Urine flow rate
Drug transporters (human peptide transporter 2 [PEPT 2], Organic anion transporter polypeptide 1A2 [OATP1A2])

collection and corresponding plasma sample is considered by many clinicians to be the most accurate test of renal function. In the clinical setting, the time delay and the difficulty in obtaining the 24-hour creatinine collection limit the utility of the 24-hour urine collection. A primary concern is an inaccurate urine collection, often due to accidental discard of a sample, or the time of collection being shorter or longer than requested.[6,7] This incomplete collection can lead to an underestimation of renal function. Because decisions about drug dosing must often be made quickly, clinicians often use equations to estimate Cl_{Cr} at the bedside, as described later in this chapter.

CREATININE PHARMACOKINETICS

The pharmacokinetics of creatinine is presented in far more detail elsewhere,[6-12] but a brief overview is necessary. Creatinine is a metabolic by-product of muscle, and its rate of formation (R_A) is primarily determined by an individual's muscle mass or lean body weight (LBW). It varies, therefore, with age (lower in older adults) and gender (lower in females).[11-14] For any given individual, the rate of creatinine production is assumed to be constant. Once creatinine is released from muscle into plasma, it is eliminated largely by glomerular filtration. A smaller component is eliminated by tubular secretion via drug transporters such as the organic cation transporter-2 (OCT2, also referred to as Solute Carrier Family 22 member 2 or SLC22A2) and the multidrug and toxin extrusion protein (MATE1, also referred to as SLC47A1). Thus, observed elevations in serum creatinine (SCr) because of drug-creatinine interactions must be evaluated in each patient. For example, elevated SCr values have been observed during administration of cobicistat, a CYP3A inhibitor used as a booster with HIV integrase inhibitors, without a reduction in measured GFR. The mechanism has been identified as an inhibition of OCT2- and MATE1-mediated tubular secretion of creatinine.[15] Any decrease in the GFR ultimately results in a rise in the SCr level until a new steady state is reached and the amount of creatinine cleared per day equals the rate of production. In other words, at steady state, the rate in must equal the rate out. Because the rate of creatinine production remains constant even when renal clearance diminishes, the SCr must rise until the product of the clearance and the SCr again equals the rate of production. This concept is represented by Equation 3.1:

$$\leftrightarrow R_A = (\downarrow Cl)(\uparrow C_{ss\,ave}) \qquad \text{(Eq. 3.1)}$$

where $\leftrightarrow R_A$ is a constant rate of creatinine production, $\downarrow Cl$ the decreased Cl_{Cr}, and $\uparrow C_{ss\,ave}$ the increased average steady-state serum creatinine level or SCr_{ss}, such that when steady state is achieved, the product of ($\downarrow Cl)(\uparrow C_{ss\,ave}$) will be equal to the R_A or production rate of creatinine.

ESTIMATING CREATININE CLEARANCE FROM STEADY-STATE SERUM CREATININE CONCENTRATIONS (STABLE KIDNEY FUNCTION)

The degree to which a steady-state SCr rises is inversely proportional to the decrease in Cl_{Cr}. Therefore, the new Cl_{Cr} can be estimated by multiplying a normal Cl_{Cr} value by the fractional change in the SCr: normal SCr/patient's serum creatinine at steady-state (SCr_{ss}). For a man weighing 70 kg, it can be assumed that the normal SCr is 1.0 mg/dL and the corresponding Cl_{Cr} is 120 mL/min.

$$\text{New } Cl_{cr} = (120 \ \text{mL/min}) \left[\frac{1 \ \text{mg/dL}}{SCr_{ss}} \right] \qquad \text{(Eq. 3.2)}$$

Based on this concept, as SCr doubles, Cl_{Cr} falls by half and small changes in SCr at low concentrations are of much greater consequence than equal changes in SCr at high concentrations. To illustrate if a patient with a normal SCr of 1.0 mg/dL is reported to have a new SCr_{ss} of 2.0 mg/dL, the estimated Cl_{Cr} has decreased from 120 to 60 mL/min. However, if a patient with CKD has a baseline SCr of 4.0 mg/dL ($Cl_{Cr} = 30$ mL/min), a similar 1.0 mg/dL increase in SCr to 5.0 mg/dL would result in a small drop in the Cl_{Cr} (6 mL/min) and a new clearance value of 24 mL/min. However, at some point, even small changes in Cl_{Cr} can be physiologically significant to the patient. As an example, for a patient with Cl_{Cr} of 100 mL/min, a 10 mL/min (or 10%) reduction in kidney function is of very little clinical consequence. However, for a patient with Cl_{Cr} of 20 mL/min, a 10 mL/min decrease (or 67%) would likely change their clinical status from CKD stage 4 to CKD stage 5, requiring dialysis.

The estimation of Cl_{Cr} from SCr_{ss} alone is reasonably satisfactory as long as the patient's daily creatinine production is average (ie, 20 mg/kg/d); the patient weighs approximately 70 kg, and the SCr is at steady state (ie, either rising or falling). These conditions are usually present in young healthy adults, but young healthy adults are not the typical patients for whom pharmacokinetic manipulations are most useful.

Adjusting to Body Size: Weight or Body Surface Area

To account for any changes in creatinine production and clearance that may result from a difference in body size, Equation 3.2 can be modified to compensate for any deviation in body surface area (BSA) from the typical 70-kg patient ($1.73 \ \text{m}^2$):

The patient's BSA can be obtained from a nomogram (see Appendix II), estimated from Equation 1.17:

$$\text{BSA in m}^2 = \left(\frac{\text{Patient's weight in kg}}{70 \ \text{kg}} \right)^{0.7} (1.73 \ \text{m}^2)$$

or calculated from the following equation[16]:

$$BSA \text{ in } m^2 = (Weight^{0.425})(Height^{0.725})0.007184 \qquad \text{(Eq. 3.3)}$$

where the BSA is in meters squared (m^2), weight in kilograms, and patient's height in centimeters.

A disadvantage of using only weight or BSA is that the older adults or patients who are emaciated and have a reduced muscle mass may not have a typical steady-state SCr value of 1.0 mg/dL. For this reason, it may be erroneous to assume that a SCr of 1.0 mg/dL is "normal" and indicative of a Cl_{Cr} of 120 mL/min in these individuals.

On average, as patients age, their muscle mass represents a smaller proportion of their total weight and creatinine production is decreased (Table 3.2). There are a number of equations that consider age, gender, body size, and SCr when calculating or estimating Cl_{Cr} for adults.[13,17,18] Although all these methods are similar and equivalent in clinical practice, the most common method used by clinicians is probably the one proposed by Cockcroft and Gault.[17]

$$Cl_{Cr} \text{ for males (mL/min)} = \frac{(140 - Age)(Weight)}{(72)(SCr_{ss})} \qquad \text{(Eq. 3.4)}$$

$$Cl_{Cr} \text{ for females (mL/min)} = (0.85)\frac{(140 - Age)(Weight)}{(72)(SCr_{ss})} \qquad \text{(Eq. 3.5)}$$

TABLE 3.2   Expected Daily Creatinine Production for Males[14]

AGE (YR)	DAILY CREATININE PRODUCTION (MG/KG/D)
20-29	24[a]
30-39	22
40-49	20
50-59	19
60-69	17
70-79	14
80-89	12
90-99	9

[a]Daily creatinine production for females would be expected to be 85% of the abovementioned values.

where age is in years, weight is in kg, and SCr is in mg/dL. Equations 3.4 and 3.5 calculate Cl_{Cr} as mL/min for the patient's characteristics entered into the equation.

The two most critical factors to consider when using the abovementioned equations are the assumptions that the SCr is at steady state and the weight, age, and gender of the individual reflect normal muscle mass. In patients with obesity, most commonly defined by the World Health Organization as having a body mass index (BMI) of 30 kg/m^2 or more (obese) and BMI 40 kg/m^2 or more (morbidly obese), weight adjustments for estimating Cl_{Cr} are recommended. Here, BMI is calculated using Equation 3.6 as follows:

$$BMI = \frac{Weight\ (kg)}{Height^2\ (m)} \qquad \text{(Eq. 3.6)}$$

It is well known that the use of total body weight (TBW) can lead to significant overestimation of Cl_{Cr} in patients who are obese. To adjust for this extra non-LBW when estimating Cl_{Cr} in this population, alternative measures of weight such as ideal body weight (IBW), adjusted body weight (AdjBW), and LBW have been proposed.

Here, IBW is calculated as follows:

$$\text{Ideal body weight for males in kg} = 50 + (2.3)\ (\text{Height in inches} > 60) \qquad \text{(Eq. 3.7)}$$

$$\text{Ideal body weight for females in kg} = 45 + (2.3)\ (\text{Height in inches} > 60) \qquad \text{(Eq. 3.8)}$$

AdjBW is calculated as follows:

$$\text{Adjusted body weight} = IBW + 0.4\ (TBW - IBW) \qquad \text{(Eq. 3.9)}$$

LBW[19] is calculated as follows:

$$LBW_{Male}: (9{,}270 \times TBW)/(6{,}680 + 216 \times BMI) \qquad \text{(Eq. 3.10)}$$

$$LBW_{Female}: (9{,}270 \times TBW)/(8{,}780 + 244 \times BMI) \qquad \text{(Eq. 3.11)}$$

To address the question "what weight do I use when estimating Cl_{Cr} in obesity?," one study was conducted by the *Food and Drug Administration* based on a review of new drug applications that included renal pharmacokinetic studies. The results showed that for patients with BMI greater than 30 (obese), it is generally acceptable to use either TBW or AdjBW in the Cockcroft and Gault equation to estimate Cl_{Cr}. In patients with BMI 40 or more (morbidly obese), it is recommended that the LBW equation be used,[20] although AdjBW has been reported to provide similar results when compared to LBW in this population.[21] There are other factors not considered in these equations that could account for additional weight in patients with BMI greater than 30. For example, it has been suggested to use the de-indexed four-variable Modification of Diet in Renal Disease (MDRD) or Chronic Kidney Disease Epidemiology Collaboration (CKD-EPI) equations (these equations are discussed later in this chapter) in place of the Cockcroft-Gault equation for drug dosing in patients who are extremely obese with stable kidney function.[22] The best approach will require clinical judgment, taking into account the limitations of any creatinine-based equations to estimate kidney function. As an example, in patients with an extensive third spacing of fluid (ie, edema or ascites), the liters (kilograms) of excess third-space fluid should not be included in the patient's estimate of TBW. In a simulated patient case, consider a 5-ft 4-inch male patient weighing 75 kg and having an estimated 15 kg of edema and ascitic fluid. To avoid assumptions associated with using weight-based indices such as IBW or LBW in this patient, it is recommended to conduct an accurately timed and measured 24-hour Cl_{Cr} for the purpose of renal drug dose adjustment.

In terms of drug dose individualization in this population, it is known that significant third-space fluid does contribute to the apparent volume of distribution for some drugs (see Chapter "Aminoglycoside Antibiotics") but is unlikely to be an important contributor to volume of distribution if the apparent volume of distribution is large (eg, digoxin) or if there is significant plasma protein binding (eg, phenytoin, cyclosporine, lidocaine).

Third-space fluid weight is unlikely to contribute to and should not be used when initial estimates of clearance are made. However, although not directly influencing clearance, it is possible that the presence of ascites or edema may indicate the presence of a hepatobiliary disease process that is known to alter drug clearance.

Patients with very low BMI who are emaciated also require special consideration when estimating kidney function. Although it may seem counterintuitive, a Cl_{Cr} calculated for an emaciated subject using the patient's weight tends to overpredict the patient's Cl_{Cr}. This is because patients who are emaciated tend to have a disproportionally greater loss in muscle mass than TBW, often accompanied by low values of SCr. Consequently, SCr_{ss} in the denominator of Equations 3.4 and 3.5 may decrease more than the weight in the numerator, resulting in an overestimate of Cl_{Cr}. In such cases, it has been suggested that when SCr values are very low (<1.0 mg/dL), an upward adjustment of creatinine to an arbitrary value may help to downwardly "correct" the Cl_{Cr}. This suggestion is based on the assumption that low SCr values are related to small muscle mass and a decreased creatinine production rather than to an unusually large Cl_{Cr}. However, the practice of using "corrected" or arbitrary values for SCr is not supported by scientific literature, and in fact, there are data indicating that correction of low SCr values up to 1.0 mg/dL falsely lowers Cl_{Cr} in older adults.[23] Because of the inherent difficulty in estimating Cl_{Cr} accurately in some populations, it is important to use clinical judgment in evaluating the risk versus benefit of drug therapy. Here, the most reliable approach, that is least susceptible to assumptions related to body weight and SCr, would be to conduct an accurately timed 24-hour measured Cl_{Cr}.

Pediatric Patients

Estimation of kidney function in children is inherently difficult. There are several approaches,[24-26] and the fact that muscle mass and kidney function continue to mature for the first year of life makes the infant especially challenging. Hence, estimation methods for infants below 1 year old are not elusive.[27] One of the more commonly used equations to estimate GFR for children aged 1 to 18 years is as follows[24,28]:

$$\text{GFR (mL/min/1.73 m}^2) = \frac{(K)(\text{Height in cm})}{SCr_{ss}} \qquad \textbf{(Eq. 3.12)}$$

where the K value is based on the infant's/child's age.

AGE	K
Preterm infants up to 1 yr	0.33
Full-term infants up to 1 yr	0.45
1-12 yr	0.55
13-21 yr female	0.55
13-21 yr male	0.70

A newer version of this equation was developed from a population of children with mild-to-moderate CKD enrolled in the Chronic Kidney Disease in Children (CKiD) study.[29] This simplified equation is commonly referred to as the Schwartz "Bedside" equation:

$$\text{GFR (mL/min/1.73 m}^2) = \frac{(0.41)(\text{Height in cm})}{SCr_{ss}} \qquad \textbf{(Eq. 3.13)}$$

It has been reported that this equation performs better than the original Schwartz equation for patients with mild-to-moderate CKD, although the accuracy in subpopulations is yet to be fully determined. An update to the equation was suggested in 2012 measuring serum cystatin C by immunonephelometry and showing improved precision and accuracy.[30] The Schwartz-Lyon equation is an adaptation of the bedside equation (Equation 3.13), which showed an improved accuracy and decreased bias when accounting for differences in sex and between children and adolescents.[31] The 2012 Kidney Disease Improving Global Outcomes (KDIGO) guidelines recommend the use of Schwartz bedside equation and serum cystatin C–based estimation when dosing drugs with a narrow therapeutic range or when SCr estimates may be assumed to be unreliable (although serum cystatin C measurements lack standardization in pediatrics and are limited by increased costs).[32]

The abovementioned equations estimate GFR, not Cl_{Cr}, in children based on standardization to 1.73 m². Although these equations do not calculate the Cl_{Cr} for the child, it is useful as a guide to the child's relative renal function; values near 100 mL/min/1.73 m² would be considered relatively normal, and many dosing guides express Cl_{Cr} in this way.

The principles and cautions to be exercised when estimating GFR and Cl_{Cr} in children are the same as in adults. The SCr should be at steady state, and the muscle mass should be close to average for the child's age, gender, and size. In cases where extremes in body weight are expected, a measured 24-hour Cl_{Cr} should be employed.

ESTIMATING TIME TO REACH STEADY-STATE SERUM CREATININE

All the previous methods for estimating Cl_{Cr} require a steady-state SCr concentration. When a patient's renal function suddenly changes, some period of time will be required to achieve a new SCr_{ss}. In this situation, it is important to be able to estimate how long it will take for the SCr to reach a steady state. If a rising SCr is used in any of the previous equations, the patient's Cl_{Cr} will be overestimated.

As presented earlier, the half-life is a function of both the volume of distribution and the clearance. If the volume of distribution of creatinine $(0.5-0.7 \text{ L/kg})^{33,34}$ is assumed to remain constant, the time required to reach 90% of steady state in patients with normal renal function is less than 1 day.[33,35] As an example, the average 70-kg patient with a Cl_{Cr} of 120 mL/min (7.2 L/hr) with a volume of distribution for creatinine of 45.5 L (0.65 L/kg) would be expected to have a creatinine $t_{1/2}$ of 4.4 hours as calculated by Equation 3.14:

$$t_{1/2} = \frac{0.693(V)}{Cl}$$

$$= \frac{0.693\,(45.5\,\text{L})}{7.2\,\text{L/hr}} \qquad \text{(Eq. 3.14)}$$

$$= 4.4\,\text{hr}$$

Under these conditions, 90% of steady state should be achieved in approximately 15 hours (3.3 $t_{1/2}$s). However, if the same patient had a Cl_{Cr} of 10 mL/min (0.6 L/hr), the creatinine $t_{1/2}$ would be 52.5 hours and more than a week would be required to ensure that a steady state had been achieved. One useful approach that helps clinicians to make relatively rapid assessments of SCr is to remember that because a drug (in this case, creatinine) concentration is accumulating toward steady state, half of the total change will occur in the first half-life. Therefore, two SCr concentrations obtained several hours apart (8-12 hours) that appear to be similar (ie, not increasing or declining significantly) and that represent reasonably normal renal function probably represent steady-state conditions. As renal function declines, proportionately longer intervals between creatinine measurements are required to ensure that steady-state conditions exist.

In clinical practice, patients occasionally have a slowly increasing SCr. As an example, a patient might have the following SCr concentrations on 4 consecutive days: 1, 1.2, 1.6, and 1.8 mg/dL. First, it should be recognized that the increase in SCr from day 1 to day 2 could be caused by assay error alone because the absolute error for most creatinine assays is ±0.1 to 0.2 mg/dL. In addition, given that the $t_{1/2}$ of creatinine at concentrations in the range of 1 to 2 mg/dL is approximately 4 to 8 hours, steady state should have been achieved on the first day. Therefore, the continued increase in SCr probably reflects ongoing changes in Cl_{Cr} over the 4 days. The difficult clinical issue is not what the Cl_{Cr} is on each of the 4 days, but rather what it will be tomorrow, what is the cause, and how to prevent or minimize the ongoing renal damage.

ESTIMATING CREATININE CLEARANCE FROM NON–STEADY-STATE SERUM CREATININE

Using non–steady-state SCr values to estimate Cl_{Cr} is difficult, and a number of approaches have been proposed.[9,10] Equation 3.15 is an example of how to estimate Cl_{Cr} when steady-state conditions have not been achieved.

$$Cl_{Cr} \, mL/min = \frac{\left(\dfrac{\text{Production of creatinine}}{\text{in mg/d}} \right) - \left[\left(\dfrac{(SCr_2 - SCr_1)(V_{Cr})}{t} \right)(10 \, dL/L) \right]}{(SCr_2)(10 \, dL/L)} \times \left(\dfrac{1,000 \, mL/L}{1,440 \, min/d} \right)$$ (Eq. 3.15)

The daily production of creatinine in milligram is calculated by multiplying the daily production value in mg/kg/d from Table 3.2 by the patient's weight in kilogram. The SCr values in Equation 3.15 are expressed in units of mg/dL; t is the number (or fraction) of days between the first serum creatinine measurement (SCr_1) and the second serum creatinine measurement (SCr_2). The volume of distribution for creatinine (V_{Cr}) is calculated by multiplying the patient's weight in kilogram times 0.65 L/kg. Equation 3.15 is essentially a modification of the mass balance Equation 3.16.

$$Cl = \frac{(S)(F)(\text{Dose}/\tau) - \dfrac{(C_2 - C_1)(V)}{t}}{C_{ss \, ave}}$$ (Eq. 3.16)

where the daily production of creatinine in milligram has replaced the dosing input rate of the drug and the second serum creatinine value replaced $C_{ss \, ave}$, S and F are the salt form and the bioavailability of the drug. The second serum creatinine is used primarily because Equation 3.15 is most commonly applied when Cl_{Cr} is decreasing (rising SCr) and using the higher of the two SCr values results in a lower, more conservative estimate of renal function. Some have suggested that the iterative search process, as represented by Equation 3.17, be used:

$$C^2 = (C)(e^{-Kt}) + \frac{(S)(F)(\text{Dose}/\tau)}{Cl}(1 - e^{-Kt_1})$$ (Eq. 3.17)

where C_2 represents SCr_2, and C represents SCr_1. Here, $(S)(F)(\text{Dose}/\tau)$ represents the daily production of creatinine, and t represents the time interval between the first and second serum creatinine concentrations. Cl represents the creatinine clearance with the corresponding elimination rate constant K being Cl/V or the creatinine clearance divided by the creatinine volume of distribution. As discussed previously (see Interpretation of Plasma Drug Concentrations: Non–Steady-State Revision of Clearance [Iterative Search] in Chapter 2), the solution would require an iterative search, and the inherent errors in the calculation process likely do not warrant this type of calculation.

The use of Equation 3.15 can be illustrated by considering a 45-year-old, 70-kg man who has a SCr concentration of 1.0 mg/dL on day 1 and a concentration of 2.0 mg/dL 24 hours later on day 2. Using Table 3.2, the expected daily production of creatinine for this patient would be 1,400 mg/d (20 mg/kg/d × 70 kg). The volume of distribution for creatinine is 45.5 L (0.65 L/kg × 70 kg), and the time between samples (t) is 1 day. Using these values, Equation 3.15 estimates Cl_{Cr} of 32.8 mL/min.

$$Cl_{Cr}\ mL/min = \frac{\left(\begin{array}{c}\text{Production of}\\ \text{creatinine in mg/d}\end{array}\right) - \left[\left(\dfrac{(SCr_2 - SCr_1)(V_{Cr})}{t}\right)(10\ dL/L)\right]}{(SCr_2)(10\ dL/L)}$$

$$\left(\dfrac{1,000\ mL/L}{1,440\ min/d}\right)$$

$$= \frac{(1,400\ mg/d) - \left[\left(\dfrac{\left(2\ mg/dL - 1\ mg/dL\right)\left(45.5\ L\right)}{1\ d}\right)(10\ dL/L)\right]}{(2\ mg/dL)(10\ dL/L)}$$

$$\left(\dfrac{1,000\ mL/L}{1,440\ min/d}\right)$$

$$= \frac{(1,400\ mg/d) - (455\ mg/d)}{(2\ mg/L)(10)}\left(0.694\ \dfrac{mL/L}{min/d}\right)$$

$$= 47.25\ L/d\left(0.694\ \dfrac{mL/L}{min/d}\right)$$

$$= 32.8\ mL/min$$

Although Equation 3.15 can be used to estimate a patient's Cl_{Cr} when a patient's SCr is rising or falling, there are potential problems associated with this and all other approaches using non–steady-state SCr values. First, a rising SCr may represent a continually declining renal function. To help compensate for the latter possibility, the SCr_2 rather than the average is used in the denominator of Equation 3.15. Furthermore, there are nonrenal routes of creatinine elimination that become significant in patients with significantly diminished renal function.[33] Because as much as 30% of a patient's daily creatinine excretion is the result of dietary intake, the ability to predict a patient's daily creatinine production in the clinical setting is limited.[35] One should also consider the potential errors in estimating creatinine production for patients who are the critically ill, the errors in SCr measurements, and the uncertainty in the volume of distribution estimate for creatinine. Estimating Cl_{Cr} in a patient with a rising or falling SCr should be viewed as a best guess under difficult conditions, and ongoing reassessment of the patient's renal function is warranted.

MEASURING CREATININE CLEARANCE: URINE COLLECTIONS

As noted earlier, in cases where the underlying assumptions of estimating Cl_{Cr} cannot be met, it may be most appropriate to conduct a measured Cl_{Cr}. This approach often used in early (phase 1) pharmacokinetic studies conducted during new drug development often utilize 24-hour measured Cl_{Cr} as the primary index for stratifying patients into renal function categories. The accuracy of a measured Cl_{Cr} highly depends on the complete and accurate measurement of creatinine concentration and urine volume over a specified time period. Errors in the collection process should always be considered, especially when collections are made in the ambulatory or unobserved setting.

To check the completeness of a timed (24-hour) urine collection, the predicted amount of creatinine produced or excreted for the patient (considering age, gender, weight, and body stature) should be compared with the amount of creatinine collected in the urine sample. At steady state, the rate in (creatinine production) equals the rate out (creatinine excretion). If the amount collected differs significantly from the patient's predicted production, the reported Cl_{Cr} is likely to be inaccurate. The patient's age, gender, and muscle mass should be considered when estimating the amount of creatinine produced. Increasing age and smaller muscle mass will reduce the expected amount of creatinine produced (see Table 3.2).

This principle will be illustrated using the following example. The following data were reported for a 55-year-old, 50-kg male patient for whom a 24-hour urine collection for Cl_{Cr} was ordered.

Total collection time	24 hr
Urine volume	1,200 mL
Urine creatinine concentration	42 mg/dL
Serum creatinine	1.5 mg/dL
Creatinine clearance	23 mL/min (uncorrected)
	30 mL/min (corrected)

The Cl_{Cr} of 23 mL/min (uncorrected) represents the patient's Cl_{Cr} as calculated from the urine collection. The Cl_{Cr} of 30 mL/min (corrected) represents what the patient's Cl_{Cr} would have been if the patient were 70 kg or 1.73 m². This "corrected" value is most useful as a relative estimate of renal function when the patient is substantially smaller or larger than our average 70-kg, 1.73 m² patient.

The uncorrected Cl_{Cr} was calculated using the following equation:

$$Cl_{Cr} = \frac{(U)(V)}{P}$$

(Eq. 3.18)

where U is the urine creatinine concentration in mg/dL, V the volume of urine per time of collection in mL/min, and P the plasma creatinine concentration in mg/dL. Equation 3.18 results in a Cl_{Cr} in the units of mL/min.

$$Cl_{Cr} = \frac{(U)(V)}{P}$$

$$= \frac{\left(42 \text{ mg/dL}\right)\left(1,200 \text{ mL/1,440 min}\right)}{1.5 \text{ mg/dL}}$$

$$= 23 \text{ mL/min}$$

The laboratory computer performs these calculations of the uncorrected or corrected Cl_{Cr}. By performing this calculation, all we have checked is the math skill of the computer and not the validity of the collection.

To determine whether the collection was complete, the total amount of creatinine collected in the 24-hour period should be calculated.

Because the patient weighs 50 kg, the apparent creatinine production per day can be calculated using the urine collection data and the appropriate conversion factors as follows:

$$\frac{\text{Apparent rate of}}{\text{creatinine production}} = \frac{\text{Amount of creatinine extracted per day in mg}}{\text{Patient's weight in kg}} = \frac{(U)(V)}{\text{Patient's weight in kg}} \quad \text{(Eq. 3.19)}$$

$$= \frac{(42 \text{ mg/dL})(1,200 \text{ mL/d})(1 \text{ dL/100 mL})}{50 \text{ kg}}$$

$$= 10.08 \text{ mg/kg/d}$$

This apparent production rate of creatinine of 10 mg/kg/d is considerably less than the normal production rate of 19 mg/kg/d as estimated from Table 3.2 for a 55-year-old man. Therefore, one possibility is that the urine collection was incomplete, and the reported value for Cl_{Cr} is much less than the patient's actual Cl_{Cr}. However, if the patient has a smaller-than-average muscle mass, the urine collection may be considered adequate and the reported Cl_{Cr} of 23 mL/min is the best estimate of the patient's renal function. In clinical practice, it is important to evaluate the patient for their "body composition." Patients who have a muscle mass that is less than average usually appear emaciated or very thin and/or have been physically inactive for a prolonged period (eg, patients who are bedridden secondary to chronic illness or a spinal cord injury). Whether to accept the 24-hour urine collection as complete would depend on our assessment of the patient's physical stature.

An alternative approach to evaluating the 24-hour urine collection could be to compare the Cl_{Cr} as calculated from Cockcroft and Gault, Equation 3.4, to the uncorrected Cl_{Cr} from the 24-hour urine collection.

$$Cl_{Cr} \text{ for males}(mL/min) = \frac{(140 - Age)(Weight)}{(72)(SCr_{ss})}$$

$$= \frac{(140 - 55)(50)}{(72)(1.5 \text{ mg/dL})}$$

$$= 39.4 \text{ mL/min}$$

In this case, Equation 3.4 calculated a Cl_{Cr} of approximately 40 mL/min and the 24-hour urine collection as a value of 23 mL/min. Clearly, they both cannot be correct. Because both Equation 3.4 and the 24-hour collection used the SCr of 1.5 mg/dL, the difference must be the rate of creatinine production. Equation 3.4 assumes that the average creatinine production for a 55-year-old man is about 19 mg/kg/d (see Table 3.2). This is in contrast to the creatinine in the 24-hour collection, suggesting a production rate of about 10 mg/kg/d. Which is correct? As previously stated, if the patient has an unusually small muscle mass for their size, age, and gender, one might conclude that Equation 3.4 overestimated the production rate and the Cl_{Cr}. If this were the case, the 24-hour urine collection would be the most reasonable estimate of the patient's Cl_{Cr}. However, if the patient appears to have a normal amount of muscle mass (ie, average physical stature for a 55-year-old man), then one might conclude that the 24-hour collection was inadequate and has underestimated the patient's creatinine production rate and, therefore, the Cl_{Cr}. If this were the case, the Cl_{Cr} of 40 mL/min from Equation 3.4 might be considered the better estimate of the patient's renal function. It is always important when determining renal function, either by use of an equation or by collecting urine, that the results be evaluated in the context of the patient's muscle mass.

ESTIMATING GLOMERULAR FILTRATION RATE (eGFR)

Another method to estimate kidney function is to use eGFR equations that were developed by public health researchers for the purpose of categorizing or staging CKD. This approach is recommended by international kidney disease organizations, such as the National Kidney Foundation (NKF) and the KDIGO, aimed to characterize and stage the patients with CKD.

The eGFR equation was originally derived from the MDRD study, with a four-variable version that was validated to estimate GFR in patients with a GFR of less than 60 mL/min/1.73 m^2. However, at higher eGFR values, it was found that this equation loses its accuracy and could lead to overestimation of GFR in some patients. It is for this reason that calculated eGFR values over 60 mL/min/1.73 m^2 are not reported and may appear in the electronic medical record (EMR) as "eGFR >60 mL/min/1.73 m^2."

$$\text{eGFR (mL/min/1.73 m}^2) = 175 \times (SCr)^{-1.154} \times (Age)^{-0.203} \times (0.742 \text{ if female}) \times (1.21 \text{ if Black}) \quad \textbf{(Eq. 3.20a)}$$

where SCr is in mg/dL and age in years.

In 2012, a newer eGFR equation was developed, based on further analysis of the MDRD study along with other pooled clinical trial data. This equation is called the Chronic Kidney Disease Epidemiology Study equation, or CKD-EPI.[36] Derivatives of this equation were recently developed based on cystatin C, another endogenous biomarker of kidney function (CKD-EPI$_{Cystatin\ C}$) and based on a cystatin C-creatinine combination (CKD-EPI$_{combined}$) which was reported to perform better than the creatinine-based CKD-EPI.[37]

CKD-EPI:

$$eGFR\ (mL/min/1.73\ m^2) = 141 \times \min\ (SCr/\kappa, 1)^{\alpha} \times \max\ (SCr/\kappa, 1)^{-1.209}$$
$$\times 0.993^{Age} \times [1.018\ if\ female] \times [1.159$$
$$if\ African\ American]$$

(Eq. 3.20b)

where SCr is serum creatinine in mg/dL, κ is 0.7 for females and 0.9 for males, α is −0.329 for females and −0.411 for males, min indicates the minimum of SCr/κ or 1, and max indicates the maximum of SCr/κ or 1.

Although both eGFR equations (MDRD and CKD-EPI) are meant to be used for staging patients with CKD, to date, these equations have not been shown to be superior to the Cockcroft and Gault equation for dosing drugs that are renally cleared. Because of the large body of evidence and experience with Cockcroft and Gault, it is recommended that these eGFR equations not be used for the dosing of drugs until studies are preformed to document the accuracy of MDRD for dose adjustment of renally cleared drugs.[38,39] This is an important issue because many hospitals and health care systems automatically calculate and display an eGFR that is calculated from the MDRD equation (see Equation 3.20a). Although the use of the CKD-EPI equation for automated reporting of eGFR is recommended, it is considered optional and has not been widely implemented at this time. Because eGFR values reported in the EMR are based on the MDRD equation, a patient with a calculated eGFR of 72 mL/min/1.73 m^2 will have an EMR-reported value of ">60 mL/min/1.73 m^2."

Furthermore, the use of a race correction in both eGFR equations (MDRD and CKD-EPI) has recently been challenged. Several studies have shown that the inclusion of a race factor does not improve accuracy in estimating GFR among Black individuals in countries outside the United States, suggesting that this correction factor may be only reflective of those African Americans with CKD who were included in the study population. To address this controversy, a joint task force of the NKF and the American Society of Nephrology is reviewing the impact of the inclusion of race as a variable in eGFR equations.[40-43]

When estimating Cl$_{Cr}$ for dosing of renally cleared drugs, it is recommended that the Cockcroft and Gault equation be used. When comparing the results of estimated Cl$_{Cr}$ and eGFR, in most cases, the estimates will be similar, especially for patients with BSA close to 1.73 m^2. The reason for this is that the units of the MDRD equation are in mL/min/1.73 m^2. Thus, back-calculation of the eGFR value to obtain the unit of mL/min is required for direct comparison with Cl$_{Cr}$, as shown in the following example:

$$\frac{\text{eGFR for patient}}{\text{mL/min}} = \frac{\text{eGFR}}{\text{mL/min/1.73 m}^2}\left(\frac{\text{BSA}}{1.73\text{ m}^2}\right) \qquad \textbf{(Eq. 3.21)}$$

or the ratio of weight/70 kg to the power 0.7

$$\frac{\text{eGFR for patient}}{\text{mL/min}} = \frac{\text{eGFR}}{\text{mL/min/1.73 m}^2}\left(\frac{\text{Weight in kg}}{70\text{ kg}}\right)^{0.7} \qquad \textbf{(Eq. 3.22)}$$

In some cases, even when the kidney function has been adjusted for the patient's size, the difference in estimated renal function can be significant. As an example, a 76-year-old, 52.3-kg African American male with an SCr of 1.0 mg/dL would have the following estimates of kidney function.

Using Cockcroft and Gault equation (Equation 3.4):

$$\text{Cl}_{\text{Cr}}\text{ for males (mL/min)} = \frac{(140 - \text{Age})(\text{Weight})}{72 \times \text{SCr}_{ss}}$$

$$= \frac{(140 - 76)\,52.3}{72 \times 1}$$

$$= 46.5\text{ mL/min}$$

Using the MDRD equation (Equation 3.20a):

$$\text{eGFR (mL/min/1.73 m}^2) = 175 \times (\text{SCr})^{-1.154} \times (\text{Age})^{-0.203}$$

$$\times [0.742\text{ if female}] \times [1.21\text{ if Black}]$$

Again substituting 1 for 0.742 if female:

$$= 175 \times (1)^{-1.154} \times (76)^{-0.203} \times 1$$
$$\times [1.21\text{ if Black}]$$
$$= 87.9\text{ mL/min/1.73 m}^2$$

Adjusting for the patient's size using Equation 3.22:

$$\frac{\text{eGFR for patient}}{\text{mL/min}} = \frac{\text{eGFR}}{\text{mL/min/1.73 m}^2}\left(\frac{\text{Weight in kg}}{70\text{ kg}}\right)^{0.7}$$

$$= \frac{87.9}{\text{mL/min/1.73 m}^2}\left(\frac{52.3\text{ kg}}{70\text{ kg}}\right)^{0.7}$$

$$= \frac{87.9}{\text{mL/min/1.73 m}^2}(0.815)$$

$$= 71.6\text{ mL/min}$$

Using the CKD-EPI equation (Equation 3.20b):

$$\text{eGFR} = 141 \times (1 \text{ mg/dL/0.9 for males})^{-0.411} \times (1 \text{ mg/dL/0.9})^{-1.209}$$
$$\times 0.993^{76 \text{ yr old}} \times 1.159 \text{ (AA)}$$
$$= 141 \times 0.9576 \times 1 \times 0.586 \times 1.159$$
$$= 91.7 \text{ mL/min/1.73 m}^2$$

When adjusting this eGFR value based on the patient's size, using Equation 3.22:

$$91.7 \times (0.815) = 74.7 \text{ mL/min}$$

In reviewing the range of values calculated in this example, it is notable that an error in comparing Cockcroft-Gault and eGFR equations is a failure to adjust for the patient's size (ie, comparing mL/min vs mL/min/1.73 m^2). In this example, after adjustment for the patient's BSA, the estimates of kidney function are significantly different depending on which equation is used, and the results from the eGFR equations appear to be much higher than expected, for this 52.3-kg, 76 year old man. This cautionary example illustrates the necessity of calculating Cl_{Cr} using the Cockcroft-Gault equation for all patients, even in cases where the laboratory computer indicates that eGFR as ">60 mL/min/1.73 m^2." Again, until specific information is known about the utility of eGFR equations (MDRD or CKD-EPI), it is recommended that Cockcroft and Gault, Equations 3.4 and 3.5 for adults or Schwartz, and Equation 3.13 for pediatrics be used when calculating dosing regimens for renally cleared drugs.

Adjusting Drug Dose Based on Kidney Function

In cases where clinical pharmacokinetic studies and renal dosing recommendations may not be readily available, calculation of dose adjustment factors based on kidney function may be needed. Because the kidneys and liver function independently, it is assumed that a change in one does not affect the other. Thus, Cl_t can be estimated in the presence of renal or hepatic failure or both. Because the metabolic function is difficult to quantitate, Cl_t is most commonly adjusted when there is decreased renal function:

$$Cl\text{ adjusted} = (Cl_m) + \left[(Cl_r) \left(\frac{\text{Fraction of normal renal}}{\text{function remaining}} \right) \right] \qquad \textbf{(Eq. 3.23)}$$

A clearance that has been adjusted for kidney function can be used to estimate the maintenance dose for a patient with stable CKD (see Equation 1.16). This adjusted clearance equation, however, is only valid if the drug's metabolites are inactive and if the metabolic clearance is indeed unaffected by kidney disease as assumed. A decrease in the function of an organ of elimination is most significant when that organ serves as the primary route of drug elimination. However, as the major elimination pathway becomes increasingly compromised, the "minor" pathway becomes more significant because it assumes a greater proportion of the total clearance. For example, a drug that is usually 67% eliminated by the renal route and 33% by the hepatic route will be 100%

metabolized in the event of complete renal failure; the total clearance, however, will only be one-third of the normal value.

As an alternative to adjusting Cl_t to calculate the dosing rate, one can substitute fraction of the total clearance that is metabolic and renal for Cl_m and Cl_r. Using this technique, the following equation can be derived.

Dosing rate adjustment factor =

$$\left(\begin{array}{c}\text{Fraction eliminated} \\ \text{metabolically}\end{array}\right) + \left[\left(\begin{array}{c}\text{Fraction eliminated} \\ \text{renally}\end{array}\right)\left(\begin{array}{c}\text{Fraction of normal renal} \\ \text{function remaining}\end{array}\right)\right] \quad \text{(Eq. 3.24)}$$

The dosing rate adjustment factor can be used to adjust the maintenance dose for a patient with altered renal function.

As an example, take a drug that is 25% metabolized and 75% renally cleared and normally administered as 100 mg every 12 hours. If this drug were to be given to a patient who has only 33% of normal renal function, the dosing rate adjustment factor would be 0.5.

Dosing rate adjustment factor =

$$\left(\begin{array}{c}\text{Fraction eliminated} \\ \text{metabolically}\end{array}\right) + \left[\left(\begin{array}{c}\text{Fraction eliminated} \\ \text{renally}\end{array}\right)\left(\begin{array}{c}\text{Fraction of normal renal} \\ \text{function remaining}\end{array}\right)\right]$$

$$= (0.25) + [(0.75)(0.33)]$$

$$= (0.25) + [0.25]$$

$$= 0.5$$

The dosing rate adjustment factor of 0.5 suggests that the drug should be administered at half the usual rate. This could be accomplished by decreasing the dose and maintaining the same interval (eg, 50 mg every 12 hours) or by maintaining the same dose and increasing the interval (eg, 100 mg every 24 hours). Depending on the situation and therapeutic intent, either method (or a combination of dose and dosing interval adjustment) might be appropriate.

Dialysis of Drugs

PHARMACOKINETIC MODELING: HEMODIALYSIS

The pharmacokinetic model for drugs in patients undergoing intermittent hemodialysis generally follows one of two patterns. In Figure 3.1, a maintenance drug dose produces plasma concentrations that are relatively constant between dialysis periods. This plasma concentration of drug represents the steady-state condition with very little fluctuation of the drug concentration between doses. This pattern occurs when the input is continuous (intravenous [IV] or oral sustained release) or the dosing interval

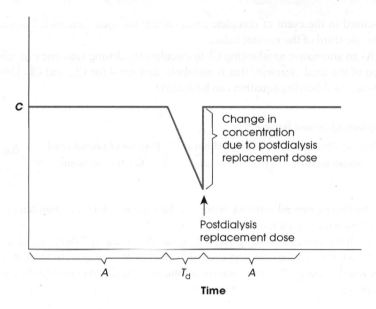

FIGURE 3.1 Plasma concentration curve between dialysis procedures. This figure represents a plasma concentration curve for a patient receiving a maintenance dose of a drug between dialysis procedures at intervals that result in small fluctuations in plasma concentration. The dosing interval during the interdialysis period (A) is arbitrary but should be less than the half-life of the drug. During the intradialysis period (T_d), the drug is rapidly removed by the dialysis procedure. The subsequent increase in the plasma concentration of drug is because of the postdialysis replacement dose. This model assumes that the drug is significantly removed during dialysis and does not include the distribution phase following the postdialysis replacement dose.

is much less than the drug half-life (ie, $\tau < \frac{1}{3}t_{\frac{1}{2}}$). The rapid decline in the drug concentration corresponds to periods of hemodialysis when the drug is being rapidly removed, and the rapid return of the plasma drug concentration to steady state reflects the administration of a postdialysis replacement dose. This pattern can be represented by the following equations:

$$Cl_{pat} = Cl_m + Cl_r \tag{Eq. 3.25}$$

$$C_{ss\,ave} = \frac{(S)(F)(Dose/\tau)}{Cl_{pat}} \tag{Eq. 3.26}$$

$$Dose = \frac{(C_{ss\,ave})(Cl_{pat})(\tau)}{(S)(F)} \tag{Eq. 3.27}$$

where Cl_{pat} is the patient's intrinsic drug clearance during nondialysis periods and is the sum of the patient's metabolic clearance (Cl_m) and any residual renal clearance (Cl_r). S and F are the salt form and bioavailability of the drug, respectively, and

τ is the dosing interval. Equation 3.26 may be used to predict the $C_{ss\,ave}$, and Equation 3.27 may be used to calculate the maintenance dose based on the estimated Cl_{pat} and the desired $C_{ss\,ave}$. In addition to the maintenance dose, the patient may also require additional doses following dialysis to replace the drug lost during the dialysis period.

$$\begin{array}{c}\text{Postdialysis}\\\text{replacement} =\\\text{dose}\end{array} \begin{bmatrix}\text{Amount of drug}\\\text{in the body}\\\text{prior to dialysis}\end{bmatrix}\begin{bmatrix}\text{Fraction of drug}\\\text{lost during dialysis}\end{bmatrix}$$

$$\begin{array}{c}\text{Postdialysis}\\\text{replacement} = (V)(C_{ss\,ave})\left(1 - e^{-\left(\frac{Cl_{pat}\,+Cl_{dial}}{V}\right)(T_d)}\right)\\\text{dose}\end{array} \qquad \text{(Eq. 3.28)}$$

$$\begin{array}{c}\text{Postdialysis}\\\text{replacement} = (V)(C_{ss\,ave})\left(1 - e^{-K_{dial}(T_d)}\right)\\\text{dose}\end{array} \qquad \text{(Eq. 3.29)}$$

In these equations, $(V)(C_{ss\,ave})$ is the amount of drug in the body at the beginning of dialysis, and the elimination rate constant during the dialysis (K_{dial}) represents the sum of the patient's intrinsic clearance and the clearance by dialysis divided by the volume of distribution $[(Cl_{pat} + Cl_{dial})/V]$. T_d is the duration of dialysis. If the patient's maintenance dose is given in divided daily doses or once daily, the patient's dose would be calculated using Equation 3.27 on nondialysis days. On dialysis days, the patient would receive, in addition to the maintenance dose, a postdialysis replacement dose as calculated by Equation 3.28 or 3.29.

The second pharmacokinetic model for drug dosing in patients undergoing hemodialysis is depicted in Figure 3.2. In this model, a single dose is given at the conclusion of each dialysis period. Significant amounts of drug are lost between dialysis periods, and the additional drug is lost during dialysis. In this model, the dose administered at the end of dialysis replaces all of the drug lost by the patient's intrinsic clearance, as well as by dialysis clearance, and returns the drug level to a targeted "peak" concentration. This replacement dose can be calculated by use of Equation 3.30 or 3.31:

$$\begin{array}{c}\text{Postdialysis}\\\text{replacement} = (V)(C_{ss\,peak})\left(1 - \left[\left(e^{-\left(\frac{Cl_{pat}}{V}\right)(t_1)}\right)\left(e^{-\left(\frac{Cl_{pat}\,+Cl_{dial}}{V}\right)(T_d)}\right)\right]\right)\\\text{dose}\end{array} \qquad \text{(Eq. 3.30)}$$

$$\begin{array}{c}\text{Postdialysis}\\\text{replacement} = (V)(C_{ss\,peak})\left(1 - \left[\left(e^{-(K_{pat})(t_1)}\right)\left(e^{-(K_{dial})(T_d)}\right)\right]\right)\\\text{dose}\end{array} \qquad \text{(Eq. 3.31)}$$

where t_1 is the interdialysis period or the period from the peak concentration to the beginning of dialysis, and T_d the dialysis period or the time interval from the beginning to

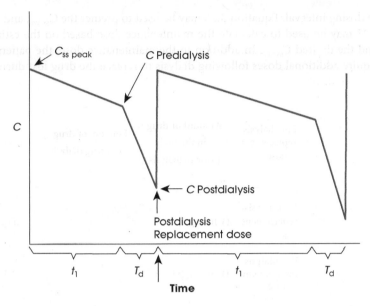

FIGURE 3.2 Plasma profile for a drug administered only at the postdialysis period for a patient receiving intermittent hemodialysis. The interdialysis period (t_1) represents the time from the steady-state peak concentration to the beginning of dialysis and may vary according to the number of days between each hemodialysis period. The intradialysis period is represented by T_d. The postdialysis dose represents the amount of drug that is lost from the body because of the patient's clearance during the interdialysis period and the dialysis clearance during the intradialysis period. This model assumes that the drug is significantly removed during dialysis and does not include the distribution phase following the postdialysis replacement dose.

the end of the dialysis procedure. K_{pat} is the elimination rate constant during the interdialysis period where drug loss is caused by Cl_{pat} alone, and K_{dial} is the elimination rate constant during the dialysis period where drug loss is the result of both Cl_{pat} and Cl_{dail}.

In some cases, it may be appropriate to calculate the drug concentrations at the beginning and end of the dialysis period. This can be accomplished using Equations 3.32 and 3.33.

$$\text{Predialysis concentration} = (C_{ss\,peak})\left(e^{\left(-\frac{Cl_{pat}}{V}\right)(t_1)} \right) \tag{Eq. 3.32}$$

$$\text{Postdialysis concentration} = \left(\text{Predialysis concentration} \right)\left(e^{\left(-\frac{Cl_{pat}+Cl_{dial}}{V}\right)(T_d)} \right) \tag{Eq. 3.33}$$

These equations are used when there are specifically targeted peak and/or trough concentrations or when transient declines in the plasma concentrations might result in therapeutic failures, as with antiarrhythmics or anticonvulsant agents. Depending on the therapeutic intent, the specific drug concentrations may be of more or less interest. As an example, in the case of aminoglycoside antibiotics, the predialysis and not the postdialysis concentration should be thought of as the "trough" in assessing the risk of aminoglycoside toxicity. This is because the pattern of decay is more rapid during the intradialysis period and as a result, the postdialysis aminoglycoside "trough" concentration is transient and does not easily translate into drug exposure and risk of toxicity (see Figure 3.2). Given that the interval between dialysis runs is often about 48 hours, it is not possible to dose aminoglycosides in a way that will achieve the usually targeted high peak and low trough concentrations in the patient who need dialysis. For these patients, the usual gentamicin/tobramycin steady-state peak and predialysis trough concentration are approximately 5 and 2 mg/L, respectively. Because of this, the risk of aminoglycoside toxicity may be greater in patients who require dialysis.

ESTIMATING DRUG DIALYZABILITY

To calculate dosing requirements for patients undergoing intermittent hemodialysis, the dialysis clearance must be known. Although several general references are available,[11,12,44-51] it is frequently difficult to find information on specific drugs, especially for drugs that are poorly dialyzable. To determine the dialyzability of a drug, the apparent volume of distribution, plasma protein binding, the patient's intrinsic clearance, and the drug's half-life should be considered as follows:

1. Divide the volume of distribution by fu or the usual free fraction to calculate the apparent unbound volume of distribution. It is only the unbound drug that can pass through the dialysis membrane, and therefore, it is the unbound volume of distribution against which the drug will be dialyzed. If the unbound volume of distribution exceeds 3.5 L/kg or approximately 250 L/70 kg, it is unlikely that a significant amount of drug will be removed by dialysis.

$$\text{Unbound volume of distribution} = \frac{V}{fu} \qquad \text{(Eq. 3.34)}$$

2. Estimate the patient's intrinsic clearance (Cl_m + residual Cl_r). If this value is greater than 10 mL/min/kg or 700 mL/min/70 kg, it is unlikely that hemodialysis will add significantly to the patient's intrinsic drug elimination or Cl_{pat}. This is because most drugs have a hemodialysis clearance of less than 150 mL/min.
3. If the usual dosing interval is much greater than the drug's $t_{1/2}$ in patients with end-stage renal failure, it is unlikely that hemodialysis will significantly alter the dosing regimen. The key here is to schedule the drug administration shortly after rather than shortly before dialysis, so that even if the drug is dialyzable, very little remains to be removed by dialysis.
4. Drugs with a low molecular weight are more likely to be removed significantly by dialysis. Drugs with a molecular weight of greater than 1,000 Da are unlikely to be removed by low-flux hemodialysis. High-flux hemodialysis can remove molecules with a molecular weight of 1,000 Da (see Low-Flux versus High-Flux Hemodialysis).

For almost all drugs, if any one of the abovementioned criteria is met, it is unlikely that the drug in question will be significantly removed by hemodialysis.

However, if a drug has an unbound volume of less than 3.5 L/kg, a clearance of less than 10 mL/min/kg, a τ that is not significantly greater than the drug's $t_{1/2}$, and a molecular weight of less than 1,000 Da if low flux or less than 5,000 Da if high flux, it is possible, but not a certainty, that hemodialysis will significantly alter the drug elimination pattern. In these cases, it is necessary to review the literature to establish whether the drug is significantly removed by hemodialysis. If Cl_{dial} adds significantly to the patient's intrinsic clearance, then additional drug replacement following hemodialysis may be appropriate.

As an additional check, the drug half-life during the dialysis period can be calculated:

$$t_{1/2} \text{ during hemodialysis} = \frac{(0.693)(V)}{(Cl_{pat} + Cl_{dial})} \qquad \text{(Eq. 3.35)}$$

If the $t_{1/2}$ during hemodialysis greatly exceeds the duration of dialysis, very little drug will be removed during any individual period of dialysis.

Whereas the techniques outlined previously can be used to estimate the dialyzability of drugs and thereby model their pharmacokinetic behavior during dialysis, there are a number of potential limitations. For many drugs, relatively little is known about either the activity or dialyzability of their metabolites. In addition, these guidelines must be used cautiously in acute overdose situations because the saturation of plasma and tissue binding as well as possible alterations in the pathways for elimination may occur when drug concentrations are very high. Considerable differences in dialysis equipment, the types of membranes used in hemodialysis, and the duration of dialysis can result in data that may not be applicable to all dialysis situations.[52]

Although it would be ideal to have data derived from the specific dialysis equipment used for the patient in question, this will not be the case in most instances. Instead, one must rely on the data in the literature to estimate the average amount of drug that most likely would be removed during the patient's hemodialysis.

Dialysis procedures also vary in duration and effectiveness, but most patients receive hemodialysis 3 times a week, with each dialysis period being approximately 3 to 4 hours. The duration of dialysis can usually be found on the hemodialysis record sheets and should be checked to be certain that the initial plans for dialysis were successfully completed. In some cases, because of hypotension, lack of venous access, or equipment malfunction, dialysis is not completed as planned, either in the duration of the dialysis or the ability to maintain the patient's blood flow through the artificial kidney (dialysis membrane) during the dialysis period. As stated earlier, the usual duration of dialysis is 3 hours, and the usual blood flow through the artificial kidney is 200 to 350 mL/min. If the usual dialysis parameters are not met, the estimated drug loss during dialysis is probably less than expected.

The uncertainties and potential problems associated with predictions of drug levels during hemodialysis suggest that plasma drug concentrations guide the approach to therapy when possible. When plasma samples are obtained, the distribution phase associated with IV drug administration, as well as the transient period of disequilibrium between the plasma and tissue compartments associated with the hemodialysis process, should be avoided. The disequilibrium between plasma and tissue occurs to varying degrees with most drugs because as the drug is removed from the plasma by dialysis, additional time is required for the drug in the tissue to reequilibrate with the decreased plasma concentration. Although the time required to reestablish equilibrium between the tissue and plasma is not documented for most drugs, it would seem reasonable to wait at least 60 minutes following the end of hemodialysis if postdialysis plasma samples are to be obtained.

LOW-FLUX VERSUS HIGH-FLUX HEMODIALYSIS

High-flux or high-efficiency hemodialysis refers to a dialysis process that utilizes a dialysis membrane that has larger pores through which both solvent (water) and solute (electrolytes, drugs, etc.) can pass.[11,12] Because the pore size is larger, high-flux hemodialysis is more efficient in removing smaller compounds and can remove some larger compounds that low-flux hemodialysis cannot remove. High-flux dialysis is more efficient than low-flux dialysis, thereby making the earlier techniques to estimate dialyzability less reliable as a predictor, but not invalid. To illustrate, vancomycin with its large molecular weight (~1,450 Da) is relatively unaffected by low-flux hemodialysis. This is because the pore size associated with the low-flux hemodialysis membranes only allows the passage of compounds with a molecular weight of less than 1,000 Da and has a limited ability to remove drugs with a molecular weight between 500 and 1,000 Da. However, when a high-flux dialysis membrane is used, the large pore size allows compounds of greater than 1,000 Da to pass through and be eliminated. As a result, during a usual 3-hour high-flux hemodialysis run, there is a rapid drop in the vancomycin drug concentrations followed by a postdialysis rebound in concentration, indicating that approximately 17% of the body stores of vancomycin is removed.[52-55]

For those compounds that are eliminated to a significant extent during low-flux dialysis, more drug is eliminated during high-flux hemodialysis. However, the differences in elimination are usually one of degree and not in most cases as significant as seen with vancomycin.

CONTINUOUS RENAL REPLACEMENT THERAPY

Continuous renal replacement therapy (CRRT) utilizes an ultrafiltration process with a large pore membrane similar to those in high-flux hemodialysis to filter free water and solute, including unbound drug. The rate of plasma filtration is commonly 1 L/hr but ranges from 0.5 to 2 L/hr. Of course, patients could not tolerate this rate of fluid removal unless the vast majority of fluid being removed was continuously being replaced. Dialysate is sometimes added to the ultrafiltration process, which can further increase solute and drug elimination through a passive diffusion process. Total CRRT output (ultrafiltration + dialysate) is usually in the range of 1 to 2 L/hr. The advantage of CRRT is that it is more hemodynamically forgiving than hemodialysis and is used in patients who are critically ill and who cannot tolerate intermittent hemodialysis, usually because of hypotension.[11,12,56-58] CRRT can be performed using several techniques or modes of therapy based on the method of solute removal. These techniques include continuous arteriovenous hemofiltration (CAVH) or continuous venovenous hemofiltration (CVVH). When dialysate is added to the process, it is referred to as continuous arteriovenous hemodialysis (CAVHD), continuous venovenous hemodialysis (CVVHD), continuous arteriovenous hemodiafiltration (CAVHDF), or continuous venovenous hemodiafiltration (CVVHDF). CRRT with or without dialysate is well documented to remove vancomycin and other drugs.[59-63] Although the absolute clearance of CRRT is not high, it is continuous and can add significantly to the elimination of some drugs.

One approach to identifying which drugs might be significantly influenced by CRRT is to calculate the maximum CRRT dialysis clearance (Cl_{CRRT}). Because the CRRT membranes, like low- and high-flux membranes, do not allow plasma proteins to pass through, only the unbound drug (Cu) can be removed by CRRT. One method of estimating the maximum Cl_{CRRT} is to multiply the total CRRT flow rate (volume of ultrafiltrate + volume of dialysate per interval of time) by the fraction of unbound drug in plasma (fu). This process assumes that the ultrafiltrate and the dialysate will be at equilibrium with plasma and have a concentration of drug that is equal to the concentration of unbound drug in plasma. This assumption is probably true because most drugs have a molecular weight that is less than 2,000 Da. Although the molecular weight "cutoff" for CRRT membranes is in the range of 30,000 Da, large molecules are not likely to be able to pass through the membrane and be cleared. However, molecules with a molecular weight of less than 5,000 and almost certainly less than 2,000 Da should be able to be efficiently filtered and come to equilibrium.

$$Cl_{CRRT} \text{ maximum} = (fu)\,(CRRT \text{ flow rate}) \qquad \text{(Eq. 3.36)}$$

In Equation 3.36, fu is the fraction of drug unbound in plasma, and CRRT flow rate is the average volume output of ultrafiltration + dialysate per unit of time. Units for CRRT flow rate are usually expressed as mL/min or L/hr depending on the preference of the clinician. If the Cl_{CRRT} maximum is 25% or less of the patient's residual intrinsic clearance (Cl_{pat}), then CRRT does not add significantly to the patient's drug elimination process, and no dose adjustment would be necessary relative to the presence or absence of CRRT. If Cl_{CRRT} maximum adds significantly to the patient's intrinsic clearance, then the literature will have to be reviewed to identify either Cl_{CRRT} values or recommended replacement doses for patients undergoing CRRT.[58,60-66]

Dose calculations are similar to the usual methods because the CRRT process is intended to be continuous. In many cases, the $t_{1/2}$ is extended, even when the patient is receiving CRRT, and doses can be calculated using Equation 3.37:

$$\text{Maintenance dose} = \frac{(Cl_{pat} + Cl_{CRRT})(C_{ss\,ave})(\tau)}{(S)(F)} \qquad \text{(Eq. 3.37)}$$

where $C_{ss\,ave}$ is the average targeted steady-state concentration, Cl_{pat} the metabolic clearance (Cl_m) plus an estimate of the patient's residual renal clearance (Cl_r), and Cl_{CRRT} an estimate of the CRRT clearance from one of the literature sources or

Equation 3.36. When there is likely to be significant fluctuation in drug concentration between doses (ie, $\tau > \frac{1}{3}t_{\frac{1}{2}}$), the following equation can be used:

$$\text{Dose} = \frac{(C_{ss1})(V)(1-e^{-K_{CRRT}\tau})}{(S)(F)(e^{-K_{CRRT}t_1})} \qquad \text{(Eq. 3.38)}$$

where C_{ss1} is the desired drug concentration, usually $C_{ss\,max}$ or $C_{ss\,min}$, t_1 the time interval from the dose to C_{ss1}, and K_{CRRT} represents the elimination rate constant consisting of Cl_{pat} ($Cl_m + Cl_r$) plus Cl_{CRRT} divided by the drug's volume of distribution.

As with hemodialysis, patients undergoing CRRT need to be monitored to ensure that the CRRT process is proceeding as planned. Because patients receiving CRRT are critically ill and the process is complex, CRRT is often adjusted on an hour-by-hour and day-by-day basis. The two most important issues to consider are whether the CRRT process has been interrupted and/or whether the CRRT flow rate has been significantly altered. Small changes in CRRT flow rates are normal, but if the patient's CRRT vascular access fails or, for some other reason, the process is discontinued or the flow rates changed, then many of the drug dosing recommendations will also have to be altered.

PERITONEAL DIALYSIS

Peritoneal dialysis, and especially continuous ambulatory peritoneal dialysis (CAPD), is occasionally used as an alternative to intermittent hemodialysis. This technique takes advantage of the large semipermeable surface area of the intraperitoneal space and is performed by instilling dialysis fluid via a catheter into the peritoneal space. The dialysate is allowed to equilibrate with the surrounding tissue vasculature and then is removed. This creates a clearance mechanism for solutes, including body waste products and drugs. The usual volume instilled into the peritoneal space for an adult is approximately 2 L, although this can vary somewhat depending on the size of the patient and the intent of dialysis. The efficiency of peritoneal dialysis in removing both drugs and body waste products depends on a number of factors. Assuming that the solute in plasma comes to equilibrium with the dialysate fluid, one would expect the concentration of drug in the dialysate to equal the unbound plasma drug concentration. Therefore, the maximum expected CAPD clearance (Cl_{CAPD}) would be approximately equal to the following:

$$Cl_{CAPD}\,\text{maximum} = (fu)\left(\frac{\text{Volume of dialysate}}{T_D}\right) \qquad \text{(Eq. 3.39)}$$

where fu is the fraction of unbound drug in plasma, volume of dialysate is the peritoneal exchange volume, and T_D the dwell time or the time the dialysate is allowed to remain in the peritoneal space before removal.

Using the usual volume of dialysate instilled into the peritoneal space of approximately 2,000 mL, the usual exchange or dwell time (T_D) of approximately 6 hours, and if fu is assumed to be 1 (no plasma binding), the expected Cl_{CAPD} maximum for solute and drugs would be approximately 5.5 mL/min.

$$Cl_{CAPD} \text{ maximum} = (fu)\left(\frac{\text{Volume of dialysate}}{T_D}\right)$$

$$= (1)(2 \text{ L/6 hr})$$

$$= 0.333 \text{ L/hr}$$

or

$$= (0.333 \text{ L/hr})(1{,}000 \text{ mL/L})(1 \text{ hr}/60 \text{ min})$$

$$= 5.5 \text{ mL/min}$$

Drugs with a residual Cl_{pat} substantially greater than 5.5 mL/min or 0.333 L/hr will not be significantly influenced by peritoneal dialysis. As a general guideline, if the Cl_{CAPD} maximum is less than 25% of the patient's residual intrinsic clearance (Cl_{pat}), one would not anticipate a need to adjust a drug's dose if peritoneal dialysis is initiated or discontinued. One of the assumptions in Equation 3.39 is that equilibrium is achieved between the unbound plasma drug concentration (Cu) and the dialysate fluid. This assumption is probably true for drugs of relatively low molecular weight (ie, <500 Da). Larger compounds may not come to equilibrium within the usual 6-hour dwell time, and very large molecules (eg, proteins) cannot diffuse across the peritoneal cell walls. Some of the plasma proteins do cross into the peritoneal space, and although it can be an issue with regard to protein loss, it is not significant in regard to drug elimination.

In theory, the Cl_{CAPD} for larger compounds could be calculated by taking into account the fraction of steady-state equilibrium achieved in the dialysate dwell time as follows:

$$Cl_{CAPD} \approx (fu)\left(\frac{\text{Volume of dialysate}}{T_D}\right)\left(1 - e^{-(K_{eq})(T_D)}\right) \qquad \text{(Eq. 3.40)}$$

where fu is the free fraction in plasma of the compound or drug in question, T_D the dwell time of the dialysate, K_{eq} the equilibrium rate constant for the equilibrium between the unbound drug in plasma and the dialysate, and $\left(1 - e^{-(K_{eq})(T_D)}\right)$ the fraction of equilibrium achieved during the dialysate dwell time (T_D). Whereas the fu is available for many drugs, it should be recognized that in renal disease, the fu is often increased. Also, the equilibrium rate constant (K_{eq}) is not generally available for most drugs. The fraction of equilibrium achieved can be estimated, however, based on the molecular weight of a drug. For example, urea and creatinine, with molecular weights of approximately 60 and 113 Da, respectively, appear to come to equilibrium relatively rapidly. The average equilibrium half-time for urea and creatinine appears to be approximately 0.66 and 2 hours, respectively.

Therefore, in the usual 6-hour exchange, urea has essentially reached equilibrium, and creatinine is approximately 85% of equilibrium.[11,67] Interestingly, the aminoglycoside antibiotics with fu approximately 1 and molecular weight of approximately 500 Da have a CAPD clearance that approaches the dialysis exchange rate when the dwell time (T_D) is approximately 6 hours.[67-69] If equilibrium is approached in 6 hours, this suggests that the equilibrium half-time is probably in the range of 2 hours. Vancomycin, on the other hand, has a peritoneal dialysis clearance of only 1 to 3 mL/min. Given that vancomycin has a fu approaching 1,[59,70,71] this low Cl_{CAPD} suggests that equilibrium between plasma and dialysate is not achieved within the usual 6-hour dwell time. This observation is consistent with the fact that vancomycin is a large molecule with a molecular weight of approximately 1,450 Da.

The significance of high plasma protein binding on drug clearance is fairly obvious. Compounds that are extensively bound to plasma proteins and have low free concentrations are not likely to be significantly cleared by peritoneal dialysis unless their residual clearance is exceedingly low. The influence of molecular weight and time to reach equilibrium on a drug's dialyzability is less well understood because relatively few data are available. However, the clearance of compounds that appear to come to equilibrium rapidly is likely to be altered if the dwell time is changed. For example, if a patient is taking a drug that has a low molecular weight, more drugs will be removed if the peritoneal dialysate fluid is exchanged more frequently as predicted by Equation 3.39. As a result, replacement doses of a drug that is necessitated by dialysis are likely to be influenced by the dialysate exchange rate. In contrast, replacement doses of drugs with high molecular weights are not likely to be significantly influenced by the exchange rate. This is because an increase in the exchange rate is offset by the decrease in dwell time and the fraction of equilibrium achieved. Consequently, the total calculated clearance by Equation 3.39 would tend to overestimate Cl_{CAPD}, and, if possible, Equation 3.40 should be used for these larger, more slowly equilibrating compounds.

Because the surface area of the peritoneal membrane is large and peritoneal infections are frequent, it has become a common practice to administer antibiotics directly into the peritoneal space.[72-76] When administered by the peritoneal route, the drug does not remain in the peritoneal space but diffuses from the high concentration in the dialysate fluid to the plasma and systemic circulation. The most common antibiotics administered intraperitoneally are cephalosporins, aminoglycosides, and vancomycin. Techniques used to administer these drugs vary from intermittently adding large doses of drug to a single dialysate exchange on a daily or weekly basis, to the addition of smaller amounts of drug in each individual exchange. When drugs are placed in the peritoneal dialysate fluid either intermittently or with each exchange, the ability to achieve peak and trough concentrations is limited (for usual dosing recommendations see Chapters 8 and 16).

REFERENCES

1. Rowland M. Drug administration and regimens. In: Melmon K, Morelli H, eds. *Clinical Pharmacology and Therapeutics*. 2nd ed. Macmillan; 1978:25-70

2. Rowland M, Tozer TN. *Clinical Pharmacokinetics: Concepts and Applications*. 2nd ed. Lea & Febiger; 1989.

3. George JA, Gounden V. Novel glomerular filtration markers. *Adv Clin Chem*. 2019;88:91-119.

4. Teaford HR, Barreto JN, Vollmer KJ, Rule AD, Barreto EF. Cystatin C: a primer for pharmacists. *Pharmacy (Basel)*. 2020;8(1):35.

5. Luft FC. Biomarkers and predicting acute kidney injury. *Acta Physiol (Oxf)*. 2021;231(1):e13479.

6. Garg N, Poggio ED, Mandelbrot D. The evaluation of kidney function in living kidney donor candidates. *Kidney360*. 2021;2(9):1523-1530.

7. Toto RD. Conventional measurement of renal function utilizing serum creatinine, creatinine clearance, inulin and para-aminohippuric acid clearance. *Curr Opin Nephrol Hypertens*. 1995;4(6):505-509.

8. Levey AS, Inker LA. GFR as the "gold standard": estimated, measured, and true. *Am J Kidney Dis*. 2016;67(1):9-12.

9. Lott RS, Hayton WL. Estimation of creatinine clearance from serum creatinine concentration: a review. *Drug Intell Clin Pharm*. 1978;12(3):140-150.

10. Bjornsson TD. Use of serum creatinine concentrations to determine renal function. *Clin Pharmacokinet*. 1979;4(3):200-222.

11. Daugirdas JT, Blake PG, Ing TS. *Handbook of Dialysis*. Lippincott Williams & Wilkins; 2001.

12. Henrich W. *Principles and Practice of Dialysis*. Lippincott Williams & Wilkins; 1998.

13. Jelliffe RW. Letter: Creatinine clearance: bedside estimate. *Ann Intern Med*. 1973;79(4):604-605.

14. Siersbaek-Nielson K, Hansen JM, Kampmann J, et al. Rapid evaluation of creatinine clearance [letter]. *Lancet*. 1971;1:1133-1134.

15. Lepist EI, Zhang X, Hao J, et al. Contribution of the organic anion transporter OAT2 to the renal active tubular secretion of creatinine and mechanism for serum creatinine elevations caused by cobicistat. *Kidney Int*. 2014;86(2):350-357.

16. Lentner C, Lentner C, Wink A, eds. *Geigy Scientific Tables. Body Surface of Children/Adults*. Ciba-Geigy; 1981:226-227.

17. Cockcroft DW, Gault MH. Prediction of creatinine clearance from serum creatinine. *Nephron*. 1976;16(1):31-41.

18. Hernandez de Acevedo L, Johnson CE. Estimation of creatinine clearance in children: comparison of six methods. *Clin Pharm*. 1982;1(2):158-161.

19. Janmahasatian S, Duffull SB, Ash S, Ward LC, Byrne NM, Green B. Quantification of lean bodyweight. *Clin Pharmacokinet*. 2005;44(10):1051-1065.

20. Park EJ, Pai MP, Dong T, et al. The influence of body size descriptors on the estimation of kidney function in normal weight, overweight, obese, and morbidly obese adults. *Ann Pharmacother*. 2012;46(3):317-328.

21. Bouquegneau A, Vidal-Petiot E, Moranne O, et al. Creatinine-based equations for the adjustment of drug dosage in an obese population. *Br J Clin Pharmacol*. 2016;81(2):349-361.

22. Erstad BL, Nix DE. Assessment of kidney function in patients with extreme obesity: a narrative review. *Ann Pharmacother*. 2021;55(1):80-88.

23. Dowling TC, Wang ES, Ferrucci L, Sorkin JD. Glomerular filtration rate equations overestimate creatinine clearance in older individuals enrolled in the Baltimore longitudinal study on aging: impact on renal drug dosing. *Pharmacotherapy*. 2013;33(9):912-921.

24. Schwartz GJ, Brion LP, Spitzer A. The use of plasma creatinine concentration for estimating glomerular filtration rate in infants, children and adolescents. *Pediatr Clin North Am*. 1987;34(3):571-590.

25. Schwartz GJ, Haycock GB, Edelmann CM Jr, Spitzer A. A simple estimate of glomerular filtration rate in children derived from body length and plasma creatinine. *Pediatrics*. 1976;58(2):259-263.

26. Schwartz GJ, Feld LG, Langford DJ. A simple estimate of glomerular filtration rate in full-term infants during the first year of life. *J Pediatr*. 1984;104(6):849-854.

27. Kastl JT. Renal function in the fetus and neonate—the creatinine enigma. *Semin Fetal Neonatal Med*. 2017;22(2):83-89.

28. Schwartz GJ, Gauthier B. A simple estimate of glomerular filtration rate in adolescent boys. *J Pediatr*. 1985;106(3):522-526.

29. Schwartz GJ, Muñoz A, Schneider MF, et al. New equations to estimate GFR in children with CKD. *J Am Soc Nephrol*. 2009;20(3):629-637.

30. Schwartz GJ, Schneider MF, Maier PS, et al. Improved equations estimation GFR in children with chronic kidney disease using an immunonephelometric determination of cystatin C. *Kidney Int.* 2012;82(4):445-453.

31. De Souza VC, Rabilloud M, Cochat P, et al. Schwartz formula: is one k-coefficient adequate for all children? *PLOS ONE.* 2012;7(12):e53439.

32. Levin A, Stevens PE, Bilous RW, et al. Kidney Disease: Improving Global Outcomes (KDIGO) CKD Work Group, KDIGO 2012 clinical practice guidelines for the evaluation and management of chronic kidney disease. *Kidney Int Suppl.* 2013;3(1):1-150.

33. Mitch WE, Collier VU, Walser M. Creatinine metabolism in chronic renal failure. *Clin Sci (Lond).* 1980;58(4):327-335.

34. Chow MS, Schweizer R. Estimation of renal creatinine clearance in patients with unstable serum creatinine concentrations: comparisons of multiple methods. *Drug Intell Clin Pharm.* 1985;19(5):385-390.

35. Bleiler RE, Schedl HP. Creatinine excretion: variability and relationships to diet and body size. *J Lab Clin Med.* 1962;59:945-955.

36. Levey AS, Stevens LA, Schmid CH, et al; CKD-EPI (Chronic Kidney Disease Epidemiology Collaboration). A new equation to estimate glomerular filtration rate. *Ann Intern Med.* 2009;150(9):604-612.

37. Seape T, Gounden V, van Deventer HE, Candy GP, George JA. Cystatin C- and creatinine-based equations in the assessment of renal function in HIV-positive patients prior to commencing highly active antiretroviral therapy. *Ann Clin Biochem.* 2016;53(Pt 1):58-66.

38. Eppenga WJ, Kramers C, Derijks HK, Wensing M, Wetzels JF, De Smet PA. Individualizing pharmacotherapy in patients with renal impairment: the validity of the modification of diet in renal disease formula in specific patient populations with a glomerular filtration rate below 60 mL/min. A systematic review. *PLOS ONE.* 2015;10(3):e011640.

39. Melloni C, Peterson ED, Chen AY, et al. Cockcroft-Gault versus modification of diet in renal disease: importance of glomerular filtration rate formula for classification of chronic kidney disease in patients with non-ST-segment elevation acute coronary syndromes. *J Am Coll Cardiol.* 2008;51(10):991-996.

40. Flamant M, Vidal-Petiot E, Metzger M, et al; NephroTest Study Group. Performance of GFR estimating equations in African Europeans: basis for a lower race-ethnicity factor than in African Americans. *Am J Kidney Dis.* 2013;62(1):182-184.

41. Rocha AD, Garcia S, Santos AB, et al. No race-ethnicity adjustment in CKD-EPI equations is required for estimating glomerular filtration rate in the Brazilian population. *Int J Nephrol.* 2020;2020:2141038.

42. Moodley N, Hariparshad S, Peer F, Gounden V. Evaluation of the CKD-EPI creatinine based glomerular filtration rate estimating equation in Black African and Indian adults in KwaZulu-Natal, South Africa. *Clin Biochem.* 2018;59:43-49.

43. Delgado C, Baweja M, Crews DC, et al. A unifying approach for GFR estimation: recommendations of the NKF-ASN task force on reassessing the inclusion of race in diagnosing kidney disease. *Am J Kidney Dis.* 2022;79(2):268-288.e1.

44. Aweeka FT. Appendix: drug reference table. In: Schrier RW, Gambertoglio JG, eds. *Handbook of Drug Therapy in Liver and Kidney Disease.* Little, Brown and Co.; 1991.

45. Takki S, Gambertoglio JG, Honda DH, Tozer TN. Pharmacokinetic evaluation of hemodialysis in acute drug overdose. *J Pharmacokinet Biopharm.* 1978;6(5):427-442.

46. Lee CS, Marbury TC. Drug therapy in patients undergoing haemodialysis. Clinical pharmacokinetic considerations. *Clin Pharmacokinet.* 1984;9(1):42-66.

47. Maher JF. Pharmacokinetics in patients with renal failure. *Clin Nephrol.* 1984;21(1):39-46.

48. Gokal R, Hutchison A. Dialysis therapies for end-stage renal disease. *Semin Dial.* 2002;15(4):220-226.

49. Pallotta KE, Manley HJ. Vancomycin use in patients requiring hemodialysis: a literature review. *Semin Dial.* 2008;21(1):63-70.

50. Israni RK, Kasbekar N, Haynes K, Berns JS. Use of antiepileptic drugs in patients with kidney disease. *Semin Dial.* 2006;19(5):408-416.

51. Aronoff GR, Bennett WM, Berns JS, et al. *Drug Prescribing in Renal Failure: Dosing Guidelines for Adults and Children.* American College of Physicians; 2007.

52. Decker BS, Mueller BA, Sowinski KM. Drug dosing considerations in alternative hemodialysis. *Adv Chronic Kidney Dis*. 2007;14(3):e17-e26.

53. Lanese DM, Alfrey PS, Molitoris BA. Markedly increased clearance of vancomycin during hemodialysis using polysulfone dialyzers. *Kidney Int*. 1989;35(6):1409-1412.

54. Pollard TA, Lampasona V, Akkerman S, et al. Vancomycin redistribution: dosing recommendations following high-flux hemodialysis. *Kidney Int*. 1994;45(1):232-237.

55. Zoer J, Schrander-van der Meer AM, van Dorp WT. Dosage recommendation of vancomycin during haemodialysis with highly permeable membranes. *Pharm World Sci*. 1997;19(4):191-196.

56. Golper TA. Continuous arteriovenous hemofiltration in acute renal failure. *Am J Kidney Dis*. 1985;6(6):373-386.

57. Pattison ME, Lee SM, Ogden DA. Continuous arteriovenous hemodiafiltration: an aggressive approach to the management of acute renal failure. *Am J Kidney Dis*. 1988;11(1):43-47.

58. Pea F, Viale P, Pavan F, Furlanut M. Pharmacokinetic considerations for antimicrobial therapy in patients receiving renal replacement therapy. *Clin Pharmacokinet*. 2007;46(12):997-1038.

59. Bickley SK. Drug dosing during continuous arteriovenous hemofiltration. *Clin Pharm*. 1988;7(3):198-206.

60. Davies JG, Kingswood JC, Sharpstone P, Street MK. Drug removal in continuous haemofiltration and haemodialysis. *Br J Hosp Med*. 1995;54(10):524-528.

61. Bugge JF. Pharmacokinetics and drug dosing adjustments during continuous venovenous hemofiltration or hemodiafiltration in critically ill patients. *Acta Anaesthesiol Scand*. 2001;45(8):929-934.

62. Böhler J, Donauer J, Keller F. Pharmacokinetic principles during continuous renal replacement therapy: drugs and dosage. *Kidney Int Suppl*. 1999;(72):S24-S28.

63. Reetze-Bonorden P, Böhler J, Keller E. Drug dosage in patients during continuous renal replacement therapy: pharmacokinetic and therapeutic considerations. *Clin Pharmacokinet*. 1993;24(5):362-379.

64. Golper TA, Marx MA. Drug dosing adjustments during continuous renal replacement therapies. *Kidney Int Suppl*. 1998;66:S165-S168.

65. Domoto DT, Brown WW, Bruggensmith P. Removal of toxic levels of N-acetylprocainamide with continuous arteriovenous hemofiltration or continuous arteriovenous hemodiafiltration. *Ann Intern Med*. 1987;106(4):550-552.

66. Fissell WH. Antimicrobial dosing in acute renal replacement. *Adv Chronic Kidney Dis*. 2013;20(1):85-93.

67. Lamier N, Bogaert M. Peritoneal pharmacokinetics and pharmacological manipulation of peritoneal transport. In: Gokal R, ed. *Continuous Ambulatory Peritoneal Dialysis*. Churchill Livingstone; 1986:56-93.

68. Matzke GR, Millikin SP. Influence of renal function and dialysis on drug disposition. In: Evans WE, Schentag JJ, Jusko WJ, eds. *Applied Pharmacokinetics: Principles of Therapeutic Drug Monitoring*. 3rd ed. Applied Therapeutics; 1992.

69. Mars RL, Moles K, Pope K, Hargrove P. Use of bolus intraperitoneal aminoglycosides for treating peritonitis in end-stage renal disease patients receiving continuous ambulatory peritoneal dialysis and continuous cycling peritoneal dialysis. *Adv Perit Dial*. 2000;16:280-284.

70. Thummel KE, Shen DD. Appendix II: design and optimization of dosage regimens: pharmacokinetic data. In: Hardman JG, ed. *Goodman and Gilman's the Pharmacologic Basis of Therapeutics*. 10th ed. McGraw-Hill; 2001:1917-2023.

71. Matzke GR. Vancomycin. In: Evans WE, Schentag JJ, Jusko WJ, eds. *Applied Pharmacokinetics: Principles of Therapeutic Drug Monitoring*. 3rd ed. Applied Therapeutics; 1992.

72. O'Brien MA, Mason NA. Systemic absorption of intra-peritoneal antimicrobials in continuous ambulatory peritoneal dialysis. *Clin Pharm*. 1992;11(3):246-254.

73. Voinescu CG, Khanna R. Peritonitis in peritoneal dialysis. *Int J Artif Organs*. 2002;25(4):249-260.

74. Keller E, Reetze P, Schollmeyer P. Drug therapy in patients undergoing continuous ambulatory peritoneal dialysis. Clinical and pharmacokinetic considerations. *Clin Pharmacokinet*. 1990;18(2):104-117.

75. Keane WF, Everett ED, Golper TA, et al. Peritoneal dialysis-related peritonitis treatment recommendations 1993 update. The Ad Hoc Advisory Committee on Peritonitis Management. International Society for Peritoneal Dialysis. *Perit Dial Int*. 1993;13(1):14-28.

76. Wiggins KJ, Craig JC, Johnson DW, Strippoli GF. Treatment for peritoneal dialysis-associated peritonitis. *Cochrane Database Syst Rev*. 2008;23(1):CD005284.

4

OBESITY

Manjunath P. Pai

Learning Objectives

By the end of the obesity chapter, the learner shall be able to:

1. Explain the strengths and limitations of body mass index as a metric to define obesity.
2. Describe the physiology-based pharmacokinetic effects of obesity.
3. Comprehend the basis, risks, and benefits of weight-based and non–weight-based drug dosing.
4. Describe the principles of scaling drug dosing across the obesity body size distribution.
5. Explain the origin, strengths, and limitations of alternate body size descriptors.
6. Compare potential drug doses in patients with obesity based on scaling and alternate body size descriptors.
7. Recall examples where a fixed weight-based dose may or may not be appropriate in patients with obesity.
8. Describe alternate emerging technologies and metrics that may improve drug dosing in patients with obesity.

Obesity is a medical condition of excessive accumulation of body fat and resultant ill health.[1] Technological advancements of the 18th century and onward have improved the quantity, quality, and accessibility of high-calorie foods.[2] An imbalance between energy consumption and expenditure leads to fat accumulation within and around organs as well as subcutaneously. Obesity contributes to heart disease, stroke, diabetes, high blood pressure, hypercholesterolemia, asthma, sleep apnea, gallstones, kidney stones, infertility, breast cancer, colon cancer, and eight other cancers.[3] Consequently, the healthcare cost burden of obesity is estimated to be $147 to $210 billion per year.[4,5] Sadly, public health strategies to reduce obesity have largely failed as seen by a tripling in adult prevalence in the U.S. adult population from ~15% to ~45% over 40 years and projected to be 50% by 2030.[6] These trends are not limited to the United States, and similar increases are being recorded across the globe.[7] While the focus of this chapter is not on the pediatric population, a rise in obesity among children is of grave concern to the future health and well-being of the nation.[8]

As noted, patients with obesity have multiple comorbid conditions that require pharmacotherapy. As a consequence, clinicians commonly face the challenge of defining the optimal drug dose in patients with obesity. Obesity is presently not regarded as a specific population by regulatory agencies, and so no systematic studies are required in this patient population to ensure pharmacokinetic (PK) or pharmacodynamic bioequivalence.[9] Patients with cancer who are obese are often underrepresented in randomized trials.[10] The discovery therefore of a need for altered drug dosing in the population relies on population PK analyses, differential outcomes in phase 3 studies, postmarketing studies, or pharmacovigilance programs. Early phase clinical trials often exclude this patient population because of comorbid conditions that may raise the risk profile of a drug with no benefit to the volunteer.[11] This has created a major gap in our knowledge on how best to dose drugs in patients with obesity and made us reliant on scaling PK parameters such as volume of distribution (V_d) and clearance (Cl) to body size.[12] These principles of scaling or generation of alternate body size descriptors currently use measured height and weight and not body composition.[13] As expected, this approach is not consistently reliable due to the physiochemical properties of the drug molecule. This chapter will overview our current understanding of the effects of obesity on pharmacokinetics and review approaches to dose selection in this patient population.

DEFINING OBESITY AND DRUG-DOSING BREAK POINTS

We currently rely on the body mass index (BMI) to classify individuals as obese or nonobese.[14] The BMI or Quetelet index was introduced in 1835 by a mathematician who sought to develop a population-level tool to assist with government resource allocation and predict criminal behavior.[15] The introduction and application of this index in medicine were made by Dr Ancel Keys, a physiologist interested in the effects of diet on health.[14] The BMI is calculated based on body weight (in kg) divided by the square of height (in m) (kg/m^2), where obesity in adults is defined as a BMI ≥ 30 kg/m^2. As expected with any population-level metric, this tool does not consistently classify patients accurately. Models of body composition have included compartmentalization into two to six components, with the simplest being fat mass and fat-free mass and the most complex being fat mass, water, protein, bone mineral content, non–bone mineral content, and glycogen.[16] Since weight is a summation of these components, this relationship between BMI and obesity improves as fat mass increases. The correlation of percent fat to BMI is good especially in patients with high BMI values but not as strong in normal weight, overweight-to-obese class 1 group.[17]

Individuals with high muscle mass and shorter stature are more likely to be incorrectly classified in the overweight-to-obese class 1 group (BMI 25-35 kg/m^2).[18] Likewise, there are ethnic, sex, and age-related (sarcopenia) differences in body composition that can misclassify individuals based solely on BMI.[19] Breakpoints that predict risk for development of diabetes may be different by genetic ancestry but at present are neatly divided into 5-point BMI units out of simplicity. Ultimately, this metric is applied because it is simple and cheap to compute relative to more accurate and costly measurement tools.[20] Alternative indices that account for body shape, waist, and hip circumferences exist but have not been applied to drug-dosing considerations.[21] Figure 4.1 illustrates the relationship of the waist-to-hip ratio with overweight and BMI and shows that although a relationship exists, marked interindividual variability in central

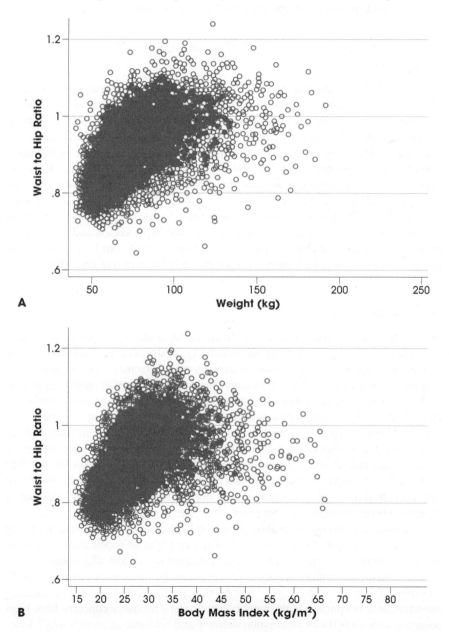

FIGURE 4.1   Scatter plot of the waist-to-hip ratio to weight **(A)** and body mass index (BMI) **(B)** illustrating the large interindividual variability of central adiposity compared with these common body size metrics. Data are transformed from the 2017-2020 National Health and Nutrition Examination Survey.

adiposity is not well characterized by height and weight. Despite this limitation, selection of alternate dosing strategies presently follow existing BMI breakpoints of dosing based on individuals 30 to 39.9 kg/m^2 and ≥40 kg/m^2. Alternatively, drug product labels select pragmatic cut-off values above 100 kg, 120 kg, or 150 kg, for example, to either recommend capping the dose to a maximum, using an adjusted dose, or suggestions for use of an alternate agent due to lack of information.

PHYSIOLOGY-BASED PHARMACOKINETIC EFFECTS OF OBESITY

A number of physiologic changes occur in obesity such as an increase in body volume, relative increase in adipose tissues, significant increase in inflammation secondary to increase adiposity, endocrine changes and associated metabolic syndrome, comparative decrease in lung volume, and reduced tissue perfusion due to limited cardiac output compared with normal-weight individuals.[22] A compensatory increase in cardiac output leads to an increase in renal blood flow, and liver blood flow is seen.[23] However, over time liver blood flow can decrease due to the development of nonalcoholic fatty liver disease (NAFLD) that can progress to steatosis and steatohepatitis (NASH).[24] Likewise, the early increase in kidney function can decline over time at a more rapid rate due to comorbid conditions such as diabetes and hypertension and the development of focal segmental glomerulosclerosis.[25] Overall, obesity can have time-varying effects on absorption, distribution, metabolism, and elimination of drugs that are detailed in the following sections.[26]

Absorption

Systematic studies to fully characterize the influence of obesity on oral and subcutaneous drug absorption are lacking. No reduction in oral absorption has been reported in studies comparing drugs such as midazolam, moxifloxacin, trazodone, and cyclosporine in obese compared with nonobese participants.[26] Use of the gastric-emptying probe substrate acetaminophen has shown a tendency for a delay in time to maximum concentration (T_{max}). However, a pooled analysis of gastric emptying suggests a marginal (6-10 minute) difference in gastric emptying when evaluating both solids and liquids.[27] Likewise, studies evaluating enterocyte metabolism that could alter prehepatic clearance and bioavailability are limited to the evaluation of cytochrome P450 (CYP) 3A4. The bioavailability of midazolam was observed to be 60% compared with 28% in patients with class 2 and 3 obesity as against normal-weight individuals.[28] However, a reproducible demonstration of this potential difference has not been confirmed.

In contrast, subcutaneous absorption may be decreased in patients with obesity and intramuscular depot injections need to ensure adequate needle depth to ensure proper administration. Insulin absorption is delayed in patients with obesity and is attributed to lower capillary density in subcutaneous fat tissue as this increases in dimension.[29] Entry of a wide range of new biotherapeutics requiring subcutaneous administration is of concern in this population. To date, no major concerns have been observed with COVID-19 vaccination delivery and response as an example.[30] Likewise, the use of epinephrine autoinjectors for immediate hypersensitivity reactions does not indicate a need for dosage adjustment.[31] Additional work is necessary with monoclonal antibody–based therapeutics that may or may not require dose adjustment due to altered absorption. Overall, the data to date suggest the potential for an alteration in the rate of absorption but not the extent of absorption in patients with obesity compared with those without.

Distribution

The biodistribution of most drugs is characterized in rodents and rarely in clinical studies before approval. As a result, our ideas about drug-specific biodistribution are often grounded on physiochemical properties of molecules and plasma or serum concentration-time profiles. The maximum concentration and the shape of the concentration-time curve are characterized by the volume of distribution (V_d), either noncompartmentally or compartmentally.[32] The V_d is therefore an apparent value or a proportionality constant that gives us a sense of whether a drug remains in the plasma (because this is what is measured) or distributes out of plasma into tissue. The term "tissue" here could be blood cell components or specific organs that can only be confirmed by measurement. This direct tissue measurement is rarely possible, and so as a general rule, we expect the drug to primarily be in the blood compartment when the V_d is less than 15 L and in tissues when the V_d is larger than this value.[32] As expected, the lipophilicity, charge, and flexibility of a molecule impact the V_d.[33] Molecules that are acidic tend to have a smaller V_d (as they bind to plasma proteins) than those that are basic (retained intracellularly).[33] The V_d of neutral and zwitterionic molecules is harder to predict.[33]

All these have an important bearing on patients with obesity because we practice scaling V_d to body weight. This value is often reported on a liter-per-kilogram basis for comparison but leads to confusion because it assumes that this value increases proportionately with weight. The molecule vancomycin, for example, has a reported V_d of 0.7 L/kg (similar to total body water). However, the absolute V_d of vancomycin is not twice as high in a 150-kg compared with a 75-kg patient, which would be computed if 0.7 L/kg were used in both scenarios.[34] The V_d in the 150-kg patient is closer to 0.5 L/kg (75 L) compared with 0.7 L/kg (52.5 L) in the 75-kg patient.[34] This 2-fold difference in weight equates to a 1.4-fold increase in V_d. This is because an increase in adipose tissue weight does not translate into a proportional increase in V_d for either hydrophilic or lipophilic drugs in a consistent manner. We expect an increase but the amount of increase tends to be drug specific.

The "free-drug" theory assumes that only drugs not bound to proteins such as albumin, lipoproteins, and α1-acid glycoprotein are active and can traverse cell membranes.[35] Studies do not consistently show changes in the absolute amount and relative composition of these blood protein concentrations.[36] The evidence to date also does not support altered unbound concentrations of drugs in individuals with class 3 obesity compared with normal-weight adults.

Poor tissue perfusion and reduced blood flow to extremities are common problems in obesity.[37] In addition, patients who are obese also have poor lymphatic drainage that contributes to tissue inflammation leading to further limitation of tissue perfusion.[37,38] Studies evaluating interstitial fluid concentrations suggest that lower concentrations are observed in patients who are obese when compared with those who are not.[39] This difference may be most relevant for compounds that have extracellular pharmacologic effects such as some antibiotics. A higher initial dose or a loading dose may be necessary to ensure adequate concentrations within these target tissue sites of infection. Limited tissue perfusion of antibiotics in patients who are obese is most important in skin and soft-tissue infections, deep-seated infections such as necrotizing pancreatitis and localized abscess, pneumonia, and surgical prophylaxis.[40]

Metabolism

The liver is a key organ for drug metabolism, and this process is dependent on intrinsic clearance (Cl_{int}) and liver blood flow (Q_l). Transporters on the cell membrane and drug metabolic enzymes drive Cl_{int}, which coupled with Q_l and plasma protein binding impact liver drug clearance. Fat deposition and inflammation of the liver are common in patients with obesity because of nonalcoholic fatty liver disease (NFLD). Patients who are obese are 3 times more likely to develop NFLD when compared with those who not.[41] Apart from metabolic complications associated with NFLD, studies have shown that NFLD can significantly affect the metabolism of various medications.[42,43] The extent of the variability in the drug metabolism in NFLD is dependent on the type of drug-metabolizing enzyme involved.[42,43]

Drugs that are metabolized via the CYP3A4 pathway are likely to have lower metabolic clearance in patients who are obese compared with the normal-weight subjects.[42] This downregulations of activity is primarily driven by the degree of liver inflammation rather than diet alone, which has shown mixed results. Similarly, CYP1A2 activity is also shown to decrease but is difficult to deconvolute from the effects of diet since this isoenzyme system is tightly regulated by food intake. Nevertheless, these changes in metabolism as measured by the area under the curve (AUC) of probe substrates indicate a 20%-to-40% reduction in Cl. The least ambiguous pathway include drugs that are the substrate of CYP2E1 and that which undergo xanthine oxidase or N-acetyl transferases reactions that have higher metabolic clearance in patients who are obese versus those who are not.[42] Drugs that may require dose adjustment due to enhanced CYP2E1 metabolism include anesthetics, acetaminophen (transformation to toxic metabolite), chlorzoxazone, and phenobarbital.

Elimination

The relationship between kidney function and obesity is complex and dependent on age as well as comorbid conditions such as hypertension and diabetes. The kidneys use three individual yet interdependent processes to eliminate waste and excrete drugs from the body, namely, glomerular filtration, tubular secretion, and tubular reabsorption.[44] Though limited information is available regarding the effect of obesity on tubular secretion and reabsorption, obesity has shown to increase the estimated glomerular filtration rate (eGFR) up to 62%.[45] Given the relatively higher incidence of proteinuria and chronic kidney disease in patients who are obese when compared with normal-weight individuals,[46,47] the possibility of reduced tubular functions cannot be ruled out in patients with obesity. Kidney function using eGFR or as estimated creatinine clearance (eCl_{cr}) is the only quantitative organ function presently used to define drug-dosing regimens. In clinical practice, this elimination process is estimated using the serum biomarker creatinine that is now assay-standardized internationally.

Alternative biomarkers such as cystatin C can improve the precision of eGFR but is not readily available across the globe.[48]

As noted, patients with obesity can have kidney function values that are 50% to 75% higher than the typical value for a normal-weight individual of similar age.[45] This is especially true in male adult patients under the age of 40 that experience physical trauma.[49] In these complex patients, measurement of kidney function through 8- to 24-hour urine collections to measure Cl_{cr} may be necessary to better define this parameter. The clinical pharmacy and regulatory approach has historically included eCl_{cr} using the Cockcroft-Gault formula.[50] This formula includes weight as a parameter and so is confounded in patients with obesity, especially those in class 2 and class 3. A common approach to reduce the bias of overestimation is the use of an alternate body weight descriptor.[45] These approaches have been tested and developed predominantly with compounds that are not metabolized and instead eliminated unchanged in urine, such as antibiotics vancomycin and aminoglycosides.[51,52] However, this estimation affects dose estimation of several other important cardiovascular medications such as direct oral anticoagulants, dofetilide, gabapentin, and several other narrow-therapeutic-index drugs.

WEIGHT- AND NON–WEIGHT-BASED DOSING

Preclinical models remain a cornerstone of drug development and rely on the advancement of molecules from in vitro systems to mouse models. Drug dose scaling then extends to larger and larger species before being used in human studies.[53] This dose translation occurs on a weight basis, for example, from a 25-g mouse, 250-g rat, 1-kg guinea pig, 2.5-kg rabbit, 8-to-10-kg dog or monkey to a 65-kg human adult. This translation is made based on allometry and scaled to the exponent of 0.67.[53] The basis for this exponent is the surface law hypothesis that dates back over 150 years and is based on Euclidean geometric transformation of weight into the surface area (see next section for details).[54] The resultant effect of this approach leads to the selection/testing of a weight-based dose for certain compounds purely out of this tradition.[13] Most often this weight-based dosing is retained for injectable drug products because the dose can be fractionated easily, which can be useful but also contribute to unnecessary waste of drugs due to available vial sizes.[13,55] Dose fractionation of solid oral drug products is less feasible and so much more expensive (need to develop multiple formulations) to do for drug development that converges to fixed-dose selection. The classic examples of this discordance include weight-based doses of trimethoprim/sulfamethoxazole and ganciclovir when administered IV but use of fixed doses when given by mouth (use of valganciclovir).

An adult weight range of 40 to 200 kg likely encompasses 99% of the U.S. population, which is a 5-fold range of weight. If a drug is approved on a weight basis, for example, 10 mg/kg once daily without any caveats for dose adjustment in patients with obesity, a clear problem emerges. The 40-kg patient would receive 400 mg and the 200-kg patient would receive 2,000 mg. As noted in this chapter, body composition and organ function do not scale proportionately to weight and so we all intuitively recognize that we may be overdosing the patient with obesity. The reality is that we are likely failing at both extremes because the typical patient evaluated in drug development is 80 kg, for an average dose of 800 mg (in this case). If drug clearance does not scale with weight, then weight-based dosing will underdose the 40-kg patient and overdose the 200-kg patient.[13,52] Likewise, use of a fixed dose of 800 mg in both the 40- and 200-kg patients may have the reverse consequence.[13,52] This concern is remarkably clear in cancer drug development and is the basis for body surface area (BSA) as a scalar for dosing.[56] Ultimately, weight is one of several covariates such as age, sex, pharmacogenetics, organ function, and disease condition that can impact empirical dose selection. Dose individualization based on an exposure or response measure is essential because neither weight nor non–weight-based dosing will be universally optimal.

DRUG DOSE SCALING

The principles of drug dose scaling are based on our understanding of metabolic rate differences across body sizes.[13] In principle, the larger the animal the smaller the per-kilogram dose that is necessary. A classic example of the failure to understand this principle contributed to the death of an elephant at the Oklahoma zoo in the 1960s due to the use of a psychotropic drug dose (mg/kg basis) directly from that used in cats.[57] Scaling information across species is a common feature in biology and is known as allometry when applied to the growth of body parts and changes to body proportions. These relationships have been extended to physiologic differences such as cardiac output, kidney function, and metabolism. When these relationships are plotted in the logarithmic scale (to linearize the relationship), the slope (β) represents the scaling exponent with an intercept term (α). A representative example of this relationship is given below for Cl as a function of weight that can be centered to a median value of 80 kg, for example.

$$Cl = \alpha \times (\text{Weight}/80)^{\beta} \qquad \textbf{(Eq. 4.1)}$$

$$\text{Log}\left(Cl\right) = \log\left(\alpha\right) + \beta \times \log(\text{Weight}/80)$$

In 1883, Max Rubner estimated this slope when evaluating heat production/loss in dogs that were starved to lose weight and found this slope to be close to 0.67.[58] Because heat loss is dependent on the surface area, this scaling principle of transforming weight (density × volume), where volume is a three-dimensional term, into a two-dimensional term (area) is achieved by raising the weight to the power of 0.67. This was referred to as the two-third power law or surface law hypothesis. Work by Max Kleiber on metabolism across species using radiotracers led to the observation that this slope is closer to 0.75.[58] Several mechanistic theories have been advanced to justify this three-quarter power law, but this area remains controversial when attempting to explain biology across the entire species continuum.[59,60] In practical terms, Figure 4.2 illustrates what happens when you scale information based purely on weight (slope = 1), surface law (slope = 0.67), Kleiber's law (slope = 0.75), and the square root of weight (slope = 0.5). This approach has been used to scale drug clearance in several population PK studies. A systematic review of the identified slopes show that this parameter has a distribution with a modal value close to 0.65.[61] As a result, when no information is available for a particular drug, dosing on BSA is likely better than

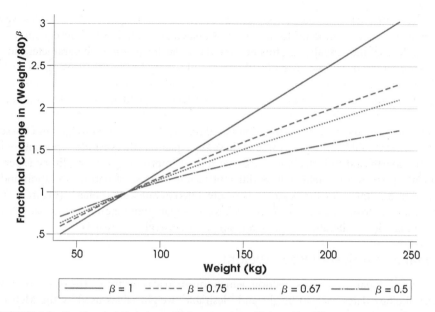

FIGURE 4.2 Fractional change in weight centered on 80 kg with different exponents that are analogous with current weight, allometry, and surface area–based scaling principles.

weight as a general rule. The use of alternate weight descriptors serves a similar purpose and is detailed in the next section.[52]

ALTERNATE BODY SIZE DESCRIPTORS

Numerous alternate body size descriptors derived by transforming height and weight measurements have been used.[13] This is a critical mathematical point that escapes many in clinical pharmacology largely in part due to scientific jargon. Given the broad use of these equations, this section is divided into the major groups of BSA and alternate weight descriptors.

Body Surface Area

What does your skin surface have to do with drug metabolism and clearance? The answer is nothing mechanistically for most drugs and so the design and generation of sophisticated technologies to measure this parameter for drug dosing is actually not useful for pharmacologic application.[62] We compute this parameter as a scalar to capture nonlinear PK changes with increasing body size. The earliest equation that was used to justify BSA dosing of cancer chemotherapy (based on animal data) was the Meeh equation that simply translated weight to BSA using the 0.67 exponents.[56] Du Bois and Du Bois published data from an experiment that included using papier-mâché to cover the bodies of nine individuals, unwrapping them, photographing them, and computing the surface area.[63] As noted in their publication from 1916, they sought to ensure that the equation that they generated obeyed Euclidean geometry and used weight and height for this function.[63] The exponent above weight was 0.725 and that above height was 0.425. Because weight is a three-dimensional term and height is a one-dimensional term, it is no coincidence that $0.725 \times 3 + 0.425 \times 1 = 2$, as that was the intent (transforming m^3 to m^2). They evaluated and "validated" their equation in 23 additional individuals, and this became the scalar for physiologic parameters and pharmacology over time. The idea that we could/should base drug dosing on such limited data is unsettling. Gehan and George attempted to improve this function for cancer chemotherapy dosing.[64] Likewise, Haycock et al argued that validation was necessary for infants, children, and adults.[65] Livingston and Lee adapted the Meeh equation approach and specified a function based on weight for normal weight and obese individuals.[66] Table 4.1 shows some of these key equations that include exponents out to the fourth and fifth decimal place that impart improved precision. Every experiment in nature will yield slightly different results because of natural variation and error, and so these equations are numerically different but scale similarly (Figure 4.3). Ultimately, Mosteller's adaptation that relies on a square root function to estimate BSA dominates in the literature because it is simple and useful (Figure 4.3).[67]

Ideal and Adjusted Body Weight

The term "ideal" imparts perfection, which this metric is far from. The origin of this terminology dates back to height and "desirable" weight tables used by the Metropolitan Life Insurance company to inform mortality risk.[68] The equation used in the pharmacy and clinical pharmacology literature was based on uncited work by Prof Benjamin Devine on how to dose gentamicin. This equation transforms height into weight, has an adjustment for sex, and is a simple rule of thumb that existed in the nutrition literature.[68] Our natural human tendency to count by the number 5 (five fingers in each hand) is the basis for this rule. This ideal body weight (IBW) rule when developed assumes males are 10 pounds heavier than females and both gain 5 pounds for every inch gain in height. At face value, this seems nonsensical because dosing on IBW is really dosing an individual on height. However, IBW remains in use for drug-dosing decisions today because the IBW distribution values generated by this metric are narrow (because most adults are between 5 and 6 ft in height) and thereby reduces the risk of overdosing. For example, a 5-ft and 6-ft male would have

TABLE 4.1   Key Body Surface Area Equations

AUTHOR(S)	EQUATION
Meeh	$BSA\ (m^2) = k \times Wt^{0.667}$
Du Bois and Du Bois	$BSA\ (m^2) = Wt\ (kg)^{0.425} \times Ht\ (cm)^{0.725} \times 0.007184$
Gehan and George	$BSA\ (m^2) = Wt\ (kg)^{0.51456} \times Ht\ (cm)^{0.42246} \times 0.0235$
Haycock et al	$BSA\ (m^2) = Wt\ (kg)^{0.5378} \times Ht\ (cm)^{0.3964} \times 0.024265$
Mosteller	$BSA\ (m^2) = ((Ht\ (cm) \times Wt\ (kg))/3{,}600)^{0.5z}$
Livingston and Lee	$BSA\ (m^2) = k \times Wt^{0.6466}$

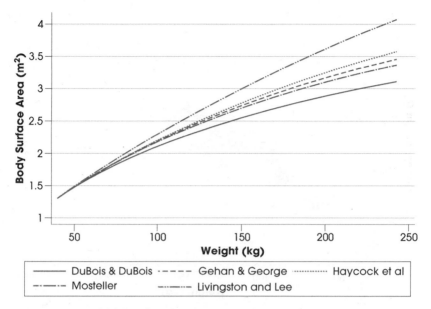

FIGURE 4.3 Estimated body surface area over weight illustrating the similarity in the nonlinear scaling of weight as body surface area or through use of a power function. Data are transformed from the 2017-2020 National Health and Nutrition Examination Survey.

IBW of 50 and 77.6 kg, respectively, and so leads to doses on an mg/kg basis that are within an ~1.5-fold range when this metric is used. The size and function of human kidneys also correlate with height, which is why pediatric eGFR equations are height or length based.[69]

As may be expected, the use of IBW instead of weight for drug dosing will bias toward lower doses when the same mg/kg value is used. This deficit was recognized with the dosing of aminoglycosides and was corrected by adding a fraction of the difference between weight and IBW and IBW.[70] This correction factor or adjustment leads to the calculation of adjusted body weight (AdjBW). The correction factor has a wide range of values and has typically been in the range of 0.3 to 0.5. Our need to simplify has led to the use of a factor of 0.4 as a common value to aid the estimation of this value.[70] In practice, a combination of IBW, weight, and AdjBW are used to dose individuals across the weight spectrum. One rule that has been applied to the aminoglycosides has been the use of weight when weight is less than IBW, use of IBW when IBW is less than weight, and use of AdjBW when IBW is 1.25- to 1.30-fold higher than weight.[70] This combination is sometimes referred to as dosing weight.[71]

This dosing weight scales information similar to allometric and BSA-based approaches. Figure 4.4 is a scatter plot of the dosing weight estimated with the foregoing rule using National Health and Nutrition Examination Survey height, weight, and sex data. When dosing weight is fit as a power function of weight, the exponent estimated is ~0.72 or between the two aforementioned power-law paradigms. So these alternate weight descriptors allow us to achieve the same goal of not overdosing drugs in patients with obesity on an empirical basis.

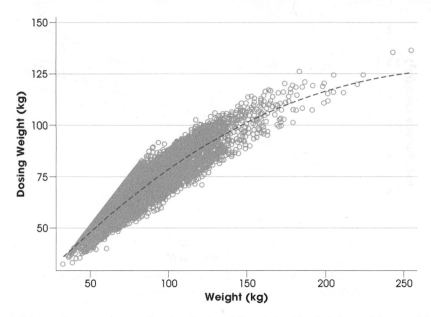

FIGURE 4.4   Scatter and power function fit plot of the relationship of dosing weight to weight using data transformed from the 2017-2020 National Health and Nutrition Examination Survey.

Lean Body Weight and Fat-Free Weight

Our underlying assumption is that fat weight has limited drug metabolic purpose. Semantically, lean body weight (LBW) and fat-free weight (FFW) are comparable terms used to characterize weight responsible for metabolism and elimination.[12] We expect and have observed a better correlation of Cl with this body size parameter for some drugs.[61] Measurement of LBW and FFW is feasible through numerous technologies, though, in practice, DEXA and bioelectric impedance analysis predominate. Multiple equations have been developed to estimate LBW and have been shown to better covariate of anesthetic Cl than weight.[61,72] Table 4.2 includes the four dominant equations used to estimate this value. As illustrated in Figure 4.5, in some instances (James equation) these equations estimate lower values with increasing body size because they are quadratic functions. The LBW equations generate numerically lower values compared with IBW and AdjBW and are more difficult to recall in clinical practice.

If LBW is used to scale drug doses, then higher mg/kg dose values are necessary with this metric than the likely approved weight-based dose. This is a confusing concept for most clinicians and also makes it challenging to implement in practice because the use of a higher mg/kg dose than the label is perceived to be risky. As a simple example, tobramycin dosing has evolved from 1 mg/kg thrice daily to 7 to 10 mg/kg once daily in patients with normal kidney function.[70] If a patient with obesity is dosed with this drug, then 7 to 10 mg/kg based on AdjBW is reasonable. However, if LBW is used then 9 to 12 mg/kg on this scalar may be necessary.[73] The difference with LBW is that this modification may be useful across the whole adult weight spectrum.[73] Ultimately, equations used to estimate LBW are like BSA in that they are simply mathematical

TABLE 4.2   Key Alternate Body Size Descriptor Equations

NAME	EQUATION
Ideal Body Weight (IBW)	Males = 50 kg + 2.3 × (Number of inches over 60 inches in Ht) Females = 45.5 kg + 2.3 × (Number of inches over 60 inches in Ht)
Adjusted Body Weight (AdjBW)	IBW + (Wt − IBW) × 0.4
Dosing Weight (DW)	Use IBW or Wt if less than IBW or AdjBW if Wt > 1.25 × Wt
Lean Body Weight (LBW) Boer Formula	Males = 0.407 × Wt (kg) + 0.267 × Ht (cm) − 19.2 Females = 0.252 × Wt (kg) + 0.473 × Ht (cm) − 48.3
James Formula	Males = 1.1 × Wt (kg) − 128 × (Wt/Ht)^2 Females = 1.07 × Wt (kg) − 148 × (Wt/Ht)^2
Hume Formula	Males = 0.32810 × Wt (kg) + 0.33929 × Ht (cm) − 29.5336 Females = 0.29569 × Wt (kg) + 0.41813 × Ht (cm) − 43.2933
Janmahasatian Formula	Males = (9,270 × Wt (kg)) / (6,680 + 216 × BMI) Females = (9,270 × Wt (kg)) / (8,780 + 244 × BMI)

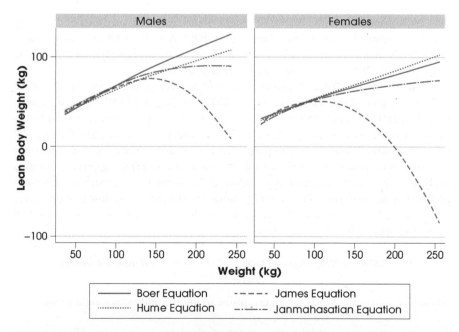

FIGURE 4.5 Median-predicted plot of the estimated lean body weight or fat-free weight using common equation used to estimate this parameter in males and females using data transformed from the 2017-2020 National Health and Nutrition Examination Survey.

transformations of height and weight. So, using them as a dosing metric limits the dose to a 2-to-2.5-fold range across the expected adult weight distribution.

CASE EXAMPLE—VANCOMYCIN DOSING IN OBESITY

Vancomycin is a common antibiotic used empirically in the hospital setting, and the recommended dosage is based on body weight and an estimate of kidney function. A 57-year-old, 143-kg, 170-cm male patient with a serum creatinine of 1.5 mg/dL is to be initiated on vancomycin. The recommended loading dose for this agent is 20 to 25 mg/kg, followed by a maintenance regimen of 15 to 20 mg/kg with a frequency-dependent on estimated kidney function.[74] For this exercise, let us assume that the maintenance dose frequency is to be every 8 hours if eCl_{cr} >90 mL/min, every 12 hours if 60 to 90 mL/min, and every 24 hours if 30 to 59 mL/min. The maximum dose of this agent is typically capped at 3 g for a loading dose and 2 g for each maintenance dose with doses rounded to the nearest 250 mg.

What doses would be estimated if weight and alternate weight descriptors were used?

METRIC	15 MG/KG	20 MG/KG	25 MG/KG
Weight = 143 kg	2,145 mg	2,860 mg	3,575 mg
IBW = 65.9 kg	989 mg	1,318 mg	1,648 mg
AdjBW = 96.7 kg	1,450 mg	1,934 mg	2,418 mg
LBW= 76.3 kg	1,145 mg	1,526 mg	1,908 mg

A loading dose of 3,000 mg (21 mg/kg) and maintenance doses of 2,000 mg (14 mg/kg) would be selected based on actual weight. A similar answer would be computed for the maintenance dose if AdjBW is used at 20 mg/kg but a higher mg/kg dose is necessary if LBW or IBW is used as the dosing scalar.

If the Cockcroft-Gault equation is used for eCL_{cr}, the estimates would be 110, 51, 74, and 59 mL/min if the weight, IBW, AdjBW, and LBW are used, respectively.[50] A clear conundrum arises because different dosing frequencies would be selected based on weight (every 8 hours), AdjBW (every 12 hours), and IBW or LBW (every 24 hours). In the case of this particular drug, maintenance doses over 4,500 mg/day have been associated with kidney injury.[74] As a result, a 2,000 mg every 12 hours is likely to be the empiric regimen that is selected. An alternative approach for this compound may be the use of a population PK model to estimate a daily dose that optimizes the exposure for this compound.[75] Multiple models exist but one such model based on an obese population is detailed below:

$$Cl = 9.656 - (0.078 \times Age) - (2.009 \times SCr) \times (1.09 \times 1 \text{ if male, 0 if female}) + (0.04 \times Wt^{0.75})$$

where, age is in years, SCr is serum creatinine in mg/dL, and Wt is weight in kg.

$$Cl = 9.656 - (0.078 \times 57) - (2.009 \times 1.5) + 1.09 \times 1 + 0.04 \times 143^{0.75}$$

$$Cl = 9.656 - 4.45 - 3.01 + 1.09 + 1.65 = 4.94 \text{ L/h}$$

The target exposure for this drug is an AUC of 400 to 600 h mg/L, so a point estimate of 500 h mg/L is reasonable.

$$\text{Daily dose} = \text{Target AUC} \times \text{Cl}$$

$$\text{Daily dose} = 500 \times 4.94 = 2{,}470 \text{ mg}$$

So in this case, a maintenance dose of 1,250 mg every 12 hours may be selected. As shown, the "correct" dose is not knowable until concentrations are measured. For vancomycin, however, assays are available and allow for measurement and confirmation of whether the optimal dose is 2,000 mg every 12 hours or 1,250 mg every 12 hours. The severity of illness may drive the choice here as clinicians have to weigh the risk and benefit of these two choices.

For the sake of illustration, let us assume in the above case scenario that the individual was 72 kg instead of 143 kg (~half in size). Then,

$$\text{Cl} = 9.656 - (0.078 \times 57) - (2.009 \times 1.5) + 1.09 \times 1 + 0.04 \times 72^{0.75}$$

$$\text{Cl} = 9.656 - 4.45 - 3.01 + 1.09 + 0.99 = 4.28 \text{ L/h}$$

$$\text{Daily dose} = 500 \times 4.94 = 2{,}138 \text{ mg}$$

So in this case, 2,000 mg/day or 1,000 mg every 12 hours would be selected and illustrates that only a 500-mg difference (20%) in dose would be predicted despite a nearly 100% difference in body weight. This would equate to 14 mg/kg every 12 hours (2,000 mg/day) and 9 mg/kg every 12 hours (2,500 mg/kg) if dosed on weight illustrating the need to require a lower mg/kg dose as one increases in body size.

CASE EXAMPLE: DAPTOMYCIN—DOSING IN OBESITY

As shown in the earlier example, selection of the optimal empiric dose when weight based can be unsettling in a patient with obesity. This uncertainty can be rectified in practice with a drug like vancomycin because of the availability of therapeutic drug monitoring. Antibiotics are delayed-response drugs, that is, the need for a few days of treatment before efficacy is quantifiable.[76] This contrasts with drugs with more easily measurable responses such as blood pressure, heart rate, pain scores, anesthesia, and so forth. For the antibiotic daptomycin, which is weight based, a clear discordance between the label and conventional dosing approach helps to serve as an illustrative example. This drug was originally developed to be administered every 8 to 12 hours on a 1 to 2 mg/kg basis.[77] This approach failed due to an increased risk of skeletal muscle toxicity. Preclinical work in dogs helped to demonstrate that once-daily administration could reduce this toxicologic risk. The drug was subsequently studied as 4 and 6 mg/kg once daily and approved for administration in this manner.[77] Clinical experience and observational studies have led experts in the field to suggest the use of higher doses of 8 to 10 mg/kg or about twice the approved dose.[78] This is a 2-fold difference from the label in a regular-sized individual (80 kg), what dose should one select in a 120-kg adult female (63 inches in height) with normal kidney function receiving daptomycin for a bloodstream infection approved at 6 mg/kg?

METRIC	6 MG/KG	8 MG/KG	10 MG/KG
Weight = 120 kg	720 mg	960 mg	1,200 mg
IBW = 52.4 kg	314 mg	419 mg	524 mg
AdjBW = 79.4 kg	476 mg	635 mg	794 mg
LBW = 55 kg	330 mg	440 mg	550 mg

The approved product label dose is 6 mg/kg on weight, and so 720 mg may be selected in this 120-kg patient. If institutional policies recommend the use of an alternate weight descriptor, then a dose of 314 to 476 mg (<500 mg) would be selected. Key questions that should be considered when making a dose selection are: (1) What would the typical dose be in an average patient such as an 80-kg adult? (2) What is the available drug product formulation and can a pragmatic dosing regimen be designed? (3) What is the risk of underdosing versus overdosing? The typical dose in an 80-kg individual enrolled in the registrational trial would have been 6 mg/kg or 480 mg (close to the 500-mg single-use IV dose vial) that this product is available as. Therefore, the use of IBW or LBW would likely underdose this individual unless 10 mg/kg were used with these scalars. Alternatively, AdjBW will lead to the calculation of a dose that is similar to the typical dose or higher between 6 and 10 mg/kg. This is a key reason why AdjBW is often selected as a scalar when shifting from one weight metric to the other.[52] When IBW or LBW is used to dose patient who is obese, the risk of underdosing these individuals is likely unless the mg/kg dose is also increased.[52]

CASE EXAMPLE: EDOXABAN—DOSING IN OBESITY

Edoxaban is a selective inhibitor of factor Xa that is used as an oral administered anticoagulant to reduce the risk of stroke and systemic embolism in patients with nonvalvular atrial fibrillation. In registrational clinical trials, an increased risk of ischemic stroke was observed in patients with an estimated creatinine clearance >95 mL/min and may not be simply exposure related.[79] It, therefore, carries a black-box warning on its label stating that the drug not be used in patients with creatinine clearance >95 mL/min. The label recommends the use of the Cockcroft-Gault equation and weight to determine eCl_{cr}. Your hospital electronic medical system presently uses the Chronic Kidney Disease-Epidemiology (CKD-EPI) equation to estimate the glomerular filtration rate (eGFR) reported in mL/min/1.73 m^2. Given the plethora of equations to estimate kidney function, your hospital clinicians frequently rely on eGFR, which is automatically reported to make dosing decisions. For a 65-year-old male patient of East Indian ancestry with a height of 172 cm and 100 kg, serum creatinine of 1.0 mg/dL is to be initiated on edoxaban. Should the drug be prescribed in this case based on the label warning?

$$eCl_{cr} = (140 - Age\,(years)) \times \frac{weight}{72 \times Serum\ creatinine \left(\frac{mg}{dL}\right)} \times 0.85\,(if\ female) \qquad \textbf{(Eq. 4.2)}$$

$$eCl_{cr} = (140 - 65) \times \frac{100}{72 \times 1} = 104\ mL/min$$

So, based on the label this patient should not receive edoxaban. Some pharmacy systems use alternate weight descriptors to estimate kidney function.

$$IBW = 50\ kg + 2.3 \times (Height\ (inches) - 60)\ kg \qquad \text{(Eq. 4.3)}$$

$$IBW = 50\ kg + 2.3 \times \left(\left(\frac{\frac{172}{2.54}\ cm}{inch}\right) - 60\right) kg$$

$$IBW = 50\ kg + 17.7\ kg$$

$$IBW = 67.7\ kg$$

$$AdjBW = IBW + 0.4 \times (Weight - IBW) \qquad \text{(Eq. 4.4)}$$

$$AdjBW = 67.7 + 0.4 \times (100 - 67.7)$$

$$AdjBW = 80.6\ kg$$

So in this case if alternate weights were used to estimate eCl_{cr}, then you would estimate:

$$eCl_{cr}\text{-}IBW = (140 - 65) \times \frac{67.7}{72 \times 1} = 70.5\ mL/min \qquad \text{(Eq. 4.5)}$$

$$eCl_{cr}\text{-}AdjBW = (140 - 65) \times \frac{80.6}{72 \times 1} = 84.0\ mL/min \qquad \text{(Eq. 4.6)}$$

These estimates are less than 95 mL/min, and so you would now select use of edoxaban in this case. What would be the case if eGFR was used directly from the electronic medical record?

The CKD-EPI equation for this particular case scenario is[80]:

$$eGFR_{CKD\text{-}EPI} = 141 \times \left(\frac{Serum\ creatinine\left(\frac{mg}{dL}\right)}{0.9}\right)^{-0.9209} \times (0.993)^{Age(years)} \qquad \text{(Eq. 4.7)}$$

$$eGFR_{CKD\text{-}EPI} = 141 \times \left(\frac{1\left(\frac{mg}{dL}\right)}{0.9}\right)^{-1.209} \times (0.993)^{65}$$

$$eGFR_{CKD\text{-}EPI} = 141 \times 0.88 \times 0.633$$

$$eGFR_{CKD\text{-}EPI} = 78.6 \text{ mL/min/1.73 m}^2$$

Given the difference in units, a consideration may be to transform these values into mL/min for fair comparison with eCl_{Cr}.

$$BSA = \sqrt{\frac{\text{Height (cm)} \times \text{Weight (kg)}}{3,600}} \qquad \textbf{(Eq. 4.8)}$$

$$BSA = \sqrt{\frac{170 \times 100}{3,600}}$$

$$BSA = \sqrt{\frac{170 \times 100}{3,600}}$$

$$BSA = \sqrt{4.72}$$

$$BSA = 2.17 \text{ m}^2$$

$$eGFR_{CKD\text{-}EPI} = 78.6 \text{ mL/min/1.73 m}^2 \qquad \textbf{(Eq. 4.9)}$$

$$= 45.5 \text{ mL/min/m}^2 \times 2.17 \text{ m}^2$$

$$= 98.6 \text{ mL/min}$$

So to summarize the results of the estimated kidney function in this case and the potential drug selection decision that may be made,

EQUATION	VALUE	ADMINISTER EDOXABAN
Cockcroft-Gault (weight)	104 mL/min	No
Cockcroft-Gault (IBW)	70.5 mL/min	Yes
Cockcroft-Gault (AdjBW)	84.0 mL/min	Yes
CKD-EPI with BSA	78.6 mL/min/1.73 m²	Yes
CKD-EPI without BSA	98.6 mL/min	No

At present, FDA-approved drug product labels have the potential to include one of the above scenarios for different drugs. This lack of homogeneity is challenging as health systems often report a single kidney function estimate in the electronic medical record. The drug product labels for most dose adjustments are also geared toward patients with chronic kidney function and not the alternate scenario (above-average kidney function) as presented in this case and plausible in obesity. As shown, it is important to pay attention to the approved drug label as conflicting decisions are plausible.

EMERGING TECHNOLOGIES FOR DRUG DOSING IN OBESITY

The cases in this chapter help illustrate a fundamental challenge that we face when dosing patients with obesity. We use height and weight to generate scalars to prevent overdosing patients with obesity. In most instances, an average empirical estimate is that a 150-kg patient may need a ~50% higher daily dose than a 75-kg patient. Differences in pharmacogenetics, organ function, and other intrinsic variables can increase or decrease this average expectation. Body size correlates with body composition, but there is a great deal of interindividual variability that limits direct translation. Measurement of body composition would be ideal but is not cost-effective and may not be feasible in patients that are acutely ill. One emerging option is the repurposing of existing radiologic imaging data into human phenotype information, a discipline known as morphomics.

Morphomics relies on the translation of computed tomography (CT) images or magnetic resonance imaging (MRI) into body composition.[81] For reference, 70 million CT scans and 40 million MRI scans are performed each year. Several studies have shown that CT data across the third lumbar (L3) or twelfth thoracic (T12) vertebrae can be used to generate morphomic data that may be useful for PK applications. Regional image analysis can compartmentalize this image into adipose, fascia, muscle, and bone tissue based on density relative to water. This density information measured in Hounsfield units can also provide information on muscle density as a surrogate measure of age-related changes. This is particularly helpful to qualify individuals with sarcopenia, or age-related loss of skeletal muscle mass.[82] Kidney function correlates with skeletal muscle mass, and so this tool may be particularly helpful to characterize age-related loss of kidney function. Other parameters such as subcutaneous fat volume, visceral fat volume, skeletal muscle area, low- and high-density muscle area, body depth, body circumference, and the like are examples of measurements that may correlate with drug Cl and V_d. This population-level information can then be scaled and normalized by age to generate expected distributions for a given population to better identify specific phenotypes of patients who are obese that require dose adjustment. Figure 4.6 provides an illustrative example of the various measurements that can be generated through morphomic analysis.

Recently, morphomic information has been used to understand the correlation of these parameters to drug PK properties.[83-85] A study of 335 patients with a median (minimum, maximum) age, height, and weight of 57 (21, 93) years, 170 (145, 203) centimeters, and 81 (42, 187) kg compared morphomics with body weight as predictors of aminoglycoside PK.[85] Skeletal muscle area and volume explained more of the interindividual variability in Cl than weight or sex. Higher precision was observed using a modified Cockcroft-Gault equation with skeletal muscle area at L3 ($R^2 = 0.38$) than the standard Cockcroft-Gault equation using body weight ($R^2 = 0.22$).[85] Similarly, vancomycin clearance was associated with total psoas muscle area and age.[83] A better correlation between the central compartment volume and T12-to-L4 torso volume than bodyweight was also demonstrated.[83] These findings have recently been extended to the anticancer agent paclitaxel, which is associated with significant peripheral neuropathy.[86] This probability for the occurrence of this toxicity is associated with the maximum concentration. Skeletal muscle area measured through morphomics was

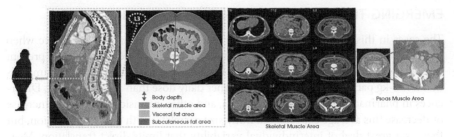

Body depth
Skeletal muscle area
Visceral fat area
Subcutaneous fat area

Skeletal Muscle Area

Psoas Muscle Area

FIGURE 4.6   Illustration of key body dimensions, fat, and muscle areas that can be derived through analytic morphomics of computed tomography images.

identified as a better covariate of paclitaxel volume of distribution. A prospective study to test different rates of infusion to lower the maximum concentration based on skeletal muscle area stratified groups is underway. Reproducibility of this approach by other research groups is the essential next step along with a determination of clinical feasibility. Improving drug dosing in patients with obesity will require continued efforts to better characterize this population phenotype to someday replace body size as the singular metric to scale drug doses.

REFERENCES

1. Apovian CM. Obesity: definition, comorbidities, causes, and burden. *Am J Manag Care.* 2016;22(7 suppl):S176-S185.

2. Suminska M, Podgorski R, Bogusz-Gorna K, Skowronska B, Mazur A, Fichna M. Historical and cultural aspects of obesity: from a symbol of wealth and prosperity to the epidemic of the 21st century. *Obes Rev.* 2022;23(6):e13440.

3. Visscher TL, Seidell JC. The public health impact of obesity. *Annu Rev Public Health.* 2001;22:355-375.

4. Biener AI, Cawley J, Meyerhoefer C. The medical care costs of obesity and severe obesity in youth: an instrumental variables approach. *Health Econ.* 2020;29(5):624-639.

5. Cawley J, Meyerhoefer C. The medical care costs of obesity: an instrumental variables approach. *J Health Econ.* 2012;31(1):219-230.

6. Ward ZJ, Bleich SN, Cradock AL, et al. Projected U.S. state-level prevalence of adult obesity and severe obesity. *N Engl J Med.* 2019;381(25):2440-2450.

7. NCD Risk Factor Collaboration. Worldwide trends in body-mass index, underweight, overweight, and obesity from 1975 to 2016: a pooled analysis of 2416 population-based measurement studies in 128.9 million children, adolescents, and adults. *Lancet.* 2017;390(10113):2627-2642.

8. Skinner AC, Ravanbakht SN, Skelton JA, Perrin EM, Armstrong SC. Prevalence of obesity and severe obesity in US children, 1999-2016. *Pediatrics.* 2018;141(3):e20173459.

9. Grimsrud KN, Sherwin CM, Constance JE, et al. Special population considerations and regulatory affairs for clinical research. *Clin Res Regul Aff.* 2015;32(2):47-56.

10. Pestine E, Stokes A, Trinquart L. Representation of obese participants in obesity-related cancer randomized trials. *Ann Oncol.* 2018;29(7):1582-1587.

11. De Vries R. A tale of two bioethics. *Perspect Biol Med.* 2022;65(1):133-142.

12. Green B, Duffull SB. What is the best size descriptor to use for pharmacokinetic studies in the obese? *Br J Clin Pharmacol.* 2004;58(2):119-133.

13. Pai MP. Drug dosing based on weight and body surface area: mathematical assumptions and limitations in obese adults. *Pharmacotherapy.* 2012;32(9):856-868.

14. Keys A, Fidanza F, Karvonen MJ, Kimura N, Taylor HL. Indices of relative weight and obesity. *J Chronic Dis.* 1972;25(6):329-343.

15. Eknoyan G. Adolphe Quetelet (1796-1874)—the average man and indices of obesity. *Nephrol Dial Transplant.* 2008;23(1):47-51.

16. Wang ZM, Deurenberg P, Guo SS, et al. Six-compartment body composition model: inter-method comparisons of total body fat measurement. *Int J Obes Relat Metab Disord.* 1998;22(4):329-337.

17. Meeuwsen S, Horgan GW, Elia M. The relationship between BMI and percent body fat, measured by bioelectrical impedance, in a large adult sample is curvilinear and influenced by age and sex. *Clin Nutr.* 2010;29(5):560-566.

18. Rothman KJ. BMI-related errors in the measurement of obesity. *Int J Obes (Lond).* 2008;32(suppl 3): S56-S59.

19. Gallagher D, Visser M, Sepulveda D, Pierson RN, Harris T, Heymsfield SB. How useful is body mass index for comparison of body fatness across age, sex, and ethnic groups? *Am J Epidemiol.* 1996;143(3):228-239.

20. Duren DL, Sherwood RJ, Czerwinski SA, et al. Body composition methods: comparisons and interpretation. *J Diabetes Sci Technol.* 2008;2(6):1139-1146.

21. Christakoudi S, Tsilidis KK, Muller DC, et al. A Body Shape Index (ABSI) achieves better mortality risk stratification than alternative indices of abdominal obesity: results from a large European cohort. *Sci Rep.* 2020;10(1):14541.

22. Ferrannini E. Physiological and metabolic consequences of obesity. *Metabolism.* 1995;44(9 suppl 3): 15-17.

23. Aurigemma GP, de Simone G, Fitzgibbons TP. Cardiac remodeling in obesity. *Circ Cardiovasc Imaging.* 2013;6(1):142-152.

24. Farrell GC, Teoh NC, McCuskey RS. Hepatic microcirculation in fatty liver disease. *Anat Rec (Hoboken).* 2008;291(6):684-692.

25. Cortinovis M, Perico N, Ruggenenti P, Remuzzi A, Remuzzi G. Glomerular hyperfiltration. *Nat Rev Nephrol.* 2022;18(7):435-451.

26. Smit C, De Hoogd S, Bruggemann RJM, Knibbe CAJ. Obesity and drug pharmacology: a review of the influence of obesity on pharmacokinetic and pharmacodynamic parameters. *Expert Opin Drug Metab Toxicol.* 2018;14(3):275-285.

27. Lu CX, An XX, Yu Y, et al. Pooled analysis of gastric emptying in patients with obesity: implications for oral absorption projection. *Clin Ther.* 2021;43(10):1768-1788.

28. Brill MJ, Valitalo PA, Darwich AS, et al. Semiphysiologically based pharmacokinetic model for midazolam and CYP3A mediated metabolite 1-OH-midazolam in morbidly obese and weight loss surgery patients. *CPT Pharmacometrics Syst Pharmacol.* 2016;5(1):20-30.

29. Gradel AKJ, Porsgaard T, Lykkesfeldt J, et al. Factors affecting the absorption of subcutaneously administered insulin: effect on variability. *J Diabetes Res.* 2018;2018:1205121.

30. Townsend MJ, Kyle TK, Stanford FC. COVID-19 vaccination and obesity: optimism and challenges. *Obesity (Silver Spring).* 2021;29(4):634-635.

31. Rudders SA, Geyer BC, Banerji A, Phipatanakul W, Clark S, Camargo CA Jr. Obesity is not a risk factor for repeat epinephrine use in the treatment of anaphylaxis. *J Allergy Clin Immunol.* 2012;130(5):1216-1218.

32. Toutain PL, Bousquet-Melou A. Volumes of distribution. *J Vet Pharmacol Ther.* 2004;27(6):441-453.

33. Holt K, Nagar S, Korzekwa K. Methods to predict volume of distribution. *Curr Pharmacol Rep.* 2019;5(5):391-399.

34. Dunn RD, Crass RL, Hong J, Pai MP, Krop LC. Vancomycin volume of distribution estimation in adults with class III obesity. *Am J Health Syst Pharm.* 2019;76(24):2013-2018.

35. Summerfield SG, Yates JWT, Fairman DA. Free drug theory—no longer just a hypothesis? *Pharm Res.* 2022;39(2):213-222.

36. Cominetti O, Nunez Galindo A, Corthesy J, et al. Obesity shows preserved plasma proteome in large independent clinical cohorts. *Sci Rep.* 2018;8(1):16981.

37. Levy BI, Schiffrin EL, Mourad JJ, et al. Impaired tissue perfusion: a pathology common to hypertension, obesity, and diabetes mellitus. *Circulation.* 2008;118(9):968-976.

38. Brook RD, Bard RL, Bodary PF, et al. Blood pressure and vascular effects of leptin in humans. *Metab Syndr Relat Disord.* 2007;5(3):270-274.

39. Simon P, Petroff D, Busse D, et al. Meropenem plasma and interstitial soft tissue concentrations in obese and nonobese patients—a controlled clinical trial. *Antibiotics (Basel).* 2020;9(12):931.

40. Huttunen R, Syrjanen J. Obesity and the risk and outcome of infection. *Int J Obes (Lond).* 2013; 37(3):333-340.

41. Wei JL, Leung JC, Loong TC, et al. Prevalence and severity of nonalcoholic fatty liver disease in non-obese patients: a population study using proton-magnetic resonance spectroscopy. *Am J Gastroenterol.* 2015;110(9):1306-1314.

42. Brill MJ, Diepstraten J, van Rongen A, van Kralingen S, van den Anker JN, Knibbe CA. Impact of obesity on drug metabolism and elimination in adults and children. *Clin Pharmacokinet.* 2012;51(5):277-304.

43. Merrell MD, Cherrington NJ. Drug metabolism alterations in nonalcoholic fatty liver disease. *Drug Metab Rev.* 2011;43(3):317-334.

44. Hall JE, Guyton AC. *Guyton and Hall Textbook of Medical Physiology.* Elsevier; 2011.

45. Pai MP. Estimating the glomerular filtration rate in obese adult patients for drug dosing. *Adv Chronic Kidney Dis.* 2010;17(5):e53-e62.

46. Alicic RZ, Patakoti R, Tuttle KR. Direct and indirect effects of obesity on the kidney. *Adv Chronic Kidney Dis.* 2013;20(2):121-127.

47. Amann K, Benz K. Structural renal changes in obesity and diabetes. *Semin Nephrol.* 2013;33(1):23-33.

48. Inker LA, Schmid CH, Tighiouart H, et al. Estimating glomerular filtration rate from serum creatinine and cystatin C. *N Engl J Med.* 2012;367(1):20-29.

49. Dickerson RN, Crawford CN, Tsiu MK, et al. Augmented renal clearance following traumatic injury in critically ill patients requiring nutrition therapy. *Nutrients.* 2021;13(5):1681.

50. Cockcroft DW, Gault MH. Prediction of creatinine clearance from serum creatinine. *Nephron.* 1976;16(1):31-41.

51. Pai MP. Antimicrobial dosing in specific populations and novel clinical methodologies: kidney function. *Clin Pharmacol Ther.* 2021;109(4):952-957.

52. Pai MP. Antimicrobial dosing in specific populations and novel clinical methodologies: obesity. *Clin Pharmacol Ther.* 2021;109(4):942-951.

53. Nair A, Morsy MA, Jacob S. Dose translation between laboratory animals and human in preclinical and clinical phases of drug development. *Drug Dev Res.* 2018;79(8):373-382.

54. McMahon T. Size and shape in biology. *Science.* 1973;179(4079):1201-1204.

55. Shortliffe EH, Lyman GH, Amankwah FK. Medications in single-dose vials and implications of discarded injectable drugs: a national academies report. *JAMA.* 2021;325(15):1507-1508.

56. Pinkel D. The use of body surface area as a criterion of drug dosage in cancer chemotherapy. *Cancer Res.* 1958;18(7):853-856.

57. West LJ, Pierce CM, Thomas WD. Lysergic acid diethylamide: its effects on a male Asiatic elephant. *Science.* 1962;138(3545):1100-1103.

58. White CR, Seymour RS. Mammalian basal metabolic rate is proportional to body mass$^{2/3}$. *Proc Natl Acad Sci U S A.* 2003;100(7):4046-4049.

59. West GB, Brown JH, Enquist BJ. A general model for ontogenetic growth. *Nature.* 2001;413(6856):628-631.

60. Agutter PS, Wheatley DN. Metabolic scaling: consensus or controversy? *Theor Biol Med Model.* 2004;1:13.

61. McLeay SC, Morrish GA, Kirkpatrick CM, Green B. The relationship between drug clearance and body size: systematic review and meta-analysis of the literature published from 2000 to 2007. *Clin Pharmacokinet.* 2012;51(5):319-330.

62. Villa C, Primeau C, Hesse U, Hougen HP, Lynnerup N, Hesse B. Body surface area determined by whole-body CT scanning: need for new formulae? *Clin Physiol Funct Imaging.* 2017;37(2):183-193.

63. Du Bois D, Du Bois EF. A formula to estimate the approximate surface area if height and weight be known. 1916. *Nutrition.* 1989;5(5):303-311; discussion 312-313.

64. Gehan EA, George SL. Estimation of human body surface area from height and weight. *Cancer Chemother Rep.* 1970;54(4):225-235.

65. Haycock GB, Schwartz GJ, Wisotsky DH. Geometric method for measuring body surface area: a height-weight formula validated in infants, children, and adults. *J Pediatr.* 1978;93(1):62-66.

66. Livingston EH, Lee S. Body surface area prediction in normal-weight and obese patients. *Am J Physiol Endocrinol Metab.* 2001;281(3):E586-E591.

67. Mosteller RD. Simplified calculation of body-surface area. *N Engl J Med.* 1987;317(17):1098.

68. Pai MP, Paloucek FP. The origin of the "ideal" body weight equations. *Ann Pharmacother.* 2000;34(9):1066-1069.

69. Schwartz GJ, Munoz A, Schneider MF, et al. New equations to estimate GFR in children with CKD. *J Am Soc Nephrol.* 2009;20(3):629-637.

70. Pai MP, Rodvold KA. Aminoglycoside dosing in patients by kidney function and area under the curve: the Sawchuk-Zaske dosing method revisited in the era of obesity. *Diagn Microbiol Infect Dis.* 2014;78(2):178-187.

71. Traynor AM, Nafziger AN, Bertino JS Jr. Aminoglycoside dosing weight correction factors for patients of various body sizes. *Antimicrob Agents Chemother.* 1995;39(2):545-548.

72. Janmahasatian S, Duffull SB, Ash S, Ward LC, Byrne NM, Green B. Quantification of lean bodyweight. *Clin Pharmacokinet.* 2005;44(10):1051-1065.

73. Pai MP, Nafziger AN, Bertino JS Jr. Simplified estimation of aminoglycoside pharmacokinetics in underweight and obese adult patients. *Antimicrob Agents Chemother.* 2011;55(9):4006-4011.

74. Rybak MJ, Le J, Lodise TP, et al. Therapeutic monitoring of vancomycin for serious methicillin-resistant *Staphylococcus aureus* infections: a revised consensus guideline and review by the American Society of Health-System Pharmacists, the Infectious Diseases Society of America, the Pediatric Infectious Diseases Society, and the Society of Infectious Diseases Pharmacists. *Am J Health Syst Pharm.* 2020;77(11):835-864.

75. Crass RL, Dunn R, Hong J, Krop LC, Pai MP. Dosing vancomycin in the super obese: less is more. *J Antimicrob Chemother.* 2018;73(11):3081-3086.

76. Pai MP, Crass RL. Translation of pharmacodynamic biomarkers of antibiotic efficacy in specific populations to optimize doses. *Antibiotics (Basel).* 2021;10(11):1368.

77. Eisenstein BI, Oleson FB Jr, Baltz RH. Daptomycin: from the mountain to the clinic, with essential help from Francis Tally, MD. *Clin Infect Dis.* 2010;50(suppl 1):S10-S15.

78. Liu C, Bayer A, Cosgrove SE, et al. Clinical practice guidelines by the Infectious Diseases Society of America for the treatment of methicillin-resistant *Staphylococcus aureus* infections in adults and children. *Clin Infect Dis.* 2011;52(3):e18-e55.

79. Yin O, Kakkar T, Duggal A, et al. Edoxaban exposure in patients with atrial fibrillation and estimated creatinine clearance exceeding 100 mL/min. *Clin Pharmacol Drug Dev.* 2022;11(5):666-674.

80. Inker LA, Eneanya ND, Coresh J, et al. New creatinine- and cystatin C-based equations to estimate GFR without race. *N Engl J Med.* 2021;385(19):1737-1749.

81. Krishnamurthy V, Zhang P, Ethiraj S, et al. Use of analytic morphomics of liver, spleen, and body composition to identify patients at risk for cirrhosis. *Clin Gastroenterol Hepatol.* 2015;13(2):360-368.e5.

82. Lee JS, He K, Harbaugh CM, et al. Frailty, core muscle size, and mortality in patients undergoing open abdominal aortic aneurysm repair. *J Vasc Surg.* 2011;53(4):912-917.

83. Pai MP, Derstine BA, Lichty M, et al. Relationships of vancomycin pharmacokinetics to body size and composition using a novel pharmacomorphomic approach based on medical imaging. *Antimicrob Agents Chemother.* 2017;61(11):e01402-17.

84. Pai MP, Debacker KC, Derstine B, Sullivan J, Su GL, Wang SC. Comparison of body size, morphomics, and kidney function as covariates of high-dose methotrexate clearance in obese adults with primary central nervous system lymphoma. *Pharmacotherapy.* 2020;40(4):308-319.

85. Crass RL, Ross BE, Derstine BA, et al. Measurement of skeletal muscle area improves estimation of aminoglycoside clearance across body size. *Antimicrob Agents Chemother.* 2018;62(6):e00441-18.

86. Hertz DL, Chen L, Henry NL, et al. Muscle mass affects paclitaxel systemic exposure and may inform personalized paclitaxel dosing. *Br J Clin Pharmacol.* 2022;88(7):3222-3229.

5

PEDIATRICS

Irving Steinberg

Learning Objectives

By the end of the pediatrics chapter, the learner shall be able to:

1. Provide overarching perspective on the needs for specific pediatric pharmacokinetic (PK) studies and clinical application concepts and differences between children and adults.
2. Describe physiologic and pathophysiologic factors affecting the absorption of drugs from various routes of administration in different age groupings, including transporter maturation and genetic expression, and provide examples of specific drugs affected.
3. Detail the influence of size maturation, fluid compartment developmental changes, physicochemical properties, and protein-binding variations on volume of distribution of drugs in children, and describe population PK models for these parameters.
4. Specify differences in protein-binding affinity and capacity in children versus adults that affects serum and tissue binding and drug distribution.
5. Delineate the ontogeny of phase 1 and phase 2 metabolism and hepatic clearance, and provide specific examples of drugs where age-dependent clearance and pharmacogenetic expression impact the dosing and effect of therapeutic agents throughout childhood and in contrast to adults.
6. Explain the developmental and pathophysiologic aspects of renal drug clearance through early postnatal life and the impact on dosage regimen design through infancy and childhood.
7. Comprehend the need for and application of proper size scaling of PK parameters and resultant dosing in infants, children, and adolescents, and describe how scaling is incorporated into pediatric population PK modeling.
8. Provide examples where weight-based dosing or body surface area (BSA) dosing is preferred.

9. Illustrate the incorporation of size, maturation, organ function, disease, genetics, and other components into population models for initiation/ modification of dosage regimens to target goal concentrations or systemic exposure in children, and demonstrate calculation competency in applying such modeled PK parameters.
10. Note selected differences in pharmacodynamics between children and adults, and assess the PK-guided dosing in treating pediatric disease states.

The days of describing pediatric patients as "therapeutic orphans," and when insufficient study of pediatric drug therapy was common, are effectively ending, if not already over. As of this writing, pediatric studies represent 20% of the total number and 11% of the pharmacokinetic (PK) trials, as listed on ClinicalTrials.gov.[1] Yet, many children are still exposed to unlicensed or off-label drugs, with a greater chance of such exposure with polypharmacy and long hospitalizations.[2] The Best Pharmaceuticals for Children Act—Pediatric Trials Network, the Obstetric and Pediatric Pharmacology and Therapeutics Branch of the Eunice Kennedy Shriver National Institute of Child Health and Human Development, the Global Research in Paediatrics initiative, the Maternal and Pediatric PRecisioN In Therapeutics (MPRINT) Hub, and other research, regulatory, and practice initiatives in pediatric clinical pharmacology[3] have provided the incentive, funding, and practical information needed to escalate the rate of discovery and optimized usage of medications specific to the needs of children.[4,5] Within that framework are the constant need to "get the dose right" for children[6,7] and the requirement for study designs to address this need.[8]

Adverse drug effects may often be linked to PK and pharmacodynamic issues unique to the pediatric patient. Decades ago, the fatal toxicity of the antibiotic chloramphenicol seen in neonates when adult dosages were being used was discovered to be due to immaturity of glucuronidation pathways. This led to initiatives of size and maturation adjustments in dosing and the initial therapeutic drug monitoring efforts to individualize the dose to reach safe therapeutic target concentrations.

PK inference via descriptive and population PK data and modeling has added to the sophistication of translational efforts toward precision dosing strategies for drugs to treat children with acute and chronic diseases effectively and safely. Furthermore, correlative studies of PK behavior linked to the pharmacodynamics and pharmacogenetics of the drug,[4,9] the disease state and physiologic alterations,[10] and the patient demographics and laboratory information create further dosing precision to obtain the desired therapeutic outcomes. Although the same is held true for adults, in children, the complexities of maturation or organ function, changes in size and body habitus, differing manifestations of disease states and laboratory abnormalities, and drug receptor avidity and sensitivity are among features that impose six or seven overlapping PK and therapeutic populations, from the preterm neonate to the older adolescent. Unique medical conditions and interventions[11-13] impose additional sources of variability in drug disposition. Efforts to model these group differences and the continuum of ontogeny in the kinetic behavior of drugs add pharmacometric precision toward managing the most vulnerable of patients through their illness and assist regulatory agencies to approve drugs and biologic agents for pediatric use with translational data applied to practice.[14]

DRUG DISPOSITION AND ELIMINATION IN PEDIATRICS

Absorption

Absorption rate and/or extent of drugs from all extravascular administration modes tend to vary depending on gestational and postnatal age, physiologic and anatomic maturation,[15,16] pathophysiology,[17] and the characteristics of the biopharmaceutical formulations developed for children.[16,18]

At birth, newborns have a more neutral to alkaline gastric pH (pH 6-8) because of residual amniotic fluid in the stomach and the inability of the stomach to express acid (achlorhydria). Gastric acid production increases over the next 24 to 48 hours to achieve adult pH levels but then declines over the following week, and acidity remains relatively low in the first months of life.[19] Slow maturation of gastric acid secretion progresses through infancy until adult production is reached at around 2 years of age. Therefore, penicillins will have greater stomach epithelial permeation and decreased decomposition and, consequently, higher concentration in preterm and term neonates compared to older children. In contrast, decreased oral bioavailability of weak acids (eg, phenobarbital,[11] phenytoin) and weak bases with low pKa (eg, itraconazole) is observed.[19] Slower rates of absorption in neonates may be accounted for by delayed biphasic gastric emptying (not >2.5 hours,[20] with adult values reached at about 6-8 months of age), irregular peristalsis, or by outlet obstructions, such as pyloric stenosis. Gastric-emptying time is slower for preterm compared with term infants and is more than halved from postconceptional age (PCA) of 28 to 36 weeks until 42 to 54 weeks. Therefore, prolonged drug action within a dosing interval may result from a longer time to maximum concentration. In addition, shorter bowel length than adults can diminish the capability to fully absorb sustained-release medications.

Reduced exocrine function occurs in newborns with low lipase production, and despite increased circulating bile acids, there is immature transporter-mediated secretion resulting in low biliary canalicular transport and intestine luminal bile acid concentrations, which can limit oral absorption of fat-soluble drugs such as oral corticosteroids. In addition, pediatric diseases of exocrine function (eg, cystic fibrosis) or biliary disruption (eg, biliary atresia) are conditions where fat malabsorption of nutrients (eg, vitamins A, D, E, and K) and lipid-soluble drugs is expected.[17]

Other transporter maturation and intestinal metabolic and functional status influence absorption and disposition. The iron transporter DMT1 increases linearly with age in children, with the percent of iron absorbed being the lowest in those less than 6 months old,[21] who utilize maternal iron stored during pregnancy.[22] Immaturity of gastrointestinal MDR1 efflux leads to higher zidovudine bioavailability in the first 14 days of life (89%) compared to those older than 14 days to 12 years (61%).[23] Intestinal efflux proteins p-glycoprotein and BCRP abundance and expression are reduced in infants compared to adolescents and adults, allowing greater oral bioavailability for substrates of these transport pumps.[24] Intestinal activity of CYP1A1, CYP3A4, and

UGT1A1 appears to increase with age, with less presystemic intestinal clearance in young children. In contrast, OATP2B1 expression is increased in young infants, with greater bioavailability for substrates such as oral methotrexate.[25] Likewise, CYP2C19 and UGT2B7 located in the ileum show a negative correlation with age.[24] Although, clearly, knowledge has been gained regarding intestinal drug transporter maturation in children, it is much less than the better studied ones in the liver and kidney.

In addition, degradation by intestinal flora, as for digoxin, is already evident in infancy and is age dependent, as the gut microbiome changes.[26] Sepsis, short-gut syndrome, and administration via jejunostomy tube are additional situations where oral bioavailability may be compromised for some drugs. Intramuscular absorption may be variable and ineffective in neonates because of autonomic and vasomotor instability, with relative regional blood flow changes, and inefficient muscular contractions. However, in infants, drugs such as epinephrine, cephalosporins, and aminoglycosides can achieve adequate peak concentrations when given intramuscularly, relying on the 25% to 50% increase in capillary density.[27] Rectal uptake of drugs in neonates and infants is reliable in providing systemic concentrations adequate for clinical effect (eg, acetaminophen, diazepam).[28] Skin penetration of many topically administered drugs often exceeds that in adults, with the hydration of the skin and thinness of the stratum corneum being fundamental to allowing more diffusion through the skin barrier compared with older children and adults.[29] Toxic exposure can result. Methemoglobinemia seen more frequently with EMLA (topical prilocaine and lidocaine eutectic mixture),[30] adverse systemic effects of topical antihistamines[31] and corticosteroids, and topical anesthetic toxicity are examples of the greater risk seen in young infants because of enhanced percutaneous absorption.

Distribution and Protein Binding

Generally, drugs have a wider range of weight-normalized distribution volumes in pediatric patients than in adults. One of the major differentiating factors among pediatric and adult patients across the age span is the continual changes in body composition, especially body fluid compartments and the influence this creates on the distribution volume of medications (Figure 5.1).[11-14] Additional alterations from pathophysiologic states that augment fluid and tissue compartments, electrolyte and extracellular fluid protein content, and inflammation and capillary integrity can be observed to alter the PK disposition of drugs in a similar manner, if not magnitude, as in adults. Premature neonates have the highest body water to total body weight ratio, and the same is true for their extracellular fluid-to-weight relationship. The former has implication for drugs that distribute to a space commensurate with total body water (eg, phenytoin, 1-1.5 L/kg in neonates) and the latter to those distributing to extracellular fluid spaces (eg, aminoglycosides, 0.4-0.5 L/kg). The progressive decreases in the weight ratio of these fluid compartments with age will translate to linear or exponential decreases in the volume of distribution normalized to the body weight of these drugs as the child matures to adolescence. Therefore, incremental doses standardized to body weight for drugs such as gentamicin (eg, 4-5 mg/kg) and vancomycin (eg, 15-20 mg/kg) will be higher in the neonate and infant in order to reach similar peak concentrations as those obtained at lower per kg doses in adolescents and adults (gentamicin dose = 1.5-2.5 mg/kg; vancomycin dose = 8-15 mg/kg).

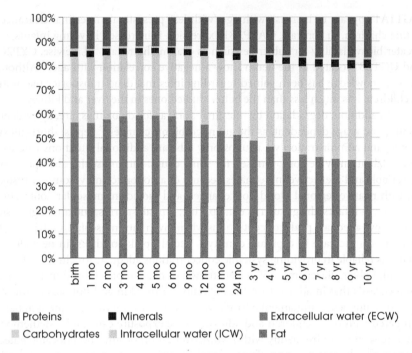

FIGURE 5.1 Changes in body composition over time during childhood. (From Jong G. Pediatric development: physiology. Enzymes, rug metabolism, pharmacokinetics and pharmacodynamics. In: Bar-Shalom D, Rose K, eds. *Pediatric Formulations: A Roadmap.* Springer; 2014:9-23. *AAPS Advances in the Pharmaceutical Sciences Series* 11.)

Serum protein binding in children may also play a role in the comparative differences seen in the volume of distribution (V_d), with more unbound drugs available to leave the intravascular space and bind with receptor and nonreceptor tissues.[32,33] In neonates, reduced albumin-binding capacity results from lower quantity (eg, 2-3 g/dL) and retained fetal albumin, which has less affinity for binding than normal albumin. Cefazolin has twice the average unbound fraction in neonates compared to adults,[34] and saturability of albumin binding is seen for this drug in neonates, but not typical of adults.[35] Similar observations have been made for vancomycin where lower binding in children is noted and the unbound fraction in neonates and young infants is dependent on the total vancomycin level and the albumin concentration; therefore, some nonlinearity of binding may exist.[36] Disease states occurring predominantly in pediatric patients, such as nephrotic syndrome, protein-losing enteropathy, and Kawasaki disease, demonstrate significant hypoalbuminemia and diminished drug-protein binding, potentially altering the kinetics and dynamics of drugs, such as furosemide, mycophenolic acid, and aspirin.

Likewise, lower concentration of α_1-acid glycoprotein (AAG) in infancy is responsible for reduced protein binding of basic drugs (eg, meperidine, methadone, fentanyl, propranolol, and lidocaine).[37] This allows for more free drugs to interact with receptors and increases the potency of effect for any given weight-based dose when compared with older children and adults. This must be factored into assessing dosage needs to meet therapeutic end points. Some drugs, such as clindamycin, show impact of reductions in both albumin and AAG quantity, and resultant reduced protein binding, on the V_d in infants.[38] For clearance, simple linear size scaling of pediatric patients to adult values is inaccurate for drugs that are highly bound to AAG.[39]

In children with sickle cell disease, increases in AAG as a result of pain crises can yield less analgesic effect of meperidine at customary doses because the higher binding will produce less unbound meperidine.[40] Yet, the need for higher doses is met with a higher repository of bound meperidine for conversion to the neurotoxic normeperidine metabolite that can cause seizures (particularly in those patients with renal compromise who accumulate normeperidine while on patient-controlled analgesia). Accordingly, most pediatric centers restrict the use of meperidine.[41]

Similarly, postoperative increases in AAG concentrations in children as an acute-phase reaction after 48 hours can also alter the short-term kinetics and dynamics of intermittently dosed methadone.[42] Blood levels for R- and S-isomers increase in correlation with the rise in AAG concentrations, whereas an inverse relationship is found for the primary metabolite concentrations with AAG. The clinical impact is seen with the pain scores also correlating to AAG, reflecting the lesser amount of free drug available to pain receptors and liver metabolism. The consequent need for addition opioids, computed as morphine equivalence, correlates with greater scores for nausea and vomiting.[42]

Other binding capacity differences may comparatively reduce serum protein binding in pediatric patients. Vancomycin was shown to have lower serum binding than three groups of adults with critical care, orthopedic, and hematologic diseases.[43] Unbound fractions averaged 81% in the pediatric group versus 56% to 62% among the adult groups. Multivariate modeling revealed total vancomycin and albumin concentrations as expected predictors of unbound concentration in all four groups, but immunoglobulin A (IgA) concentration was a significant variable only for the adult patient groups, where the IgA concentrations were 3- to 7.5-fold higher than in the pediatric patients. Lower trough level targets of 7 to 10 mg/L are seen as beneficial in achieving pharmacodynamics end points (eg, area under the curve to minimum inhibitory concentration [AUC/MIC] ratio $\geq$400) in children when compared to those suggested for adults.[44] The higher unbound fraction may contribute to the clinical and microbiologic success of vancomycin therapy at these serum concentration and systemic exposure measures. Another illustration showed variable but lower protein binding of vancomycin in critically ill children (median free fraction = 71%).[45] The target of AUC/MIC of 400 or higher for total drug and 200 or more for free drug (assumed from typical adult value for protein binding of 50%) reached 54% and 83% of the patients, respectively, with 8 of 11 patients achieving the target free systemic exposure even when the total AUC/MIC was less than 400. The free level could be computed from the total vancomycin and total protein concentrations as follows[45]:

$$C_{\text{unbound mg/L}} = 5.38 + (0.71 \times C_{\text{total mg/L}}) - (0.085 \times C_{\text{total protein g/dL}})$$

Binding interactions of particular concern in pediatrics include the disruption of the albumin binding of high concentrations of bilirubin (and the potential risk of kernicterus) in the young infant by highly bound drugs, such as ibuprofen, salicylates, sulfisoxazole, and ceftriaxone.[46] The greatest risk for concern with ibuprofen and ceftriaxone is reserved for the premature or low birth weight neonate.[47,48]

Tissue-binding differences can also translate into altered pharmacodynamic response.[33] Infants have 3-fold greater number of erythrocyte (and by association, myocardial) receptors for digoxin and a 2 times higher dissociation constant, leading to relative insensitivity compared with older children and adults.[49] In addition, greater tissue binding leads to a volume of distribution of digoxin averaging 12.8 L/kg in patients aged 2 to 3 months and 16.2 L/kg in 1.3- to 5-year-old (compared with a typical 7 L/kg in adults).[50] Therefore, doses of digoxin to treat cardiac arrhythmias or heart failure in young infants are 8 to 15 µg/kg/d, as compared with 2 to 4 µg/kg/d for adults.

Hepatic Metabolism

Maturation of phase 1 and phase 2 metabolic pathways occurs at differing rates in neonates, infants, and children until adult rates are achieved or, for some pathways, surpassed.[51-53] Evidence of primordial drug metabolic enzymes and activity exists in the fetus. CYP3A7 is the fetal isoform that is present in utero at 50 to 60 days PCA, peaks within 1 week postnatal age and then diminishes rapidly to be replaced with developing levels of the similar-acting CYP3A4. This creates a developmental shift in the dominant metabolite of male hormones before and after birth.[54] Whereas CYP2E1, CYP2C19, and CYP2D6 show activity within hours to days, CYP2C9, CYP3A4, and CYP1A2 are delayed in onset of activity and maturation (see Figure 5.2).[51] Note that the capacity for CYP3A4, CYP3A5, CYP2C9, CYP2C19, and CYP1A2 reaches 150% to

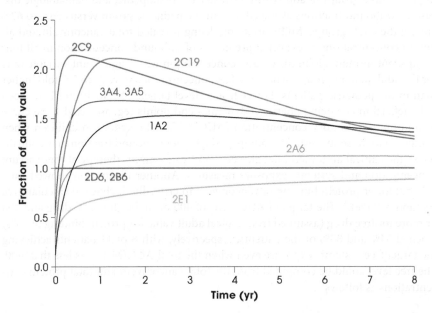

FIGURE 5.2 Maturations rates of noted cytochrome P450 enzymes as a percentage of adult activity. Data represent meta-analysis of in vivo determinations from multiple sources. (From Upreti VV, Wahlstrom JL. Meta-analysis of hepatic cytochrome P450 ontogeny to underwrite the prediction of pediatric pharmacokinetics using physiologically based pharmacokinetic modeling. *J Clin Pharmacol.* 2016;56(3):266-283.)

200% of adult values in early childhood. Probe drugs such as theophylline provide useful examples of the maturation of drug metabolism. With CYP2E1 functional early in postnatal life, the major metabolite of theophylline is 1,3-dimethyluric acid, with more primitive pathways such a methylation represented (producing the active metabolite caffeine early in postnatal life), along with reliance on unchanged drug elimination via the kidney (Table 5.1).[55] With maturation, these latter pathways reduce or disappear, and the enhancement of 1,3-dimethyluric acid is observed with the contributions of the later-developing CYP1A2 and CYP3A4 pathways; the former isoenzyme also contributing to 1-methyluric acid and 3-methylxanthine metabolite production, and the less unchanged drug being renally excreted.[55] Similarly, phenobarbital metabolism is slow in the neonate and young infant because of the immaturity of CYP2C9 and CYP2C19 oxidation pathways, with elimination half-lives in the range of 100 to 140 hours, and decaying by an average of 4.6 hours/d to a half-life of 60 to 70 hours by 4 weeks postnatal age.[56]

Dextromethorphan is another probe drug to examine the ontogeny of metabolism. Because CYP2D6 matures faster than CYP3A4, the O-demethylation of dextromethorphan exceeds that of N-demethylation derived from CYP3A4 metabolism during the first 2 to 3 months of infancy. These pathways produce these metabolites equivalently after 4 months, and by 1 year, the CYP3A4 products exceed those of CYP2D6.[57] Although CYP3A4 becomes a more dominant pathway in the maturing child for substrate drugs such as midazolam, critical illness may temporally negatively affect this metabolic potential.[51] Factors and time patterns of hepatic enzyme maturation in pediatrics can be accurately modeled using sophisticated neural network computing.[58] Proteomics has also been applied to quantify enzyme functional drug metabolism maturation of the liver and kidney.[59]

Even anatomy may define differing clearance values. Liver weight-to-body weight ratio is higher in children than in adults, peaking at 2 to 3 years of age. Therefore, it is not surprising that with a full complement of liver microsomal enzymes and wild-type genetic expression, the metabolic clearance of many drugs when standardized to body weight is higher in ages 2 years to preadolescence than in adults. Warfarin clearance is a good example of this, where prepubertal children are observed to have higher body weight–standardized clearances than adults, but when standardized to

TABLE 5.1 Molar Mean % Recovery of Theophylline and Its Metabolites in Urine and Clearance Values After Multiple Doses Given to Infants

POSTCONCEPTIONAL AGE (WK)	THEO	3-MX	1-MU	1,3-DIMU	CAFFEINE	CLEARANCE (ML/HR/KG)
30-40	55.2	1.4	8.2	24.0	8.5	21.5
40-50	32.6	5.0	11.1	42.3	3.3	30.3
>50	17.9	12.8	22.0	43.7	0.8	60.7

1,3-diMU, 1,3-dimethyluric acid; 1-MU, 1-methyluric acid; 3-MX, 3-methylxanthine.
Kraus DM, Fischer JH, Reitz SJ, et al. Alterations in theophylline metabolism during the first year of life. *Clin Pharmacol Ther.* 1993;54(4):351-359.

liver weight, as assessed by ultrasonography, these clearances were not significantly different.[60] Other hepatically cleared drugs have also shown no relationship between liver weight–normalized clearance and age.[61] This provides partial reasoning for allometric or other scaling methods related to body weight as a preferable size function to quantitatively relate to clearance (see further discussion).[62-64] Moreover, the efficiency of metabolism may be reduced for numerous enzyme pathways in obese pediatric patients as exemplified by the diminished CYP2C19 conversion of voriconazole to its N-oxide metabolite of obese children undergoing hematopoietic stem cell transplant compared to normal weight counterparts.[65] Similar data showing unbound intrinsic clearance negatively correlated with several obesity indices are noted in adults.[66]

Phase 2 metabolism is mostly subject to maturation influences. Sulfation and acetylation capacity are present very early in life.[67] Modeling of metabolite formation clearances in neonates of varying gestational ages demonstrated at an average of 1 week postnatal age a clearance by sulfation of 0.21 L/hr, by glucuronidation of 0.049 L/hr, and by oxidation of 0.058 L/hr. The fraction by oxidation increased by less than 15% through the restricted PCA range studied.[68] The efficiency of metabolism in young children is noted by the comparative lack of toxicity from an acetaminophen acute overdose because of the protection of higher conjugation capacity (sulfation and glucuronidation). The balance of predominant sulfation to mostly glucuronidation of acetaminophen shifts during childhood, making older children and adolescents more vulnerable to acute overdose toxicity. This is contrasted by the greater risk of severe toxicity from chronic supratherapeutic dosing in the toddler to young child age group owing to higher P450 enzyme metabolism and continued production of the liver toxic intermediate, combined with less conjugation if the child's illness is sustained and if not ingesting adequate food substrate.[69] Age dependence of acetylation can be seen for isoniazid where both slow and fast acetylator status create a lower metabolic ratio for young infants compared to older children.[70] Therefore, the particular metabolic pathway, its efficiency, and the production of active versus inactive metabolites must be evaluated for the individual drug and assessed for age and maturation.

UGT1A1 matures fairly early; bilirubin conjugation is only 1% of adult values at gestational ages of 30 to 40 weeks (hence the risk of unconjugated hyperbilirubinemia and kernicterus in that age group early after birth), which then accelerates rapidly to adult values obtained at 2 to 4 months.[71] Slightly more delayed are UGT1A6 and UGT2B7, which mature with half-maximal adult values at 50.1 and 54.6 weeks postmenstrual age.[72,73] UGT2B7-mediated glucuronidation of the antiretroviral zidovudine increases rapidly after 40 weeks PCA, with adult clearance value of around 20 mL/min/kg reaching at 46 to 52 weeks PCA and full maturation values occurring in the first 2 years of life.[74,75] Slower maturation rates are seen in premature infants.[75] In addition, the expression of transporters that allow incorporating of drugs into or pumping out of organs of elimination or receptor sites, such as OCT1, OATP1B3, and p-glycoprotein, is low in neonates and steadily increases during childhood, gaining near-adult values during adolescence.[25,76] This, combined with immaturity in pathways expression, may diminish metabolism and conversion to active and inactive metabolites.

As an example, morphine clearance ranges from 1.7 mL/min/kg in premature neonates at 24 weeks PCA weighing 0.5 kg, to 2.5 mL/min/kg in a 1-kg neonate at

28 weeks PCA, to 3.5 mL/min/kg in a 2-kg infant at 32 weeks PCA.[77] Morphine is metabolized to morphine-6-glucuronide (M6G) through the action of UGT, and its developmental immaturity yields lower production in young infants.[78] Because M6G is 3 to 5 times more potent as an analgesic but the production is less, more of the analgesic effect must come from the parent drug, and, therefore, despite an immature blood-brain barrier, the morphine EC50 is (paradoxically) higher in neonates than in older children and adults.[78] However, with continued therapy, the immature renal function begins to play a larger role, and any formation of M6G is inadequately cleared, accumulates, and begins to contribute to the overall pharmacodynamic effect. Moreover, immature p-glycoprotein expression and diminished blood-brain barrier protection enhance brain sensitivity to morphine.[25] Therefore, morphine dosing later in therapy may need to be reduced if accumulation of M6G creates a toxicity risk. Additional PK variability results from hemodynamic changes and interventions altering cardiac performance and blood flow to the liver.[79-81]

In addition, lower OCT1 activity (responsible for drug transport into the liver cell) would predict decreased incorporation into the liver for glucuronidation,[82] further limiting M6G production.[79] Pharmacogenetic influence of OCT1 alleles does not affect morphine clearance in premature neonates, but show growing differences in clearance values based on the genotype may be seen in 34- to 40-week and 40- to 58-week postmenstrual age groups.[83] This is true not only for young infants but exists with the pharmacogenetic differences observed between African American and Caucasian children. Decreased function of OCT1 alleles are more common in Caucasian children,[84] and with the demonstrated comparatively diminished clearance, the potential for more adverse reactions in Caucasian children could be anticipated. This may account for African American children needing significantly more analgesic interventions and having higher maximum pain scores and opioid requirements than Caucasian children in a large study of post-tonsillectomy pain.[85] Despite lower opioid doses, the Caucasian children had greater opioid-related adverse effects and longer postanesthesia care required.[86]

Concerns over pharmacogenetically endowed CYP2D6 activity with codeine use, especially in ultrafast metabolizers, have resulted in restricted use[87] and contraindication in pediatric patients.[88] Ultrafast CYP2D6 metabolizers of codeine can more quickly convert codeine into the more potent morphine, risking exaggerated response and toxicity (eg, respiratory depression), whereas poor functioning alleles promote ineffective analgesic response with the inadequate conversion to morphine.[89] Deaths were reported in breastfeeding infants of mothers with alleles for ultrafast conversion and augmented p-glycoprotein activity[63] and for children with these alleles exposed to codeine after tonsillectomy and adenoidectomy,[64] when the child's airway is more vulnerable to respiratory depression.

An extensive description of the age dependence of pharmacogenetic expression and the impact of polymorphisms on the kinetics of phase 1 and phase 2 processes in children is presented elsewhere.[90] There is a knowledge gap in pharmacogenetics and its impact on pharmacotherapy within the pediatric practitioner community.[91,92] The pediatric clinical pharmacist can add greatly to such knowledge and implementation toward precision dosing in children. Pharmacogenetic genotypes can be mathematically incorporated into employed pediatric population models, as has been performed for warfarin,[93,94] tacrolimus,[95,96] and voriconazole,[97,98] with varying genetic penetrance, clearance influence, and clinical implementation.[90] Selectively applied pharmacogenetic testing and proper interpretation of allele activity in real time can assist providers in the selection and dosing of a variety of agents used in children.[89,99,100]

Renal Elimination

Renal elimination begins in utero with the development of renal structures and urine production as early as at 9 weeks. The number of nephrons is dependent on gestational age and birth weight.[101] Full nephrogenesis occurs at 34 to 36 weeks, and those born prematurely will need to complete development ex utero.[102] Postnatal glomerular filtration rate (GFR) development has a flatter upward trajectory in lower birth weight preterm neonates than those with higher birth weight, and steeper still in full-term newborns.[101,102] Small-for-gestational-age neonates have a reduced GFR and renal drug clearance compared to normal weight neonates of comparable gestational age.[103] Three- to 4-fold increases in GFR (from 15 to 20 increases to 60 mL/min/1.73 m^2) are seen in full-term normally developed neonates during the first month of life,[101] because increases in cardiac output and renal blood flow and diminished renovascular resistance lead to more peripheral glomerular perfusion to the more abundant cortical nephrons. Perinatal sepsis or hypoxia can stunt this maturation and further delay the renal elimination of drugs. Models to describe the nonlinear increases in GFR during the first months of life have been developed.[104] The postmenstrual age at which GFR reaches 50% of adult values is estimated at 47.7 weeks (or about 8 weeks postnatal age in a full-term infant), with continued increases during infancy, achieving maximum values for body surface area (BSA)-normalized GFR at 2 to 6 years of age. Consequently, the elimination half-life of the renally cleared drug acyclovir falls from approximately 13 hours in infants of 26 weeks postmenstrual age to 4 hours at 40 weeks postmenstrual age.[105] As with the liver, kidney weight-to-body weight ratio also peaks at 2 to 3 years of age,[106] forecasting that the fastest half-lives of drugs, such as cephalosporins, aminoglycosides, vancomycin, levetiracetam, and acyclovir, are observed in early childhood. Renal impairment will predictably slow elimination as in adults, and doses can be tailored to estimated or measured creatinine clearance,[107] with the estimation methods less accurate for children in the pediatric intensive care unit (PICU) with augmented renal function.[108,109] There are a large number of equations used to calculate creatinine clearance in children, from linear to power function to quadratic formulae, with widely varying precision, and used in first approximations of GFR and renal drug clearance.[107] The more commonly used equation for estimated GFR (eGFR) in children is the original Schwartz equation and its modified or "bedside" version. The versions share the structure of eGFR = k × height in cm/ SCr in mg/dL, where the k constant varies with age and sex. However, when used as a predictor for renally excreted drug clearance, these forms of the equation consistently overestimate clearance, especially in infants with low SCr.[110] A k constant of 0.296 used in 1- to 12-year-old aligns more closely with drug clearance compared to 0.55 in the original Schwartz equation and 0.413 in the modified version. This may create problems with the application for pediatric dosing and may have implications for the definition of augmented renal clearance (see later discussion). Other equations and modifications with the addition of cystatin C measurements more accurately assess eGFR,[111] and maturation models of eGFR can more precisely compute drug clearance.[112]

Although higher in output quantity, tubular secretion maturation rate initially lags behind that of GFR maturation, but equals or exceeds it after 2 to 3 months postnatal age, and until adult values reached at 1 year of age.[102,106] Tubular secretion can also be induced when young infants are exposed to drugs using the carboxylic acid secretion pathway for clearance (eg, penicillin, furosemide).[113]

Gestational age, postnatal age, weight, and serum creatinine (SCr) all can have individual or collective influence on the ability of infants and children to eliminate drugs renally (though the maternal contribution of creatinine during the first couple of days of postnatal life may create a falsely low drug clearance to creatinine clearance relationship).[114] It is best to consider the individual magnitude of each maturational component in influencing creatinine clearance in young infants.[115] As an example, fluconazole population PK modeling in infants 23 to 40 weeks of gestation and less than 120 days postnatal age revealed that all four of the abovementioned factors were statistically significant in predicting drug clearance.[116] Many such population models exist for commonly used drugs in pediatric patients, and further construction and applications of these models are discussed later in this chapter.

Combining these clinical factors with those of maturation milestones gives a more comprehensive evaluation of clearance. As can be seen in Figure 5.3, the aminoglycoside antibiotic amikacin clearance develops through renal maturation on both a gestational (or antenatal) and postnatal development basis.[117] If ibuprofen is given to an infant for the indication of patent ductus arteriosus, this can reduce renal

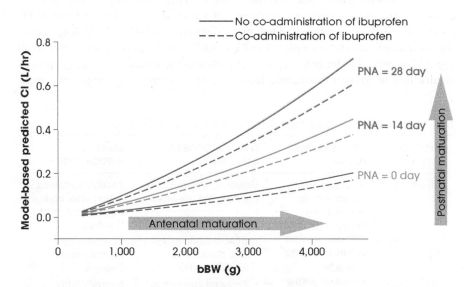

FIGURE 5.3 Amikacin clearance in neonates as a function of antenatal and postnatal maturation and influence of ibuprofen on renal elimination. PNA, postnatal age. (Shakhnovich V, Hornik CP, Kearns GL, Weigel J, Abdel-Rahman SM. How to conduct clinical trials in children: a tutorial. *Clin Transl Sci.* 2019;12(3):218-230; Capparelli EV, Englund JA, Connor JD, et al. Population pharmacokinetics and pharmacodynamics of zidovudine in HIV-infected infants and children. *J Clin Pharmacol.* 2003;43(2):133-140.)

blood flow and blunt the magnitude increase in clearance within each developmental time period. Furthermore, augmented renal clearance (often defined as an eGFR $\geq$ 130 mL/min/1.73 m^2 or $\geq$ 160 mL/min/1.73 m^2; other cutoff values exist) has been studied in children,[118] with more rapid clearance observed for vancomycin,[119,120] aminoglycosides,[121] and β-lactams such as cefepime,[122] piperacillin,[123] meropenem,[124] as well as for acyclovir,[125] ganciclovir,[126] and levetiracetam,[127,128] and seen in patients with neurotrauma, cancer, critically ill children, and potentially other disease states featuring glomerular hyperfiltration (eg, sickle cell disease, diabetic nephropathy, morbid obesity). This requires increases in dosage or more frequent administration (eg, continuous infusion of β-lactams) to meet target concentrations or exposure to avoid the risk of clinical failure in the most severely ill children.[122,128,129]

PEDIATRIC DOSING: PHARMACOKINETIC SCALING AND MODELING

Extrapolation procedures endorsed by the Food and Drug Administration (FDA) attempting to leverage drug effectiveness in adults to improve pediatric labeling require adjusted pediatric dosing to attempt to match systemic exposures associated with response.[130] It is obvious that some method of downsizing doses from adults to children is necessary to provide that systemic exposure, though linear proportions are less likely to meet the need. Mathematically accounting for variables such as weight, BSA, age, organ function, disease, and genetics of the child are among the properties to examine toward assigning the proper dose to be administered.[62] These variables, their expression and maturation over time, and their manifold changes during the composite of childhood must be assessed for their linear and nonlinear properties in relation to PK parameters, such as clearance and volume of distribution (Table 5.2). Linkage across the life span has also been employed in PK modeling of drugs commonly used in all ages.[131] This will allow for better a priori estimation of these parameters, and improved empiric dosing, to meet therapeutic, laboratory, or other measured targets of efficacy

TABLE 5.2 Pharmacokinetic Alterations in Childhood

PHYSIOLOGIC SYSTEM	TRENDS RELATED TO AGE	PHARMACOKINETIC IMPLICATION	CLINICAL IMPLICATIONS
GI tract	Neonates and young infants: reduced and irregular peristalsis followed by slow gastric emptying Neonates: increased gastric pH (>4) in relation to infants Infants: increased motility of lower GI	Slower absorption of the drug (eg, elevated T_{max}) • Faster absorption of acid-labile drugs (eg, penicillin G, erythromycin) • Reduced absorption of weak acid drugs (eg, phenobarbital, phenytoin) • Decreased retention of suppositories	Possible sustained action after oral administration of the drug Possible altered bioavailability ↓ Rectal bioavailability

TABLE 5.2   Pharmacokinetic Alterations in Childhood (*continued*)

PHYSIOLOGIC SYSTEM	TRENDS RELATED TO AGE	PHARMACOKINETIC IMPLICATION	CLINICAL IMPLICATIONS
Skin	Neonates and young infants: a thinner stratum corneum (neonates), increased skin perfusion, increased water content, and higher BSA-to-weight ratio	• ↑ Rate and extent of absorption through the skin during infancy • Higher systemic exposure to drugs for topical use in relation to adults (eg, corticosteroids)	Increased bio-availability and potential toxicity of drugs applied topically; need for a reduced amount of the drug applied to the skin and care in application
Muscle tissue	Neonates: reduction in muscle perfusion, decreased muscle contractility Infants: higher density of capillaries in skeletal muscles	Neonates: poor perfusion limits the absorption, unpredictable PK Infants: ↑ absorption	Neonates: avoid IM administration of drugs Infants: effectiveness of drugs applied IM is higher (eg, epinephrine)
Spatial compartments	Neonates and infants: lower proportion of adipose tissue (10%), ↓ muscle mass, ↑ amount of water related to the body weight (80%), and ↑ proportion of the extracellular fluid (45%) as compared to the intracellular fluid	Neonates: ↑ V_d for water-soluble drugs (eg, gentamicin), and a reduced V_d of drugs that bind to muscles and adipose tissue (eg, morphine, propofol)	Necessary to adjust the loading/maintenance dosing (mg/kg) to achieve therapeutic concentrations of drug in plasma
Plasma protein binding	Neonates: reduced concentrations of albumin and α_1-acid glycoprotein, with a decreased drug protein–binding affinity relative to children and adults; residual fetal albumin in early neonatal period less capable of binding drugs	Increased plasma concentration of unbound drug, with increased V_d and the possibility of occurrence of toxic effects; lower total plasma concentration for low-extraction ratio drugs in children with efficient intrinsic metabolism	For drugs with high binding affinity for proteins (eg, >80%), it is necessary to adjust the dose to maintain the drug levels in the plasma close to the lower limit of the recommended therapeutic range

(*continued*)

TABLE 5.2   Pharmacokinetic Alterations in Childhood (*continued*)

PHYSIOLOGIC SYSTEM	TRENDS RELATED TO AGE	PHARMACOKINETIC IMPLICATION	CLINICAL IMPLICATIONS
Drug metabolism	Neonates and young infants: immature isoform of cytochrome P450 and phase 2 enzymes with harsh developmental expression Children aged 1-6 yr: apparent increased activity of certain enzymes over the normal values for adults	Neonates and young infants: reduced hepatic drug metabolism, with increase in half-life Children aged 1-6 yr: enhanced drug clearance (eg, decrease in half-life) for the specific pharmacologic substrates	Neonates and young infants: increase dosage interval of drug and/or reduce maintenance dose Children aged 1-6 yr: for certain drugs, it is necessary to increase the dose and/or reduce the dosage interval compared to recommended adult dose
Renal drug excretion	Neonates and young infants: decreased GFR (first 6 mo) and active tubular secretion (first 12 mo). Adult values are achieved by the 24th month of life	Neonates and young infants: accumulation of drugs that are secreted via the kidneys and/or the active metabolite; ↓ plasma clearance and ↑ half-life during early infancy	Neonates and young infants: ↑ dosage interval and/or reduce maintenance dose during early infancy

BSA, body surface area; GFR, glomerular filtration rate; GI, gastrointestinal; IM, intramuscular; PK, pharmacokinetic.
Modified from Samardzic J, Allegaert K, Bajcetic M. Developmental pharmacology: a moving target. *Int J Pharm.* 2015;492(1-2):335-337. Copyright 2015, with permission from Elsevier.

while avoiding toxicity. Unique pharmacodynamics in children may further pose differences between adult and pediatric dose scaling.[132]

Weight-based dosing (eg, mg/kg) is a logical first step toward downsizing, but still needs to be related in many cases to maturation, organ function, and other variables in order to more precisely assign the dose needed.[133] The Joint Commission requires weight-based dosing drug protocols in all accredited hospitals treating children. However, as shown earlier for theophylline, digoxin, and aminoglycosides, weight-normalized clearance values vary by age, and the selection of a weight-based daily dose often needs to be grouped by ages sharing similar average standardized clearance values (eg, mL/min/kg). Even for the long-time commonly used over-the-counter ibuprofen, four studies inclusive of obese children with different dosage regimens (low mg/kg, fixed based on age, and adjusted weight) provided no consensus on safe and effective dosing recommendations for these children.[134] Nonstandardized drug clearances (eg, mL/min) are generally not linear with weight or age, and the efficiency of metabolism and renal elimination of many drugs chronologically matures, peaks, and deceases across the pediatric and adolescent age spectrum (see Figure 5.4). Alternate expressions of size attempt to encompass more patients across pediatrics age groups.

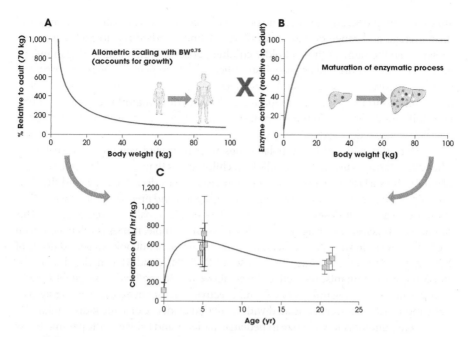

FIGURE 5.4 Influence of scaling of size and maturation of elimination pathways create typical pattern of drug clearance manifested throughout childhood. Pharmacogenetic expression may be more significant than maturation in determining transporter, metabolic, and elimination pathway efficiencies than maturation as the child develops. (From Samant TS, Mangal N, Lukacova V, et al. Quantitative clinical pharmacology for size and age scaling in pediatric drug development: a systematic review. *J Clin Pharmacol.* 2015;55(11):1207-1217, with permission.)

BSA dosing in children has been used successfully for more fat-soluble drugs with wide distribution volumes and hepatic metabolism and is traditionally applied to numerous antineoplastic agents.[135-137] The use of BSA for PK parameterization follows similar standardization of physiologic parameters, such as cardiac output and GFR, and attempts to reduce age-related differences in clearance values correlate better with the kinetic parameter and minimize the variability (eg, coefficient of variation) around the mean value of the kinetic parameters in comparison to body weight standardization. For some agents, such as the antiarrhythmic sotalol, the volume of distribution and clearance both correlate best with BSA, and dosing per BSA can be used throughout childhood and adolescence for those greater than 0.33 m², providing the same AUC as seen in adults.[138] Likewise, population PK modeling showed a statistical preference for a clearance model incorporating BSA for the antifungal caspofungin when validated in children.[139] The use of BSA may, however, provide for imprecise dosing in morbidly obese patients where drugs may only have fractional penetration into adipose tissue,[64] reduced enzymatic clearances impacted by nonalcoholic fatty liver disease,[140] or alterations in clearance of active metabolites, as is seen for with a 30% reduced clearance in obese children of doxorubicinol, a cardiotoxic metabolite of doxorubicin.[141] Adjustments of antineoplastic drug dosing from BSA to weight based are recommended for children less than 3 years to avoid hepatotoxicity and vaso-occlusive disease.[142] However, although initial concerns for neurotoxicity with BSA-dosed vincristine in infants and their average and range of clearances of vincristine standardized to BSA have been shown to be the same as those of older children, doses less than 0.05 mg/kg in infants have reduced exposure and antineoplastic efficacy.[143] Therapeutic drug monitoring and CYP3A5 genotyping can enhance dosing precision. Likewise, a randomized trial of children with nephrotic syndrome comparing daily doses of 60 mg/m^2 with 2 mg/kg found no significant differences in time to remission, but more hypertension was observed in the BSA-adjusted dose group.[144]

More difficulty exists for polar drugs with restricted volumes of distribution when BSA dosing is utilized, particularly in children less than 2 years. In these younger children, the surface area-to-volume ratio increases with decreased age, and the relationship of weight to BSA shifts with age. Bias is highest and precision is least when BSA is used to scale adult doses to infants for water-soluble, renally cleared drugs.[145] This can prove dangerous for drugs like acyclovir. As an example, if BSA is calculated from the 50th percentile weights and heights for age in boys, handbook-suggested doses of 1,500 mg/m^2/d would yield acyclovir doses of 89.5, 84.2, and 81.1 mg/kg/d in 1-, 2-, and 3-month-old infants, respectively, well above the 60 mg/kg/d dose established in clinical studies in young infants as safe and effective.[146] Doses in excess of 60 mg/kg/d or 1,500 mg/m^2/d have been associated with increased evidence of acute kidney injury.[147]

Better attempts to scale size in pediatric patients and bridge to PK parameter estimates in pediatric age groups and extrapolate to adults are through the use of allometric scaling, in analogy to interspecies scaling performed to assign initial drug doses in human trials based on the physiologic and PK animal study.[62] The general expression for this using clearance as the parameter is a power model:

$$Cl = a \cdot (Wt)^b$$

where a is the coefficient and b is the exponent that relates size (in this case, weight) to clearance. This can be expanded and related to adults as follows:

$$Cl_{child} = Cl_{adult} (Wt_{child}/Wt_{adult})^{0.75}$$

Although 0.75 is commonly used and validated as a workable exponent,[62] this applies best when relating a child's clearance to that of an adult for more renally cleared drugs and in children aged 1 year or older. For hepatically eliminated agents, 0.75 consistently provided little prediction error when used in children aged 2 years and older.[148] As simulations and compiled data reveal, the exponent for clearance can deviate moderately or greatly away from 0.75 for certain drugs and approaches 1 to 1.2 in infants and neonates.[149] Those investigations suggest age-related allometric exponents ($\leq$3 months = 1.1; 3 months to 2 years = 1.0; $\geq$2 years to 5 years = 0.9; $\geq$5 years = 0.75) that project drug clearance similar to values derived from full physiologically based PK models.[150]

Serum protein binding and alterations in hepatic enzyme and drug transporter performance can further modify this exponent relationship.[148] Therefore, deriving the specific exponent for clearance of each drug may ultimately be more useful for empiric and Bayesian dosing of that drug in individual patients. An exponent of approximately 1 is often acceptable for most drugs for volume of distribution (ie, a linear function of weight).

The selection and application of allometric exponents, or other size descriptors, can be used more effectively when other maturation and organ function variables are added to the model.[151] Maturation parameters can be added to size descriptors to produce useful models for infants.

Example—Maturation Model

A 4.5-month-old 7-kg infant with a normal-for-age SCr of 0.35 mg/dL, born at 8 months of gestation, is given vancomycin attempting to target an AUC_{24hr} of 400 mg · hr/L to provide effective therapy of staphylococcal bacteremia. What dose would you empirically start?

$$Cl_{child} = Cl_{adult} \times \left(\frac{Wt}{70}\right)^{0.75} \times \frac{(PCA)^{\Theta}}{(PCA)^{\Theta} + (TM_{50})^{\Theta}} \qquad \text{(Eq. 5.1)}$$

Vancomycin maturation parameters[152]:

Cl_{adult} = 93.5 mL/min/70 kg

PCA = Gestational + postnatal ages
TM_{50} = PCA at which Cl is 50% of adult values = 9.5 months
Θ = Hill coefficient ≈ 3.4

$$Cl_{child} = 93.5 \times \left(\frac{7}{70}\right)^{0.75} \times \frac{(12.5)^{3.4}}{(12.5)^{3.4} + (9.5)^{3.4}}$$

$$= 93.5 \times 0.1778 \times 0.7177$$

$$= 11.93 \text{ mL/min}$$

$$= 0.716 \text{ L/hr}$$

The dose can then be calculated using Equation 5.2 to achieve the targeted AUC.

$$\text{Dose (mg)} = Cl \text{ (L/hr)(Target } AUC_{24hr} \text{ in mg·hr/L)} \qquad \text{(Eq. 5.2)}$$

$$= 0.716 \text{ L/hr} \times 400 \text{ mg·hr/L}$$

$$= 286.3 \text{ mg/d}$$

$$= 40.9 \text{ mg/kg/d}$$

Likewise, the mathematical description of the function of the organs of elimination provides numeric input for calculating drug clearance and the dose needed to reach target exposure. For example, valganciclovir for cytomegalovirus prophylaxis in solid organ transplant patients was one of the first examples of a package insert containing a population PK model to calculate the dose of a drug for a pediatric patient:

$$\text{Pediatric dose (mg)} = 7 \times BSA \times Cl_{Cr} \text{ (in mL/min/1.73 m}^2).$$

The essence of PK modeling is to find statistically associated variables that best explain the kinetic parameters and their variability in a group or population, and mathematically quantify these relationships. In pediatrics, because of the clinical and ethical limits on drawing blood, having validated population PK models that can be used in a Bayesian framework, without and then with serum concentration feedback, can provide for more assured initial and adjusted dosing of drugs in children, particularly where a narrow therapeutic range and therapeutic drug monitoring apply. Microdosing (ultralow dose, radiolabeled medication)[153] and microsampling (utilizing dried blood spots)[154] are techniques that have been applied to infants and children to model kinetic parameters while sparing potentially toxic exposure and multiple blood draws.[155]

Taking into account the features of size, maturation and organ function provide for a general approach to modeling clearance in infants and children that can be linked to the adult or standard clearance, but with function parameterization analyzed and itemized to the data (expressed as linear, exponential, power, hyperbolic, etc), and with additional factors (disease, pharmacogenetics, etc) incorporated[6,7]:

$$Cl_{child} = Cl_{adult} \cdot (f_{size}) \cdot (f_{maturation}) \cdot (f_{organ\,function}) \cdot (f_{genetic\,typing}) \cdot (f_{disease\,severity/intervention})$$

Examples of disease states or interventions that may markedly alter the PK in children of various drugs include therapeutic hypothermia, extracorporeal membrane oxygenation, HIV infection, burns, and other critical care conditions.

We can use the abovementioned infant data calculating vancomycin dosing using this modeling approach, with a published pediatric model derived from a one-compartment data fit.[121]

Example—Population Pharmacokinetic Model

$$Cl\ (L/hr) = 0.248 \times Wt^{0.75} \times (0.48/SCr)^{0.361} \times [\ln(Age)/7.8]^{0.995} \qquad \textbf{(Eq. 5.3)}$$

where weight is in kg, SCr is the serum creatinine in mg/dL, and postnatal age in days (4.5 months = 135 days).

$$= 0.248 \times 4.304 \times 1.1208 \times 0.6303$$

$$= 0.7541\ L/hr$$

$$= 1.8\ mL/min/kg$$

The dose can then be calculated using Equation 5.2.

$$Dose = Cl \times Target\ AUC_{24hr}$$

$$= 0.7541\ L/hr \times 400\ mg \cdot hr/L$$

$$= 301.64\ mg/d$$

$$= 42.9\ mg/kg/d$$

Note that this model gives a similar calculated daily dose as the maturation model used previously.

Although no model is perfect in construction or application,[156] the advances in population modeling in pediatrics, with extension to pharmacodynamic linkage,[157] allow further refinement of dose and effect prediction and advise on study design and the potential for extrapolation from adults to children.

PHARMACODYNAMICS AND PHARMACOKINETICALLY DIRECTED DOSING

For most drugs, the extrapolation of effect and a PK search of the correct dose in children and adolescents to provide a pharmacologic effect can initially be derived from studies and experiences in adults and are mostly similar.[158] An antihypertensive medication in adults is expected to have similar blood pressure–reducing effects in children, but finding the dose (total and weight adjusted) to provide a similar percentage decrease in systolic and diastolic pressures may take further PK and pharmacodynamic investigation. However, precise efficacy and adverse effect profiles may differ in children in relationship to dose depending on the comorbidities and indication circumstances.[132] Unique pharmacodynamic effects exist for some immunosuppressive agents with qualitative and quantitative differences between children and adults in cellular and humoral immune systems. Age-varying vitamin K–dependent clotting factor concentrations impact the amount of warfarin needed for therapeutic anticoagulation. And sotalol has different QTc prolongation potential relative to the serum concentration, with greater sensitivity seen in neonates than infants, and in infants more than in children and adolescents, because of the immaturity of potassium channels in the former age groups.[159] In addition, the parameters garnered from population PK modeling may provide biologic relevance to the therapeutic outcome. An elegant example is in the use of infliximab in the management of pediatric Crohn disease, where early clearance determination via a population model and related to the degree of inflammation and tissue uptake of drug was predictive of remission response over a year after initiating the medication, and more so than the trough level or dose.[160]

Finding the proper pediatric dosing can often be challenging depending on the target response sought. While with antimicrobials, the target response is generally set to adult microbiologic and clinical end points (eg, AUC-to-MIC ratio, peak concentration-to-MIC ratio, time above the MIC, quantitative pathogen eradication), the target may move with time and organism resistance. Fluoroquinolones are secondary agents in the management of community-acquired pneumonia (CAP) owing to adverse effects that may be more worrisome in children.[161] Dosing calculations derived from a pediatric population model for levofloxacin based on a goal of unbound serum concentration AUC-to-MIC ratio of 33.7 mg·hr/L (published breakpoint for success against *Streptococcus pneumoniae*) challenge the pediatric CAP guidelines.[162] Clearance (mL/min/kg) was determined to be equal to:

$$\alpha \cdot (Wt)^{\beta} \cdot \frac{Age}{Age + A_{50}}$$

where $\alpha = 1.5 \pm 0.06$ mL/min/kg, $\beta = 0.43 \pm 0.06$, and $A_{50} = 0.32 \pm 0.18$ years.

The volume of distribution was 1.4 to 1.6 L/kg for the five evaluated age groups. Projected AUCs using these parameter estimates revealed that the doses suggested by the pediatric CAP guidelines[163] would provide low target responses of 50% to 60% among 5- to less than 10-year-olds and 76% to 81% among 10- to 16-year-olds.[162] In order to ensure a greater than 90% success, the doses would need to be raised to 12 mg/kg every 12 hours in those 6 months to less than 5-year-olds and 8 mg/kg every 12 hours in 5- to less than 14-year-olds, which are higher than the current guideline doses of 10 mg/kg every 12 hours for patients 6 months to less than 5-year-olds and 10 mg/kg every 24 hours for 5- to 16-year-olds. Similarly, based on the construction of a population PK model, more aggressive doses than the currently recommended 50 mg/kg every 8 or 12 hours for cefepime may be necessary in pediatric patients when simulating the effect against a gram-negative rod with an MIC of 8 mg/L.[164]

Example—Dose Derivation for Newer Clinical Challenge

VR is an 8-week-old, 5.5-kg female born at 38 weeks of gestation to a mother with gestational diabetes and hypertension. The infant is now suffering from a fever and increased respiratory distress at home after having been exposed to family members with COVID-19–positive antigen tests. The infant has mild bilateral ground-glass opacities on chest x-ray (CXR) but needs mechanical ventilation and a positive severe acute respiratory syndrome coronavirus 2 (SARS-CoV-2) polymerase chain reaction (PCR) test along with elevated C-reactive protein (CRP), ferritin, interleukin-6 (IL-6) levels, and lymphopenia, all suggestive of severe COVID-19. Remdesivir is ordered. What dose should be given to provide an AUC reflecting similar systemic exposure to that in treated adults?

FDA dosing: Neonates weighing 3.5 kg or more: intravenous (IV) loading dose: 5 mg/kg on day 1; followed by 2.5 mg/kg/dose once daily 5 to 10 days

$$CL = \text{Dose} \, (F)/\text{AUC} = a \, (\text{Wt})^b$$

$$CL_{\text{child}} = CL_{\text{adult}} \, (\text{Wt}_{\text{child}}/\text{Wt}_{\text{adult}})^b$$

Assuming the goal AUC is the same in the child as in the adult ($\approx$4,500 ng·hr/mL), then:

$$\text{Dose}_{\text{child}} = \text{Dose}_{\text{adult}} \, (\text{Wt}_{\text{child}}/\text{Wt}_{\text{adult}})^b$$

Using 70 kg weight for the adult and the recommended 200 mg remdesivir loading dose and 100 mg daily maintenance dose, and using an exponent of 1.1 for an infant less than 3 months as described earlier,[150] the loading dose for this child is calculated as follows:

$$\text{Dose}_{\text{child}} = 200 \, (5.5/70)^{1.1} = 12.18 \text{ mg} = 2.21 \text{ mg/kg}$$

And the maintenance dose would be half of that, or 1.1 mg/kg every 24 hours, providing systemic exposure equivalent to 100 mg every 24 hours as recommended in adults. This is consistent with a published simulation of remdesivir dosing for children and adolescents by weight category.[165] These doses are in contrast to the higher doses in the FDA recommendations.

More investigation of pharmacodynamic differences between children and adults and guidance of dosing using population PK with Bayesian adjustment based on individual parameter estimates subsequently modified by concentration feedback should assist both the practical application to individualize dosing for optimal response and the development and approval of new drug entities with optimized doses for the targeted age group of children and adolescents (see Figure 5.5).[5,111] Physiologically

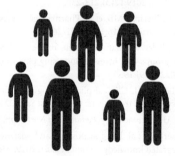

Drug-related considerations
- Lipophilicity
- Protein binding
- Degree of renal elimination
- Metabolism
- Molecular size

Dosing considerations
- Age grouping
- Body size metric (for weight-based dosing)
- Dose capping
- Recommended therapeutic range
- Available formulations
- Dosing route

Physiologic considerations
- Body size
- Binding-protein concentrations
- Blood flow
- Organ size
- Body fat
- GFR
- Metabolic enzymes
- Transporters

Methodological considerations
- Variability in sampling and dosing schemes
- Heterogeneity in underlying patient population
- Sample size
- Covariate selection
- Timing with drug development process

Patient population considerations
- Age range
- Dosing
- Concomitant drugs
- Comorbidities
- Pharmacogenetics
- Disease state

FIGURE 5.5 Factors to include in parameter derivation, assessment, and modeling for precision dosing in pediatric patients via population and physiologic pharmacokinetic methods. GFR, glomerular filtration rate. (From Gerhart JG, Balevic S, Sinha J, et al. Characterizing pharmacokinetics in children with obesity-physiological, drug, patient, and methodological considerations. *Front Pharmacol.* 2022;13:818726.)

based PK modeling, with full or limited parameterization, adds to the tools useful for initial prediction and pharmacometrics-guided dosing and precision medicine for pediatric patients.[62,166-169]

REFERENCES

1. ClinicalTrials.gov. What's new. Accessed January 31, 2023. https://clinicaltrials.gov/ct2/about-site/new

2. Moulis F, Durrieu G, Lapeyre-Mestre M. Off-label and unlicensed drug use in children population. *Therapie*. 2018;73(2):135-149.

3. Harrill AH, Samedy-Bates LA, Pawlyk AC, Ren Z. Advances in maternal, fetal, and pediatric safety and precision therapeutics supported by programs at the National Institute of Child Health and Human Development. *J Clin Pharmacol*. 2022;62(suppl 1):S9-S11.

4. Rieder MJ, Elzagallaai AA. Pharmacogenomics in children. *Methods Mol Biol*. 2022;2547:569-593.

5. Veluvolu SM, Grohar PJ. Importance of pharmacologic considerations in the development of targeted anticancer agents for children. *Curr Opin Pediatr*. 2023;35(1):91-96.

6. Vinks AA, Emoto C, Fukuda T. Modeling and simulation in pediatric drug therapy: application of pharmacometrics to define the right dose for children. *Clin Pharmacol Ther*. 2015;98(3):298-308.

7. Vinks AA, Barrett JS. Model-informed pediatric drug development: application of pharmacometrics to define the right dose for children. *J Clin Pharmacol*. 2021;61(suppl 1):S52-S59.

8. Shakhnovich V, Hornik CP, Kearns GL, Weigel J, Abdel-Rahman SM. How to conduct clinical trials in children: a tutorial. *Clin Transl Sci*. 2019;12(3):218-230.

9. Maagdenberg H, Vijverberg SJ, Bierings MB, et al. Pharmacogenomics in pediatric patients: towards personalized medicine. *Paediatr Drugs*. 2016;18(4):251-260.

10. Allegaert K, Abbasi MY, Michelet R, Olafuyi O. The impact of low cardiac output on propofol pharmacokinetics across age groups—an investigation using physiologically based pharmacokinetic modelling. *Pharmaceutics*. 2022;14(9):1957.

11. Tang F, Ng CM, Bada HS, Leggas M. Clinical pharmacology and dosing regimen optimization of neonatal opioid withdrawal syndrome treatments. *Clin Transl Sci*. 2021;14(4):1231-1249.

12. Valentine K, Kummick J. PICU pharmacology. *Pediatr Clin North Am*. 2022;69(3):509-529.

13. Raffaeli G, Pokorna P, Allegaert K, et al. Drug disposition and pharmacotherapy in neonatal ECMO: from fragmented data to integrated knowledge. *Front Pediatr*. 2019;7:360.

14. Standing JF. Understanding and applying pharmacometric modelling and simulation in clinical practice and research. *Br J Clin Pharmacol*. 2017;83(2):247-254.

15. Neal-Kluever A, Fisher J, Grylack L, Kakiuchi-Kiyota S, Halpern W. Physiology of the neonatal gastrointestinal system relevant to the disposition of orally administered medications. *Drug Metab Dispos*. 2019;47(3):296-313.

16. Johnson TN, Bonner JJ, Tucker GT, Turner DB, Jamei M. Development and applications of a physiologically-based model of paediatric oral drug absorption. *Eur J Pharm Sci*. 2018;115:57-67.

17. Stillhart C, Vučićević K, Augustijns P, et al. Impact of gastrointestinal physiology on drug absorption in special populations—an UNGAP review. *Eur J Pharm Sci*. 2020;147:105280.

18. Malkawi WA, AlRafayah E, AlHazabreh M, AbuLaila S, Al-Ghananeem A.M. Formulation challenges and strategies to develop pediatric dosage forms. *Children*. 2022;9(4):488.

19. Khan D, Kirby D, Bryson S, Shah M, Rahman Mohammed A. Paediatric specific dosage forms: patient and formulation considerations. *Int J Pharm*. 2022;616:121501.

20. Lee JJ, Price JC, Duren A, et al. Ultrasound evaluation of gastric emptying time in healthy term neonates after formula feeding. *Anesthesiology*. 2021;134(6):845-851.

21. Garrick MD. Human iron transporters. *Genes Nutr*. 2011;6(1):45-54.

22. Helman SL, Anderson GJ, Frazer DM. Dietary iron absorption during early postnatal life. *Biometals*. 2019;32(3):385-393.

23. Mirochnick M, Capparelli E, Connor J. Pharmacokinetics of zidovudine in infants: a population analysis across studies. *Clin Pharmacol Ther.* 1999;66(1):16-24.

24. Kiss M, Mbasu R, Nicolai J, et al. Ontogeny of small intestinal drug transporters and metabolizing enzymes based on targeted quantitative proteomics. *Drug Metab Dispos.* 2021;49(12):1038-1046.

25. Rodieux F, Gotta V, Pfister M, van den Anker JN. Causes and consequences of variability in drug transporter activity in pediatric drug therapy. *J Clin Pharmacol.* 2016;56(suppl 7):S173-S192.

26. Zhang X, Han Y, Huang W, Jin M, Gao Z. The influence of the gut microbiota on the bioavailability of oral drugs. *Acta Pharm Sin B.* 2021;11(7):1789-1812.

27. Tom-Revzon C. Erratic absorption of intramuscular antimicrobial delivery in infants and children. *Expert Opin Drug Metab Toxicol.* 2007;3(5):733-740.

28. Hua S. Physiological and pharmaceutical considerations for rectal drug formulations. *Front Pharmacol.* 2019;10:1196.

29. Mancini AJ. Skin. *Pediatrics.* 2004;113(4 suppl):1114-1119.

30. Kuiper-Prins E, Kerkhof GF, Reijnen CG, van Dijken PJ. A 12-day-old boy with methemoglobinemia after circumcision with local anesthesia (lidocaine/prilocaine). *Drug Saf Case Rep.* 2016;3(1):12.

31. Turner JW. Death of a child from topical diphenhydramine. *Am J Forensic Med Pathol.* 2009; 30(4):380-381.

32. Celestin MN, Musteata FM. Impact of changes in free concentrations and drug-protein binding on drug dosing regimens in special populations and disease states. *J Pharm Sci.* 2021;110(10):3331-3344.

33. Deb PK, Al-Attraqchi O, Prasad MR, Tekade RK. Protein and tissue binding: implication on pharmacokinetic parameters. In: Tekade RK, ed. *Dosage Form Design Considerations.* Academic Press; 2018:371-399.

34. Smits A, Roberts JA, Vella-Brincat JW, Allegaert K. Cefazolin plasma protein binding in different human populations: more than cefazolin-albumin interaction. *Int J Antimicrob Agents.* 2014;43(2):199-200.

35. De Cock RF, Smits A, Allegaert K, et al. Population pharmacokinetic modelling of total and unbound cefazolin plasma concentrations as a guide for dosing in preterm and term neonates. *J Antimicrob Chemother.* 2014;69(5):1330-1338.

36. Smits A, Pauwels S, Oyaert M, et al. Factors impacting unbound vancomycin concentrations in neonates and young infants. *Eur J Clin Microbiol Infect Dis.* 2018;37(8):1503-1510.

37. McNamara PJ, Meiman D. Predicting drug binding to human serum albumin and alpha one acid glycoprotein in diseased and age patient populations. *J Pharm Sci.* 2019;108(8):2737-2747.

38. Gonzalez D, Delmore P, Bloom BT, et al. Clindamycin pharmacokinetics and safety in preterm and term infants. *Antimicrob Agents Chemother.* 2016;60(5):2888-2894.

39. Krekels EHJ, Calvier EAM, van der Graaf PH, Knibbe CAJ. Children are not small adults, but can we treat them as such? *CPT Pharmacometrics Syst Pharmacol.* 2019;8(1):34-38.

40. Perlman KM, Myers-Phariss S, Rhodes JC. A shift from Demerol (meperidine) to Dilaudid (hydromorphone) improves pain control and decreases admissions for patients in sickle cell crisis. *J Emerg Nurs.* 2004;30(5):439-446.

41. Benner KW, Durham SH. Meperidine restriction in a pediatric hospital. *J Pediatr Pharmacol Ther.* 2011;16(3):185-190.

42. Sadhasivam S, Aruldhas BW, Packiasabapathy S, et al. A novel perioperative multidose methadone-based multimodal analgesic strategy in children achieved safe and low analgesic blood methadone levels enabling opioid-sparing sustained analgesia with minimal adverse effects. *Anesth Analg.* 2021; 133(2):327-337.

43. Oyaert M, Spriet I, Allegaert K, et al. Factors impacting unbound vancomycin concentrations in different patient populations. *Antimicrob Agents Chemother.* 2015;59(11):7073-7079.

44. Le J, Bradley JS, Murray W, et al. Improved vancomycin dosing in children using area under the curve exposure. *Pediatr Infect Dis J.* 2013;32(4):e155-e163.

45. De Cock PA, Desmet S, De Jaeger A, et al. Impact of vancomycin protein binding on target attainment in critically ill children: back to the drawing board? *J Antimicrob Chemother.* 2017;72(3):801-804.

46. Amin SB. Bilirubin binding capacity in the preterm neonate. *Clin Perinatol.* 2016;43(2):241-257.

47. Lee ZM, Yang YH, Chang LS, Chen CC, Yu HR, Kuo KC. Increased total serum bilirubin level post-ibuprofen use is inversely correlated with neonates' body weight. *Children.* 2022;9(8):1184.

48. Amin SB. Bilirubin-displacing effect of ceftriaxone in infants with unconjugated hyperbilirubinemia born at term. *J Pediatr.* 2023;254:91-95.

49. Kearin M, Kelly JG, O'Malley K. Digoxin "receptors" in neonates: an explanation of less sensitivity to digoxin than in adults. *Clin Pharmacol Ther.* 1980;28(3):346-349.

50. Gong Y, Chen Y, Li Q, Li Z. Population pharmacokinetic analysis of digoxin in Chinese neonates and infants. *J Pharmacol Sci.* 2014;125(2):142-149.

51. Upreti VV, Wahlstrom JL. Meta-analysis of hepatic cytochrome P450 ontogeny to underwrite the prediction of pediatric pharmacokinetics using physiologically based pharmacokinetic modeling. *J Clin Pharmacol.* 2016;56(3):266-283.

52. Sadler NC, Nandhikonda P, Webb-Robertson BJ, et al. Hepatic cytochrome P450 activity, abundance, and expression throughout human development. *Drug Metab Dispos.* 2016;44(7):984-991.

53. van Groen BD, Nicolai J, Kuik AC, et al. Ontogeny of hepatic transporters and drug-metabolizing enzymes in humans and in nonclinical species. *Pharmacol Rev.* 2021;73(2):597-678.

54. Lacroix D, Sonnier M, Moncion A, Cheron G, Cresteil T. Expression of CYP3A in the human liver— evidence that the shift between CYP3A7 and CYP3A4 occurs immediately after birth. *Eur J Biochem.* 1997;247(2):625-634.

55. Kraus DM, Fischer JH, Reitz SJ, et al. Alterations in theophylline metabolism during the first year of life. *Clin Pharmacol Ther.* 1993;54(4):351-359.

56. Pacifici GM. Clinical pharmacology of phenobarbital in neonates: effects, metabolism and pharmaco-kinetics. *Curr Pediatr Rev.* 2016;12(1):48-54.

57. Blake MJ, Gaedigk A, Pearce RE, et al. Ontogeny of dextromethorphan O- and N-demethylation in the first year of life. *Clin Pharmacol Ther.* 2007;81(4):510-516.

58. Matlock MK, Tambe A, Elliott-Higgins J, Hines RN, Miller GP, Swamidass SJ. A time-embedding network models the ontogeny of 23 hepatic drug metabolizing enzymes. *Chem Res Toxicol.* 2019;32(8):1707-1721.

59. Streekstra EJ, Russel FGM, van de Steeg E, de Wildt SN. Application of proteomics to understand mat-uration of drug metabolizing enzymes and transporters for the optimization of pediatric drug therapy. *Drug Discov Today Technol.* 2021;39:31-48.

60. Takahashi H, Ishikawa S, Nomoto S, et al. Developmental changes in pharmacokinetics and pharma-codynamics of warfarin enantiomers in Japanese children. *Clin Pharmacol Ther.* 2000;68(5):541-555.

61. Kanamori M, Takahashi H, Echizen H. Developmental changes in the liver weight- and body weight-normalized clearance of theophylline, phenytoin and cyclosporine in children. *Int J Clin Phar-macol Ther.* 2002;40(11):485-492.

62. van Rongen A, Krekels EH, Calvier EA, de Wildt SN, Vermeulen A, Knibbe CA. An update on the use of allometric and other scaling methods to scale drug clearance in children: towards decision tables. *Expert Opin Drug Metab Toxicol.* 2022;18(2):99-113.

63. Germovsek E, Barker CIS, Sharland M, Standing JF. Pharmacokinetic-pharmacodynamic modeling in pediatric drug development, and the importance of standardized scaling of clearance. *Clin Pharma-cokinet.* 2019;58(1):39-52.

64. Gerhart JG, Balevic S, Sinha J, et al. Characterizing pharmacokinetics in children with obesity-physiological, drug, patient, and methodological considerations. *Front Pharmacol.* 2022;13:818726.

65. Takahashi T, Smith AR, Jacobson PA, Fisher J, Rubin NT, Kirstein MN. Impact of obesity on voriconazole pharmacokinetics among pediatric hematopoietic cell transplant recipients. *Antimicrob Agents Chemother.* 2020;64(12):e00653-20.

66. Krogstad V, Peric A, Robertsen I, et al. Correlation of body weight and composition with hepatic activities of cytochrome P450 enzymes. *J Pharm Sci.* 2021;110(1):432-437.

67. Olafuyi O, Abbasi MY, Allegaert K. Physiologically based pharmacokinetic modelling of acetamino-phen in preterm neonates—the impact of metabolising enzyme ontogeny and reduced cardiac output. *Biopharm Drug Dispos.* 2021;42(9):401-417.

68. Cook SF, Stockmann C, Samiee-Zafarghandy S, et al. Neonatal maturation of paracetamol (Acetaminophen) glucuronidation, sulfation, and oxidation based on a parent-metabolite population pharmacokinetic model. *Clin Pharmacokinet.* 2016;55(11):1395-1411.

69. Acheampong P, Thomas SHL. Determinants of hepatotoxicity after repeated supratherapeutic paracetamol ingestion: systematic review of reported cases. *Br J Clin Pharmacol.* 2016;82(4):923-931.

70. Zhu R, Kiser JJ, Seifart HI, et al. The pharmacogenetics of NAT2 enzyme maturation in perinatally HIV exposed infants receiving isoniazid. *J Clin Pharmacol.* 2012;52(4):511-519.

71. Krekels EH, Danhof M, Tibboel D, Knibbe CA. Ontogeny of hepatic glucuronidation; methods and results. *Curr Drug Metab.* 2012;13(6):728-743.

72. Anderson BJ, Holford NHG. Mechanistic basis of using body size and maturation to predict clearance in humans. *Drug Metab Pharmacokinet.* 2009;24(1):25-36.

73. Anderson BJ, Larsson P. A maturation model for midazolam clearance. *Paediatr Anaesth.* 2011;21(3):302-308.

74. Capparelli EV, Englund JA, Connor JD, et al. Population pharmacokinetics and pharmacodynamics of zidovudine in HIV-infected infants and children. *J Clin Pharmacol.* 2003;43(2):133-140.

75. Capparelli EV, Mirochnick M, Dankner WM, et al; Pediatric AIDS Clinical Trials Group 331 Investigators. Pharmacokinetics and tolerance of zidovudine in preterm infants. *J Pediatr.* 2003;142(1):47-52.

76. Elmorsi Y, Barber J, Rostami-Hodjegan A. Ontogeny of hepatic drug transporters and relevance to drugs used in pediatrics. *Drug Metab Dispos.* 2016;44(7):992-998.

77. Anand KJ, Anderson BJ, Holford NH, et al. Morphine pharmacokinetics and pharmacodynamics in preterm and term neonates: secondary results from the NEOPAIN trial. *Br J Anaesth.* 2008;101(5):680-689.

78. Pacifici GM. Metabolism and pharmacokinetics of morphine in neonates: a review. *Clinics.* 2016;71(8):474-480.

79. Emoto C, Johnson TN, Neuhoff S, Hahn D, Vinks AA, Fukuda T. PBPK model of morphine incorporating developmental changes in hepatic OCT1 and UGT2B7 proteins to explain the variability in clearances in neonates and small infants. *CPT Pharmacometrics Syst Pharmacol.* 2018;7(7):464-473.

80. Yalcin N, Surmelioglu N, Allegaert K. Population pharmacokinetics in critically ill neonates and infants undergoing extracorporeal membrane oxygenation: a literature review. *BMJ Paediatr Open.* 2022;6(1):e001512.

81. Favie LMA, Groenendaal F, van den Broek MPH, et al; PharmaCool Study Group. Pharmacokinetics of morphine in encephalopathic neonates treated with therapeutic hypothermia. *PLoS One.* 2019;14(2):e0211910.

82. Hahn D, Emoto C, Vinks AA, Fukuda T. Developmental changes in hepatic Organic Cation Transporter OCT1 protein expression from neonates to children. *Drug Metab Dispos.* 2017;45(1):23-26.

83. Hahn D, Emoto C, Euteneuer JC, Mizuno T, Vinks AA, Fukuda T. Influence of OCT1 ontogeny and genetic variation on morphine disposition in critically ill neonates: lessons from PBPK modeling and clinical study. *Clin Pharmacol Ther.* 2019;105(3):761-768.

84. Fukuda T, Chidambaran V, Mizuno T, et al. OCT1 genetic variants influence the pharmacokinetics of morphine in children. *Pharmacogenomics.* 2013;14(10):1141-1151.

85. Sadhasivam S, Chidambaran V, Ngamprasertwong P, et al. Race and unequal burden of perioperative pain and opioid related adverse effects in children. *Pediatrics.* 2012;129(5):832-838.

86. Balyan R, Zhang X, Chidambaran V, et al. OCT1 genetic variants are associated with postoperative morphine-related adverse effects in children. *Pharmacogenomics.* 2017;18(7):621-629.

87. Livingstone MJ, Groenewald CB, Rabbitts JA, Palermo TM. Codeine use among children in the United States: a nationally representative study from 1996 to 2013. *Paediatr Anaesth.* 2017;27(1):19-27.

88. Tobias JD, Green TP, Cote CJ; Section on Anesthesiology and Pain Medicine; Committee on Drugs. Codeine: time to say "No". *Pediatrics.* 2016;138(4):e20162396.

89. Crews KR, Monte AA, Huddart R, et al. Clinical pharmacogenetics implementation consortium guideline for CYP2D6, OPRM1, and COMT genotypes and select opioid therapy. *Clin Pharmacol Ther.* 2021;110(4):888-896.

90. Yalcin N, Flint RB, van Schaik RHN, Simons SHP, Allegaert K. The impact of pharmacogenetics on pharmacokinetics and pharmacodynamics in neonates and infants: a systematic review. *Pharmgenomics Pers Med.* 2022;15:675-696.

91. Rahawi S, Naik H, Blake KV, et al. Knowledge and attitudes on pharmacogenetics among pediatricians. *J Hum Genet.* 2020;65(5):437-444.

92. Tang Girdwood SC, Rossow KM, Van Driest SL, Ramsey LB. Perspectives from the Society for Pediatric Research: pharmacogenetics for pediatricians. *Pediatr Res.* 2022;91(3):529-538.

93. Marek E, Momper JD, Hines RN, et al. Prediction of warfarin dose in pediatric patients: an evaluation of the predictive performance of several models. *J Pediatr Pharmacol Ther.* 2016;21(3):224-232.

94. Hamberg AK, Hellman J, Dahlberg J, Jonsson EN, Wadelius M. A Bayesian decision support tool for efficient dose individualization of warfarin in adults and children. *BMC Med Inform Decis Mak.* 2015;15:7.

95. Jacobo-Cabral CO, Garcia-Roca P, Romero-Tejeda EM, et al. Population pharmacokinetic analysis of tacrolimus in Mexican paediatric renal transplant patients: role of CYP3A5 genotype and formulation. *Br J Clin Pharmacol.* 2015;80(4):630-641.

96. Huang Q, Lin X, Wang Y, et al. Tacrolimus pharmacokinetics in pediatric nephrotic syndrome: a combination of population pharmacokinetic modelling and machine learning approaches to improve individual prediction. *Front Pharmacol.* 2022;13:942129.

97. Teusink A, Vinks A, Zhang K, et al. Genotype-directed dosing leads to optimized voriconazole levels in pediatric patients receiving hematopoietic stem cell transplantation. *Biol Blood Marrow Transplant.* 2016;22(3):482-486.

98. Wu Y, Lv C, Wu D, et al. Dosage optimization of voriconazole in children with haematological malignancies based on population pharmacokinetics. *J Clin Pharm Ther.* 2022;47(12):2245-2254.

99. Ramsey LB, Prows CA, Chidambaran V, et al. Implementation of CYP2D6-guided opioid therapy at Cincinnati Children's Hospital Medical Center. *Am J Health Syst Pharm.* 2023;zxad025.

100. Roberts TA, Wagner JA, Sandritter T, Black BT, Gaedigk A, Stancil SL. Retrospective review of pharmacogenetic testing at an Academic Children's Hospital. *Clin Transl Sci.* 2021;14(1):412-421.

101. Iacobelli S, Guignard JP. Maturation of glomerular filtration rate in neonates and infants: an overview. *Pediatr Nephrol.* 2021;36(6):1439-1446.

102. Correa LP, Gatto FR, Bressani GYS, Lanza K, Simoes ESAC. Nephrogenesis, renal function, and biomarkers in preterm newborns. *Curr Med Chem.* 2022;29(23):4097-4112.

103. Allegaert K, Anderson BJ, van den Anker JN, Vanhaesebrouck S, de Zegher F. Renal drug clearance in preterm neonates: relation to prenatal growth. *Ther Drug Monit.* 2007;29(3):284-291.

104. Rhodin MM, Anderson BJ, Peters AM, et al. Human renal function maturation: a quantitative description using weight and postmenstrual age. *Pediatr Nephrol.* 2009;24(1):67-76.

105. Sampson MR, Bloom BT, Lenfestey RW, et al; Best Pharmaceuticals for Children Act–Pediatric Trials Network. Population pharmacokinetics of intravenous acyclovir in preterm and term infants. *Pediatr Infect Dis J.* 2014;33(1):42-49.

106. Goldman J, Becker ML, Jones B, Clements M, Leeder JS. Development of biomarkers to optimize pediatric patient management: what makes children different? *Biomark Med.* 2011;5(6):781-794.

107. Pottel H. Measuring and estimating glomerular filtration rate in children. *Pediatr Nephrol.* 2017;32(2):249-263.

108. Dhont E, Windels C, Snauwaert E, et al. Reliability of glomerular filtration rate estimating formulas compared to iohexol plasma clearance in critically ill children. *Eur J Pediatr.* 2022;181(11):3851-3866.

109. André P, Chtioui H, Dao K, et al. Estimating glomerular filtration rate from serum creatinine concentration in children with augmented renal clearance: all formulas are equivocal, but some are more equivocal than others. *Kidney Int.* 2023;103(1):225-226.

110. Zhang Y, Sherwin CM, Gonzalez D, et al. Creatinine-based renal function assessment in pediatric drug development: an analysis using clinical data for renally eliminated drugs. *Clin Pharmacol Ther.* 2021;109(1):263-269.

111. Llanos-Paez CC, Staatz C, Lawson R, Hennig S. Comparison of methods to estimate glomerular filtration rate in paediatric oncology patients. *J Paediatr Child Health*. 2018;54(2):141-147.

112. Cristea S, Krekels EHJ, Allegaert K, Knibbe CAJ. The predictive value of glomerular filtration rate-based scaling of pediatric clearance and doses for drugs eliminated by glomerular filtration with varying protein-binding properties. *Clin Pharmacokinet*. 2020;59(10):1291-1301.

113. Cristea S, Krekels EHJ, Rostami-Hodjegan A, Allegaert K, Knibbe CAJ. The influence of drug properties and ontogeny of transporters on pediatric renal clearance through glomerular filtration and active secretion: a simulation-based study. *AAPS J*. 2020;22(4):87.

114. Rodieux F, Wilbaux M, van den Anker JN, Pfister M. Effect of kidney function on drug kinetics and dosing in neonates, infants, and children. *Clin Pharmacokinet*. 2015;54(12):1183-1204.

115. Salem F, Johnson TN, Hodgkinson ABJ, Ogungbenro K, Rostami-Hodjegan A. Does "Birth" as an event impact maturation trajectory of renal clearance via glomerular filtration? Reexamining data in preterm and full-term neonates by avoiding the creatinine bias. *J Clin Pharmacol*. 2021;61(2):159-171.

116. Wade KC, Wu D, Kaufman DA, et al. Population pharmacokinetics of fluconazole in young infants. *Antimicrob Agents Chemother*. 2008;52(11):4043-4049.

117. De Cock RF, Allegaert K, Schreuder MF, et al. Maturation of the glomerular filtration rate in neonates, as reflected by amikacin clearance. *Clin Pharmacokinet*. 2012;51(2):105-117.

118. Rhoney DH, Metzger SA, Nelson NR. Scoping review of augmented renal clearance in critically ill pediatric patients. *Pharmacotherapy*. 2021;41(10):851-863.

119. Shimamoto Y, Verstegen RHJ, Mizuno T, Schechter T, Allen U, Ito S. Population pharmacokinetics of vancomycin in paediatric patients with febrile neutropenia and augmented renal clearance: development of new dosing recommendations. *J Antimicrob Chemother*. 2021;76(11):2932-2940.

120. Scully PT, Lam WM, Coronado Munoz AJ, Modem VM. Augmented renal clearance of vancomycin in suspected sepsis: single-center, retrospective pediatric cohort. *Pediatr Crit Care Med*. 2022;23(6):444-452.

121. Avedissian SN, Rohani R, Bradley J, Le J, Rhodes NJ. Optimizing aminoglycoside dosing regimens for critically ill pediatric patients with augmented renal clearance: a convergence of parametric and non-parametric population approaches. *Antimicrob Agents Chemother*. 2021;65(4):e02629-20.

122. de Cacqueray N, Hirt D, Zheng Y, et al. Cefepime population pharmacokinetics and dosing regimen optimization in critically ill children with different renal function. *Clin Microbiol Infect*. 2022;28(10):1389.e1-1389.e7.

123. Beranger A, Benaboud S, Urien S, et al. Piperacillin population pharmacokinetics and dosing regimen optimization in critically ill children with normal and augmented renal clearance. *Clin Pharmacokinet*. 2019;58(2):223-233.

124. Avedissian SN, Skochko SM, Le J, et al. Use of simulation strategies to predict subtherapeutic mero-penem exposure caused by augmented renal clearance in critically ill pediatric patients with sepsis. *J Pediatr Pharmacol Ther*. 2020;25(5):413-422.

125. Abdalla S, Briand C, Oualha M, et al. Population pharmacokinetics of intravenous and oral acyclovir and oral valacyclovir in pediatric population to optimize dosing regimens. *Antimicrob Agents Chemother*. 2020;64(12):e01426-20.

126. Nguyen T, Oualha M, Briand C, et al. Population pharmacokinetics of intravenous ganciclovir and oral valganciclovir in a pediatric population to optimize dosing regimens. *Antimicrob Agents Chemother*. 2021;65(3):e02254-20.

127. Klein P, Herr D, Pearl PL, et al. Results of phase II pharmacokinetic study of levetiracetam for prevention of post-traumatic epilepsy. *Epilepsy Behav*. 2012;24(4):457-461.

128. Surtees TL, Kumar I, Garton HJL, et al. Levetiracetam prophylaxis for children admitted with traumatic brain injury. *Pediatr Neurol*. 2022;126:114-119.

129. Andre P, Diezi L, Dao K, et al. Ensuring sufficient trough plasma concentrations for broad-spectrum beta-lactam antibiotics in children with malignancies: beware of augmented renal clearance! *Front Pediatr*. 2021;9:768438.

130. Samuels S, Park K, Bhatt-Mehta V, et al. Pediatric efficacy extrapolation in drug development submitted to the US Food and Drug Administration 2015-2020. *J Clin Pharmacol*. 2023;63(3):307-313.

131. Colin PJ, Allegaert K, Thomson AH, et al. Vancomycin pharmacokinetics throughout life: results from a pooled population analysis and evaluation of current dosing recommendations. *Clin Pharmacokinet.* 2019;58(6):767-780.

132. Mulla H. Understanding developmental pharmacodynamics: importance for drug development and clinical practice. *Paediatr Drugs.* 2010;12(4):223-233.

133. Pan SD, Zhu LL, Chen M, Xia P, Zhou Q. Weight-based dosing in medication use: what should we know? *Patient Prefer Adherence.* 2016;10:549-560.

134. Shamsaee E, Huws A, Gill A, McWilliam SJ, Hawcutt DB. Ibuprofen efficacy, tolerability and safety in obese children: a systematic review. *Arch Dis Child.* 2023;108(1):67-71.

135. Chatelut E, Puisset F. The scientific basis of body surface area-based dosing. *Clin Pharmacol Ther.* 2014;95(4):359-361.

136. Bins S, Ratain MJ, Mathijssen RH. Conventional dosing of anticancer agents: precisely wrong or just inaccurate? *Clin Pharmacol Ther.* 2014;95(4):361-364.

137. Nijstad AL, Barnett S, Lalmohamed A, et al. Clinical pharmacology of cytotoxic drugs in neonates and infants: providing evidence-based dosing guidance. *Eur J Cancer.* 2022;164:137-154.

138. Saul JP, Ross B, Schaffer MS, et al. Pharmacokinetics and pharmacodynamics of sotalol in a pediatric population with supraventricular and ventricular tachyarrhythmia. *Clin Pharmacol Ther.* 2001;69(3):145-157.

139. Yang XM, Leroux S, Storme T, et al. Body surface area-based dosing regimen of caspofungin in children: a population pharmacokinetics confirmatory study. *Antimicrob Agents Chemother.* 2019;63(7):e00248-19.

140. Murphy WA, Adiwidjaja J, Sjostedt N, et al. Considerations for physiologically based modeling in liver disease: from nonalcoholic fatty liver (NAFL) to nonalcoholic steatohepatitis (NASH). *Clin Pharmacol Ther.* 2023;113(2):275-297.

141. Thompson PA, Rosner GL, Matthay KK, et al. Impact of body composition on pharmacokinetics of doxorubicin in children: a Glaser Pediatric Research Network study. *Cancer Chemother Pharmacol.* 2009;64(2):243-251.

142. Arndt C, Hawkins D, Anderson JR, Breitfeld P, Womer R, Meyer W. Age is a risk factor for chemotherapy-induced hepatopathy with vincristine, dactinomycin, and cyclophosphamide. *J Clin Oncol.* 2004;22(10):1894-1901.

143. Barnett S, Hellmann F, Parke E, et al. Vincristine dosing, drug exposure and therapeutic drug monitoring in neonate and infant cancer patients. *Eur J Cancer.* 2022;164:127-136.

144. Raman V, Krishnamurthy S, Harichandrakumar KT. Body weight-based prednisolone versus body surface area-based prednisolone regimen for induction of remission in children with nephrotic syndrome: a randomized, open-label, equivalence clinical trial. *Pediatr Nephrol.* 2016;31(4):595-604.

145. Johnson TN. The problems in scaling adult drug doses to children. *Arch Dis Child.* 2008;93(3):207-211.

146. Steinberg I, Kimberlin DW. Acyclovir dosing and acute kidney injury: deviations and direction. *J Pediatr.* 2015;166(6):1341-1344.

147. Rao S, Abzug MJ, Carosone-Link P, et al. Intravenous acyclovir and renal dysfunction in children: a matched case control study. *J Pediatr.* 2015;166(6):1462-8.e1-4.

148. Calvier EA, Krekels EH, Valitalo PA, et al. Allometric scaling of clearance in paediatric patients: when does the magic of 0.75 fade? *Clin Pharmacokinet.* 2017;56(3):273-285.

149. Mahmood I. Prediction of drug clearance in premature and mature neonates, infants, and children $</=2$ years of age: a comparison of the predictive performance of 4 allometric models. *J Clin Pharmacol.* 2016;56(6):733-739.

150. Mahmood I, Tegenge MA. A comparative study between allometric scaling and physiologically based pharmacokinetic modeling for the prediction of drug clearance from neonates to adolescents. *J Clin Pharmacol.* 2019;59(2):189-197.

151. Anderson BJ, Holford NH. Understanding dosing: children are small adults, neonates are immature children. *Arch Dis Child.* 2013;98(9):737-744.

152. Lu H, Rosenbaum S. A model for maturation of renal function in pediatric population developed from the clearance of vancomycin and gentamicin. *J Pharmacokinet Pharmacodyn.* 2013;40:S51.

153. Roth-Cline M, Nelson RM. Microdosing studies in children: a US regulatory perspective. *Clin Pharmacol Ther.* 2015;98(3):232-233.

154. Moorthy GS, Vedar C, Downes KJ, Fitzgerald JC, Scheetz MH, Zuppa AF. Microsampling assays for pharmacokinetic analysis and therapeutic drug monitoring of antimicrobial drugs in children: a critical review. *Ther Drug Monit.* 2021;43(3):335-345.

155. Altamimi MI, Choonara I, Sammons H. Invasiveness of pharmacokinetic studies in children: a systematic review. *BMJ Open.* 2016;6(7):e010484.

156. Germovsek E, Barker CI, Sharland M, Standing JF. Scaling clearance in paediatric pharmacokinetics: all models are wrong, which are useful? *Br J Clin Pharmacol.* 2017;83(4):777-790.

157. Brussee JM, Calvier EA, Krekels EH, et al. Children in clinical trials: towards evidence-based pediatric pharmacotherapy using pharmacokinetic-pharmacodynamic modeling. *Expert Rev Clin Pharmacol.* 2016;9(9):1235-1244.

158. Mulugeta Y, Barrett JS, Nelson R, et al. Exposure matching for extrapolation of efficacy in pediatric drug development. *J Clin Pharmacol.* 2016;56(11):1326-1334.

159. Laer S, Elshoff JP, Meibohm B, et al. Development of a safe and effective pediatric dosing regimen for sotalol based on population pharmacokinetics and pharmacodynamics in children with supraventricular tachycardia. *J Am Coll Cardiol.* 2005;46(7):1322-1330.

160. Chung A, Carroll M, Almeida P, et al. Early infliximab clearance predicts remission in children with Crohn's disease. *Dig Dis Sci.* 2022;68(5):1995-2005.

161. Patel K, Goldman JL. Safety concerns surrounding quinolone use in children. *J Clin Pharmacol.* 2016;56(9):1060-1075.

162. Courter JD, Nichols KR, Kazazian C, Girotto JE. Pharmacodynamically guided levofloxacin dosing for pediatric community-acquired pneumonia. *J Pediatric Infect Dis Soc.* 2017;6(2):118-122.

163. Bradley JS, Byington CL, Shah SS, et al. The management of community-acquired pneumonia in infants and children older than 3 months of age: clinical practice guidelines by the Pediatric Infectious Diseases Society and the Infectious Diseases Society of America. *Clin Infect Dis.* 2011;53(7):e25-e76.

164. Shoji K, Bradley JS, Reed MD, van den Anker JN, Domonoske C, Capparelli EV. Population pharmacokinetic assessment and pharmacodynamic implications of pediatric cefepime dosing for susceptible-dose-dependent organisms. *Antimicrob Agents Chemother.* 2016;60(4):2150-2156.

165. Maharaj AR, Wu H, Hornik CP, et al; Best Pharmaceuticals for Children Act–Pediatric Trials Network Steering Committee. Simulated assessment of pharmacokinetically guided dosing for investigational treatments of pediatric patients with coronavirus disease 2019. *JAMA Pediatr.* 2020;174(10):e202422.

166. Allegaert K, Abbasi MY, Annaert P, Olafuyi O. Current and future physiologically based pharmacokinetic (PBPK) modeling approaches to optimize pharmacotherapy in preterm neonates. *Expert Opin Drug Metab Toxicol.* 2022;18(5):301-312.

167. Freriksen JJM, van der Heijden JEM, de Hoop-Sommen MA, Greupink R, de Wildt SN. Physiologically Based Pharmacokinetic (PBPK) model-informed dosing guidelines for pediatric clinical care: a pragmatic approach for a special population. *Paediatr Drugs.* 2023;25(1):5-11.

168. Mahmood I. Prediction of total and renal clearance of renally secreted drugs in neonates and infants (</=3 months of age). *J Clin Transl Res.* 2022;8(6):445-452.

169. van Groen BD, Pilla Reddy V, Badee J, et al. Pediatric pharmacokinetics and dose predictions: a report of a satellite meeting to the 10th juvenile toxicity symposium. *Clin Transl Sci.* 2021;14(1):29-35.

6

PHARMACOGENETICS

Reginald F. Frye and Scott A. Mosley

Learning Objectives

By the end of the chapter on pharmacogenetics, the learner shall be able to:

1. Summarize how genetic variation in drug-disposition proteins affects therapeutic effectiveness and toxicity.
2. Describe the molecular basis for a genetic variation influencing the functional activity of drug-disposition proteins.
3. Discuss the clinical relevance of genetic polymorphisms of important drug-disposition proteins.
4. Explore the potential applications of pharmacogenetics to tailor drug therapy in the context of therapeutic drug management.

Variability in drug response has long been recognized. While differences in drug response based on hereditary have been described by ancient civilizations, Professor Friedrich Vogel, a human geneticist, first published the term "pharmacogenetics" in 1959 when describing clinical relationships between pharmacology and genetics.[1] Inherent differences in pharmacokinetics, pharmacodynamics, or both contribute to the variability, and therapeutic drug monitoring (TDM) emerged in the 1970s as a means to individualize (or personalize) therapy for a patient. In addition to patient factors, such as adherence, age, sex, weight, and renal function, the observed variability in drug response may result from genetic variation in genes that encode for drug-disposition proteins (ie, drug-metabolizing enzymes and drug transporters) and drug-target proteins (eg, receptors). Studies in this field have evolved from examining genetic variants within one or more candidate genes (pharmacogenetics) to studies evaluating multiple genes or the entire genome (pharmacogenomics). This chapter reviews clinically relevant consequences of common genetic variation in drug-disposition proteins on drug pharmacokinetics and describes how this information provides the foundation for pharmacogenetics-informed therapeutic considerations and drug monitoring.

PHARMACOGENETICS AND DRUG DISPOSITION

Most marketed drugs are metabolized by oxidative metabolism, which is primarily mediated by enzymes in the cytochrome P450 (CYP) family.[2] The expression and metabolic activity of these enzymes are modulated by many nongenetic factors, including age, concomitant drugs or dietary supplements, sex, disease states (eg, liver disease, kidney disease, or inflammatory conditions), and environmental influences (eg, smoking).[2] In addition, genetic variation in genes that encode for drug-metabolizing enzymes may contribute substantially to variability in pharmacokinetics. The net effect is that CYP enzyme activity has been reported to vary substantially between individuals, yielding potentially large differences in drug clearance and corresponding steady-state drug concentrations, which, in turn, may influence therapeutic effect (eg, adverse events and therapeutic failure).[3]

The standard nomenclature for individual CYP enzymes includes the root "CYP," followed by an Arabic number designating the enzyme family (based on sequence homology), a letter for the enzyme subfamily, and another number denoting the individual CYP enzyme (eg, CYP2D6). For each enzyme, the reference or "wild-type" allele is denoted as *1. Allelic variants (ie, alleles having one or more single-nucleotide polymorphisms [SNPs]) are sequentially numbered as identified (ie, *2, *3, etc).[4] Throughout this chapter, consistent with formatting in published literature, genes are italicized, whereas enzymes resulting from gene expression are not. A comprehensive listing of pharmacogenetic variants is available at https://www.pharmvar.org/.

SNP, a common type of genetic variation in the human genome, may contribute significantly to variability in drug response owing to effects on the expression or function of drug-disposition proteins and corresponding effects on drug pharmacokinetics. An SNP in a gene that encodes for a drug-disposition protein, such as a CYP enzyme, may cause changes in the amino acid sequence, yielding a nonsynonymous protein with altered function, that is, an enzyme with decreased (most common) or increased metabolic activity. For some enzymes, allelic variants result from SNPs that create an altered splice site, frameshift mutation, premature stop codon, or gene deletion, each of which produces a nonfunctional (or loss-of-function) allele. These variations can have a profound impact on the ability of an individual to metabolize some drugs; carriers of these alleles may be at risk for toxicities associated with high drug concentrations, particularly with narrow therapeutic index drugs that are metabolized by a single enzyme.[5] In contrast, some CYP genes exhibit gene duplication events, whereby an individual carries multiple functional copies of the gene. These individuals may demonstrate substantially increased drug metabolism that results in therapeutic failure owing to lower-than-expected drug concentrations.

CYP ENZYMES

Genetic variation has been described for each of the major CYP enzymes that contribute to human drug metabolism.[2,5,6] The genes that encode for some CYP enzymes (eg, CYP1A2, CYP2E1, CYP3A4) are fairly well conserved with few or no clinically relevant polymorphisms reported. However, other CYP-encoding genes (eg, *CYP2B6, CYP2C9, CYP2C19, CYP2D6*) are highly polymorphic, and variants having substantial functional consequences are known. The CYP enzymes that mediate the majority of drug metabolism in humans are in the subfamilies CYP2C, CYP2D, and CYP3A.

CYP2D6

The gene that encodes the CYPD6 enzyme is one of the best characterized *CYP* genes with more than 130 known allelic variants. Early studies in large populations showed that clearance for some CYP2D6-metabolized drugs is an inherited trait.[7] For example, metabolism of the antihypertensive and CYP2D6 substrate drugs debrisoquine and sparteine was shown to be an inherited trait and most notably absent in up to 10% of the population.[8] It is interesting to note that in drug metabolism pharmacogenetics research, the phenotype typically preceded the genotype, meaning that the phenotype (eg, drug clearance) was used to categorize individuals into activity or "phenotype groups" originally defined as "extensive metabolizers" or "poor metabolizers" (PMs).[9] It was several years later that the genetic basis for the observation of clearance as an inherited trait was linked to an SNP in the *CYP2D6* gene.[7,8] Though subsequent research included additional CYP2D6 substrates, phenotypes were further divided to reflect more granular differences in metabolite ratios and are currently described as PMs, intermediate, normal (NMs), and ultrarapid metabolizers (UM). For example, only individuals who lacked any ability to metabolize a CYP2D6 substrate are currently labeled as PMs.

The CYP2D6 enzyme constitutes only 2% to 4% of the total CYP protein content in the human liver, but this enzyme metabolizes 25% to 30% of all clinically used drugs.[2] Substrates include antiarrhythmics, antidepressants, antipsychotics, β-blockers, and codeine.[2] About 5% to 10% of whites and 1% of Asians exhibit the PM phenotype.[3,10] The most common nonfunctional alleles are *CYP2D6*3, CYP2D6*4, CYP2D6*5,* and *CYP2D*6.* The PM phenotype results when an individual is homozygous for loss-of-function alleles, which may be the same or different alleles (eg, *CYP2D6*4/*4* or *CYP2D6*4/*6*). There are also three common variant alleles that have been associated with decreased catalytic activity: *CYP2D6*10,* found predominantly in Asians; *CYP2D6*17,* found in blacks; and *CYP2D6*41,* found in whites and blacks. In addition to NMs, some individuals (up to 5% of whites) exhibit greatly enhanced clearance, termed *ultrarapid metabolizers* (UMs), because they carry multiple copies of the *CYP2D6* gene (ie, gene duplication). The nomenclature for *CYP2D6* gene duplication is *CYP2D6** × *N,* where *N* indicates the presence of two or more copies of the gene on the same chromosome, resulting in the UM phenotype.[10] Adding to the complexity of interpreting *CYP2D6* genotype–derived phenotype, clinically relevant drug interactions (eg, CYP2D6 inhibitors) can alter the observed phenotype so that the genotype-based phenotype does not match the clinical phenotype, leading to a gene-drug-drug interaction termed "phenoconversion."[11]

A broad range of substrates are metabolized by CYP2D6, and as it is with other enzymes, the clinical consequence of *CYP2D6* genetic variation depends on the characteristics of the drug and the extent to which CYP2D6 metabolizes it. In general, compared with NMs, PMs exhibit much higher plasma drug concentrations, whereas UMs exhibit much lower plasma drug concentrations. If the parent drug is active and inactive metabolite formed via CYP2D6, then a PM is at risk of an exaggerated pharmacodynamic effect and adverse effects and a UM is at risk of therapeutic failure. If the drug administered is a prodrug converted to an active metabolite (eg, codeine to morphine or tramadol to O-desmethyltramadol), then a PM is at risk of therapeutic failure and a UM is at greater risk of adverse effects owing to respective low and high concentrations of the active metabolite.[12] For example, because CYP2D6 mediates the metabolism of codeine to the active moiety morphine, PMs will not experience the expected therapeutic effect. Conversely, UMs exhibit increased formation of morphine, which can result in an augmented pharmacodynamic effect and severe adverse effects, including respiratory depression and death.[10]

CYP2B6

The CYP2B6 enzyme constitutes 3% to 6% of total hepatic CYP content.[13] CYP2B6 plays an important role in the metabolism of cyclophosphamide, diazepam, efavirenz, and nevirapine. Nonsynonymous polymorphisms in the CYP2B6 gene that are functionally relevant include CYP2B6*4, CYP2B6*5, CYP2B6*6, CYP2B6*9, and CYP2B6*18.[13,14] The nonsynonymous SNP at position 516 (G>T) causes decreased CYP2B6 expression and activity through aberrant splicing and reduced functional messenger RNA (mRNA); this polymorphism is part of the CYP2B6*6, CYP2B6*7, CYP2B6*9, CYP2B6*13, CYP2B6*19, and CYP2B6*20 alleles.[14]

Genetic variation in CYP2B6 contributes to clinically relevant differences in systemic exposure for efavirenz, which has a narrow therapeutic index.[15] The CYP2B6 rs4803419 (g.15582C>T) has been independently associated with higher efavirenz estimated C_{min} values.[16] In addition, homozygous 516T carriers may have 2- to 3-fold higher area under the curve values than 516G carriers.[14,15]

CYP2C9

The major CYP2C enzyme found in the human liver is CYP2C9, which mediates the metabolism of several clinically important drugs, including the narrow therapeutic index drugs phenytoin and warfarin.[17,18] Sixty variant alleles have been identified in the CYP2C9 gene (https://www.pharmvar.org/), many of which have clinically important racial differences in allele frequencies. SNPs within the coding region produce the variant alleles CYP2C9*2 and CYP2C9*3, which are found in up to 35% of whites but are much less prevalent in blacks and Asians; the CYP2C9*5 allele is found only in blacks.[18]

The clinical relevance of CYP2C9 polymorphisms stems primarily from the contribution of CYP2C9 to the metabolism of the narrow therapeutic index drugs phenytoin and warfarin. The CYP2C9 variant alleles that have been identified are associated with decreased enzyme activity, though the magnitude of effect is substrate dependent. For warfarin, a strong relationship between the CYP2C9 genotype and S-warfarin pharmacokinetics has been demonstrated. The impact of CYP2C9 genotype on S-warfarin pharmacokinetics affects the daily dose of warfarin required to obtain a target international normalized ratio (INR). While CYP2C9 has been described as having the greatest genetic impact on variability, other pharmacokinetic (CYP4F2) and pharmacodynamic (VKORC1) genes are also known to contribute to variability in response to dose.[18]

Phenytoin is primarily metabolized by CYP2C9 and, to a lesser extent, CYP2C19. Even modest changes in CYP2C9 activity are likely to be clinically relevant with phenytoin because of its nonlinear pharmacokinetics. The dose required to achieve a therapeutic concentration is smaller in variant *CYP2C9* allele carriers compared with patients having the *CYP2C9*1/*1* genotype. In addition, patients with one or more variant alleles appear to be more susceptible to concentration-related adverse events, particularly during therapy initiation.[17]

CYP2C19

CYP2C19 is involved in the metabolism of drugs, such as citalopram, clopidogrel, diazepam, escitalopram, proton-pump inhibitors (PPIs) (eg, lansoprazole, omeprazole, and pantoprazole), sertraline, and voriconazole. Nonfunctional variants of *CYP2C19* are associated with the PM phenotype, which occurs in 1% to 3% of whites and 13% to 23% of Asians.[19] The most common allelic variants are *CYP2C19*2* and *CYP2C19*3*, which together account for about 95% of PMs. An SNP in the promoter region of the *CYP2C19* gene (*CYP2C19*17*) confers ultrarapid enzyme activity because of enhanced enzyme expression; the allele is relatively common, occurring at a frequency of up to 25% in whites.[2,6,19]

The presence of *CYP2C19* loss-of-function alleles can not only increase the risk of concentration-related adverse effects but may also lead to diminished response or treatment failure with drugs that require activation by CYP2C19. For example, the oral antiplatelet drug clopidogrel is a prodrug that undergoes a two-step activation process in which about 15% of the dose is converted to an active metabolite. Substantial evidence indicates that clopidogrel activation is critically dependent on CYP2C19 activity.[20]

The *CYP2C19*17* allele causes increased enzyme expression that results in rapid CYP2C19 activity. The increased expression yields higher metabolism and increased clearance, which may result in treatment failure for drugs such as voriconazole and PPIs. Indeed, voriconazole exposure in *CYP2C19*17* carriers was 52% of that achieved in CYP2C19 NMs and 15% of that achieved in CYP2C19 PMs.[19] Pharmacokinetic studies evaluating pantoprazole, a first-generation PPI, demonstrated that individuals who were homozygous for CYP2C19*17 had lower plasma concentrations, compared to NMs.[21] These lower plasma levels were clinically significant as they correlated with decreased rates of successful acid suppression (pH > 4) for *CYP2C19*17* carriers.[22]

CYP3A4 and CYP3A5

CYP3A enzymes are the most abundantly expressed enzymes in both the liver and the intestine. CYP3A enzymes constitute 30% and 70% of the total CYP enzyme content in the human liver and intestine, respectively, and are responsible for the metabolism of almost 50% of marketed drugs. CYP3A4 is considered the most abundant and clinically significant enzyme in human drug metabolism; CYP3A5 is important for some drugs because it is polymorphically expressed.[2,6]

Over 30 allelic variants of *CYP3A4* have been identified (https://www.pharmvar.org/gene/CYP3A4), but none of the variants identified are considered a loss-of-function allele and nonsynonymous polymorphisms are rare. In vitro and in vivo studies have demonstrated that *CYP3A4*22* is associated with reduced hepatic expression of CYP3A4 mRNA and CYP3A4 metabolic activity, but the clinical impact of these variants is unclear.[23,24] The most common variant is *CYP3A4*1B*, which is an SNP in the promoter region that has a modest functional consequence. However, a loss-of-function allele has been identified in the gene that encodes for CYP3A5 that creates an aberrant splice site and results in a truncated, non-functional protein (*CYP3A5*3* allele).[25] Identification of this SNP explains some variability in CYP3A5 expression—only people who carry at least one copy of the *CYP3A5*1* allele express CYP3A5. Only 20% of whites and 75% of blacks express CYP3A5.[25]

There is tremendous interindividual variability in CYP3A-mediated metabolism, with the clearance of some substrate drugs varying up to 20-fold. However, it appears that environmental influences affecting gene expression (eg, inhibition or induction), rather than genetic variation, are the most important factors contributing to variability in CYP3A4 activity. CYP3A5 may be important with respect to interindividual variability in CYP3A-mediated metabolism. It is estimated that CYP3A5 accounts for up to 50% of the total CYP3A content in people with at least one *CYP3A5*1* allele. The only drug for which *CYP3A5* genotype has consistently been shown to be clinically important is the immunosuppressant tacrolimus.[25] The dose required to achieve target therapeutic plasma concentrations in adult and pediatric transplant patients is typically 1.5- to 2-fold higher in CYP3A5 expressers (*CYP3A5*1/*1*) compared with nonexpressers (*CYP3A5*3/*3*).[25,26]

PHARMACOGENETICS-INFORMED THERAPEUTIC DRUG MONITORING

One goal of precision medicine is to utilize genetic results and other patient-specific factors to select drug therapies and dosing regimens to maximize effectiveness and minimize toxicity, thereby avoiding therapeutic misadventures and achieving optimal therapeutic outcomes. Traditional TDM has a similar goal and accounts for nongenetic and genetic factors that contribute to pharmacokinetic and pharmacodynamic variability. However, pharmacogenetics can be used to provide information that may be used before the initiation of therapy to decide the appropriateness and risk of drug therapy.

Drugs that have a narrow therapeutic index and are extensively or exclusively metabolized by a polymorphic enzyme (eg, CYP2C9, CYP2D6, CYP3A5) are ideal candidates for this approach. Preemptive genotyping for variants of drug-metabolizing enzymes may help guide successful treatment, such as through the development of dosing recommendations for different genetic subpopulations of patients. For example, the Clinical Pharmacogenetics Implementation Consortium (CPIC) has developed a guideline for *CYP3A5* genotype–guided dosing regimens for tacrolimus (Figure 6.1).[25] The genotype-guided dose is intended to help achieve a therapeutic concentration earlier in therapy; traditional concentration monitoring then ensures that the target concentration is achieved or the dose is adjusted accordingly.[27] Although there is evidence to support this approach, prospective clinical studies to assess outcomes and costs are required to support the implementation of this approach in clinical practice.

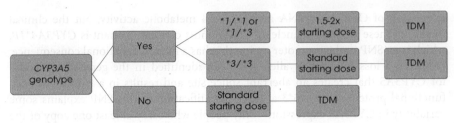

FIGURE 6.1 Pharmacogenetics-informed therapeutic drug monitoring: genotype-guided dosing for tacrolimus based on *CYP3A5* genotype. TDM, therapeutic drug monitoring.

CLINICAL PHARMACOGENETICS IMPLEMENTATION CONSORTIUM

The CPIC (https://cpicpgx.org/) is a collaboration of international pharmacogenetics experts and was formed in 2009 with a primary goal to address barriers to implementation of pharmacogenetic tests into clinical practice.[28] CPIC publishes guidelines that advise on how best to use genetic information, such as *CYP3A5* genotype, in clinical practice to guide drug therapy (eg, tacrolimus). The guidelines do not make recommendations regarding whether genetic testing should be performed, but rather advise on how to use existing genetic information to support clinical decision-making. The guidelines are peer reviewed, published as open access, and updated regularly. The CPIC website (https://cpicpgx.org/) provides a valuable resource for additional information about specific gene-drug pairs and recommendations for drug therapy management. The guidelines have a standardized format that includes background information on genetic variability and its relevance to the drug, genotype function translation tables, and, importantly, a summary of the levels of evidence and strength of recommendation for dosing recommendations. The CPIC guidelines are used by some institutions as the rationale and justification for implementing pharmacogenetic testing. In this text, pharmacogenomic information is included, and the CPIC guidelines are noted when relevant in the individual drug chapters—*CYP2C9*/phenytoin,[17] *CYP2C19*/voriconazole,[19] and *CYP3A5*/tacrolimus.[25]

Patient Case

SA is a 70-year non-Hispanic Black male with a history of hypertension and type 2 diabetes mellitus. He presents to the emergency department complaining of occasional palpitations that have been going on and off for 5 days. He has not noticed any signs of dizziness, lightheadedness, or weakness.

SA is diagnosed with new onset valvular atrial fibrillation and was started on metoprolol tartrate 25 mg by mouth twice daily. The patient agrees with his medical team's decision to begin anticoagulant therapy with warfarin before attempting an elective cardioversion as an outpatient. He will be considered a new patient and has not taken any doses of warfarin yet.

His current INR is 1.1. He reports that he has never smoked and drinks one to two alcoholic drinks per week. His home medications include losartan 25 mg by mouth once daily, atorvastatin 20 mg by mouth once daily, and metformin 1,000 mg by mouth twice daily.

Objective:

Weight:	86 kg
Height:	178 cm
Blood pressure:	132/83 mm Hg
Heart rate:	129 beats per minute

His full genotype results are included in the electronic health record, and results pertinent to initial warfarin dosing are provided as follows:

GENETIC MARKER	RESULT
VKORC1-1639/3673	GG
CYP4F2 V433M	CT
GGCX rs11676382	CC
CYP2C9*2	CC
CYP2C9*3	AA
CYP2C9*5	CG
CYP2C9*6	AA

Instructions:
Use the patient characteristics, labs, and genetic report to determine an appropriate starting dose of warfarin for this patient (question 1). Use the dosing calculator at http://www.warfarindosing.org/Source/InitialDose.aspx to determine the suggested starting daily dose of warfarin to maintain an average target INR of 2.5 (INR range 2-3).

Question 1   *What starting dose (estimated mini-loading dose) of warfarin you would recommend for this patient based on the calculator including genetic factors?*

A. 1 mg
B. 4 mg
C. 6 mg
D. 9 mg

Correct answer: C. 6 mg
Answer C, 6 mg, is correct because the estimated mini-loading dose is 6.1 mg, and warfarin is supplied as oral tablets in 1-mg increments (with a 2.5-mg tablet and a 7.5-mg tablet available). Therefore, a reasonable starting (loading) dose would be 6 mg.

Answer A is incorrect.
Answer B is incorrect because 4.3 mg (~4 mg/d) is the estimated therapeutic dose.

Answer D is incorrect because 9 mg is approximately 50% more than the mini-loading dose. This would be a recommended dose if the clinical goal is to have the INR rise quickly for the initial 1 or 2 days.

For additional practice, use the calculator to change individual genetic results (can use back function in a browser without losing other parameters) to see how they affect dose recommendations.

Question 2 *How would the starting dose (mini-loading dose) and estimated therapeutic dose for warfarin change if the patient was taking an azole antifungal, like fluconazole? Why is the coadministration of azole antifungals a factor in warfarin dosing? Explore the "Recommendations" at the bottom of the results page.*

Correct answer:
If this patient was taking fluconazole at the time of warfarin initiation, the estimated mini-loading dose is unchanged (6.1 mg) and the estimated therapeutic dose is decreased by half (2.2 mg). The developers note in their recommendation below the results that this may still be an excessive estimate, though.

As you notice in the warfarin calculator, pharmacogenomics factors are only part of the clinical equation. Drug-drug interactions like CYP2C9 inhibition by fluconazole influence warfarin metabolism. In this case, warfarin plasma concentrations are higher at a given dose, compared to those not taking fluconazole, and may increase the risk for complications like bleeding.

Therefore, the manufacturer's labeling for warfarin advises to consider reducing the warfarin dose by 10% to 20% if combined with fluconazole and closely monitor for increased anticoagulant effects (ie, increased INR, bleeding) to guide further dose adjustments.

Question 3 *How would the starting dose (mini-loading dose) and therapeutic dose for warfarin change if the patient had preexisting liver disease (but not taking fluconazole)? Why is liver function considered in dosing and monitoring warfarin? Explore the "Recommendations" at the bottom of the results page and the "Hemorrhage Risk" tab on the left-hand side of the calculator for a detailed list of clinical factors that predict bleeding risk.*

Correct answer:
Preexisting liver diseases do not change the starting dose or therapeutic dose predicted by the calculator, but the developers note in their recommendation that the estimated therapeutic dose is too high and a lower warfarin dose should be prescribed.

As you notice in the warfarin calculator, pharmacogenomics factors are only part of the clinical equation. Comorbid diseases, such as liver disease, do not change the recommended dosing for warfarin (per the calculator or in the manufacturer's labeling) but may increase the risk for complications like bleeding. Preexisting liver disease, such as cirrhosis or hepatitis, increases the risk for both bleeding and thrombosis. This is due, in part, to the liver's role in synthesizing vitamin K–dependent clotting factors.

Therefore, based on clinical judgment and goals of care decided by the patient and healthcare provider, a lower starting dose may be warranted with adjustments based on TDM (INR). The developers recommend, "To get a better estimate, save this record and return to this site after 3 warfarin doses to enter the INR on the 4th morning." Laboratory (INR) and clinical symptoms of bleeding should be closely monitored for patients with hepatic disease and taking warfarin.

REFERENCES

1. Vogel F. Moderne problem der humangenetik. *Ergeb Inn Med U Kinderheilk.* 1959;12:52125.

2. Zanger U, Schwab M. Cytochrome P450 enzymes in drug metabolism: regulation of gene expression, enzyme activities, and impact of genetic variation. *Pharmacol Ther.* 2013;138(1):103-141.

3. Sim S, Kacevska M, Ingelman-Sundberg M. Pharmacogenomics of drug-metabolizing enzymes: a recent update on clinical implications and endogenous effects. *Pharmacogenomics J.* 2013;13(1):1-11.

4. Nelson D, Koymans L, Kamataki T, et al. P450 superfamily: update on new sequences, gene mapping, accession numbers and nomenclature. *Pharmacogenetics.* 1996;6(1):1-42.

5. Zhang G, Nebert D. Personalized medicine: genetic risk prediction of drug response. *Pharmacol Ther.* 2017;175:75-90.

6. Pinto N, Dolan M. Clinically relevant genetic variations in drug metabolizing enzymes. *Curr Drug Metab.* 2011;12(5):487-497.

7. Nebert D, Zhang G, Vesell E. From human genetics and genomics to pharmacogenetics and pharmacogenomics: past lessons, future directions. *Drug Metab Rev.* 2008;40(2):187-224.

8. Relling MV, Evans WE. Pharmacogenomics in the clinic. *Nature.* 2015;526(7573):343-350.

9. Brøsen K, Gram L. Clinical significance of the sparteine/debrisoquine oxidation polymorphism. *Eur J Clin Pharmacol.* 1989;36(6):537-547.

10. Crews K, Caudle K, Dunnenberger H, Sadhasivam S, Skaar T. Considerations for the utility of the CPIC guideline for CYP2D6 genotype and codeine therapy. *Clin Chem.* 2015;61(5):775-776.

11. Cicali E, Smith D, Duong B, Kovar L, Cavallari L, Johnson J. A scoping review of the evidence behind cytochrome P450 2D6 isoenzyme inhibitor classifications. *Clin Pharmacol Ther.* 2020;108(1):116-125.

12. Crews KR, Monte AA, Huddart R, et al. Clinical pharmacogenetics implementation consortium guideline for CYP2D6, OPRM1, and COMT genotypes and select opioid therapy. *Clin Pharmacol Ther.* 2021;110(4):888-896.

13. Zanger U, Klein K, Saussele T, Blievernicht J, Hofmann M, Schwab M. Polymorphic CYP2B6: molecular mechanisms and emerging clinical significance. *Pharmacogenomics.* 2007;8(7):743-759.

14. Vo T, Varghese Gupta S. Role of cytochrome P450 2B6 pharmacogenomics in determining efavirenz-mediated central nervous system toxicity, treatment outcomes, and dosage adjustments in patients with human immunodeficiency virus infection. *Pharmacotherapy.* 2016;36(12):1245-1254.

15. Swart M, Skelton M, Ren Y, Smith P, Takuva S, Dandara C. High predictive value of CYP2B6 SNPs for steady-state plasma efavirenz levels in South African HIV/AIDS patients. *Pharmacogenet Genomics.* 2013;23(8):415-427.

16. Holzinger E, Grady B, Ritchie M, et al. Genome-wide association study of plasma efavirenz pharmacokinetics in AIDS Clinical Trials Group protocols implicates several CYP2B6 variants. *Pharmacogenet Genomics.* 2012;22(12):858-867.

17. Karnes J, Rettie A, Somogyi A, et al. Clinical Pharmacogenetics Implementation Consortium (CPIC) guideline for CYP2C9 and HLA-B genotypes and phenytoin dosing: 2020 update. *Clin Pharmacol Ther.* 2021;109(2):302-309.

18. Johnson J, Caudle K, Gong L, et al. Clinical Pharmacogenetics Implementation Consortium (CPIC) guideline for pharmacogenetics-guided warfarin dosing: 2017 update. *Clin Pharmacol Ther.* 2017;102(3):397-404.

19. Moriyama B, Obeng A, Barbarino J, et al. Clinical Pharmacogenetics Implementation Consortium (CPIC) guidelines for CYP2C19 and voriconazole therapy. *Clin Pharmacol Ther.* 2017; 102(1):45-51.

20. Lee C, Luzum J, Sangkuhl K, et al. Clinical Pharmacogenetics Implementation Consortium guideline for CYP2C19 genotype and clopidogrel therapy: 2022 update. *Clin Pharmacol Ther.* 2022; 112(5):959-967.

21. Gawrońska-Szklarz B, Adamiak-Giera U, Wyska E, et al. CYP2C19 polymorphism affects single-dose pharmacokinetics of oral pantoprazole in healthy volunteers. *Eur J Clin Pharmacol.* 2012;68(9):1267-1274.

22. Hunfeld N, Mathot R, Touw D, et al. Effect of CYP2C19*2 and *17 mutations on pharmacodynamics and kinetics of proton pump inhibitors in Caucasians. *Br J Clin Pharmacol.* 2008;65(5):752-760.

23. Wang D, Guo Y, Wrighton S, Cooke G, Sadee W. Intronic polymorphism in CYP3A4 affects hepatic expression and response to statin drugs. *Pharmacogenomics J.* 2011;11(4):274-286.

24. Moes D, Swen J, den Hartigh J, et al. Effect of CYP3A4*22, CYP3A5*3, and CYP3A combined genotypes on cyclosporine, everolimus, and tacrolimus pharmacokinetics in renal transplantation. *CPT Pharmacometrics Syst Pharmacol.* 2014;3(2):e100.

25. Birdwell K, Decker B, Barbarino J, et al. Clinical Pharmacogenetics Implementation Consortium (CPIC) guidelines for CYP3A5 genotype and tacrolimus dosing. *Clin Pharmacol Ther.* 2015; 98(1):19-24.

26. Buendia J, Bramuglia G, Staatz C. Effects of combinational CYP3A5 6986A>G polymorphism in graft liver and native intestine on the pharmacokinetics of tacrolimus in liver transplant patients: a meta-analysis. *Ther Drug Monit.* 2014;36(4):442-447.

27. Lancia P, Jacqz-Aigrain E, Zhao W. Choosing the right dose of tacrolimus. *Arch Dis Child.* 2015;100(4):406-413.

28. Relling M, Klein T. CPIC: Clinical Pharmacogenetics Implementation Consortium of the pharmacogenomics research network. *Clin Pharmacol Ther.* 2011;89(3):464-467.

7

PREGNANCY

Irving Steinberg

Learning Objectives

By the end of the pregnancy chapter, the learner shall be able to:

1. Describe specific clinical, epidemiologic, and pharmacologic issues related to pregnancy that justify and encourage more pharmacokinetic (PK) and pharmacodynamic trials.
2. List the numerous dynamic physiologic changes that occur through the trimesters of pregnancy that impact drug PK.
3. Enumerate the drug or drug classes that show dose dependency in their fetotoxic effects.
4. Discuss the alterations in body composition, pregnancy-related hormones, and laboratory parameters that affect absorption, distribution, metabolism, and clearance of various drugs during pregnancy.
5. Evaluate the physicochemical properties of selected drugs and how physiologic alterations merge with them to create changes in PK during pregnancy.
6. Suggest the reasons for and impact of serum protein–binding changes on the PK of drugs in the pregnant patient and the fetus.
7. Assess the chemical and PK factors that promote and prevent transplacental passage and the role of the placental metabolism and transporters in fetal exposure.
8. Illustrate how changes in phase 1 and phase 2 metabolism during pregnancy augment or reduce the hepatic clearance of drugs and how those changes can alter the dose-response relationships and clinical outcomes of diseases impacting the pregnant patient and fetal exposure. Provide specific drug examples.
9. Comprehend and apply renal function changes to clearance properties and dosing of drugs during pregnancy.
10. Explain the role of therapeutic drug monitoring, ex vivo and physiologically based PK modeling in parameter estimation, and dose optimization in pregnancy.

INTRODUCTION

Although the pediatric patient has often been referred to as the "therapeutic orphan," the gap in knowledge of dynamic effects and pharmacokinetics (PK) of drugs in the pregnant patient population may in fact be larger.[1-3] This is even more relevant to newer agents potentially useful in the pregnant patient where less study reduces informed use. Yet, older and commonly used agents with a known safety profile, such as acetaminophen and caffeine, have new concerns raised about use during pregnancy and safety to the fetus.[4,5] Changes in the Food and Drug Administration (FDA) required labeling of drugs for use in pregnancy to a more narrative assessment for the clinician to read and implement demands more careful study of these drugs and reliable unbiased data interpretation, taking efficacy and safety for the mother and the fetus into account.[6] Commercial interest in PK and pharmacotherapeutic discovery may be reduced because a woman will spend a relatively low percentage of a lifetime being pregnant, yet the physiologic changes and the unique gestational pathophysiologic manifestations command more study toward appropriate use and evidence-based dosing in this population.

Diseases may exist in their mostly typical forms (eg, asthma,[7] epilepsy,[8] chronic hypertension[9]) or may have unique etiologies and manifestations related to pregnancy, for example, gestational diabetes,[10,11] pregnancy-induced hypertension and preeclampsia,[12] and peripartum cardiomyopathy.[13] Drugs considered first line for management may need to yield alternative choices during pregnancy for maternal and fetal safety. Overarching considerations of drug use and investigation of ethical challenges, with the often unknown or potentially harmful fetal exposure, influence study design and increased care in therapeutic decision-making and maternal-fetal monitoring throughout pregnancy.[14] The lack of solid scientific information when applied to drug use and/or consideration for termination of the pregnancy based on the suspected but often unconfirmed fetal risk,[15] as seen for fluoroquinolones,[16] places an added burden of joint therapeutic decision-making for the provider and the patient. Many newer agents used in nonpregnant patients that might prove advantageous in the therapy of diseases in pregnant patients do not get utilized for lack of studies of efficacy, toxicity, PK, and precision dosing in this special population. This knowledge gap furthers the differences between state-of-the-art and standards of care treatments for pregnant versus nonpregnant patients.[17] Exceptional circumstances such as medical exigency of COVID-19 vaccination, with the greater severity of disease seen in pregnancy,[18] forced reliance on ongoing gathered safety and efficacy information in this population drawn mainly from post hoc analysis of clinical usage data and the hope of no long-term consequences on the fetus.[19,20] However, ethical considerations will typically limit such rapid provisional drug approval in pregnancy, if studied or approved at all in this population using traditional timelines.[21] Consideration and careful inclusion of pregnant women in therapeutic trials are advised.[22-24]

The need for specific studies of drug kinetics and dynamics in pregnancy has never been greater,[25] as these studies make up a small percentage of the studies done across all drug classes in this patient population. Dynamic changes in organ function, efficiencies, and body composition during the phases of gestation lead to corresponding PK changes that must be accounted for throughout pregnancy (as summarized in Table 7.1), during individual trimesters, and with postpartum

TABLE 7.1 Pharmacokinetic Relevant Physiologic Changes During Pregnancy

Absorption:	
Gastric emptying time	↑
Intestinal motility, acid secretion	↓
Pulmonary function	↑ (TV, MV ≈ 40%)
Cardiac output	↑ (40%-50%)
Skin blood flow	↑
Distribution:	
Plasma volume	↑ (≈50%)
ECF and total body water	↑ (33%-40%; TBW by 8 L)
Body fat	↑
Plasma proteins	↓ (via dilution → further ↑ in V_d)
Metabolism:	
Hepatic blood flow	↔, ↑ (eg, lidocaine, β-blockers)
Hepatic enzyme efficiency	↑ (CYP2D6, CYP3A4, CYP3A5, CYP2B6, CYP2A6)
	↓ (CYP2C19, CYP1A2)
Hepatic conjugation	↑ (UGT1A4, UGT1A6, UGT2B7)
	↓, ↔ (NAT2)
Extrahepatic metabolism	↑ (eg, placenta)
Plasma proteins	↓ (dilution → further ↑ V_d)
(albumin, AAG)	
Excretion:	
Renal plasma flow	↑ (20%-50% second trimester; 75% term)
Glomerular filtration	↑ (30%-50%; eg, aminoglycosides, vancomycin)
Secretion (↑ transporter	↑ P-gp, OCT2, BCRP, PEPT1
expression)	(eg, digoxin, metformin, corticosteroids, ampicillin)

AAG, α_1-acid glycoprotein; BCRP, breast cancer resistance protein; MV, minute ventilation; P-gp, p-glycoprotein; TBW, total body water; TV, tidal volume.

return to the nonpregnant state.[26] Extrapolations from adult PK studies and dosing in nonpregnant patients are often inadequate in addressing the precision dosing needs during pregnancy. Dose-normalized differences in systemic exposure are 25% to 50% lower in pregnant patients for commonly used drugs, such as oseltamivir, glyburide, and buprenorphine.[1] Therefore, stable prenatal dosing regimens may need multiple adjustments in a substantial number of pregnant patients to maintain similar serum concentrations and consistent systemic exposure to maintain disease control.[27]

For study purposes and therapeutic drug monitoring, the propriety of taking multiple samples for formal PK evaluation in pregnancy is limited due to pregnancy-associated anemia and other clinical considerations. Utility of sparse dose-concentration data collection has value in constructing and validating population PK models and physiologically based pharmacokinetic models (PBPMs) to use in Bayesian forecasting. These techniques are useful in modeling and assessing influential demographic and clinical factors for empiric dosing and regimen adjustments and for predicting tissue disposition of drugs in the maternal, placental, and fetal compartments.[26-28] The placenta and fetus as unique metabolic, drug binding, and clearance spaces add further complexity to the assessment and prediction of drug disposition in the pregnant patient and the fetoplacental compartment.[29] Consideration for the magnitude of transplacental drug exposure has become more relevant to fetopathy, with increasing evidence of maternal dose dependency for lithium,[30] antiseizure medications (ASMs),[31] and opioids.[32] Other functional adverse effects on fetal growth, prematurity, and postnatal adaptation may be drug dose related, as seen with opioids,[33] β-blockers,[34] and antidepressants.[35]

CHANGES IN PHARMACOKINETICS DURING PREGNANCY

Absorption

The continued increases in maternal progesterone levels during gestation are suggested to influence alterations in drug absorption, resulting from delay in gastric emptying, decreased production of stomach acid, and diminished gastrointestinal motility.[36] This affects the rate of oral drug absorption and time to peak concentration, so drugs with expected rapid action after oral administration may be slowed, and weak acids may have reduced bioavailability. Weak acids such as aspirin will become more ionized at the higher stomach pH and have reduced absorption, whereas weak bases such as caffeine will have increased uptake. Pregnancy-induced emesis may further cause incomplete bioavailability via a reduced fraction absorbed or lowered usage compliance. Frequently used metal-containing medications in pregnancy, such as oral iron, iron-fortified vitamins, and calcium-containing antacids, can chelate other drugs and reduce their absorption. Intrahepatic cholestasis complicating pregnancy could further impose changes in absorption rate for lipid-soluble drugs. Bioavailability may also be affected by dietary changes during pregnancy as well as the efficiency of, and gene polymorphisms in, intestinal and hepatic enzymes (discussed further under Metabolism), with potential variation in first-pass metabolism.[26] Drugs with high first-pass metabolism (eg, nifedipine, propranolol) can exhibit large variations in bioavailability during pregnancy.[37] Presystemic clearance can also limit the systemic exposure of nifedipine when applied to therapy of hypertensive disorders of pregnancy.[37]

   Altered regional blood perfusion and body fat composition during pregnancy can potentially enhance subcutaneous and intramuscular injectable drug tissue absorption, such as the more rapid uptake and shorter time to peak concentration when 17-hydroxyprogesterone caproate in castor oil intramuscular injection is given to prevent preterm labor compared to nonpregnant females for other indications.[38] A somewhat lower absorption rate constant and delayed time to peak concentrations are observed for subcutaneously administered low-molecular-weight heparin in pregnant compared to postpartum patients[39]; however, not all studies show this, and the peak is still seen at approximately 4 hours. Inhaled medication may see faster or more extensive uptake, with approximately 40% increase in tidal volume and minute ventilation during pregnancy.[36] Transcutaneous blood flow also allows for increased absorption of topically administered medications.

Volume of Distribution

Numerous factors influence changes in volume of distribution during pregnancy. The vast changes in body composition by gestation period have a clear impact on the changes in distribution volume for many drugs during pregnancy. Increases in total body water by approximately 50%, extracellular fluid by approximately 40%, and intravascular volume by approximately 45% to 50% serve to increase the volume of distribution of drugs distributing to those spaces, such as phenytoin, aminoglycosides, and heparin, respectively.[26,36,40] The growth of the placenta, development of the conceptus, expansion of the amniotic space, and enlargement of the uterine and breast tissue, along with the increases in fluid volumes and body fat, increase the volume of distribution for both water-soluble and lipid-soluble drugs. With the expansion of the intravascular and extracellular fluid space, the V_d for drugs like β-lactam antibiotics, aminoglycosides, vancomycin, lithium, low-molecular-weight heparin, and intravenous magnesium is larger than under nonpregnant conditions.[41] In the mid to late third trimester, the V_d of enoxaparin increases disproportionately to the increases in renal clearance, the half-life may increase compared to earlier in pregnancy, and the peak-to-trough concentration variability is reduced from earlier gestational weeks.[42] Increases in fat mass during pregnancy provide a repository for distribution and persistence in adipose tissue for lipid-soluble sedative agents, such as diazepam and thiopental, with increased V_d and a lengthening of the half-life and pharmacologic activity duration. In contrast to drugs with expanded distribution volume, the relative proportion of nonfat or muscle tissue to adipose tissue and total body water declines during pregnancy, yielding a decreased weight-corrected V_d for digoxin (5.7 L/kg in pregnancy compared to 7 L/kg in nonpregnant controls).[43] Alterations in serum protein binding due to diminished binding capacity from progressive reductions in albumin and α_1-acid glycoprotein (AAG) concentration during gestation will generally increase the volume of distribution for both highly bound acidic and basic drugs.[44] The fetoplacental space adds to the volume of distribution anatomically and may trap ionized drugs when weakly basic drugs such as lidocaine are introduced, as the pH is typically 0.1 to 0.15 pH units below the maternal 7.4 value. This pH difference can be greater when fetal distress occurs and fetal acidosis ensues, trapping more drug.[45]

Protein Binding

Serum and tissue protein binding can have PK influence on the volume of distribution, clearance, the magnitude and persistence of pharmacodynamic effects, as well as the interpretation of serum concentrations and therapeutic ranges of drugs.[46] These all can shift during pregnancy.[26,44] Albumin concentration progressively decreases during the three trimesters owing to dilution from the increased fluid load, whereas albumin synthesis remains stable. Albumin concentrations fall to 3.1 g/dL in the first trimester, 2.6 g/dL in the second, and 2.3 g/dL in the third. This decrease in binding capacity leads to more highly bound drugs having increased free concentration per any given total drug concentration. Higher free fatty acid concentration in the pregnant patient can also alter the albumin binding of drugs via displacement interactions. The higher unbound fraction leaves more free drug available to interact with receptor sites, to distribute to other nonreceptor tissue spaces, to be filtered and cleared through glomerular filtration, and to be subject to increased hepatic clearance for a low hepatic extraction ratio drug. Warfarin, ibuprofen, phenytoin, valproic acid, and several antiretroviral agents are examples of such drugs, with the unbound fraction of phenytoin increasing by 40%. Likewise, with the dilution of AAG throughout pregnancy, the binding of basic drugs, such as lidocaine, meperidine, propranolol, and amitriptyline, is reduced by approximately 50% by the third trimester. AAG is an acute-phase reactant and increases in numerous physiologic disease stress situations, including late pregnancy preeclampsia, thereby altering the typical pregnancy trend. These decreases in protein binding in pregnancy may be even more impactful for drugs, such as valproic acid, lidocaine, and disopyramide, that exhibit concentration-dependent protein binding within their respective therapeutic serum concentration ranges. Prednisolone also demonstrates concentration-dependent protein binding on its low-capacity binding site transcortin and added to lower albumin binding results in higher total and renal clearance.[47] While maternal drug–binding proteins are decreasing, these proteins are increasing in the fetal space during gestation, sequestering transplacentally delivered agents, and expanding the overall maternal apparent V_d.[48] The drug can then be metabolized by the fetus and circulated through the amniotic sac or cause pharmacologic benefit or harm as the fetal-to-maternal concentration ratio increases, as evident for select antiretroviral drugs.[49]

Clearance

The efficiency of drug disposition pathways and the organs of elimination change substantially during pregnancy. With the increase in cardiac output of 40% to 50% during pregnancy,[36] organ perfusion is enhanced, but it is debated whether liver blood flow is increased. Phases 1 and 2 metabolism are subject to significant changes depending on the abundance of the enzymes involved, their genetic expression and any polymorphisms, and the substrate specificity.[50] Efflux pumps and transporter proteins have a large role in differentiating drug clearance in pregnant from nonpregnant patients.

METABOLISM

Phase 1 metabolism is influenced by the elevations in pregnancy-related hormones and their enzyme–inducing effect.[51] But, the direction of the changes is enzyme and drug specific. The various cytochrome (CYP) P450 enzymes, other catalysts, and transporters responsible for the majority of drug metabolism and disposition are summarized in Table 7.2. The measured abundance of the enzymes correlates to the increase in metabolic performance seen during pregnancy. A few examples are noteworthy.

The clearance of intravenous and oral acetaminophen is seen to increase during pregnancy, and conversion to the toxic intermediate NAPQI increases during the first trimester, mainly due to the increases in CYP2E1 activity. Conjugation with sulfation and glucuronidation is accelerated during the second and third trimesters, reducing the percentage of the NAPQI metabolite toward prenatal levels. Furthermore, preterm and twin pregnancies have a 25% to 30% higher average clearance (normalized to body surface area) than comparative term and singleton pregnancies.[52] The similar

TABLE 7.2   Alterations in Metabolizing Enzymes and Transporters in Pregnancy

ENZYME	ACTIVITY CHANGE	CLINICAL EVIDENCE
CYP1A2	Decrease 30%-65%	↓ CL or ↑ metabolic ratios of caffeine, theophylline, olanzapine, clozapine
CYP2E1	Increase 1.8-fold	↑ CL of acetaminophen
CYP2B6	Increase	↑ CL of methadone
CYP2D6	Increase 1.5- to 2.8-fold	↑ CL or ↓ metabolic ratio of flu-oxetine, citalopram, metoprolol, dextromethorphan
CYP2C9	Increase 1.5-fold	↑ CL of phenytoin and glyburide
CYP2C19	Decrease	↓ CL of proguanil, methadone (polymorphisms present)
CYP3A4	Increase 90%-150%	↑ CL of midazolam, amlodipine, nifed-ipine, and indinavir
CBR1	Decrease 30%-39%	↓ CL of doxorubicin
UGT1A4	Increase 65%-264%	↑ CL of lamotrigine
TRANSPORTERS		
OCT2	Increase 25%-45%	↑ CL of metformin (renal CL by 64%)
P-gp	Increase 107%	↑ CL of digoxin
OAT1	Increase >50%	↑ CL of amoxicillin
PEPT1	Decrease	↑ CL of cephalexin, amoxicillin

CL, clearance; P-gp, p-glycoprotein.

magnitude of expansion of both V_d and clearance leaves the elimination half-life similar to that of nonpregnant women. The values of the heightened clearance of acetaminophen in pregnancy overlap with those seen in women using oral contraceptives, with both being much higher clearances from nonpregnant women not on oral contraceptives.[53] Though higher therapeutic doses of acetaminophen may be suggested to provide antipyretic and analgesic effects in the pregnant patient, caution must be considered, given multiple concerns of suspected effects in the fetus and newborn.[1,2]

The accelerated metabolism seen with other drugs creates clinical challenges. Metoprolol is subject to CYP2D6 metabolism, which increases the drug's clearance 2- to 4-fold in pregnancy for those with normal genetic expression, with a lesser magnitude impact for those with poor metabolizer genotype.[54] The dramatic increase in metoprolol clearance (361 L/hr in mid-pregnancy, 568 L/hr in late pregnancy, 195 L/hr at >3 months postpartum) signals for higher and more frequent dosing when used for hypertension, arrhythmia, or cardiomyopathy during pregnancy, and a return to standard dosing after birth. Correcting for the shifts in body mass shows the same pattern of elevated clearance when normalized to weight (4.02 L/hr/kg in mid-pregnancy, 6.37 L/hr/kg in late pregnancy, 2.41 L/hr/kg at >3 months postpartum), demonstrating that the changes in total clearance values are not merely a function of weight changes. Similar manifold increases in hepatic clearance are seen for clonidine due to induced CYP2D6 metabolism that significantly overwhelms the more typically predominant renal clearance ($Cl_{total\ pregnant}$ = 440 ± 168 mL/min, $Cl_{total\ nonpregnant}$ = 245 ± 72 mL/min; excreted unchanged pregnant = 36 ± 11%, nonpregnant = 59 ± 18%).[55] The very large reduction in area under the curve (AUC) after oral dosing of these two adrenergic blockers makes reliable use and effect more doubtful, as these may need a frequency of every 6-hour dosing to reach blood pressure (BP) and heart rate (HR) goals.[26] Sustained-release forms of these drugs, if the indication warrants, and/or other medication choices, may be preferred. The additional pharmacogenetic impact on CYP2D6 performance for poor, extensive, and ultrarapid during pregnancy has also been demonstrated, simulated, and accurately predicted for the conversion of codeine to morphine.[50]

Induced increases in clearance rates are also present for CYP3A4-, CYP3A5-, CYP2B6-, CYP2B8-, and CYP2C9-catalyzed metabolism, where the increases in messenger RNA (mRNA) and enzyme protein levels correlate with pregnancy-related hormones in a concentration-dependent manner.[56,57] The accelerated elimination of amlodipine via CYP3A4 in pregnant patients leads to an $AUC_{0-\infty}$ and elimination half-life that is one-third of that seen in normal volunteers.[58,59] The conversion of nifedipine to dehydro-nifedipine by CYP3A4 and CYP3A5 follows this pattern in pregnancy, with accelerated presystemic clearance lowering the bioavailability and systemic clearance further reducing the systemic exposure.[60] Pharmacogenetic influences are seen with polymorphisms in CYP3A5, with high (wild-type) expressers having an oral nifedipine clearance nearly 3 times higher than the genetically variant low expressers.[61] Similar differences in clearance are seen for those carrying CYP3A4*1B functional allele versus the nonfunctional allelic polymorphism.

For low extraction ratio drugs, the higher free fraction, together with the induced intrinsic clearances, combines to create the manifold increases in hepatic clearance:

$$Cl_{hepatic} \approx fu \times Cl_{int}$$

Free drug concentration measurements can be used in therapeutic drug monitoring of the pregnant patient, as well as to examine the relative contributions of protein binding and altered intrinsic clearance expected in these patients.[62]

A faster conversion of midazolam to its 1-hydroxy metabolite furnished by CYP3A4 is observed during pregnancy, and midazolam clearance is even higher when taking the pregnancy-related differences in protein binding and body weight into account.[63] This is further amplified for those pharmacogenetically found to be extensive metabolizers. Quetiapine, an antipsychotic agent mainly metabolized by CYP3A4 and CYP2D6, demonstrated decreased steady-state serum concentrations of 22%, 57%, and 76% during the first, second, and third trimesters, respectively, in 35 pregnancies with patients receiving defined daily doses of 400 mg.[64] Aripiprazole, which is prescribed for pregnant women to treat schizophrenia and bipolar disorder and has an active metabolite, showed similar decreases of 12%, 35%, and 52%, respectively, through the trimesters at a studied dose of 15 mg/d. The average third-trimester concentration would fall below the therapeutic range, and the recommended doses in pregnancy are, therefore, higher than the defined daily dose studied in this report,[65] as can be seen in Figure 7.1.

The 1.5- to 2-fold augmentation of glyburide systemic clearance in pregnancy via CYP2C9 induction halves the AUC and may require higher daily dosing to meet maternal blood glucose goals.[66] Yet, this drug has been favored over other oral hypoglycemic agents for gestational diabetes with presumed lower fetal exposure. Likewise, the unbound fraction of phenytoin, which is increased during pregnancy, is more rapidly cleared during pregnancy, with the induced CYP2C9-mediated intrinsic clearance. Even when P450 enzyme metabolic induction suggests higher drug dosing needs during pregnancy,[67] the adverse effect profile must be carefully considered as seen with methadone in opioid dependence, where doses above 100 mg/d were more likely to have prolongation of the QTc interval, particularly in the peripartum period.[68]

Although not often used during pregnancy, drugs such as clopidogrel and voriconazole must be carefully dosed as their CYP2C19-mediated metabolism is relatively diminished in the second and third trimesters. More frequently used agents such as omeprazole and esomeprazole show significant reductions in clearance during pregnancy, with the latter demonstrating potential autoinhibition of CYP2C19 metabolism with chronic dosing.[69] Caffeine may have more prominent and longer acting effects in the pregnant patient owing to reduced CYP1A2 metabolism (33%, 49%, and 65% in

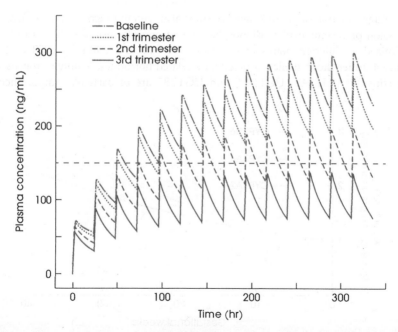

FIGURE 7.1 Plasma concentration-time profile for aripiprazole during gestational phases. (Zheng L, Tang S, Tang R, Xu M, Jiang X, Wang L. Dose adjustment of quetiapine and aripiprazole for pregnant women using physiologically based pharmacokinetic modeling and simulation. *Clin Pharmacokinet.* 2021;60(5):623-635.)

trimester 1, 2, and 3, respectively).[70] This results in increased elimination half-life by 2.5- to 4-fold compared to nonpregnant females.[71] Faster clearance and conversion to potentially harmful metabolites (eg, paraxanthine) have been associated with fetal growth restriction, and the consumption of greater than 300 mg/d and CYP1A2 rapid metabolizer polymorphism are added risks.[72,73] Inversely, faster caffeine metabolism and a higher paraxanthine-to-caffeine ratio in the second trimester were associated with a lower risk of preeclampsia versus controls.[74] Overall, careful consumption of caffeine-containing products is encouraged during pregnancy.

Many drugs have multiple pathways of metabolism, complicating the predictability of the net effect on clearance with the dynamic changes in enzyme abundance and activity throughout gestation and any polymorphisms that may inform differences in enzymatic performance. Drugs with pathways that diverge in the direction of change in metabolic efficiency during pregnancy (as illustrated in Figure 7.2)[75] may create greater variability in the clearance or serum concentration-to-dose ratios among pregnant patients. The dosing of drugs from the same pharmacologic classification must be carefully calibrated during pregnancy in relation to the metabolic path utilized. While the selective serotonin reuptake inhibitors (SSRIs) such as paroxetine and fluoxetine may require higher-than-average adult doses during pregnancy because of their prominent CYP2D6 metabolism, the highly protein bound sertraline is metabolized via the CYP2C19, CYP2B6, CYP2D6, and CYP2C9, which may either offset each other to minimize change from the second semester until postpartum or steadily augment clearance to require higher doses.[76] Population PK modeling and therapeutic drug monitoring PBPMs can be of utility in refining empiric initial and adjusted doses.[77,78]

Augmentation of phase 2 metabolism is also seen in pregnancy, with increased expression of various uridine diphosphate-glucuronosyltransferase (UGT) isoforms maximized at different points of gestation and with induction for UGT1A1 and UGT1A4 under the influence of pregnancy-related hormones, mainly estrogens and progestins.[79,80] UGT1A1, UGT1A4, and UGT2B7 are of particular importance in

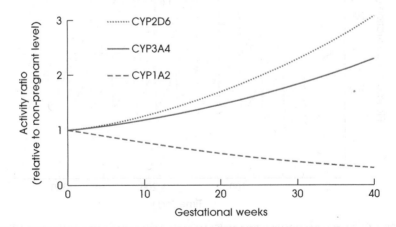

FIGURE 7.2 Changes in activity of cytochrome P450 isoforms during pregnancy. (Abduljalil K, Pansari A, Jamei M. Prediction of maternal pharmacokinetics using physiologically based pharmacokinetic models: assessing the impact of the longitudinal changes in the activity of CYP1A2, CYP2D6 and CYP3A4 enzymes during pregnancy. *J Pharmacokinet Pharmacodyn.* 2020;47(4):361-383.)

increasing the conjugation of numerous drugs. Activity of UGT1A1 and UGT1A4 increases by 200% by the second trimester and 300% by the third trimester. The combination of α- and β-blocker labetalol shows increased glucuronide formation from UGT1A1 during gestation, but the glucuronide derived from UGT2B7 decreases. Overall, the clearance of labetalol increases linearly throughout pregnancy from 40% to 70% over postpartum values, resulting in higher and more frequent doses needed to avoid therapeutic failure when treating hypertension and preeclampsia.[81] Unique stereoselective clearance is also observed that effects this drug's activity in pregnancy. The RR-isomer, which is the β-blocker component, is cleared more rapidly in pregnancy when labetalol is given orally. And in patients with gestational diabetes, the SR-isomer, which is the α-blocker component, demonstrates a lower clearance than in normal pregnancy.[82] Both circumstances should lead to greater vasodilatory antihypertensive effect and may alter the presumed relationship between intravenous to oral dose equivalencies used in nonpregnancy states.[37]

The large increases in glucuronidation can have a substantial clinical influence on drug response. Multiple studies have demonstrated large increases (up to 250% from baseline) in clearance for the ASM lamotrigine, which is a UGT1A4 substrate and is favored for its much lower rates of congenital anomalies[31] and neurodevelopmental impairment[83] among the ASMs. In one study of 60 pregnancies and 600 monitored serum levels, 77% of the women had a steep increase in mean bioavailability–corrected clearance from 2.16 L/hr at baseline to 6.88 L/hr throughout pregnancy and then an exponential drop in the peripartum and postpartum period to usual prepregnancy values within 3 weeks.[84] About one-fourth of the pregnant population with epilepsy receiving lamotrigine saw only minimal to no increases in clearance. These clearance increases in pregnancy are noted when normalized to weight or when looked at as free drug (or intrinsic) clearance.[85] Therefore, many pregnant patients are at risk for breakthrough seizures owing to augmentation of lamotrigine clearance, and that risk occurs when the individual's serum concentration falls to less than 65% of the prepregnancy or target value.[85,86] Continual increases in lamotrigine dosage during gestation are necessary to offset the increased clearance and maintain therapeutic concentrations and response.[87] Similar risks tied to falling concentrations exist for oxcarbazepine, which is converted to its active 10-monohydoxy form through a noninducible enzyme and then conjugated to two glucuronide metabolites.[88] Given the dangers of uncontrolled epilepsy to the mother and the fetus, therapeutic drug monitoring has been advocated. Simulations using population PK models can also provide useful empiric guidance based on quantifying the probability and variability of the expected PK changes, the influential variables, and validating any employed strategies.[89]

Although the metabolism of drugs that are substrates for N-acetyltransferase-2 (NAT2) is mostly determined by the genotype of acetylator status, mixed effects can be seen in the influence of pregnancy, seemingly depending on the drug studied. While a 13% reduction in caffeine metabolism is seen in the NAT2 pathway during pregnancy, no effect of pregnancy was exerted on hydralazine conversion to its major metabolite.[90] In a study evaluating the PK of isoniazid and efavirenz in women with HIV, no difference was seen in isoniazid AUC and C_{max} between pregnant and nonpregnant patients among rapid and intermediate acetylators but were significantly lower among the pregnant patients compared to nonpregnant patients having slow acetylator status, with drug clearance increased by 26% by pregnancy status alone.[91] It is important to assess acetylator status to provide more precise dosing and safety for these drugs during pregnancy.

Medications may be used during pregnancy to relieve burdensome substance habituation, allowing for a healthier pregnancy and lower short- and long-term risks to the fetus and newborn. Augmentation of phase 1 and phase 2 metabolism together during pregnancy can be seen where those pathways are operational. Pregnant patients initiating or continuing nicotine replacement therapy for withdrawal from smoking must be monitored for potential failure or reduced efficacy owing to the induction of metabolism of nicotine via CYP2C6 and UGT2B10.[92] Nicotine is metabolized to cotinine and then 3′-hydroxycotinine, and the ratio of 3′-hydroxycotinine to cotinine is a biomarker for CYP2C6 activity. That ratio goes from approximately 4:1 in early pregnancy to 5.5:1 in late pregnancy to 3:1 postpartum. Further illustrating the phase changes in metabolism, the UGT2B10-catalyzed nicotine and cotinine glucuronide conjugates significantly increase during these phases, whereas the unchanged nicotine excretion is 6%, 2%, and 11%, respectively.[93] Most clinicians encourage smoking cessation before pregnancy for healthy fetal and neonatal development, as therapies employed during pregnancy are more likely to fail, given the enhanced nicotine clearance.[92]

Similarly, buprenorphine used for opioid use disorder and to lower the risk of neonatal abstinence syndrome is simultaneously oxidized to norbuprenorphine via CYP3A4 and CYP2C8 and glucuronidated by UGT1A1, UGT1A3, and UGT2B7, with norbuprenorphine further glucuronidation via UGT1A1 and UGT1A3. Buprenorphine and norbuprenorphine AUC decreased to the same extent during the evaluated second and third trimesters compared to postpartum, whereas both metabolite to its precursor ratios were progressively elevated during gestation.[94] Dosing must be itemized carefully within designed opioid use disorder protocols to accommodate the special PK changes in the pregnant patient[95] while being mindful of the potential effects of those changes on fetal response.[96]

The combined impact of pharmacogenetic variation on the PK efficiency of metabolism and transport is demonstrated by glyburide in gestational diabetes. Examining high, intermediate, and poor functioning alleles for both CYP2C9 and the liver uptake organic acid transporter OATP1B3, pregnant patients with the wild-type allele for both had the least episodes of hypoglycemia (4.1%) and the highest dose needed for glycemic control (8.7 ± 5.7 mg), compared to those poor functioning alleles for either CYP2C9 or OATP1B3 (hypoglycemia 20%; dose 4.7 ± 3.5 mg). An intermediate functioning allele for either the enzyme or the transporter, as expected, yielded in-between results (hypoglycemia 8.1%; dose 5.7 ± 3.7 mg).[97]

RENAL ELIMINATION

The enhanced blood volume, renal collecting system dilatation, progressive increases in cardiac output (by 40%-50%), renal perfusion, and plasma flow (by 25%-50% mid-pregnancy; ≈75% near term) in the healthy pregnant patient yield large increases in glomerular filtration rate (GFR), with a peak in the second to third trimesters and a plateauing or small reduction seen in late pregnancy and at term owing to the increasing abdominal compression.[40] The peak inulin clearance averaged 155 mL/min (95% CI = 145-165) in a meta-analysis of reports on renal function during pregnancy. Serum creatinine (SCr) takes a U-shaped pattern and falls by an average of 0.4 mg/dL to a pregnancy range of 0.4 to 0.8 mg/dL, with an inverse pattern to GFR, and an increase toward prepregnancy creatinine values at term.[98] It is, therefore, important to recognize the pregnant patient among the other patient populations considered to have augmented renal clearance. Renal drug clearance is increased by the lower serum protein binding of drugs in pregnancy, with higher delivery of drugs through the glomerulus and with enhanced tubular secretion from greater renal plasma flow per the following:

$$Cl_{renal} = fu \times [(GFR + Cl_{tubular\ secretion})\ (1 - f_{reabsorbed})]$$

where fu is the fraction unbound in the serum, and $f_{reabsorbed}$ is the fraction that is reabsorbed in the kidney tubules.

The renal clearance of many water-soluble drugs and metabolites is elevated during pregnancy. Antibiotics such as β-lactams, carbapenems, aminoglycosides, and vancomycin demonstrate faster clearances during pregnancy.[99] This prompts the necessity for specific empiric doses that may be different than other adult populations but are often not regarded in general treatment protocols. The need for shorter dosage intervals or continuous infusion strategies for β-lactams to meet systemic exposure goals is relevant in this population. Cefazolin, which is used for a variety of prophylaxis and treatment indications for late pregnancy infections and before cesarean section, needs 2 g doses at more frequent intervals to provide adequate systemic exposure, surgical tissue, and maternal/fetal/neonatal free drug concentrations above the minimal inhibitory concentration (MIC) for target pathogens. Obese pregnant patients may require 3 g doses of cefazolin or earlier redosing to meet concentration targets, especially if a longer duration of surgery occurs.[100,101] Though peak concentrations are lower during pregnancy, concerns over transplacental aminoglycosides causing neonatal ototoxicity may limit the usage of once-daily dosing, yet maternal treatment requires attention to the increased distribution volume and clearance in individualizing the dose to meet concentration targets in multiple doses per day regimen. Importantly, hypertensive diseases of pregnancy including preeclampsia (hypertension, proteinuria, fluid retention, potential end-organ damage) do not necessarily have a boosted GFR as with normal pregnancy,[102] which impacts renal drug clearance, particularly in the third trimester. The added risk of drug-induced acute kidney injury in preeclampsia has significant maternal and perinatal consequences.[103,104]

Therapeutic challenges as discussed earlier for hepatically cleared lamotrigine and oxcarbazepine in treating seizure disorders during pregnancy are relevant to renally cleared ASMs.[27] Levetiracetam, whose clearance correlates with creatinine clearance, shows a more than doubling in clearance during pregnancy. When prescribed doses of levetiracetam remain at prepregnancy amounts, the likelihood of seizure breakthrough is high, with the peak risk at three to four months of gestation and late term.[88] Though blood levels are not routinely monitored for these antiseizure drugs, the invariable need for dosage adjustment may require frequent therapeutic drug monitoring to provide guidance on appropriate dosing to maintain seizure control.[105]

Magnesium sulfate at high serum levels, used for tocolysis and prevention of eclamptic seizures, is purely renally cleared, but unlike other such drugs needing dose increases in pregnancy, the clearance of magnesium can be slowed in preeclampsia by one-third, so careful monitoring based on renal function, BP end points, and serum magnesium levels is essential.[106] A variety of dosage regimen suggestions are proposed to obtain the positive tocolytic, vascular, and anti-inflammation effects of magnesium sulfate, and PK models have been proposed.[107] Numerous treatment indications exist for low-molecular-weight heparins in pregnancy. Standard dosage regimens for enoxaparin may be inadequate to reach anti-Xa assay goals for prophylaxis or treatment with both enhanced V_d and renal elimination progressively increasing during gestation, with postpartum rapid reversal of these parameters.[39,42] Caution and careful monitoring must be applied to use in obese pregnant patients as standard weight–based regimens may yield supratherapeutic levels.[108]

Tubular secretion in the previous GFR equation is increased during pregnancy by the additional activity of renal drug transporters, which are also induced. The organic cation transporter OCT2 elevates the tubular secretion clearance of metformin by 64% at term compared to nonpregnant patients with type 2 diabetes and combines with the higher GFR to raise weight-corrected Cl/F by 24%.[109] Higher bioavailability is also exhibited at 500 mg doses because of the intestinal motility–slowing effect of progesterone, which is somewhat reduced at a 1,000-mg dose. The complex PK suggest that the dosing needs of metformin when managing gestational diabetes or chronic type 2 diabetes in pregnancy with monotherapy or in combination therapy must be carefully calibrated and readjusted promptly once the patient is postpartum.[110,111] Tubular cell efflux transporters preventing reabsorption, such as p-glycoprotein (P-gp), and influx transporters like organic anion transporter polypeptides (OATPs) provide for higher intraluminal levels of digoxin. The mean tubular clearance of digoxin during gestation was nearly double that of the postpartum values (mean = 0.99 mL/min/kg vs 0.53 mL/min/kg) and, together with the enhanced GFR, raised the total renal clearance of digoxin to 2.4 mL/min/kg during gestation compared to 1.7 mL/min/kg postpartum.[63] Higher digoxin doses are, therefore, needed in the pregnant patient with a treatable arrhythmia or cardiomyopathy. Moreover, digoxin is a first-line medication for the management of fetal tachyarrhythmias where the delivery vehicle for giving the drug to the fetus is through maternal administration.[112] Because the transplacental passage of digoxin is approximately 60% to 70%, the maternal levels needed to provide fetal antiarrhythmic effect may be above 2 ng/mL. Therefore, higher-than-typical digoxin doses may be required to overcome the higher maternal clearance and the fractional transplacental passage.[26,113] Careful therapeutic drug monitoring is required, as well as for the alternative agents, flecainide and sotalol.

The combination of physiologic and PK changes during pregnancy and the need for increasing drug doses for many drugs are illustrated in Figure 7.3. Drugs where significant PK changes during pregnancy suggest the need for therapeutic drug monitoring are listed and discussed in Table 7.3.

Transplacental Passage

Clearly, the maternal PK of drugs will be a determinant in the systemic exposure within the pregnant patient and transmission to the fetus (see Figure 7.4). While teratogenic agents have their window of impact during the first trimester of drug exposure, other congenital and functional effects on the unborn come mostly with the second- and third-trimester drug exposure, and acute effects in the newborn following drugs used in labor and delivery. Although these effects and their relationship to maternal dosing

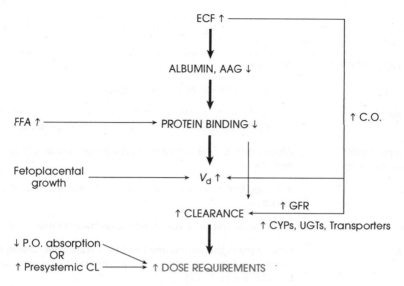

FIGURE 7.3 Impact of pregnancy-related physiologic and pharmacokinetic changes on drug dosing requirements. AAG, α_1-acid glycoprotein; CL, clearance; CYP, cytochrome; C.O., cardiac output; ECF, extracellular fluid; FFA, free fatty acids; GFR, glomerular filtration rate; UGT, uridine diphosphate-glucuronosyltransferase.

TABLE 7.3 Drugs Benefiting From Therapeutic Drug Monitoring During Pregnancy

DRUG/DRUG CLASS	COMMENT
Aminoglycosides	Augmented renal clearance from ↑GFR, large ↑ in ECF and V_d
Vancomycin	↑ in Cl_{Cr}, drug CL and V_d with gestation; goal AUC or trough concentration interpreted in context with lower albumin binding
β-Lactam antibiotics, carbapenems	Same as above with enhanced renal tubular secretion for cefazolin and piperacillin, altered protein binding; TDM needed when treating less susceptible pathogens or assuring effective continuous infusion dose and C_{ss} relative to MIC
Antiretroviral agents	Pregnancy-related changes in protein binding, metabolism, and clearance for numerous agents
Lamotrigine, oxcarbazepine, levetiracetam	Induction and progressive ↑ in glucuronidation, metabolism, and renal function, respectively, alter concentration-dose ratios (<0.65 compared to prepartum greatly enhance the risk of breakthrough seizures)
Digoxin, flecainide, sotalol	Fractional transplacental passage when treating fetal arrhythmia via maternal administration → high doses and serum levels to provide effective fetal therapy with careful monitoring for maternal toxicity
Quinidine, lidocaine, verapamil, procainamide, amiodarone	Altered protein binding and metabolic clearance

(continued)

TABLE 7.3   Drugs Benefiting From Therapeutic Drug Monitoring During Pregnancy (*continued*)

DRUG/DRUG CLASS	COMMENT
Voriconazole	Lower CYP2C19 metabolism in pregnancy
Carboplatin	Increased GFR, CL, and V_d potentially alter doses needed to meet goal AUC as determined by utilized equations, eg, Calvert formula
Antipsychotics, antidepressants	Altered metabolism → treatment resistance → dose adjustment needs
Lithium	Increased GFR and renal clearance → ↑ dose to maintain therapeutic C_{ss}
Tacrolimus	Higher unbound to whole blood concentration ratio
Warfarin	Careful use in the second and third trimesters; lower albumin protein binding and altered CYP3A4 metabolism requires consistent INR monitoring
Heparin/LMWH	Increasing V_d, especially in late pregnancy; enhanced GFR and CL
Thyroid hormone	No appreciable differences from nonpregnant state

AUC, area under the curve; CL, clearance; Cl$_{Cr}$, creatinine clearance; ECF, extracellular fluid; GFR, glomerular filtration rate; INR, international normalized ratio; LMWH, low-molecular-weight heparin; MIC, minimal inhibitory concentration; TDM, therapeutic drug monitoring.

are beyond the scope of this chapter, a review of the determinants of fetal exposure and the PK role of the placenta is important.

The placenta is a transporter of chemicals, nutrients, and drugs and controls exposure to the fetus under normal conditions. Vascular compromise, inflammation, and infection can change the delivery and permeability of drugs crossing the placenta. Similar to the pathways used by molecules to traverse cell membranes, drugs utilize simple, carrier-mediated, and active diffusion and receptor endocytosis for larger molecules, such as monoclonal antibodies and immunoglobulins.[29] Passive immunization through maternal delivery of SARS-CoV-2 antibodies to the fetus has been demonstrated after COVID vaccination.[114,115] The factors influencing transplacental passage are summarized in Table 7.4.[26] Simple diffusion follows Fick's law and is related to the concentration gradient and the surface area and inversely related to the placental membrane thickness as follows:

$$\text{Rate of diffusion} = k \times \text{surface area (maternal-fetal concentration difference)} / \text{placental membrane thickness}$$

The surface area enlarges as the placenta becomes larger with gestation. The placental membrane thickness is greatest in the first trimester when the greatest protection against teratogens is needed and thinnest (single layer of trophoblast cells) during the late third trimester when the need for nutrients and oxygen in the developing fetus is greater. Therefore, drugs will have easier access to the fetoplacental unit to create

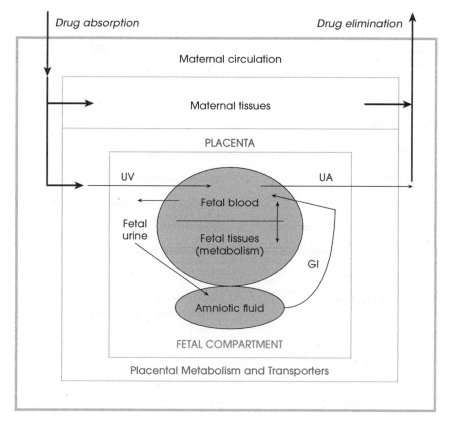

FIGURE 7.4 Compartmental schematic of drug movement during pregnancy. GI, gastrointestinal; UA, umbilical artery; UV, umbilical vein.

perinatal or postnatal pathophysiologic problems when given in late pregnancy, and the risk-benefit ratio must be carefully negotiated.

The integrity of the placenta and its perfusion is paramount in the transport of nutrients and xenobiotics. As discussed earlier, a number of forces including protein binding, pH differential, amniotic fluid circulation, and specific placental transporter function can allow for retention of drug within the fetal compartment. Vestigial fetal drug metabolism and renal elimination do not contribute greatly to the overall disposition. Placental metabolism does contribute to overall maternal drug disposition and is generally protective of the fetus in converting active drug to inactive metabolites.[116,117] Maternal enzymes such as 1A1, 2E1, 3A4, and 3A5 are present in the placenta, along with more unique ones such as CYP4B1 and CYP3A7; the latter also present in the neonate and involved in oxidizing drugs during the first month of life.[118]

As with other organs, efflux and influx transporters are important for regulating nutrient entry and drug exposure through the placenta.[119] P-gp is more abundant in the placenta during the first trimester than later in pregnancy and pumps a wide range of drug substrates against the concentration gradient and away from reaching the fetal compartment. Breast cancer resistance protein (BCRP) provides similar protection but to a lesser number of substrate drugs. These pumps are regulated by gene expression,

TABLE 7.4   Factors Affecting Transplacental Passage of Drugs

MATERNAL/FETAL	PHYSICOCHEMICAL/PHYSIOLOGIC
Pharmacokinetics in the mother	Diffusion, facilitated diffusion, carrier mediated, active transport, saturable uptake; pinocytosis, exocytosis, and endocytosis
Pharmacokinetics in the fetus	Lipid > water soluble
Integrity of the placenta	Small > large molecular weight
Gestational age	Unionized > ionized (weak bases > acids)
Membrane permeability	Maternal/fetal pH difference
Maternal and fetal blood flow rates	Altered maternal protein binding
Anatomy/geometry of vasculature	Maternal vs fetal protein binding
Interspecies differences	Maternal-fetal (uteroplacental) blood flow
Placental metabolism	Placental drug retention and metabolism (CYP450 isozymes: CYP1A1, CYP2E1, CYP3A4, CYP3A5, CYP3A7, CYP4B1 in term placenta; UGT1A1, UGT1A4, UGT1A5, UGT1A9)
Placental transporters	Drug transporters (eg, efflux pumps P-gp and BCRP)

BCRP, breast cancer resistance protein; P-gp, p-glycoprotein.

and single-nucleotide polymorphisms can impact their performance and the amount of drug transport. Gestational age (GA) dependence is seen in the protein abundance and performance of these transporters, with efflux pumps more active earlier in gestation and the organic acid transporters in the later phases.[120,121] MRP1 and MRP5 work mostly in the maternal-to-fetal direction, whereas OCT3 is more bidirectional. The transporters are also subject to chemical inhibitors and regulators, such as verapamil inhibiting P-gp and allowing more transplacental passage of digoxin and cyclosporin. Lopinavir and saquinavir show multifold increased placental passage in the presence of inhibitors.[29] Not only inhibitors, but multiple drugs such as substrates for these efflux transporters may create negative consequences. In a very large patient cohort, drugs in polytherapy given during pregnancy showed a statistically higher rate of congenital anomalies than as monotherapy (P-gp: 5.4% vs 4.6%; BCRP: 6.2 vs 5.1%).[122] Combination of P-gp and BCRP substrate drugs showed similar effects compared to monotherapy or those unexposed to such drugs. It is presumed that when paired, one or both drugs gain more fetal concentration to cause fetopathy. Other factors that can affect these efflux pumps are presented in Table 7.5.[26]

Transplacental Passage and Pharmacokinetic Prediction

Measurement of fetal concentrations is typically done opportunistically via cord blood measurements, amniocentesis, or sampling simultaneously with direct fetal space drug

TABLE 7.5 Chemical and Pathophysiologic Factors Affecting Placental Transporters

- Oxygen (variable depending on the resistance protein and O_2 tension)
- Infection: Bacterial (early) and viral (late) on P-gp and BCRP
- PGE_2 (increases BCRP expression)
- Inhibitor drug interactions (verapamil on P-gp, etc); DDIs
- Higher maternal plasma IL-1β/TNF-α concentrations → ↓ P-gp
- Obesity (inhibition of P-gp effect → ↑ fetal digoxin, quinidine)
- 17α-Ethinyl estradiol–induced intrahepatic cholestasis could ↑ P-gp
- Corticosteroids (↑ P-gp and BCRP)
- Diabetes (varying effects depending on polarity of the substrate drug)
- Polymorphisms (maternal and fetal)

BCRP, breast cancer resistance protein; DDIs, drug-drug interactions; IL, interleukin; P-gp, p-glycoprotein; TNF, tumor necrosis factor.

injection. The cord blood sample provides a point estimate of transplacental disposition only at the end of pregnancy, and the fetal-maternal concentration ratio will be somewhat dependent on when the last maternal administration of drug occurred before birth. It does not relate to exposure throughout pregnancy. Ex vivo placental perfusion studies capture the fetal-maternal concentration ratio as correlated to maternal and cord sampling at birth, and experimental conditions (eg, altering perfusion rates, pressures and direction, protein binding, pH, transporter function) can refine the estimates, mimicking pathophysiologic such as preeclampsia.[123] This methodology is also useful for comparing transplacental passage among different agents within a drug class and assessing risk, and transport using placentae harvested from premature births can evaluate earlier phases of pregnancy. In vitro methods such as the placenta-on-a-chip technology can provide "fetal" and "maternal" concentration measurements and the mechanism of transport using trophoblast-like cells with the capability to alter experimental conditions.[124]

These methods do not lend themselves easily to data determination at all time points during gestation dynamic changes in drug disposition. Population PK modeling can statistically search for the factors that influence the kinetic disposition during gestations and their magnitude, with subsequent testing and validation of the generated equations.[125] PBPM takes the physiologic flow and extraction rates; volumes and protein binding within the anatomic spaces (including the fetoplacental unit); the calculated efficiencies of metabolism and elimination for individual enzymes and transporter, combined with the physicochemical properties of the drug; and the PK parameters of nonpregnant individuals to form large mathematical models that resolve the concentration-time profile within the patient and these spaces.[2,126] This is illustrated in Figure 7.5.[127] Placental perfusion study results can be added to this model to refine fetoplacental kinetic estimates.[128] This methodology can help project the maternal PK of various established drugs and those not yet tested or extensively used in pregnant patients, to estimate and validate the quantity of exposure to the fetus at various gestation time points.[129] These models have been applied to acetaminophen,[130] opioids,[131] indomethacin,[132] quetiapine,[133] olanzapine,[134] acyclovir,[135] metoprolol,[75] theophylline,[136] caffeine,[70] metformin,[135] and a variety of antibacterial

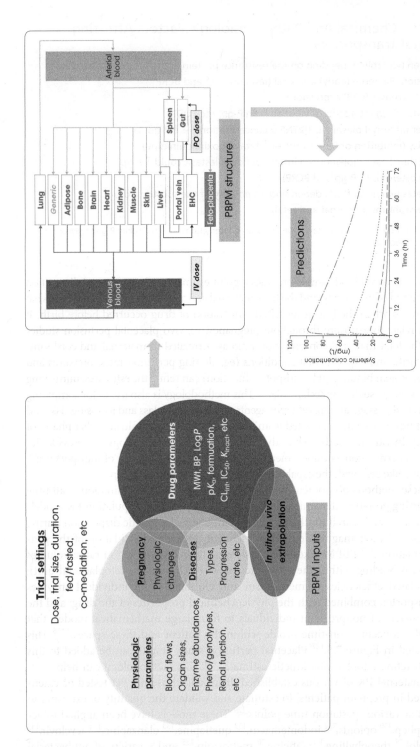

FIGURE 7.5 Physiologically based pharmacokinetic modeling (PBPM) and concentration prediction in pregnancy. BP, blood pressure; EHC, enterohepatic circulation; MW, molecular weight; IV, intravenous; PO, orally. (Abduljalil K, Badhan RKS. Drug dosing during pregnancy-opportunities for physiologically based pharmacokinetic models. *J Pharmacokinet Pharmacodyn.* 2020;47(4):319-340.)

and antiretroviral agents used in pregnancy.[137] Given the ethical and medical limitations of drug clinical trials during pregnancy, these methods are of growing important steps in predicting drug disposition for both the mother and the fetus, with validation of these predictions potentially improving the management of postnatal complications, such as neonatal opioid withdrawal syndrome.[138]

EXAMPLE

Aripiprazole is prescribed for pregnant women to treat schizophrenia and bipolar disorder. The drug is metabolized via CYP2D6 and CYP3A4, accounting for 43% and 56% of the clearance, respectively, with a small component of renal clearance. The suggested therapeutic range for the total drug is 150 to 500 ng/mL. The clearance of aripiprazole in nonpregnant women is 2.7 to 3.3 L/hr, with a renal clearance of 0.03 L/hr.

PBPM has been used to determine the magnitude of change in metabolic efficiency of the CYP450 enzymes during pregnancy, quantified based on GA in weeks.[65]

$$CYP2D6_{Pregnancy} \text{ fold-change} = 1 + (0.0163 \text{ GW}) + (0.0009 \text{ GW}^2)$$

$$CYP3A4_{Pregnancy} \text{ fold-change} = 1 + (0.0129 \text{ GW}) + (0.0005 \text{ GW}^2)$$

QUESTION 1: *Compared to nonpregnant women, what will be the computed overall percentage changes in aripiprazole metabolic clearance at 12, 25, and 40 weeks of gestation? Plot these results.*

This demands a two-step calculation: first to calculate the manifold increase in each pathway and second to calculate the contribution of each pathway based on their percent influence from each metabolic pathway and combining the result.

At 12, 25, and 40 weeks, the manifold increases in metabolism for each pathway are calculated as follows:

For CYP2D6:

$$CYP2D6_{Pregnancy} \text{ fold-change} = 1 + (0.0163 \times 12) + (0.0009 \times 12^2) = 1.325$$

$$CYP2D6_{Pregnancy} \text{ fold-change} = 1 + (0.0163 \times 25) + (0.0009 \times 25^2) = 1.970$$

$$CYP2D6_{Pregnancy} \text{ fold-change} = 1 + (0.0163 \times 40) + (0.0009 \times 40^2) = 3.092$$

For CYP3A4:

$$CYP3A4_{Pregnancy} \text{ fold-change} = 1 + (0.0129 \times 12) + (0.0009 \times 12^2) = 1.227$$

$$CYP3A4_{Pregnancy} \text{ fold-change} = 1 + (0.0129 \times 25) + (0.0009 \times 25^2) = 1.635$$

$$CYP3A4_{Pregnancy} \text{ fold-change} = 1 + (0.0129 \times 40) + (0.000 \times 40^2) = 2.315$$

Total metabolic clearance increases at 12, 25, and 40 weeks = Contribution of CYP2D6 + contribution from CYP3A4:

At 12 weeks: $(0.43 \times 1.325) + (0.56 \times 1.227) = 0.570 + 0.687$
$= 1.257\text{-fold or }126\% \text{ increase.}$

At 25 weeks: $(0.43 \times 1.970) + (0.56 \times 1.635) = 0.847 + 0.916$
$= 1.763\text{-fold or }176\% \text{ increase.}$

At 40 weeks: $(0.43 \times 3.092) + (0.56 \times 2.315) = 1.329 + 1.296$
$= 2.625\text{-fold or }263\% \text{ increase.}$

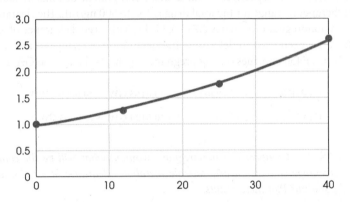

QUESTION 2: *Assuming a mean Cl of 3 L/hr in the nonpregnant state and a bioavailability of 87%, what would be the expected steady-state concentration for a 15-mg daily dose of aripiprazole given at 40 weeks? Would that dose meet therapeutic range goals?*

Metabolic Cl in nonpregnant = $Cl_{total} - Cl_{renal} = 3 - 0.03 = 2.97$ L/hr

Clearance during pregnancy will = [Manifold change in metabolic Cl] × [Metabolic Cl in nonpregnant] + Renal Cl

At 25 weeks: Cl = $2.97 + (1.763 \times 2.97) + 0.03 = 8.236$ L/hr

C_{ss} = Dose × F/Cl = 15 mg (0.87)/8.236 L/hr = 1.58 mg/L or 158 ng/mL

At 40 weeks: Cl = $2.97 + (2.62 \times 2.97) + 0.03 = 10.79$ L/hr

C_{ss} = Dose × F/Cl = 15 mg (0.87)/10.79 L/hr = 1.21 mg/L or 121 ng/mL

Therefore, a daily dose of 15 mg daily will provide a steady-state concentration at the low end of the therapeutic range at 25 weeks of gestation and falls below it at term. It is rational that recommended dose during pregnancy be increased to 30 mg daily.

EXAMPLE

NJ is a 33-year-old white woman, G3P2A1, with a history of chronic hypertension and gestational diabetes is in week 30 with increasing BP and HR. The patient was switched from enalapril to labetalol once she was aware of her pregnancy. Tight control had been initially maintained with 300 mg twice daily (BID) of labetalol in week 18, but high mean arterial pressures were consistently present afterward. The clinical concern for preeclampsia is heightened, given its presence in NJ's last pregnancy. The labetalol dose was raised to 400 mg BID, but the diastolic BP is still elevated, though increased variability is seen. HR = 95. She is 161 cm tall and weighs 95 kg (lean body weight [LBW] = 50 kg). She is also receiving low-dose aspirin for prophylaxis of preeclampsia. The following pharmacodynamic graph in the following figure shows the concentration-effect relationship for labetalol as change in systolic pressure (blue dots) and diastolic pressure (white dots) in pregnant study patients,[139] with effective concentration at 50% of maximum (EC$_{50}$) of 77 ng/mL. The relationship of maternal bioavailability–corrected clearance to GA, discussed earlier in this chapter,[81] is captured by its linear increase with time:

$$Cl_{Preg}/F \text{ in L/hr/50 kg LBW} = Cl_{nonpreg}/F + [54 \times (1 + GA/40)]$$

where $Cl_{nonpreg} = 188$ L/hr.

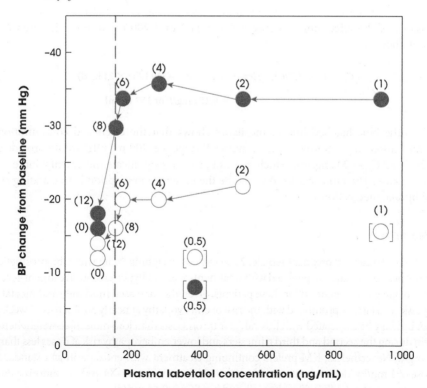

QUESTION 3:   *What therapeutic choice should be made at this time?*

a. Increase the labetalol dose to 300 mg 3 times daily (TID).
b. Increase the labetalol dose to 400 mg TID.
c. Increase the labetalol dose and frequency to 400 mg 4 times daily (QID).
d. Replace with pure β_1-blocker or central α-agonist.
e. Add a calcium channel blocker.

Although the addition of or replacement with another antihypertensive could be considered, favorable HR and racial factors for labetalol response in hypertension in pregnancy are present in this patient.[140] Adjustment of the labetalol dose is viewed as a first option in this case. Maximum daily doses suggested in various guidelines have been 1,200 to 2,400 mg. For this patient, the dose to provide a maximum likelihood of response can be computed. Using the concentration-response graph and the PK equation, a 300 mg TID would provide a steady-state level calculated as follows:

$$Cl_{Preg}/F = Cl_{nonpreg}/F\,[54 \times (1 + GA/40)] = 188 + [54 \times$$
$$(1 + 30/40)] = 329\ \text{L/hr}$$

$$C_{ss} = \text{Dose}\ (F)/Cl_{Preg}/F = 900\ \text{mg/d} \div (329\ \text{L/hr} \times 24\ \text{hr/d})$$

$$= 0.114\ \text{mg/L or }114\ \text{ng/mL}$$

As can be seen in the graph, this concentration is on the lower part of the upslope of the effect curve. Using 400 mg TID or 1,200 mg/d, the calculated C_{ss} would be:

$$C_{ss} = \text{Dose}\ (F)/Cl_{Preg}/F = 1{,}200\ \text{mg/d} \div (329\ \text{L/hr} \times 24\ \text{hr/d})$$

$$= 0.152\ \text{mg/L or }152\ \text{ng/mL}$$

The blue-hatched line in the figure shows that the calculated concentration comes closer to generating the maximum BP response. 400 mg QID would provide a calculated $C_{ss} = 203$ ng/mL, which may not provide a significant incremental increase in response. Therefore, choice B would be the preferred first option before adding an additional medication.

EXAMPLE

KM is a 35-year-old pregnant female, 20 weeks GA, weighing 90 kg with a bioprosthetic aortic heart valve and hospitalized with treatment-resistant hypertension. Treatment-level anticoagulation is required for these patients, given the increased morbidity and mortality risk. Warfarin is prohibited with the risk of embryopathy at nearly 30% at 6 to 12 weeks GA but may be associated with less valvular thrombosis than low-molecular-weight heparin during the second and third trimesters and lower embryopathy risk at doses less than 5 mg/d. Nevertheless, KM prefers continuing treatment with enoxaparin at a standard dose of 1 mg/kg/dose subcutaneously every 12 hours, with anti-Xa assay monitoring every 1 to 2 weeks. KM's is 68 inches tall, and her SCr is 0.65 mg/dL.

QUESTION 4: *What 4-hour postdose (peak) and predose (trough) steady-state anti-Xa level can be projected for KM? Do these levels meet the goals for managing pregnant patient with mechanical heart valves?*

Population PK model in pregnancy[42]:

- V_d (L) = V_d pop (Wt/70) $\times$ 1.41 (if GA > 31 weeks)
  where V_d pop = 7.81 L.
- Cl (L/hr) = Cl pop $[(Wt/SCr)/1.27]^{0.423}$
  where Cl pop = 0.781 L/hr, Wt in kg, SCr in μmol/L (88.4 μmol/L = 1 mg/dL).
- Ka = 0.56 hr^{-1}
  V_d = 7.81 (90/70) = 10.04 L
  Cl = 0.781 $[(90/0.65 \times 88.4)/1.27]^{0.423}$ = 0.8534 L/hr

Therefore, $ke = Cl/V_d$ = 0.8534/10.04 = 0.085 hr^{-1}

In order to ensure that the units are consistent with the calculation of anti-Xa assay results in IU/mL, the enoxaparin dose in mg can be converted to IU by multiplying by 100. A one-compartment absorption and elimination model is assumed.

Because $e^{-ka(\tau)}$ approaches zero, we can calculate the steady-state trough concentration as follows:

$$C_{ss\,min} = \frac{F \times Dose \times ka}{V_d \times (ka - ke)} \times \frac{e^{-ke \times \tau}}{1 - e^{-ke \times \tau}}$$

$$C_{ss\,min} = \frac{1 \times 9,000\ IU \times 0.56}{10.04\ L \times (0.56 - 0.085)} \times \frac{e^{-0.085 \times 12}}{1 - e^{-0.085 \times 12}}$$

$$C_{ss\,min} = 597.3\ IU/L = 0.6\ IU/mL$$

As the absorption half-life is = 0.693/0.56 = 1.24 hours, 3.23 half-lives ($\approx$90% toward complete absorption) have past 4 hours after the dose is administered. So, one can be fairly comfortable calculating the 4-hour postdose peak bioactivity concentration via back extrapolation of the $C_{ss\,min}$.

$$C_{ss\,max} = \frac{C_{ss\,min}}{e^{-ke \times \Delta t}} = \frac{0.597}{e^{-0.085 \times 8}}$$

$$C_{ss\,max} = 1178\ IU/L = 1.18\ IU/mL$$

One can, however, do the more rigorous calculation of the 4-hour peak:

$$C_{ss\,max} = \frac{F \times Dose \times ka}{V_d \times (ka - ke)} \times \frac{e^{-ke \times t4}}{1 - e^{-ke \times \tau}}$$

$$C_{ss\,max} = \frac{1 \times 9,000\ IU \times 0.56}{10.04\ L \times (0.56 - 0.085)} \times \frac{e^{-0.085 \times 4}}{1 - e^{-0.085 \times 12}} = 1,176\ IU/L = 1.18\ IU/mL$$

The peak and trough are within range for treating a deep vein thrombosis in an adult, and the stated range for necessary anticoagulation of pregnant patients with mechanical valves (ie, troughs > 0.6 and peaks 0.8-1.2 IU/mL for aortic valves, and >0.6 and 1.0-1.2 IU/mL, respectively, for mitral valves).[141]

KM remains on this dose until gestation week 33 with occasional anti-Xa assay checks. The patient now starts complaining of flank pain. Her weight is now 98 kg, her SCr has remained the same, but hematuria and proteinuria are now present, with an increase in BP. While considering a diagnosis of preeclampsia and labetalol initiated, a workup is begun for the hematuria.

QUESTION 5:   *How have KM's PK parameters changed? What steady-state levels would you now anticipate?*

$$V_d = 7.81 (98/70) \times 1.41 = 15.42 \text{ L}$$

$$Cl = 0.781 [(98/0.65 \times 88.4)/1.27]^{0.423} = 0.8847 \text{ L/hr}$$

Therefore, $ke = Cl/V_d = 0.8847/15.42 = 0.0574 \text{ hr}^{-1}$

$$C_{ss\,min} = \frac{1 \times 9,000 \text{ IU} \times 0.56}{15.42 \text{ L} \times (0.56 - 0.0574)} \times \frac{e^{-0.0574 \times 12}}{1 - e^{-0.0574 \times 12}} = 656 \text{ IU/L}$$

$$= 0.66 \text{ IU/mL}$$

$$C_{ss\,max} = \frac{1 \times 9,000 \text{ IU} \times 0.56}{15.42 \text{ L} \times (0.56 - 0.0574)} \times \frac{e^{-0.0574 \times 4}}{1 - e^{-0.0574 \times 12}} = 1038 \text{ IU/L}$$

$$= 1.04 \text{ IU/mL}$$

Note the peak-to-trough fluctuation is lower than at GA week 20, but level goals are still being met.

KM's hematuria intensifies, a new onset of left flank pain is noted, and the clinical team is concerned for a renal vein thrombosis, which is radiologically confirmed. Her creatinine has risen to 1.2 mg/dL, and her hemoglobin has decreased by 1.2 g/dL.

QUESTION 6:   *What would be the new steady-state peak and trough anti-Xa levels?*

Recalculating the PK parameters:

The volume of distribution stays the same, with no change in weight reported. Clearance will likely decrease with the change in renal function.

$$V_d = 7.81 (98/70) \times 1.41 = 15.42 \text{ L}$$

$$Cl = 0.781 [(98/1.2 \times 88.4)/1.27]^{0.423} = 0.6826 \text{ L/hr}$$

Therefore, $ke = Cl/V_d = 0.6826/15.42 = 0.0443 \text{ hr}^{-1}$

$$C_{ss\ min} = \frac{1 \times 9{,}000\ \text{IU} \times 0.56}{15.42\ \text{L} \times (0.56 - 0.0443)} \times \frac{e^{-0.0443 \times 12}}{1 - e^{-0.0443 \times 12}} = 903\ \text{IU/L}$$

$$= 0.90\ \text{IU/mL}$$

$$C_{ss\ max} = \frac{1 \times 9{,}000\ \text{IU} \times 0.56}{15.42\ \text{L} \times (0.56 - 0.0443)} \times \frac{e^{-0.0443 \times 4}}{1 - e^{-0.0443 \times 12}} = 1{,}287\ \text{IU/L}$$

$$= 1.29\ \text{IU/mL}$$

As the patient's GFR has notably decreased, and with the gestational expansion of the volume of distribution, the peak and trough have risen beyond the goal, though a clear upper limit for the trough is not elucidated. Note the further narrowing of the peak-to-trough variability resulting from the now decreased clearance and increased half-life while the dosage interval remains unchanged. The hematuria may be part of an unresolved renal vein thrombosis, but the increased anti-Xa can certainly be causative of additive, and the hemoglobin drop is further evidence for concern of overanticoagulation. While advancing a decision of thrombolysis and endovascular treatment, it is decided to maintain the enoxaparin, and a once-daily dose is requested to provide a trough closer to 0.6 and a peak of 0.8 to 1.2 IU/mL.

Setting the goal of the $C_{ss\ min}$ of 0.6 IU/mL (or 600 IU/L), we can rearrange the previous equation and solve for the dose at an interval of every 24 hours.

$$\text{Dose} \times ka = C_{ss\ min} \times V_d \times (ka - ke) \times \frac{1 - e^{-ke \times 24}}{e^{-ke \times 24}}$$

$$\text{Dose} \times ka = 600 \times 15.42 \times (0.56 - 0.0443) \times \frac{1 - e^{-0.0443 \times 24}}{e^{-0.0443 \times 24}}$$

$$\text{Dose} \times ka = 4{,}771 \times \frac{0.6547}{0.3453} = 9{,}044.4$$

$$\text{Dose} = 9{,}044.4 \div 0.56 = 16{,}150\ \text{IU or }160\ \text{mg every 24 hours}$$

With the longer elimination phase, we can calculate T_{max}:

$$T_{max} = \ln \frac{ka}{ke \times (1 - e^{-ke \times \tau})} \div (ka - ke)$$

$$T_{max} = \ln \frac{0.56}{0.0443 \times (1 - e^{-0.0443 \times 24})} \div (0.56 - 0.0443) = 5.74\ \text{hours}$$

$$C_{ss\ max} = \frac{1 \times 16{,}000\ \text{IU} \times 0.56}{15.42\ \text{L} \times (0.56 - 0.0443)} \times \frac{e^{-0.0443 \times 4}}{1 - e^{-0.0443 \times 24}} = 1{,}441\ \text{IU/L or }1.44\ \text{IU/mL}$$

Through back extrapolation, virtually the same answer is computed, with C_{ss} 4-hour peak = 1.45 IU/mL.

Therefore, it may be seen as unachievable to meet these simultaneous trough and peak goals on the 24-hour dosage interval despite the lowered $C_{ss\,min}$ goal. Staying with an every 12-hour regimen, a linear proportionality can be used from the earlier calculation:

$$\text{Dose} = \frac{C_{ssmin}\text{goal}}{C_{ssmin}\text{prior}} \times \text{Prior dose} = \frac{0.6}{0.903} \times 90 \text{ mg} = 59.8 \text{ or } 60 \text{ mg every 12 hours}$$

On this dose, the C_{ss} 4-hour peak = 1.287 IU/mL × 0.6/0.9 = 0.86 IU/mL.

The peak still meets the goal of preventing an aortic valve thrombosis pending further therapy for KM's renal vein thrombosis.

REFERENCES

1. Caritis SN, Venkataramanan R. Obstetrical, fetal, and lactation pharmacology-a crisis that can no longer be ignored. *Am J Obstet Gynecol.* 2021;225(1):10-20.

2. Chaphekar N, Dodeja P, Shaik IH, Caritis S, Venkataramanan R. Maternal-fetal pharmacology of drugs: a review of current status of the application of physiologically based pharmacokinetic models. *Front Pediatr.* 2021;9:733823.

3. Eke AC, Dooley KE, Sheffield JS. Pharmacologic research in pregnant women—time to get it right. *N Engl J Med.* 2019;380(14):1293-1295.

4. McCulley DJ, Jensen EA, Sucre JMS, et al. Racing against time: leveraging preclinical models to understand pulmonary susceptibility to perinatal acetaminophen exposures. *Am J Physiol Lung Cell Mol Physiol.* 2022;323(1):L1-L13.

5. Bauer AZ, Swan SH, Kriebel D, et al. Paracetamol use during pregnancy—a call for precautionary action. *Nat Rev Endocrinol.* 2021;17(12):757-766.

6. Byrne JJ, Saucedo AM, Spong CY. Evaluation of drug labels following the 2015 pregnancy and lactation labeling rule. *JAMA Netw Open.* 2020;3(8):e2015094.

7. Shebl E, Chakraborty RK. Asthma in Pregnancy. In: *StatPearls* [Internet]. StatPearls Publishing; 2022.

8. Li Y, Meador KJ. Epilepsy and pregnancy. *Continuum.* 2022;28(1):34-54.

9. Tita AT, Szychowski JM, Boggess K, et al. Treatment for mild chronic hypertension during pregnancy. *N Engl J Med.* 2022;386(19):1781-1792.

10. Pham S, Churruca K, Ellis LA, Braithwaite J. A scoping review of gestational diabetes mellitus healthcare: experiences of care reported by pregnant women internationally. *BMC Pregnancy Childbirth.* 2022;22(1):627.

11. Mukherjee SM, Dawson A. Diabetes: how to manage gestational diabetes mellitus. *Drugs Context.* 2022;11:2021-9-12.

12. Longhitano E, Siligato R, Torreggiani M, et al. The hypertensive disorders of pregnancy: a focus on definitions for clinical nephrologists. *J Clin Med.* 2022;11(12):3420.

13. Hoevelmann J, Engel ME, Muller E, et al. A global perspective on the management and outcomes of peripartum cardiomyopathy: a systematic review and meta-analysis. *Eur J Heart Fail.* 2022;24(9):1719-1736.

14. Kaye DK. The moral imperative to approve pregnant women's participation in randomized clinical trials for pregnancy and newborn complications. *Philos Ethics Humanit Med.* 2019;14(1):11.

15. Widnes SF, Schjøtt J. Risk perception regarding drug use in pregnancy. *Am J Obstet Gynecol.* 2017; 216(4):375-378.

16. Acar S, Keskin-Arslan E, Erol-Coskun H, Kaya-Temiz T, Kaplan YC. Pregnancy outcomes following quinolone and fluoroquinolone exposure during pregnancy: a systematic review and meta-analysis. *Reprod Toxicol.* 2019;85:65-74.

17. Thiele L, Thompson J, Pruszynski J, Spong CY. Gaps in evidence-based medicine: underrepresented populations still excluded from research trials following 2018 recommendations from the Health and

Human Services Task Force on Research Specific to Pregnant Women and Lactating Women. *Am J Obstet Gynecol.* 2022;227(6):908-909.

18. Jering KS, Claggett BL, Cunningham JW, et al. Clinical characteristics and outcomes of hospitalized women giving birth with and without COVID-19. *JAMA Intern Med.* 2021;181(5):714-717.

19. Fell DB, Dimanlig-Cruz S, Regan AK, et al. Risk of preterm birth, small for gestational age at birth, and stillbirth after Covid-19 vaccination during pregnancy: population based retrospective cohort study. *BMJ.* 2022;378:e071416.

20. Rubin R. Pregnant people's paradox-excluded from vaccine trials despite having a higher risk of Covid-19 complications. *JAMA.* 2021;325(11):1027-1028.

21. Wesley BD, Sewell CA, Chang CY, Hatfield KP, Nguyen CP. Prescription medications for use in pregnancy-perspective from the US Food and Drug Administration. *Am J Obstet Gynecol.* 2021;225(1):21-32.

22. LaCourse S, John-Stewart G, Adams Waldorf KM. Importance of inclusion of pregnant and breast-feeding women in COVID-19 therapeutic trials. *Clin Infect Dis.* 2020;71(15):879-881.

23. Badell ML, Dude CM, Rasmussen SA, Jamieson DJ. Covid-19 vaccination in pregnancy. *BMJ.* 2022;378:e069741.

24. David AL, Ahmadzia H, Ashcroft R, Bucci-Rechtweg C, Spencer RN, Thornton S. Improving development of drug treatments for pregnant women and the fetus. *Ther Innov Regul Sci.* 2022;56(6):976-990.

25. Avram MJ. Pharmacokinetic studies in pregnancy. *Semin Perinatol.* 2020;44(3):151227.

26. Steinberg I. Pharmacokinetics of drugs in pregnancy and lactation. In: Elkayam U, ed. *Cardiac Problems in Pregnancy.* 4th ed. John Wiley & Sons, Inc; 2020:435-455.

27. Pennell PB, Karanam A, Meador KJ, et al; MONEAD Study Group. Antiseizure medication concentrations during pregnancy: results from the Maternal Outcomes and Neurodevelopmental Effects of Antiepileptic Drugs (MONEAD) Study. *JAMA Neurol.* 2022;79(4):370-379.

28. Ke AB, Greupink R, Abduljalil K. Drug dosing in pregnant women: challenges and opportunities in using physiologically based pharmacokinetic modeling and simulations. *CPT Pharmacometrics Syst Pharmacol.* 2018;7(2):103-110.

29. Tetro N, Moushaev S, Rubinchik-Stern M, Eyal S. The placental barrier: the gate and the fate in drug distribution. *Pharm Res.* 2018;35(4):71.

30. Patorno E, Huybrechts KF, Bateman BT, et al. Lithium use in pregnancy and the risk of cardiac malformations. *N Engl J Med.* 2017;376(23):2245-2254.

31. Tomson T, Battino D, Perucca E. Teratogenicity of antiepileptic drugs. *Curr Opin Neurol.* 2019;32(2):246-252.

32. Wen X, Belviso N, Murray E, Lewkowitz AK, Ward KE, Meador KJ. Association of gestational opioid exposure and risk of major and minor congenital malformations. *JAMA Netw Open.* 2021;4(4):e215708.

33. Wen X, Lawal OD, Belviso N, et al. Association between prenatal opioid exposure and neurodevelopmental outcomes in early childhood: a retrospective cohort study. *Drug Saf.* 2021;44(8):863-875.

34. Sorbye IK, Haualand R, Wiull H, Letting AS, Langesaeter E, Estensen ME. Maternal beta-blocker dose and risk of small-for gestational-age in women with heart disease. *Acta Obstet Gynecol Scand.* 2022;101(7):794-802.

35. Colombo A, Giordano F, Giorgetti F, et al. Correlation between pharmacokinetics and pharmacogenetics of selective serotonin reuptake inhibitors and selective serotonin and noradrenaline reuptake inhibitors and maternal and neonatal outcomes: results from a naturalistic study in patients with affective disorders. *Hum Psychopharmacol.* 2021;36(3):e2772.

36. Eke AC. An update on the physiologic changes during pregnancy and their impact on drug pharmacokinetics and pharmacogenomics. *J Basic Clin Physiol Pharmacol.* 2021;33(5):581-598.

37. Mulrenin IR, Garcia JE, Fashe MM, et al. The impact of pregnancy on antihypertensive drug metabolism and pharmacokinetics: current status and future directions. *Expert Opin Drug Metab Toxicol.* 2021;17(11):1261-1279.

38. Feghali M, Venkataramanan R, Caritis S. Prevention of preterm delivery with 17-hydroxyprogesterone caproate: pharmacologic considerations. *Semin Perinatol.* 2014;38(8):516-522.

39. Patel JP, Green B, Patel RK, Marsh MS, Davies JG, Arya R. Population pharmacokinetics of enoxaparin during the antenatal period. *Circulation.* 2013;128(13):1462-1469.

40. Kazma JM, van den Anker J, Allegaert K, Dallmann A, Ahmadzia HK. Anatomical and physiological alterations of pregnancy. *J Pharmacokinet Pharmacodyn*. 2020;47(4):271-285.

41. Pariente G, Leibson T, Carls A, Adams-Webber T, Ito S, Koren G. Pregnancy-associated changes in pharmacokinetics: a systematic review. *PLoS Med*. 2016;13(11):e1002160.

42. Lebaudy C, Hulot JS, Amoura Z, et al. Changes in enoxaparin pharmacokinetics during pregnancy and implications for antithrombotic therapeutic strategy. *Clin Pharmacol Ther*. 2008;84(3):370-377.

43. Azancot-Benisty A, Jacqz-Aigrain E, Guirgis NM, Decrepy A, Oury JF, Blot P. Clinical and pharmacologic study of fetal supraventricular tachyarrhythmias. *J Pediatr*. 1992;121(4):608-613.

44. Celestin MN, Musteata FM. Impact of changes in free concentrations and drug-protein binding on drug dosing regimens in special populations and disease states. *J Pharm Sci*. 2021;110(10):3331-3344.

45. Mitani GM, Steinberg I, Lien EJ, Harrison EC, Elkayam U. The pharmacokinetics of antiarrhythmic agents in pregnancy and lactation. *Clin Pharmacokinet*. 1987;12(4):253-291.

46. Roberts JA, Pea F, Lipman J. The clinical relevance of plasma protein binding changes. *Clin Pharmacokinet*. 2013;52(1):1-8.

47. Ryu RJ, Easterling TR, Caritis SN, et al. Prednisone pharmacokinetics during pregnancy and lactation. *J Clin Pharmacol*. 2018;58(9):1223-1232.

48. Abduljalil K, Jamei M, Johnson TN. Fetal physiologically based pharmacokinetic models: systems information on fetal blood components and binding proteins. *Clin Pharmacokinet*. 2020;59(5):629-642.

49. Sudhakaran S, Rayner CR, Li J, Kong DC, Gude NM, Nation RL. Differential protein binding of indinavir and saquinavir in matched maternal and umbilical cord plasma. *Br J Clin Pharmacol*. 2007;63(3):315-321.

50. Badaoui S, Hopkins AM, Rodrigues AD, Miners JO, Sorich MJ, Rowland A. Application of model informed precision dosing to address the impact of pregnancy stage and CYP2D6 phenotype on foetal morphine exposure. *AAPS J*. 2021;23(1):15.

51. Choi SY, Koh KH, Jeong H. Isoform-specific regulation of cytochromes P450 expression by estradiol and progesterone. *Drug Metab Dispos*. 2013;41(2):263-269.

52. Allegaert K, Kulo A, Verbesselt R, et al. The pharmacokinetics of a high intravenous dose of paracetamol after caesarean delivery: the effect of gestational age. *Eur J Anaesthesiol*. 2012;29(10):484-488.

53. Kulo A, Van Calsteren K, van de Velde M, et al. Weight, pregnancy and oral contraceptives affect intravenous paracetamol clearance in young women. *Eur Rev Med Pharmacol Sci*. 2014;18(5):599-604.

54. Ryu RJ, Eyal S, Easterling TR, et al. Pharmacokinetics of metoprolol during pregnancy and lactation. *J Clin Pharmacol*. 2016;56(5):581-589.

55. Buchanan ML, Easterling TR, Carr DB, et al. Clonidine pharmacokinetics in pregnancy. *Drug Metab Dispos*. 2009;37(4):702-705.

56. Jeong H. Altered drug metabolism during pregnancy: hormonal regulation of drug-metabolizing enzymes. *Expert Opin Drug Metab Toxicol*. 2010;6(6):689-699.

57. Zhang Z, Farooq M, Prasad B, Grepper S, Unadkat JD. Prediction of gestational age-dependent induction of in vivo hepatic CYP3A activity based on HepaRG cells and human hepatocytes. *Drug Metab Dispos*. 2015;43(6):836-842.

58. Morgan JL, Kogutt BK, Meek C, et al. Pharmacokinetics of amlodipine besylate at delivery and during lactation. *Pregnancy Hypertens*. 2018;11:77-80.

59. Wang T, Wang Y, Lin S, et al. Evaluation of pharmacokinetics and safety with bioequivalence of amlodipine in healthy Chinese volunteers: bioequivalence study findings. *J Clin Lab Anal*. 2020;34(6):e23228.

60. Khatri R, Kulick N, Rementer RJB, et al. Pregnancy-related hormones increase nifedipine metabolism in human hepatocytes by inducing CYP3A4 expression. *J Pharm Sci*. 2021;110(1):412-421.

61. Haas DM, Quinney SK, Clay JM, et al; Obstetric-Fetal Pharmacology Research Units Network. Nifedipine pharmacokinetics are influenced by CYP3A5 genotype when used as a preterm labor tocolytic. *Am J Perinatol*. 2013;30(4):275-281.

62. Schalkwijk S, Greupink R, Burger D. Free dug concentrations in pregnancy: bound to measure unbound? *Br J Clin Pharmacol*. 2017;83(12):2595-2598.

63. Hebert MF, Easterling TR, Kirby B, et al. Effects of pregnancy on CYP3A and P-glycoprotein activities as measured by disposition of midazolam and digoxin: a University of Washington specialized center of research study. *Clin Pharmacol Ther*. 2008;84(2):248-253.

64. Westin AA, Brekke M, Molden E, Skogvoll E, Castberg I, Spigset O. Treatment with antipsychotics in pregnancy: changes in drug disposition. *Clin Pharmacol Ther*. 2018;103(3):477-484.

65. Zheng L, Tang S, Tang R, Xu M, Jiang X, Wang L. Dose adjustment of quetiapine and aripiprazole for pregnant women using physiologically based pharmacokinetic modeling and simulation. *Clin Pharmacokinet*. 2021;60(5):623-635.

66. Hebert MF, Ma X, Naraharisetti SB, et al. Are we optimizing gestational diabetes treatment with glyburide? The pharmacologic basis for better clinical practice. *Clin Pharmacol Ther*. 2009;85(6):607-614.

67. Jarvis MA, Wu-Pong S, Kniseley JS, Schnoll SH. Alterations in methadone metabolism during late pregnancy. *J Addict Dis*. 1999;18(4):51-61.

68. Bogen DL, Hanusa BH, Perel JM, Sherman F, Mendelson MA, Wisner KL. Corrected QT interval and methadone dose and concentrations in pregnant and postpartum women. *J Clin Psychiatry*. 2017;78(8):e1013-e1019.

69. Gebreyesus MS, Decloedt EH, Cluver CA, et al. Population pharmacokinetics of esomeprazole in patients with preterm preeclampsia. *Br J Clin Pharmacol*. 2022;88(10):4639-4645.

70. Darakjian LI, Kaddoumi A. Physiologically based pharmacokinetic/pharmacodynamic model for caffeine disposition in pregnancy. *Mol Pharm*. 2019;16(3):1340-1349.

71. Knutti R, Rothweiler H, Schlatter C. The effect of pregnancy on the pharmacokinetics of caffeine. *Arch Toxicol Suppl*. 1982;5:187-192.

72. CARE Study Group. Maternal caffeine intake during pregnancy and risk of fetal growth restriction: a large prospective observational study. *BMJ*. 2008;337:a2332.

73. Sasaki S, Limpar M, Sata F, Kobayashi S, Kishi R. Interaction between maternal caffeine intake during pregnancy and CYP1A2 C164A polymorphism affects infant birth size in the Hokkaido study. *Pediatr Res*. 2017;82(1):19-28.

74. Eichelberger KY, Baker AM, Woodham PC, Haeri S, Strauss RA, Stuebe AM. Second-trimester maternal serum paraxanthine, CYP1A2 activity, and the risk of severe preeclampsia. *Obstet Gynecol*. 2015;126(4):725-730.

75. Abduljalil K, Pansari A, Jamei M. Prediction of maternal pharmacokinetics using physiologically based pharmacokinetic models: assessing the impact of the longitudinal changes in the activity of CYP1A2, CYP2D6 and CYP3A4 enzymes during pregnancy. *J Pharmacokinet Pharmacodyn*. 2020;47(4):361-383.

76. Poweleit EA, Cinibulk MA, Novotny SA, Wagner-Schuman M, Ramsey LB, Strawn JR. Selective serotonin reuptake inhibitor pharmacokinetics during pregnancy: clinical and research implications. *Front Pharmacol*. 2022;13:833217.

77. Almurjan A, Macfarlane H, Badhan RKS. Precision dosing-based optimisation of paroxetine during pregnancy for poor and ultrarapid CYP2D6 metabolisers: a virtual clinical trial pharmacokinetics study. *J Pharm Pharmacol*. 2020;72(8):1049-1060.

78. Almurjan A, Macfarlane H, Badhan RKS. The application of precision dosing in the use of sertraline throughout pregnancy for poor and ultrarapid metabolizer CYP 2C19 subjects: a virtual clinical trial pharmacokinetics study. *Biopharm Drug Dispos*. 2021;42(6):252-262.

79. Wang ML, Tao YY, Sun XY, et al. Estrogen profile- and pharmacogenetics-based lamotrigine dosing regimen optimization: recommendations for pregnant women with epilepsy. *Pharmacol Res*. 2021;169:105610.

80. Jeong H, Choi S, Song JW, Chen H, Fischer JH. Regulation of UDP-glucuronosyltransferase (UGT) 1A1 by progesterone and its impact on labetalol elimination. *Xenobiotica*. 2008;38(1):62-75.

81. Fischer JH, Sarto GE, Hardman J, et al. Influence of gestational age and body weight on the pharmacokinetics of labetalol in pregnancy. *Clin Pharmacokinet*. 2014;53(4):373-383.

82. Carvalho TM, Cavalli Rde C, Cunha SP, et al. Influence of gestational diabetes mellitus on the stereoselective kinetic disposition and metabolism of labetalol in hypertensive patients. *Eur J Clin Pharmacol*. 2011;67(1):55-61.

83. Meador KJ, Cohen MJ, Loring DW, et al; Maternal Outcomes and Neurodevelopmental Effects of Antiepileptic Drugs Investigator Group. Two-year-old cognitive outcomes in children of pregnant women with epilepsy in the maternal outcomes and neurodevelopmental effects of antiepileptic drugs study. *JAMA Neurol.* 2021;78(8):927-936.

84. Polepally AR, Pennell PB, Brundage RC, et al. Model-based lamotrigine clearance changes during pregnancy: clinical implication. *Ann Clin Transl Neurol.* 2014;1(2):99-106.

85. Pennell PB, Peng L, Newport DJ, et al. Lamotrigine in pregnancy: clearance, therapeutic drug monitoring, and seizure frequency. *Neurology.* 2008;70(22 Pt 2):2130-2136.

86. Voinescu PE, Park S, Chen LQ, et al. Antiepileptic drug clearances during pregnancy and clinical implications for women with epilepsy. *Neurology.* 2018;91(13):e1228-e1236.

87. Ding Y, Tan X, Zhang S, Guo Y. Pharmacokinetic changes and therapeutic drug monitoring of lamotrigine during pregnancy. *Brain Behav.* 2019;9(7):e01315.

88. Yin X, Liu Y, Guo Y, Zhao L, Li G, Tan X. Pharmacokinetic changes for newer antiepileptic drugs and seizure control during pregnancy. *CNS Neurosci Ther.* 2022;28(5):658-666.

89. Bhavatharini PA, Sanghavi S, Thomas G, et al. Dosage optimization of lamotrigine in pregnancy: a pharmacometric approach using modeling and simulation. *J Clin Pharmacol.* 2022;62(12):1557-1565.

90. Han LW, Ryu RJ, Cusumano M, et al. Effect of N-acetyltransferase 2 genotype on the pharmacokinetics of hydralazine during pregnancy. *J Clin Pharmacol.* 2019;59(12):1678-1689.

91. Gausi K, Wiesner L, Norman J, et al; IMPAACT P1078 (TB APPRISE) Study Group Team. Pharmacokinetics and drug-drug interactions of isoniazid and efavirenz in pregnant women living with HIV in high TB incidence settings: importance of genotyping. *Clin Pharmacol Ther.* 2021;109(4):1034-1044.

92. Arger CA, Taghavi T, Heil SH, Skelly J, Tyndale RF, Higgins ST. Pregnancy-induced increases in the nicotine metabolite ratio: examining changes during antepartum and postpartum. *Nicotine Tob Res.* 2019;21(12):1706-1710.

93. Taghavi T, Arger CA, Heil SH, Higgins ST, Tyndale RF. Longitudinal influence of pregnancy on nicotine metabolic pathways. *J Pharmacol Exp Ther.* 2018;364(2):238-245.

94. Zhang H, Bastian JR, Zhao W, et al. Pregnancy alters CYP- and UGT-mediated metabolism of buprenorphine. *Ther Drug Monit.* 2020;42(2):264-270.

95. Caritis SN, Bastian JR, Zhang H, et al. An evidence-based recommendation to increase the dosing frequency of buprenorphine during pregnancy. *Am J Obstet Gynecol.* 2017;217(4):459.e1-459.e6.

96. Griffin BA, Caperton CO, Russell LN, et al. In utero exposure to norbuprenorphine, a major metabolite of buprenorphine, induces fetal opioid dependence and leads to neonatal opioid withdrawal syndrome. *J Pharmacol Exp Ther.* 2019;370(1):9-17.

97. Bouchghoul H, Bouyer J, Senat MV, et al. Hypoglycemia and glycemic control with glyburide in women with gestational diabetes and genetic variants of cytochrome P450 2C9 and/or OATP1B3. *Clin Pharmacol Ther.* 2021;110(1):141-148.

98. Lopes van Balen VA, van Gansewinkel TAG, de Haas S, et al. Maternal kidney function during pregnancy: systematic review and meta-analysis. *Ultrasound Obstet Gynecol.* 2019;54(3):297-307.

99. Stojanova J, Arancibia M, Ghimire S, Sandaradura I. Understanding the pharmacokinetics of antibiotics in pregnancy: is there a role for therapeutic drug monitoring? A narrative review. *Ther Drug Monit.* 2022;44(1):50-64.

100. Swank ML, Wing DA, Nicolau DP, McNulty JA. Increased 3-gram cefazolin dosing for cesarean delivery prophylaxis in obese women. *Am J Obstet Gynecol.* 2015;213(3):415.e1-415.e8.

101. Grupper M, Kuti JL, Swank ML, Maggio L, Hughes BL, Nicolau DP. Population pharmacokinetics of cefazolin in serum and adipose tissue from overweight and obese women undergoing cesarean delivery. *J Clin Pharmacol.* 2017;57(6):712-719.

102. Lafayette R. The kidney in preeclampsia. *Kidney Int.* 2005;67(3):1194-1203.

103. Conti-Ramsden FI, Nathan HL, De Greeff A, et al. Pregnancy-related acute kidney injury in preeclampsia: risk factors and renal outcomes. *Hypertension.* 2019;74(5):1144-1151.

104. Rodriguez AN, Nelson DB, Spong CY, McIntire DD, Reddy MT, Cunningham FG. Acute kidney injury in pregnancies complicated by late-onset preeclampsia with severe features. *Am J Perinatol.* 2022. doi:10.1055/s-0042-1749632

105. Nucera B, Brigo F, Trinka E, Kalss G. Treatment and care of women with epilepsy before, during, and after pregnancy: a practical guide. *Ther Adv Neurol Disord*. 2022;15:17562864221101687.

106. Brookfield KF, Su F, Elkomy MH, Drover DR, Lyell DJ, Carvalho B. Pharmacokinetics and placental transfer of magnesium sulfate in pregnant women. *Am J Obstet Gynecol*. 2016;214(6): 737.e1-737.e9.

107. da Costa TX, Azeredo FJ, Ururahy MAG, da Silva Filho MA, Martins RR, Oliveira AG. Population pharmacokinetics of magnesium sulfate in preeclampsia and associated factors. *Drugs R D*. 2020;20(3):257-266.

108. Petrie S, Barras M, Lust K, Fagermo N, Allen J, Martin JH. Evaluation of therapeutic enoxaparin in a pregnant population at a tertiary hospital. *Intern Med J*. 2016;46(7):826-833.

109. Liao MZ, Flood Nichols SK, Ahmed M, et al. Effects of pregnancy on the pharmacokinetics of metformin. *Drug Metab Dispos*. 2020;48(4):264-271.

110. Shuster DL, Shireman LM, Ma X, et al. Pharmacodynamics of glyburide, metformin, and glyburide/metformin combination therapy in the treatment of gestational diabetes mellitus. *Clin Pharmacol Ther*. 2020;107(6):1362-1372.

111. Espnes KA, Honnas A, Lovvik TS, et al. Metformin serum concentrations during pregnancy and post partum—a clinical study in patients with polycystic ovary syndrome. *Basic Clin Pharmacol Toxicol*. 2022;130(3):415-422.

112. Gozar L, Gabor-Miklosi D, Toganel R, et al. Fetal tachyarrhythmia management from digoxin to amiodarone—a review. *J Clin Med*. 2022;11(3):804.

113. Steinberg I, Mitani GM, Harrison EC, Elkayam U. Digitalis glycosides in pregnancy. In: Elkayam U, Gleicher N, eds. *Cardiac Problems in Pregnancy*. 3rd ed. Wiley-Liss Inc; 1998:419-435.

114. Atyeo C, Shook LL, Nziza N, et al. COVID-19 booster dose induces robust antibody response in pregnant, lactating, and nonpregnant women. *Am J Obstet Gynecol*. 2023;228(1):68.e1-68.e12.

115. Kugelman N, Nahshon C, Shaked-Mishan P, et al. Third trimester messenger RNA COVID-19 booster vaccination upsurge maternal and neonatal SARS-CoV-2 immunoglobulin G antibody levels at birth. *Eur J Obstet Gynecol Reprod Biol*. 2022;274:148-154.

116. Syme MR, Paxton JW, Keelan JA. Drug transfer and metabolism by the human placenta. *Clin Pharmacokinet*. 2004;43(8):487-514.

117. Kammala AK, Lintao RCV, Vora N, et al. Expression of CYP450 enzymes in human fetal membranes and its implications in xenobiotic metabolism during pregnancy. *Life Sci*. 2022;307:120867.

118. Lacroix D, Sonnier M, Moncion A, Cheron G, Cresteil T. Expression of CYP3A in the human liver—evidence that the shift between CYP3A7 and CYP3A4 occurs immediately after birth. *Eur J Biochem*. 1997;247(2):625-634.

119. Yamashita M, Markert UR. Overview of drug transporters in human placenta. *Int J Mol Sci*. 2021;22(23):13149.

120. Anoshchenko O, Prasad B, Neradugomma NK, Wang J, Mao Q, Unadkat JD. Gestational age-dependent abundance of human placental transporters as determined by quantitative targeted proteomics. *Drug Metab Dispos*. 2020;48(9):735-741.

121. Goetzl L, Darbinian N, Merabova N, Devane LC, Ramamoorthy S. Gestational age variation in human placental drug transporters. *Front Pharmacol*. 2022;13:837694.

122. Ellfolk M, Tornio A, Niemi M, Leinonen MK, Lahesmaa-Korpinen AM, Malm H. Placental transporter-mediated drug interactions and offspring congenital anomalies. *Br J Clin Pharmacol*. 2020;86(5):868-879.

123. Hutson JR, Garcia-Bournissen F, Davis A, Koren G. The human placental perfusion model: a systematic review and development of a model to predict in vivo transfer of therapeutic drugs. *Clin Pharmacol Ther*. 2011;90(1):67-76.

124. Blundell C, Yi YS, Ma L, et al. Placental drug transport-on-a-chip: a microengineered in vitro model of transporter-mediated drug efflux in the human placental barrier. *Adv Healthc Mater*. 2018;7(2):10.

125. Ke AB, Rostami-Hodjegan A, Zhao P, Unadkat JD. Pharmacometrics in pregnancy: an unmet need. *Annu Rev Pharmacol Toxicol*. 2014;54:53-69.

126. Dallmann A, Pfister M, van den Anker J, Eissing T. Physiologically based pharmacokinetic modeling in pregnancy: a systematic review of published models. *Clin Pharmacol Ther*. 2018;104(6):1110-1124.

127. Abduljalil K, Badhan RKS. Drug dosing during pregnancy-opportunities for physiologically based pharmacokinetic models. *J Pharmacokinet Pharmacodyn.* 2020;47(4):319-340.

128. Freriksen JJM, Schalkwijk S, Colbers AP, et al. Assessment of maternal and fetal dolutegravir exposure by integrating ex vivo placental perfusion data and physiologically-based pharmacokinetic modeling. *Clin Pharmacol Ther.* 2020;107(6):1352-1361.

129. Silva LL, Silvola RM, Haas DM, Quinney SK. Physiologically based pharmacokinetic modelling in pregnancy: model reproducibility and external validation. *Br J Clin Pharmacol.* 2022;88(4):1441-1451.

130. Brookhuis SAM, Allegaert K, Hanff LM, Lub-de Hooge MN, Dallmann A, Mian P. Modelling tools to characterize acetaminophen pharmacokinetics in the pregnant population. *Pharmaceutics.* 2021;13(8):1302.

131. Shum S, Shen DD, Isoherranen N. Predicting maternal-fetal disposition of fentanyl following intravenous and epidural administration using physiologically based pharmacokinetic modeling. *Drug Metab Dispos.* 2021;49(11):1003-1015.

132. Pillai VC, Shah M, Rytting E, et al. Prediction of maternal and fetal pharmacokinetics of indomethacin in pregnancy. *Br J Clin Pharmacol.* 2022;88(1):271-281.

133. Badhan RKS, Macfarlane H. Quetiapine dose optimisation during gestation: a pharmacokinetic modelling study. *J Pharm Pharmacol.* 2020;72(5):670-681.

134. Zheng L, Yang H, Dallmann A, Jiang X, Wang L, Hu W. Physiologically based pharmacokinetic modeling in pregnant women suggests minor decrease in maternal exposure to olanzapine. *Front Pharmacol.* 2021;12:793346.

135. Abduljalil K, Pansari A, Ning J, Jamei M. Prediction of maternal and fetal acyclovir, emtricitabine, lamivudine, and metformin concentrations during pregnancy using a physiologically based pharmacokinetic modeling approach. *Clin Pharmacokinet.* 2022;61(5):725-748.

136. Abduljalil K, Gardner I, Jamei M. Application of a physiologically based pharmacokinetic approach to predict theophylline pharmacokinetics using virtual non-pregnant, pregnant, fetal, breast-feeding, and neonatal populations. *Front Pediatr.* 2022;10:840710.

137. Shenkoya B, Atoyebi S, Eniayewu I, Akinloye A, Olagunju A. Mechanistic modeling of maternal lymphoid and fetal plasma antiretroviral exposure during the third trimester. *Front Pediatr.* 2021;9:734122.

138. van Hoogdalem MW, Wexelblatt SL, Akinbi HT, Vinks AA, Mizuno T. A review of pregnancy-induced changes in opioid pharmacokinetics, placental transfer, and fetal exposure: towards fetomaternal physiologically-based pharmacokinetic modeling to improve the treatment of neonatal opioid withdrawal syndrome. *Pharmacol Ther.* 2022;234:108045.

139. Saotome T, Minoura S, Terashi K, Sato T, Echizen H, Ishizaki T. Labetalol in hypertension during the third trimester of pregnancy: its antihypertensive effect and pharmacokinetic-dynamic analysis. *J Clin Pharmacol.* 1993;33(10):979-988.

140. Stott D, Bolten M, Salman M, Paraschiv D, Douiri A, Kametas NA. A prediction model for the response to oral labetalol for the treatment of antenatal hypertension. *J Hum Hypertens.* 2017;31(2):126-131.

141. Society for Maternal-Fetal Medicine (SMFM). Electronic address: pubs@smfm.org; Pacheco LD, Saade G, Shrivastava V, Shree R, Elkayam U; Publications Committee. Society for maternal-fetal medicine consult series #61: anticoagulation in pregnant patients with cardiac disease. *Am J Obstet Gynecol.* 2022;227(2):B28-B43.

II

DRUG MONOGRAPHS

The following are the goals and objectives for Part II: Drug Monographs. Although we have used words to indicate that the learner should be able to independently recall and perform pharmacokinetic calculations, in many cases, the learner should be able to identify the important issues and then be able to retrieve information and perform pharmacokinetic calculations. As an example, the expectations for the level of knowledge and immediate recall about digoxin versus vancomycin might be different depending on whether the learner would be dealing with cardiology or infectious disease patients. Also, note that we have focused on the pharmacokinetic issues and not the pharmacodynamic issues. Depending on the level of the learner, it may be appropriate to add goals and objectives on pharmacodynamics, both therapeutic and toxic.

GOALS

The learner should be able to analyze a patient history or scenario and then use that information to calculate dosing regimens using population parameters that would achieve the desired drug concentration(s). In addition, given a patient history or scenario, dosing regimen, and measured drug concentrations, the learner should be able to perform revisions of the appropriate pharmacokinetic parameter(s) and then use the revised patient-specific parameters to calculate dosing regimen that would achieve the desired drug concentration(s).

OBJECTIVES FOR EACH DRUG

After finishing each chapter in Part II, the learner shall be able to:

1. Know the therapeutic plasma concentrations, key parameters, and recommended sampling times.
2. Calculate, using the appropriate formula, a patient's expected volume of distribution, clearance, elimination rate constant, and half-life.
3. Select the appropriate equations that would be necessary to calculate an initial dose and a maintenance dosing regimen that would achieve and maintain the desired therapeutic concentrations.

4. Use the appropriate equations to calculate an initial loading (if appropriate) and maintenance dose that would achieve the desired target concentration(s)

5. Do the following if a patient history and measured plasma concentrations are given:

    a. Determine which pharmacokinetic parameter(s) can be revised.

    b. Use the appropriate equation(s) to revise the pharmacokinetic parameter(s).

    c. Use the revised pharmacokinetic parameter(s) to design a new dosing strategy to achieve the desired plasma concentrations(s).

6. Identify and know the direction of effect for the known disease and drug interactions. For the most common disease and drug interactions, the learner shall be able to adjust the appropriate pharmacokinetic parameter to account for the disease or drug interaction.

7. Defend, using pharmacokinetic principles, why a specific equation was used to design the dosing regimen—for example, why steady state versus non–steady state, a continuous versus intermittent input model, and so on.

8

AMINOGLYCOSIDE ANTIBIOTICS

Emily Han

Learning Objectives

By the end of the aminoglycoside antibiotics chapter, the learner shall be able to:

1. Define the relationship between serum aminoglycoside concentrations and clinical/microbiologic outcomes as well as the risk for the development of nephrotoxicity and ototoxicity.
2. List the patient factors and other drugs that are known to alter the volume of distribution or clearance of aminoglycosides.
3. State the optimal sampling times to determine the therapeutic efficacy and safety of a dosing regimen.
4. Calculate an initial dosing regimen to achieve targeted serum concentrations, given patient demographics and clinical characteristics.
5. Determine individualized pharmacokinetic parameters based on measured serum concentrations and develop a revised dosing regimen to achieve therapeutic drug concentrations.
6. Design a sampling scheme to enable dosage adjustment in a patient with changing renal function.
7. Calculate an appropriate dosage regimen for patients receiving hemodialysis, peritoneal dialysis, or continuous renal replacement therapy (CRRT).

Aminoglycosides are bactericidal antibiotics used to treat serious gram-negative infections. Because absorption from the gastrointestinal tract is poor, the aminoglycosides must be administered parenterally to achieve therapeutic concentrations in the systemic circulation. In most instances, aminoglycosides are administered by intermittent intravenous (IV) infusions. The dose of aminoglycoside is influenced by the specific agent (eg, gentamicin vs amikacin), infection (eg, site and organism), renal function, and weight or body composition of the patient. The most commonly monitored aminoglycoside antibiotics are gentamicin, tobramycin, and amikacin. The usual dose for gentamicin and tobramycin is 5 to 7 mg/kg/d, administered over 30 to 60 minutes as a single daily dose or in divided doses every 8 to 12 hours; the dose of amikacin is 15 to 20 mg/kg/d, administered over 30 to 60 minutes as a single daily dose or in divided doses every 8 to 12 hours. The clearance, volume of distribution, and half-life of all aminoglycosides are similar.[1] Therefore, the same pharmacokinetic model can be used for all the aminoglycosides, and the principles described in this chapter for any given aminoglycoside generally apply to the others as well.

PHARMACODYNAMICS OF AMINOGLYCOSIDES

Traditionally, aminoglycosides have been dosed multiple times a day. Investigations into the pharmacodynamic properties of aminoglycosides have yielded data that favor extended-interval administration. Bactericidal activity of the aminoglycosides has been demonstrated to be concentration dependent (ie, plasma concentrations that exceed 10 times the minimum inhibitory concentration [MIC] for a given bacteria are more effective than concentrations just above the MIC).[2-5] Aminoglycosides exhibit a postantibiotic effect that results in depressed bacterial growth after plasma concentrations have fallen below the MIC.[2,6,7] Taken together, the pharmacodynamic properties of aminoglycosides suggest that less frequent administration of larger doses can maximize bactericidal activity. In addition, saturable uptake mechanisms within the renal cortex and inner ear indicate that extended-interval dosing may also minimize the likelihood of developing nephrotoxicity and ototoxicity.[8-10] Experience from randomized controlled trials suggests that once-daily administration of aminoglycosides results in similar efficacy and perhaps a decreased risk of developing toxicities compared with traditional dosing.[11,12]

THERAPEUTIC AND TOXIC PLASMA CONCENTRATIONS

Peak plasma concentrations for gentamicin and tobramycin using extended-interval dosing (ie, 5-7 mg/kg every 24 hours) range from 20 to 30 mg/L. This peak concentration target is based on the pharmacodynamic goal of achieving a peak-to-MIC ratio of greater than 10 and the breakpoint for susceptibility of 2 mg/L.[13] Trough concentrations are below the limit of detection by design to provide a drug-free interval, which reduces the risk for the development of nephrotoxicity. Peak and trough plasma concentrations following traditional multiple-daily dosing regimens are in the range of 6 to 10 and less than 2 mg/L, respectively.[14-16] Desirable peak concentrations for traditional multiple-daily dosing of amikacin are usually 20 to 30 mg/L; trough concentrations are usually less than 10 mg/L.[1]

Most available data correlating aminoglycoside concentrations with ototoxicity and nephrotoxicity refer to trough plasma concentrations, although some data suggest a correlation between peak concentrations and toxicity.[17,18] Gentamicin trough concentrations of greater than 2 mg/L have been associated with renal toxicity; however, the high trough concentrations may be the result, and not the cause, of renal dysfunction. In fact, the use of elevated trough concentrations as an indication of early renal damage has been suggested by some investigators.[19,20] Fortunately, most patients who develop renal dysfunction during aminoglycoside therapy appear to regain normal renal function after the drug has been discontinued.[21]

Ototoxicity has been associated with trough plasma concentrations of genta-micin exceeding 4 mg/L for more than 10 days. When the trough concentration is multiplied by the number of days of therapy, the risk of ototoxicity is increased when the product exceeds 40 mg/d/L. Aminoglycoside ototoxicity also seems to be most prevalent in patients with an existing impaired renal function or who have received large doses during the treatment course.[17-19,22,23]

KEY PARAMETERS: Aminoglycosides

THERAPEUTIC SERUM CONCENTRATIONS AND AUC_{24}

Gentamicin, tobramycin		Conventional dosing	"Once-daily" dosing
	Peak	6-10 mg/L	20-30 mg/L
	Trough	<2 mg/L	Undetectable
	AUC_{24}	70-100 mg·hr/L	70-100 mg·L/hr
Amikacin			
	Peak	20-30 mg/L	60 mg/L
	Trough	<10 mg/L	Undetectable
	AUC_{24}	210-300 mg·hr/L[a]	210-300 mg·L/hr

VOLUME OF DISTRIBUTION[b] (V)

Adults, children >12 yr	0.25 L/kg
Children 5-12 yr	0.35 L/kg

CLEARANCE (Cl)

Adults, children >12 yr	Equal to Cl_{Cr}
Functionally anephric patients	0.0043 L/kg/hr
• Surgically anephric patients[c]	0.0021 L/kg/hr
• Hemodialysis[c]	6.6 L/hr
Children ≤12 yr[d]	Equal to GFR

HALF-LIFE ($t_{1/2}$)

Normal renal function	2-3 hr
Functionally anephric patients	30-60 hr
FRACTION UNBOUND IN PLASMA (fu)	>0.95

[a]Amikacin AUC_{24} is ~3 times higher than gentamicin and tobramycin AUC_{24}.
[b]Volume of distribution should be adjusted for obesity and/or alterations in extracellular fluid status.
[c]A functionally anephric patient is a dialysis patient with kidneys intact. A surgically anephric patient is a dialysis patient with kidneys removed. Hemodialysis clearance of 6.6 L/hr refers to high-flux hemodialysis.
[d]Glomerular filtration rate (GFR) calculated by modified Schwartz equation.

Although aminoglycoside peak and trough concentrations are used as predic-tors for both efficacy and toxicity, the adoption of once-daily aminoglycoside dosing at many institutions has led to less intensive monitoring of serum concentrations. The nomogram developed by Nicolau et al[13] recommends that a single level be drawn 6 to 14 hours after the dose. The nomogram then defines in a graphical form whether the dosing interval is appropriate or needs to be extended. This type of approach is much more simplified than the traditional method of determining the individualized pharmacokinetic parameters based on the measured peak and trough concentrations; however, it may not provide the same precise control of drug exposure (ie, peak, area under the curve [AUC]) in patients who exhibit altered pharmacokinetics (ie, third-space fluid, burns, cystic fibrosis, spinal cord injury). Alternatively, Barclay et al[24] have defined a method of dosage individualization of extended-interval aminoglycoside dosing based on a measured peak concentration and an estimation of the AUC. This dosing method is based on the assumption that the goal is to provide a similar degree of drug exposure as traditional daily dosing methods (ie, AUC) to minimize the risk of toxicity but provide a higher peak concentration to maximize the bactericidal activity. The target AUC_{24} range for gentamicin and tobramycin is 70 to 100 mg·hr/L.

BIOAVAILABILITY (*F*)

The aminoglycoside antibiotics are highly water-soluble and poorly lipid-soluble compounds. As a result, they are poorly absorbed when administered orally and must be administered parenterally for the treatment of systemic infections.

VOLUME OF DISTRIBUTION (*V*)

The volume of distribution of aminoglycosides is approximately 0.25 L/kg, although a relatively wide range of 0.1 to 0.5 L/kg has been reported.[25-31] Because aminoglycosides distribute very poorly into adipose tissue, lean rather than total body weight (TBW) should result in a more accurate approximation of *V* in patients with obesity.[32] The aminoglycoside volume of distribution in subjects with obesity also could be adjusted based on the patient's ideal body weight (IBW) plus 10% of their excess weight.[33,34] These adjustments in the estimation of aminoglycoside volumes of distribution in patients with obesity seem reasonable because aminoglycoside antibiotics appear to distribute into extracellular space, and the extracellular fluid volume of adipose tissue is approximately 10% of adipose weight versus 25%, which is an average for all the other tissues. Equation 8.1 can be used to approximate the volume of distribution (*V*) in patients with obesity:

Aminoglycoside *V* (patients with obesity) = (0.25 L/kg)(IBW) + 0.1(TBW − IBW)   **(Eq. 8.1)**

The nonobese or IBW can be approximated using Equations 8.2 and 8.3 (see Creatinine Clearance [Cl_{Cr}] in Chapter "Drug Dosing in Kidney Disease and Dialysis").

Ideal body weight for males in kg = 50 + (2.3) (Height in inches > 60)   **(Eq. 8.2)**

Ideal body weight for females in kg = 45 + (2.3) (Height in inches > 60)   **(Eq. 8.3)**

The volume of distribution of aminoglycosides is increased in patients with ascites, edema, or other enlarged "third-space" volume.[35,36] One approach to approximating the increased volume of distribution for patients with ascites or edema is to increase the V by 1 L for each kilogram of weight gain. This approach is based on the assumption that the volume of distribution of aminoglycoside antibiotics is approximately equal to the extracellular fluid volume. This is consistent with the low plasma protein binding[1] and the fact that aminoglycosides cross membranes very poorly.

$$\text{Aminoglycoside } V \text{ (L)} = 0.25 \text{ L/kg} \begin{pmatrix} \text{Nonobese,} \\ \text{Non–excess} \\ \text{fluid weight (kg)} \end{pmatrix} + 0.1 \begin{pmatrix} \text{Excess} \\ \text{adipose} \\ \text{weight (kg)} \end{pmatrix} + \begin{pmatrix} \text{Excess} \\ \text{third space} \\ \text{fluid} \\ \text{weight (kg)} \end{pmatrix} \quad \text{(Eq. 8.4)}$$

The volume of distribution of aminoglycosides can be estimated using Equation 8.4. The nonobese, non–excess fluid weight is usually estimated as the IBW, and the difference between the nonobese weight and the patient's total weight, without excess third-space fluid, is the excess adipose weight. The excess third-space fluid weight is estimated clinically. In cases where a rapid increase in weight has occurred over several days, this weight gain is likely to represent fluid in a third space; it is, therefore, easily estimated by taking a difference between the initial and current weights. On initial evaluation, some patients may exhibit a significant third spacing of fluids (apparent as either edema or ascites). It is most difficult to estimate an aminoglycoside V in a patient with obesity with a significant third spacing of fluid. As Equation 8.4 illustrates, assigning excess third-space fluid to adipose weight could substantially underestimate the volume of distribution. For this reason, it should be recognized that Equation 8.4 only approximates the V, and plasma concentration measurements are needed to make patient-specific adjustments.

Physiologic changes in the extracellular fluid volume occur with age in children. As the body weight increases, the percent of total body water decreases from approximately 85% in premature infants to 75% in full-term infants, to 60% in adults.[37] Accordingly, the volume of distribution of aminoglycoside continues to decline from an initial value of 0.5 L/kg to the adult value of 0.25 L/kg between birth and adolescence.[38] In children younger than 5 years, the difference in V results in aminoglycoside doses that are twice that of older children or adults to achieve similar C_{max}.[31]

$$\begin{array}{l} \text{Aminoglycoside} \\ V \text{ (L) in children} \\ 1 \text{ to 5 years} \end{array} = \left[0.5 \text{ L/kg} - \left(\frac{\text{Age in years}}{5} \times 0.25 \right) \right] \left(\frac{\text{Weight}}{\text{in kg}} \right) \quad \text{(Eq. 8.5)}$$

Because the change in volume of distribution is gradual, some clinicians have chosen to use the abovementioned algorithm to estimate the volume of distribution for patients between 1 and 5 years of age. Note that in Equation 8.5, it is assumed that the child's weight in kilogram represents a weight that is not obese and does not contain a significant excess third-space fluid. Children with obesity have a smaller-than-average volume of distribution for their age and size, which results in higher peak concentration than children with lean body weight (LBW),[31] and children with a significant third spacing of fluid should have a larger-than-average V. Pediatric patients presenting with fever and dehydration may initially have decreased V but eventually require higher aminoglycoside doses to achieve the same target peak level to account for increase V with fluid boluses.[39] In general, the volume of distribution of 0.35 L/kg is used for patients between 5 and 12 years of age, and the adult V of 0.25 L/kg is used with older children.[39,40]

The pharmacokinetics of the aminoglycoside antibiotics has been described by a two- or three-compartment model.[41,42] However, a one-compartment model has been used widely in the clinical setting to facilitate aminoglycoside pharmacokinetic calculations. The initial distribution phase following a gentamicin IV infusion is not considered when the one-compartment model is utilized for gentamicin pharmacokinetic calculations.[42-44] For this reason, reported values for plasma samples obtained near the conclusion of an IV infusion may be higher than expected. In addition, there is some evidence that the length of the distribution phase may be dose dependent.[45] These reported values probably have no correlation with the therapeutic or toxic effects of the drug; however, they are important in terms of the optimal timing and interpretation of measured serum concentrations. A third distribution phase, or γ phase, for gentamicin has also been identified.[41] This final volume of distribution phase for gentamicin is large, and because gentamicin clearance is decreased when plasma concentrations are low, the average half-life associated with this third compartment is in excess of 100 hours.[41,42] This large final volume of distribution and long terminal half-life may be significant when evaluating a patient's potential for aminoglycoside toxicity.[46]

Despite the existence of the three-compartment model for the aminoglycosides, pharmacokinetic calculations can be based on a one-compartment model that utilizes the second volume of distribution. The errors encountered when using a single-compartment model for aminoglycosides can be minimized if plasma drug concentrations are obtained at times that avoid the first and third distribution phases and at 24 hours after therapy has been initiated.[47]

CLEARANCE (Cl)

The aminoglycoside antibiotics are eliminated almost entirely by the renal route.[1,30] Because the aminoglycoside and creatinine clearances are similar over a wide range of renal function, aminoglycoside clearance can be estimated from the formulas used to estimate creatinine clearance (Equations 8.6 and 8.7).[1,25,30,42]

$$\text{Cl}_{\text{Cr}} \text{ for males (mL/min)} = \frac{(140 - \text{Age})(\text{Weight})}{(72)(\text{SCr}_{\text{SS}})} \qquad \textbf{(Eq. 8.6)}$$

$$\text{Cl}_{\text{Cr}} \text{ for females (mL/min)} = (0.85) \frac{(140 - \text{Age})(\text{Weight})}{(72)(\text{SCr}_{\text{SS}})} \qquad \textbf{(Eq. 8.7)}$$

As presented in Chapter "Drug Dosing in Kidney Disease and Dialysis," the age is in years, weight is in kg, and serum creatinine is in mg/dL. Correct estimates of creatinine clearance can only be obtained if the patient's weight represents a normal ratio of muscle mass to TBW and the serum creatinine is at steady state. For this reason, pharmacokinetic calculations for patients with obesity and patients who have a significant third spacing of fluid should take into consideration adjustments for obesity and third spacing. Although IBW, calculated from Equations 8.2 and 8.3, is generally used to calculate creatinine clearance in patients with obesity, glomerular filtration rate (GFR) has been shown to increase in proportion to the LBW, and LBW has been suggested to provide better estimation of creatinine clearance in morbidly patients with obesity (body mass index [BMI] > 40).[48] In patients who are obese (ie, BMI 30-40), creatinine clearance can be best estimated by using a weight that falls between the IBW and the TBW.[49,50] For this reason, some clinicians prefer to estimate the nonobese weight, or adjusted body weight, by using the following equation:

$$\text{Adjusted body weight} = \text{IBW} + 0.4\,(\text{TBW} - \text{IBW}) \qquad \textbf{(Eq. 8.8)}$$

where IBW is estimated by Equations 8.2 and 8.3, and TBW represents the patient's TBW without the presence of excess third-space fluid. Alternately, TBW can be used to estimate creatinine clearance in patients with BMI less than 30.

Predicted creatinine clearance is the most commonly employed method of estimating aminoglycoside clearance; however, this formula is known to be inaccurate at low creatinine concentrations. The Modification of Diet in Renal Disease (MDRD) equation was developed to provide a more accurate estimate of GFRs. Data correlating estimated GFRs using the MDRD equation and measured aminoglycoside clearance are currently limited.[51] More recently, cystatin C concentrations have been utilized to estimate glomerular filtration. Cystatin C is an endogenous protein that is constitutively expressed from all nucleated cells and is eliminated by glomerular filtration. One advantage of cystatin C is that it is unaffected by changes in muscle mass. Several studies demonstrated an improved ability to predict aminoglycoside clearance with cystatin C clearance compared with creatinine clearance, especially in older adults or critically ill patients with lower muscle mass.[52,53] Until more definitive data are available, the use of predicted creatinine clearance as a marker of aminoglycoside clearance is still recommended.

Creatinine clearance in children older than 12 years can be determined by using Equations 8.6 and 8.7, which are used to calculate creatinine clearance in adults.[54] However, in younger children, the ongoing maturation of the renal function and the hemodynamic and physiologic changes after birth lead to variable GFR at different stages of development.[37] Utilization of Equations 8.6 and 8.7 in these children will result in inaccurate creatinine clearance. For this reason, there are numerous methods trying to measure GFR in children, including allometric and quadratic formulas.[55,56] The most widely used equation to estimate renal clearance in the pediatric population is the one utilizing the child's height and plasma creatinine concentration derived by Schwartz.[57]

$$\text{GFR (mL/min/1.73 m}^2) = 0.413\left(\frac{\text{Height in cm}}{(\text{SCr})}\right) \qquad \textbf{(Eq. 8.9)}$$

Because Equation 8.9 was derived from the data in children with GFR 15 to 75 mL/min/1.73 m^2, estimated GFR greater than 75 mL/min/1.73 m^2 should be used with caution. Equation 8.9 has been shown to overestimate GFR in those patients whose Ht/Scr ratio exceeds 251, which corresponds to GFR[58] of 103 mL/min/1.73 m^2.

The evaluation of GFR should be done with caution in neonates because the maturation of kidney depends on the birth weight and postnatal age.[56] The allometric equation using the body weight scaled to adults shows that the clearance is higher in neonates and young children compared with that in older children and adults,[56] which is in accordance with greater gentamicin and tobramycin clearance seen in the first weeks of life until 1 year after birth. In these young children with changing renal function, population pharmacokinetic modeling may give a better prediction of aminoglycoside clearance.

Nonrenal Clearance

Another factor that should be considered when estimating the clearance of aminoglycosides is the nonrenal clearance, which is approximately 0.0021 L/kg/hr (or ≈2.5 mL/min/70 kg). The nonrenal clearance of aminoglycosides is generally ignored in most patients, but it is significant in patients whose renal function is remarkably diminished. In patients who are functionally anephric and receiving intermittent hemodialysis, a clearance value of approximately 0.0043 L/kg/hr (5 mL/min/70 kg) represents the residual renal clearance and the nonrenal clearance. These values, however, are only approximations; serum concentrations of aminoglycosides should be monitored in patients with poor renal function.

Penicillin Interaction

Aminoglycosides are often used in combination with β-lactam antibiotics for serious gram-negative infections. Older β-lactam antibiotics such as carbenicillin and ticarcillin have shown to chemically inactivate gentamicin and tobramycin.[59] The β-lactam ring of these penicillin compounds interacts in vivo and in vitro with one of the primary amines on gentamicin and tobramycin to form an inactive compound.[59-62] Although there may be a higher risk of inactivation in renally impaired patients where the contact time between penicillins and aminoglycosides is increased,[21,60] the rate of this interaction is generally slow and will not be clinically significant in patients with normal clearance of these drugs.[63]

In general, tobramycin interacts with penicillins the most, followed by gentamicin.[59-61,64-67] Amikacin appears to be more resistant to degradation by penicillins.[59,68] However, many of the older β-lactams agents that significantly inactivated aminoglycosides are no longer available in the United States (ie, carbenicillin, ticarcillin). The in vitro interaction between the cephalosporins (eg, cefazolin, cefamandole, cefotaxime) and the aminoglycoside antibiotics appears to be minimal.[68] Because the third-generation cephalosporin antibiotics have, to a large degree, replaced the use of penicillin derivatives, this interaction is encountered infrequently in most clinical practices.[65,69]

The lack of data on the impact of newer β-lactam antibiotics and the extended infusion of β-lactam drugs (infusing each dose over 3 hours vs 0.5 hour) on aminoglycoside antibiotics warrants close monitoring of aminoglycoside plasma levels when used together.

ELIMINATION HALF-LIFE

The elimination half-life of aminoglycoside antibiotics from the body is a function of the volume of distribution and clearance. Because renal function varies considerably among individuals, the half-life is also variable. For example, a 70-kg, 25-year-old man with a serum creatinine of 1 mg/dL will have an estimated aminoglycoside clearance of approximately 110 mL/min (6.6 L/hr). If his volume of distribution is 0.25 L/kg, the corresponding elimination half-life will be 1.8 approximately 2 hours based on Equation 8.10.

$$t_{1/2} = \frac{(0.693)(V)}{Cl} = 0.693/K \qquad \text{(Eq. 8.10)}$$

$$= \frac{(0.693)(0.25 \text{ L/kg})(70 \text{ kg})}{6.6 \text{ L/hr}}$$

$$= 1.8 \text{ hr}$$

In contrast, a 75-year-old man with a similar V and serum creatinine of 1.6 mg/dL might have an aminoglycoside clearance of approximately 40 mL/min (2.4 L/hr) and a half-life of approximately 5 hours.

$$t_{1/2} = \frac{(0.693)(V)}{Cl}$$

$$= \frac{(0.693)(0.25 \text{ L/kg})(70 \text{ kg})}{2.4 \text{ L/hr}}$$

$$= 5.1 \text{ hr}$$

For this reason, the initial aminoglycoside dose and dosing interval should be selected with care. Although initial estimates of the patient's aminoglycoside pharmacokinetic parameters may be highly variable, it is hoped that pharmacokinetic adjustments will optimize the achievement of therapeutic, yet nontoxic, concentrations of aminoglycoside antibiotics.

NOMOGRAMS AND COMPUTERS

The wide availability of nomograms to dose aminoglycosides may lead one to question the necessity for pharmacokinetic calculations.[10] One nomogram that is utilized at a number of centers is the Hartford high-dose extended-interval dosing nomogram.[13] The dose in this nomogram is 7 mg/kg, which targets a peak concentration of 20 to 30 mg/L, which is 10 times the breakpoint for susceptibility for gentamicin and tobramycin (ie, 2 μg/mL). The dosing interval is adjusted based on the degree of renal function to maintain the target peak concentration while achieving a drug-free interval of approximately 6 hours to reduce accumulation within the renal cortex and inner ear.

Hartford Nomogram for Extended-Interval Dosing

CREATININE CLEARANCE (mL/min)	INITIAL DOSE AND INTERVAL
>60	7 mg/kg every 24 hr
40-60	7 mg/kg every 36 hr
20-40	7 mg/kg every 48 hr
<20	7 mg/kg, then follow levels to determine time of the next dose (level <1 µg/mL)

The nomogram also provides the ability to adjust the dosing interval based on a measured serum concentration obtained 6 to 14 hours after a dose. Three regions defined in the nomogram correspond to the appropriate dosing interval that should be chosen based on the single measured concentration. For example, suppose a patient was initiated on a dose of 7 mg/kg every 24 hours and had a measured concentration of 8.2 mg/L approximately 9 hours after the dose. In that case, the nomogram indicates that the dosing interval should be extended to every 36 hours (see Figure 8.1).

The limitation of nomograms is that they are usually designed to achieve fixed peak and trough serum concentrations and do not allow the clinician to individualize the dosing regimens to account for the type of infection treated or the peak/MIC ratio

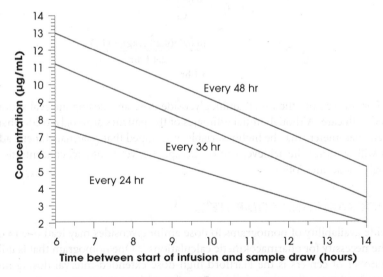

FIGURE 8.1 Gentamicin or tobramycin concentrations obtained 6 to 14 hours following a 7-mg/kg dose are plotted on the nomogram relative to the time of sampling following the dose. Concentrations that fall within the every 24-hour quadrant indicate that the dosing interval of 24 hours should be maintained. Concentrations that fall in the every 36-hour or every 48-hour quadrant indicate that the dosing interval should be extended to 36 or 48 hours. (Adapted from Nicolau D, Freeman CD, Belliveau PP, et al. Experience with a once-daily aminoglycoside program administered to 2,184 adult patients. *Antimicrob Agents Chemother*. 1995;39:650-655, with permission from the American Society for Microbiology.)

for the individual patient. Furthermore, nomograms are based on average pharmacokinetic parameters and do not provide a method for dose adjustment for unique patients (eg, individuals with obesity or those who have a significant third spacing of fluid). Patient-specific adjustments based on the measured plasma concentrations also cannot be extrapolated from these nomograms. An understanding of the basic pharmacokinetic principles used to individualize aminoglycoside doses, coupled with a rational clinical approach, will enable the clinician to provide optimal therapy for the patient.

A number of computer programs are available to help clinicians to dose aminoglycosides and other therapeutic agents. Computers tend to be more flexible than nomograms in that the user can select dosing intervals and peak or trough concentrations based on clinical judgment. In addition, they enable dosage determination based on data (including multiple sets of measurements) obtained under non–steady-state conditions, which is particularly important in patients with changing renal function. Bayesian analysis has been incorporated in most computerized pharmacokinetic programs and has been proven to provide very precise estimates of the pharmacokinetic parameters. However, one potential pitfall is that the user must be familiar with the algorithms initially used to define the expected pharmacokinetic parameters and how patient-specific parameters are revised when plasma concentrations and dosing histories are supplied. In the revision process, the user must be able to recognize data that are obviously wrong and interpret the computer output to ensure that the parameters and dosing recommendations are reasonable. The computer should be viewed as a labor-saving device, not a substitute for a thorough understanding of pharmacokinetic process.

TIME TO SAMPLE

Correct timing of the sample collection is important because aminoglycoside antibiotics have a relatively short half-life and a small but significant distribution phase. The most widely accepted guidelines recommend that samples for peak serum concentrations be obtained 1 hour after the maintenance dose has been initiated. This recommendation assumes that the drug is infused over about 30 minutes; an acceptable range for the infusion period is 20 to 40 minutes. If it is longer than 40 minutes, peak concentrations should be obtained approximately 30 minutes after the end of the infusion to ensure that distribution is complete. Others have suggested that peak measurements should be obtained later in the dosing interval to avoid the distribution phase, particularly with extended-interval dosing because of the potential dose-dependent distribution phase.[45] Trough concentrations generally should be obtained within 0.5 hour before the administration of the next maintenance dose. In cases in which the trough concentrations are expected to be lower than the assay sensitivity (particularly with extended-interval dosing), an earlier sampling time may be appropriate so that measurable trough concentration is obtained and patient-specific pharmacokinetic parameters can be derived. Ideally, the interval between the two concentration measurements should be two to four half-lives to provide more precise estimates of the half-life and reduce the potential for the later concentration to fall below the level of assay sensitivity. In all cases, the exact time of sampling and dose administration should be recorded.

When aminoglycoside plasma concentrations are sampled at a time that extends beyond the expected peak, it is possible to calculate the plasma concentration at the earlier time by simply rearranging

$$C = C_0\, e^{-Kt} \qquad \text{(Eq. 8.11)}$$

where C_0 is the initial plasma concentration and C, a concentration at some time t later, to

$$C_0 = \frac{C}{e^{-Kt}} \qquad \text{(Eq. 8.12)}$$

In this equation, t represents the time from the measured plasma concentration (C) to the earlier plasma concentration (C_0). This equation is used to back extrapolate a plasma concentration to the "clinical peak," which is 1 hour after the start of the infusion. The "clinical peak" concentration is generally used to determine aminoglycoside efficacy.

The optimal time to sample within the first 24 hours of therapy is difficult to determine. For critically ill patients, a peak and subsequent trough (or midpoint for extended-interval dosing) serum aminoglycoside concentrations obtained after the initial loading dose allow for the most rapid evaluation of patient-specific parameters and subsequent dose adjustment, if necessary. In a large number of cases, however, this early sampling may not be necessary, particularly if the expected duration of therapy is relatively short (ie, 3-5 days). The standard of practice in many institutions has been to obtain the first aminoglycoside samples after three or four doses of aminoglycoside have been administered. The majority of patients will be approaching steady state by this time; however, with the wide availability of computers and pharmacokinetic software programs, it is not absolutely necessary to wait until steady state is achieved. With extended-interval dosing, there should be no significant accumulation as observed with multiple dosing; therefore, measurements can be obtained after any dose.

Although one can estimate patient-specific pharmacokinetic parameters more accurately with three or four aminoglycoside plasma concentrations (particularly using a multicompartment model), reasonable pharmacokinetic parameters can be estimated using a one-compartment model and two plasma samples in most cases.

When aminoglycoside antibiotics are administered intramuscularly (IM), the time for absorption or drug input is less predictable; however, in most patients, plasma concentrations peak about 1 hour after the IM injection.[70] For this reason, a peak plasma concentration should be obtained 1 hour after the IM dose is administered. Because the rate of absorption is uncertain, it is difficult to know whether unusual plasma concentrations following IM administration represent delayed absorption or unusual pharmacokinetic parameters (eg, a large volume of distribution).

Question #1 *B.T. is a 50-year-old, 80-kg, nonobese man with a serum creatinine of 1.2 mg/dL. An initial gentamicin dose of 200 mg was infused IV over 0.5 hour. Calculate the plasma concentration of gentamicin 1 hour after the infusion was started (ie, 0.5 hour after the infusion was completed).*

A rough estimate of the peak gentamicin concentration can be calculated using Equation 8.13 by treating the 30-minute infusion as a bolus dose. The 200-mg dose would be divided by the literature value for the volume of distribution (≈ 0.25 L/kg or 20 L) in this 80-kg man.

$$C_1 = \frac{(S)(F)(\text{Loading dose})}{V} \qquad \text{(Eq. 8.13)}$$

$$= \frac{(1)(1)(200 \text{ mg})}{20 \text{ L}}$$

$$= 10 \text{ mg/L}$$

The salt form (S) and bioavailability (F) were both assumed to be 1, and the plasma concentration of 10 mg/L is an approximation that assumes absorption was very rapid and that no significant drug elimination took place during the time of administration. In addition, it is assumed that the drug is distributed into a single compartment. Even though there is clearly a distribution phase associated with the IV injection of aminoglycosides, the initially high drug concentration can be ignored as long as plasma sampling is avoided during this distribution phase.[29,30,44]

A more precise calculation of the plasma concentration 1 hour after the 0.5-hour infusion has been initiated would take into account the decay of gentamicin levels from the peak concentration as calculated by Equation 8.13. In Equation 8.14, t_1 is the time elapsed from the beginning of the IV infusion to the time of sampling at 1 hour when C_1 is measured, and the elimination rate constant (K) represents the clearance of gentamicin divided by its volume of distribution (V) (Equation 8.15).

$$C_1 = \frac{(S)(F)(\text{Loading dose})}{V}(e^{-Kt_1}) \qquad \text{(Eq. 8.14)}$$

$$K = \frac{\text{Cl}}{V} \qquad \text{(Eq. 8.15)}$$

A creatinine clearance (and therefore gentamicin clearance) of approximately 83.3 mL/min or 5 L/hr can be calculated for B.T., using Equation 8.6:

$$\text{Cl}_{Cr} \text{ for males (mL/min)} = \frac{(140 - \text{Age})(\text{Weight})}{(72)(\text{SCr}_{ss})}$$

$$= \frac{(140 - 50)(80)}{(72)(1.2)}$$

$$= 83.3 \text{ mL/min}$$

$$\text{Cl}_{Cr} \text{ (L/hr)} = (83.3 \text{ mL/min})\left(\frac{60 \text{ min/hr}}{1,000 \text{ mL/L}}\right)$$

$$= 4.99 \text{ L/hr}$$

Using this clearance of approximately 5 L/hr and the apparent volume of distribution of 20 L, an elimination rate constant of 0.25 hr^{-1} can be calculated using Equation 8.15. This elimination rate constant is used in Equation 8.14 to calculate the gentamicin concentration 1 hour after the initiation of the dose, resulting in a predicted concentration of 7.8 mg/L.

$$K = \frac{Cl}{V}$$

$$= \frac{5 \text{ L/hr}}{20 \text{ L}}$$

$$= 0.25 \text{ hr}^{-1}$$

$$C_1 = \frac{(S)(F)(\text{Loading dose})}{V} (e^{-Kt_1})$$

$$= (10 \text{ mg/L}) (e^{-(0.25\,hr^{-1})(1\,hr)})$$

$$= (10 \text{ mg/L})(0.78)$$

$$= 7.8 \text{ mg/L}$$

To evaluate whether the IV bolus dose model is appropriate, the duration of infusion (0.5 hour) should be compared with the apparent drug half-life. When the duration of infusion or absorption is less than one-sixth of the half-life, then the bolus dose model can be used (see Chapter "Selecting the Appropriate Equation and Interpretation of Measured Drug Concentrations"). If, however, the duration of drug input is greater than one-sixth of the half-life, then an infusion model should be used. Using Equation 8.10 and the elimination rate constant of 0.25 hr^{-1}, B.T.'s half-life is 2.8 hours as follows:

$$t_{1/2} = \frac{(0.693)(V)}{Cl}$$

$$= \frac{0.693 (20 \text{ L})}{5 \text{ L/hr}}$$

$$= 2.8 \text{ hr}$$

Question #2 *Using the clearance of 5 L/hr, the volume of distribution of 20 L, the elimination rate constant of 0.25 hr^{-1}, and the short infusion model, calculate the expected gentamicin concentration for B.T. 1 hour after initiating the 0.5-hour infusion of a 200-mg dose.*

Equation 8.16 represents the short infusion model and can be used to calculate the plasma concentration 1 hour after starting the 0.5-hour infusion. The duration of infusion or t_{in} would be 0.5 hour, and t_2, or the time of decay from the end of the infusion, would be 0.5 hour. Using these values, the plasma concentration 1 hour after initiation of the 0.5-hour infusion would be 8.4 mg/L.

$$C_2 = \frac{(S)(F)(\text{Dose}/t_{in})}{Cl} (1 - e^{-Kt_{in}})(e^{-Kt_2}) \qquad \textbf{(Eq. 8.16)}$$

$$= \frac{(1)(1)(200 \text{ mg}/0.5 \text{ hr})}{5 \text{ L/hr}} (1 - e^{-(0.25 \text{hr}^{-1})(0.5 \text{hr})})(e^{-(0.25 \text{hr}^{-1})(0.5 \text{hr})})$$

$$= (80 \text{ mg/L})(0.12)(0.88)$$

$$= 8.4 \text{ mg/L}$$

The plasma concentration of 8.4 mg/L at the end of the 0.5-hour infusion is lower than the calculated peak concentration of 10 mg/L following a bolus dose (see Question 1). This lower concentration at the end of the infusion reflects the clearance of the drug during the infusion process. Also, note that the plasma concentration of 8.4 mg/L at 1 hour calculated by the infusion model is greater than the comparable plasma concentration (7.8 mg/L) calculated by the bolus dose model in Question 1. Less drug remains in the body at this time when the bolus dose model is used because this model assumes that the entire dose entered the body at the beginning of the infusion. Therefore, the total dose has been exposed to the body's clearing mechanisms for a longer time.

Question #3   *In what types of patients is it more appropriate to use the infusion equation for the prediction of aminoglycoside concentrations? When can the bolus dose model be used satisfactorily?*

Because the difference between the results obtained from these two approaches is primarily related to the amount of drug cleared from the body during the infusion period, it is reasonable to assume that the bolus model could be used satisfactorily in patients with decreased renal function and longer aminoglycoside half-lives. In patients with good renal function (eg, young adults and children), the infusion model is more appropriate because these patients often have very short aminoglycoside half-lives.

Question #4   *B.T., the 80-kg man described in Question 1, was given 200 mg of gentamicin over 0.5 hour every 12 hours. Predict his peak and trough plasma concentrations at steady state.*

Again, one could treat this problem as if B.T. was receiving intermittent IV boluses or as if he was receiving 0.5-hour infusions every 12 hours. If the bolus dose model is applied, Equation 8.17 can be used to predict the peak levels, where t_1 represents the time interval between the start of the infusion and the time at which the "peak concentration" is sampled (1 hour), and τ is the interval between the doses (12 hours). Using the volume of distribution of 20 L and the elimination rate constant of 0.25 hr^{-1}, the calculated peak concentration would be 8.2 mg/L.

$$C_{ss1} = \frac{\frac{(S)(F)(\text{Dose})}{V}}{(1 - e^{-K\tau})} e^{-Kt_1} \qquad \text{(Eq. 8.17)}$$

$$= \frac{\dfrac{(1)(1)(200 \text{ mg})}{20 \text{ L}}(e^{-(0.25\,\text{hr}^{-1})(1\,\text{hr})})}{(1 - e^{-(0.25\,\text{hr}^{-1})(12\,\text{hr})})}$$

$$= \left(\frac{10 \text{ mg/L}}{0.95}\right)(0.78)$$

$$= 8.2 \text{ mg/L}$$

The trough concentration can also be calculated using Equation 8.17, where t_1 is the time interval between the start of the infusion and the time at which trough level is sampled (12 hours). If the trough sample is obtained just before the start of the next infusion, then Equation 8.18 for $C_{ss\,min}$ also can be used. Using the appropriate values for volume of distribution, elimination rate constant, and dosing interval, the calculated trough concentration would be 0.53 mg/L.

$$C_{ss\,min} = \frac{\dfrac{(S)(F)(\text{Dose})}{V}}{(1 - e^{-K\tau})}e^{-K\tau} \qquad \textbf{(Eq. 8.18)}$$

$$= \frac{\dfrac{(1)(1)(200 \text{ mg})}{20 \text{ L}}(e^{-(0.25\,\text{hr}^{-1})(12\,\text{hr})})}{(1 - e^{-(0.25\,\text{hr}^{-1})(12\,\text{hr})})}$$

$$= \frac{10 \text{ mg/L}}{0.95}(0.05)$$

$$= 0.53 \text{ mg/L}$$

If the infusion input model,

$$C_{t_{in}} = \frac{(S)(F)(\text{Dose}/t_{in})}{Cl}(1 - e^{-Kt_{in}}) \qquad \textbf{(Eq. 8.19)}$$

where t_{in} is the duration of the infusion, is used to replace the bolus dose model

$$\frac{(S)(F)(\text{Dose})}{V} \qquad \textbf{(Eq. 8.20)}$$

in Equations 8.17 and 8.18, the resultant substitution results in an equation describing the intermittent infusion steady-state model (also see Chapter "Selecting the Appropriate Equation and Interpretation of Measured Drug Concentrations")

$$C_{ss2} = \frac{\dfrac{(S)(F)(\text{Dose}/t_{in})}{Cl}(1 - e^{-Kt_{in}})}{(1 - e^{-K\tau})}(e^{-Kt_2}) \qquad \textbf{(Eq. 8.21)}$$

where τ is the dosing interval, and t_2 the time interval between the end of the infusion and the time at which the concentration is measured. That is, when peak concentrations are measured 1 hour after the initiation of a 0.5-hour infusion, t_2 is 0.5 hour. For trough concentrations sampled just before the start of a subsequent infusion (ie, administered on a 12-hour schedule), t_2 is 11.5 hours.

Again, assuming S and F to be 1, the infusion time to be 0.5 hour, the dosing interval (τ) to be 12 hours, the clearance (Cl) and the elimination rate constant (K) to be 5 L/hr and 0.25 hr^{-1}, respectively, the "peak" concentration 1 hour after starting the 0.5-hour infusion would be calculated using Equation 8.21 as follows:

$$C_{ss2} = \frac{\dfrac{(S)(F)(\text{Dose}/t_{in})}{\text{Cl}}(1 - e^{-Kt_{in}})}{(1 - e^{-K\tau})}(e^{-Kt_2})$$

$$= \frac{\dfrac{(1)(1)(200 \text{ mg}/0.5 \text{ hr})}{5 \text{ L/hr}}(1 - e^{-(0.25 \text{hr}^{-1})(0.5 \text{hr})})}{(1 - e^{-(0.25 \text{hr}^{-1})(12 \text{hr})})}(e^{-(0.25 \text{hr}^{-1})(0.5 \text{hr})})$$

$$= \frac{(80 \text{ mg/L})(0.12)}{0.95}(0.88)$$

$$= (10.1 \text{ mg/L})(0.88)$$

$$= 8.89 \text{ mg/L}$$

Note that this steady-state "peak concentration" is not the true peak value that would occur at the end of the infusion but a concentration obtained 1 hour after starting the infusion. It is this 1-hour value that is traditionally used to make the clinical correlation with aminoglycoside efficacy. Concentrations obtained earlier may be considerably higher because of the two-compartment modeling associated with the IV administration of the aminoglycosides.

If the trough concentration is sampled just before the start of the next infusion, a modification of Equation 8.21 can be used, where t_2 is represented by ($\tau - t_{in}$). A trough concentration of 0.6 mg/L is calculated, making the appropriate substitution of 12 hours for τ and 0.5 hour for t_{in} (Figure 8.2).

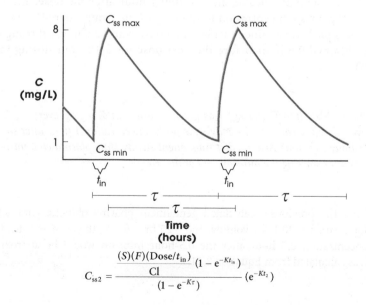

$$C_{ss2} = \frac{\dfrac{(S)(F)(\text{Dose}/t_{in})}{\text{Cl}}(1 - e^{-Kt_{in}})}{(1 - e^{-K\tau})}(e^{-Kt_2})$$

FIGURE 8.2   Intermittent intravenous infusion at steady state. The infusion is administered over t_{in} hours, and τ is the dosing interval; t_2 represents the time from the end of the infusion to the time of sampling.

$$C_{ss\,min} = \frac{\dfrac{(S)(F)(Dose/t_{in})}{Cl}(1 - e^{-Kt_{in}})}{(1 - e^{-K\tau})}(e^{-K(\tau - t_{in})}) \qquad \text{(Eq. 8.22)}$$

$$= \frac{\dfrac{(1)(1)(200 \text{ mg}/0.5 \text{ hr})}{5 \text{ L/hr}}(1 - e^{-(0.25\,hr^{-1})(0.5\,hr)})}{(1 - e^{-(0.25\,hr^{-1})(12\,hr)})}(e^{-(0.25\,hr^{-1})(12\,hr - 0.5\,hr)})$$

$$= (10.1 \text{ mg/L})(e^{-(0.25\,hr^{-1})(11.5\,hr)})$$

$$= (10.1 \text{ mg/L})(0.06)$$

$$= 0.6 \text{ mg/L}$$

Note that if the trough concentration is obtained at a time earlier than just before the next dose, Equation 8.22 should not be used. Instead, Equation 8.21 should be used where t_2 represents the time interval from the end of the infusion to the time of sampling. For example, if the trough concentration was obtained 0.5 hour before the next dose, then t_2 in Equation 8.21 would be 11 hours rather than 11.5 hours used in Equation 8.22.

Trough concentrations can also be calculated by multiplying the peak concentration 1 hour after the dose with the fraction of drug remaining at the time the trough level is sampled (Equation 8.11):

$$C = C_0 e^{-Kt}$$

where C_0 represents the peak concentration 1 hour after the dose, and t is the time from the peak concentration to the time of the trough sampling (11 hours if trough samples are obtained just before a dose, and 10.5 hours if trough samples are obtained 0.5 hour before the next dose for a 12-hour dosing interval regimen).

Question #5 *If B.T. (80 kg) was given gentamicin 7 mg/kg every 24 hours, what would be the calculated steady-state peak concentration 1 hour after starting the 0.5-hour infusion? Also predict subsequent steady-state plasma concentrations 12 hours after starting the infusion and at the trough.*

Using the previously calculated gentamicin pharmacokinetic parameters of 5 L/hr for clearance, 20 L for volume, and 0.25 hr^{-1} for K, the expected steady-state peak concentration 0.5 hour after the 0.5-hour infusion would be approximately 24 mg/L as calculated from Equation 8.21.

$$C_{ss2} = \frac{\dfrac{(S)(F)(\text{Dose}/t_{in})}{Cl}(1 - e^{-Kt_{in}})}{(1 - e^{-K\tau})}(e^{-Kt_2})$$

$$= \frac{\dfrac{(1)(1)(560 \text{ mg}/0.5 \text{ hr})}{5 \text{ L/hr}}(1 - e^{-(0.25\text{hr}^{-1})(0.5\text{hr})})}{(1 - e^{-0.25(24)})}(e^{-(0.25\text{hr}^{-1})(0.5\text{hr})})$$

$$= \frac{(224 \text{ mg/L})(0.12)}{(0.997)}(0.88)$$

$$= 23.7 \text{ mg/L}$$

The plasma concentrations at 12 and 24 hours can be estimated using Equation 8.11, where C_0 would be approximately 24 mg/L, and t would be 11 hours for the mid-concentration and 23 hours for the trough concentration.

$$C = C_0 e^{-Kt}$$

$$= (24 \text{ mg/L})(e^{-(0.25)(11\text{hr})})$$

$$= (24 \text{ mg/L})(0.064)$$

$$= 1.53 \text{ mg/L}$$

Twelve hours after starting the infusion and

$$C = (24 \text{ mg/L})(e^{-(0.25)(23\text{hr})})$$

$$= (24 \text{ mg/L})(0.0032)$$

$$= 0.08 \text{ mg/L at the trough}$$

These calculations show that the initial plasma concentrations are well above the usual accepted therapeutic range for gentamicin, and the mid-interval and trough concentrations are very low. As previously discussed, administration of aminoglycosides as a total daily dose once every 24 hours is as efficacious as the usual 8- to 12-hour divided doses and may reduce the risk of the development of nephrotoxicity. Most institutions have guidelines for the use of high-dose, once-daily aminoglycoside therapy. This type of regimen is usually restricted to patients with reasonable renal function (eg, $Cl_{Cr} > 60$ mL/min) and normal body composition (eg, not excessively obese or having excessive third-space fluid).

One common question is whether aminoglycoside plasma concentrations should be monitored in patients receiving the drug once daily. In most cases, peak concentrations will have little meaning because they are likely to be well above the usual therapeutic range: approximately 20 to 30 mg/L for gentamicin and tobramycin and about 3 times that value for amikacin. Trough plasma concentrations do not appear to be useful in that they are likely to be well below the usual detectable range and may be misinterpreted because of the tissue redistribution (γ phase). In patients with diminished renal function, plasma level monitoring may be warranted to guard against excessive drug accumulation. AUC dosing can be applied in this patient population.

With this method, serum concentrations are obtained at a peak and approximately two to four half-lives later. The two levels are used to calculate the 24-hour AUC and the extrapolated peak concentration at 1 hour into the dosing interval. The assumption with this method is that the level of drug exposure with extended-interval dosing should be the same as conventional multiple-daily dosing regimens (ie, AUC_{24} 70-100 mg·hr/L).[24]

Question #6 *Y.B., a 70-kg, 38-year-old patient with a serum creatinine of 1.8 mg/dL, has been receiving IV tobramycin, 100 mg over 0.5 hour every 8 hours, for several days. A peak plasma concentration obtained 1 hour after the start of an infusion was 8 mg/L, and a trough concentration obtained just before the initiation of a dose was 3 mg/L. Estimate the apparent elimination rate constant (K), clearance (Cl), and volume of distribution (V) for tobramycin in Y.B.*

The two reported plasma concentrations were measured from samples obtained during the elimination phase of the plasma concentration-versus-time curve. Because the 7-hour time interval between samples exceeds the half-life of tobramycin in Y.B. (ie, the trough concentration is less than one-half the measured peak concentration), the two concentrations can be used to estimate the elimination rate constant (see Elimination Rate Constant [K] and Half-Life [$t_{1/2}$] in Chapter "Pharmacokinetic Processes and Parameters" and Equation 8.23).

$$K = \frac{\ln\left(\dfrac{C_1}{C_2}\right)}{t} \qquad \text{(Eq. 8.23)}$$

$$= \frac{\ln\left(\dfrac{8}{3}\right)}{7 \text{ hr}}$$

$$= \frac{0.98}{7 \text{ hr}}$$

$$= 0.14 \text{ hr}^{-1}$$

Using the elimination rate constant of 0.14 hr^{-1}, the observed peak concentration of 8 mg/L, and the dosing regimen of 100 mg administered over 0.5 hour every 8 hours, Y.B.'s volume of distribution can be calculated by rearranging Equation 8.17 for C_{ss1}, where τ is 8 hours and the sample is obtained 0.5 hours after the end of the 0.5-hour infusion making t_1 1 hour,

$$C_{ss1} = \frac{\dfrac{(S)(F)(\text{Dose})}{V}}{(1 - e^{-K\tau})}\, e^{-Kt_1}$$

$$V = \frac{\dfrac{(S)(F)(\text{Dose})}{C_{ss1}}}{(1 - e^{-K\tau})}\, e^{-Kt_1} \qquad \text{(Eq. 8.24)}$$

$$V = \frac{\dfrac{(1)(1)(100 \text{ mg})}{8 \text{ mg/L}}}{(1 - e^{-(0.14 \text{ hr}^{-1})(8 \text{hr})})} (e^{-(0.14 \text{ hr}^{-1})(1 \text{hr})})$$

$$= \frac{12.5 \text{ L}}{0.67}(0.87)$$

$$= 16.2 \text{ L}$$

and the clearance can be calculated using a rearrangement of Equation 8.15

$$K = \frac{\text{Cl}}{V}$$

to solve for Cl.

$$\text{Cl} = (K)(V)$$
$$= (0.14 \text{ hr}^{-1})(16.2 \text{ L})$$
$$= 2.3 \text{ L/hr}$$

(Eq. 8.25)

This volume of distribution of 16.2 L corresponds to about 0.23 L/kg. The value of calculating tobramycin pharmacokinetic parameters that are specific for Y.B. is that they may now be used to calculate a dosing regimen that will produce any desired peak and trough concentrations.

Question #7 *The microbiology report reveals Pseudomonas aeruginosa with MIC of 1 µg/mL. Calculate a dosing regimen for Y.B. that will achieve a peak concentration of greater than 10 mg/L (peak: MIC > 10:1) and AUC_{24} in the range of 70 to 100 mg·hr/L.*

As before, the dose required to achieve a specific peak concentration can be calculated from Equation 8.17. To select an appropriate dosing interval, however, one should first consider Y.B.'s apparent half-life, which can be calculated using V of 16.2 L and Cl of 2.3 L/hr in Equation 8.10.

$$t_{\frac{1}{2}} = \frac{(0.693)(V)}{\text{Cl}}$$
$$= \frac{0.693 (16.2 \text{ L})}{2.3 \text{ L/hr}}$$
$$= 4.9 \text{ hr}$$

A dosing interval of approximately four to five half-lives is desirable to maximize the peak concentration and bactericidal activity while minimizing drug accumulation and potential nephrotoxicity and ototoxicity. Because Y.B.'s tobramycin half-life is approximately 5 hours, the most convenient dosing interval is 24 hours. Using this dosing interval and the appropriate volume of distribution and elimination rate constant,

Equation 8.26 (a rearrangement of Equation 8.17 to solve for dose) indicates that a dose of 180 mg administered every 24 hours should result in a peak concentration of approximately 10 mg/L 1 hour after the start of a 0.5-hour infusion.

$$\text{Dose} = \frac{(C_{ss1})(V)(1 - e^{-K\tau})}{(S)(F)(e^{-Kt_1})} \qquad \text{(Eq. 8.26)}$$

$$\text{Dose} = \frac{(10 \text{ mg/L})(16.2 \text{ L})(1 - e^{-(0.14 \text{hr}^{-1})(24 \text{hr})})}{(1)(1)e^{-(0.14 \text{hr}^{-1})(1 \text{hr})}}$$

$$= \frac{(10 \text{ mg/L})(16.2 \text{ L})(0.97)}{(1)(1)(0.87)}$$

$$= 180 \text{ mg}$$

Equation 8.11 can be used to determine the trough concentration. A t of 23 hours and a C_0 of 10 mg/L should be used.

$$C = C_0 e^{-Kt}$$

$$= (10 \text{ mg/L})(e^{-(0.14 \text{hr}^{-1})(23 \text{hr})})$$

$$= (10 \text{ mg/L})(0.04)$$

$$= 0.4 \text{ mg/L}$$

To confirm whether the level of drug exposure is in the desirable range, Equation 8.27 can be used to calculate the AUC_{24}.

$$AUC_{24} = \frac{(\text{Dose in mg})(24 \text{ hr})/\tau \text{ in hr}}{Cl \text{ in L/hr}} \qquad \text{(Eq. 8.27)}$$

$$= \frac{(180 \text{ mg})(24 \text{ hr})/24 \text{ hr}}{2.3 \text{ L/hr}}$$

$$= 78 \text{ mg} \cdot \text{hr/L}$$

Question #8 *C.I. is a 50-year-old, 60-kg man with a serum creatinine of 1.5 mg/dL, who is receiving 350 mg of amikacin IV over 0.5 hour every 8 hours at midnight, 8:00 AM, and 4:00 PM. He had a trough concentration of 6 mg/L obtained just before the 8:00 AM dose and a peak concentration of 15 mg/L obtained at 9:00 AM. Assuming these peak and trough concentrations represent steady-state levels, calculate C.I.'s elimination rate constant, clearance, and volume of distribution. Evaluate whether these parameters seem reasonable and should be used to adjust C.I.'s amikacin maintenance dose.*

The approach to calculating the revised pharmacokinetic parameters for C.I. is essentially the same as that used in the previous questions. First, the elimination rate

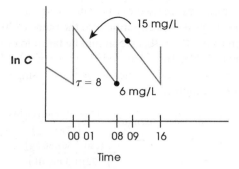

FIGURE 8.3 Calculating K by transposing $C_{ss\ max}$ into the same interval as $C_{ss\ min}$. Note that steady state must have been achieved (same dose, same interval for $>3\text{-}5t_{1/2}s$). Also, the $C_{ss\ max}$ is moved to the same time within the interval relative to the preceding dose (ie, from 09:00 in one interval to 01:00 in the preceding interval). The intermittent bolus dose model has been used for the input model, and the concentrations are ln concentrations so that the decay phase is a straight line.

constant of $0.13\ hr^{-1}$ can be calculated using Equation 8.23 and the 7-hour time interval between the peak and trough concentrations (Figure 8.3):

$$K = \frac{\ln\left(\dfrac{C_1}{C_2}\right)}{t}$$

$$= \frac{\ln\left(\dfrac{15}{6}\right)}{7\ hr}$$

$$= 0.13\ hr^{-1}$$

Next, the volume of distribution can be calculated by using Equation 8.24. A dose of 350 mg and a τ of 8 hours can be used. The latter t_1 represents the time from the beginning of the infusion to the "peak concentration" sampling time ($t_1 = 1$ hour).

$$V = \frac{(S)(F)(\text{Dose})}{\dfrac{C_{ss1}}{(1 - e^{-K\tau})}}(e^{-Kt_1})$$

$$= \frac{(1)(1)(350\ mg)}{\dfrac{15\ mg/L}{(1 - e^{-(0.13hr^{-1})(8hr)})}}(e^{-(0.13hr^{-1})(1hr)})$$

$$= \frac{(23.3\ L)(0.88)}{0.65}$$

$$= 31.5\ L$$

Using the calculated volume of distribution of 31.5 L and the elimination rate constant of $0.13\ hr^{-1}$, a clearance value of 4.1 L/hr can be calculated using Equation 8.25.

$$Cl = (K)(V)$$

$$Cl = (0.13\ hr^{-1})(31.5\ L)$$

$$= 4.1\ L/hr$$

Before these parameters are used to calculate an adjusted amikacin dosing regimen that will bring C.I.'s peak concentration into the range of 20 to 30 mg/L and the trough concentration below 10 mg/L, care should be taken to evaluate whether these parameters appear reasonable. The calculated clearance of 4.1 L/hr is slightly greater than the expected clearance of 3 L/hr, which is calculated using Equation 8.6 and C.I.'s age, weight, and serum creatinine.

$$Cl_{Cr} \text{ for males (mL/min)} = \frac{(140 - \text{Age})(\text{Weight})}{(72)(SCr_{ss})}$$
$$= \frac{(140 - 50)(60 \text{ kg})}{(72)(1.5 \text{ mg/dL})}$$
$$= 50 \text{ mL/min}$$

or

$$Cl_{Cr} \text{ (L/hr)} = 50 \text{ mL/min} \times \frac{(60 \text{ min/hr})}{(1,000 \text{ mL/L})}$$
$$= 3 \text{ L/hr}$$

Although this clearance value is greater than expected, it is not so unusual as to be considered unrealistic.

The volume of distribution value of 0.53 L/kg (31.5 L/60 kg), however, is unusually large. In general, volumes of distribution greater than 0.35 L/kg are only observed in patients who have a significant third spacing of fluid (eg, ascites or edema). If there is no evidence of any third spacing in C.I., then the volume of distribution would be unrealistically large. Therefore, the dosing history or the measured plasma concentrations are probably in error. If C.I. had received tobramycin or gentamicin, the possibility of a penicillin interaction resulting in spuriously low plasma concentrations would have to be considered; however, amikacin does not interact with penicillins to a significant extent. Therefore, this is an unlikely explanation for the unusually large volume of distribution.

When pharmacokinetic calculations lead to parameters that are very different from those expected, there may be an error in the time of sampling, assay results, or dosing history. In such cases, it may be more prudent to use the expected rather than the calculated parameters to adjust doses. In some cases, however, the patient may actually have unusual parameters. When this is suspected, the dosing history should be reevaluated and another set of plasma drug concentrations should be obtained, with special attention to precise sampling times and the dosing history.

Question #9 *D.H., a 40-year-old man, was admitted to the hospital following an automobile accident. He is 5 feet 5 inches tall and, on admission, weighed 85 kg. He was taken for abdominal surgery and postoperatively became hypotensive and required large volumes of fluid to maintain his blood pressure. Currently, he weighs 105 kg and has a serum creatinine of 2.3 mg/dL. D.H. is to receive gentamicin empirically after his abdominal surgery. Estimate his pharmacokinetic parameters and dose to achieve peak gentamicin concentrations greater than 10 mg/L and an AUC_{24} between 70 and 100 mg·hr/L.*

To calculate D.H.'s pharmacokinetic parameters, it is first necessary to identify his nonobese, excess adipose, and excess third-space fluid weight. Using Equation 8.2, D.H.'s IBW is calculated to be approximately 61.5 kg.

$$\text{Ideal body weight for males in kg} = 50 + (2.3)(\text{Height in inches} > 60)$$
$$= 50 + (2.3)(5 \text{ inches})$$
$$= 61.5 \text{ kg}$$

Assuming D.H. did not have any excess third-space fluid on admission, his excess adipose weight is approximately 23.5 kg (estimated by subtracting his IBW of 61.5 kg from his admission weight of 85 kg). D.H.'s excess third-space fluid weight of 20 kg can be estimated by subtracting his initial weight of 85 kg from his current weight of 105 kg. Using these weight estimates for his body composition, Equation 8.4 can be used to estimate an aminoglycoside volume of distribution of approximately 38 L:

$$\text{Aminoglycoside } V \text{ (L)} = 0.25 \text{ L/kg} \left(\begin{array}{c} \text{Nonobese,} \\ \text{non-excess} \\ \text{fluid weight (kg)} \end{array} \right) + 0.1 \left(\begin{array}{c} \text{Excess} \\ \text{adipose} \\ \text{weight (kg)} \end{array} \right) + \left(\begin{array}{c} \text{Excess} \\ \text{third space} \\ \text{fluid} \\ \text{weight (kg)} \end{array} \right)$$
$$= (0.25 \text{ L/kg} \times 61.5 \text{ kg}) + 0.1(23.5 \text{ kg}) + (20 \text{ kg})$$
$$= 37.7 \text{ or } 38 \text{ L}$$

Because D.H.'s BMI is greater than 30, adjusted IBW, calculated using Equation 8.8, and his current serum creatinine of 2 mg/dL should be used with Equation 8.6 to estimate gentamicin clearance.

$$\text{Adjusted body weight} = \text{IBW} + 0.4 \, (\text{TBW} - \text{IBW})$$
$$= 61.5 \text{ kg} + 0.4 \, (85 \text{ kg} - 61.5 \text{ kg})$$
$$= 70.9 \text{ kg}$$

$$\text{Cl}_{\text{Cr}} \text{ for males (mL/min)} = \frac{(140 - \text{Age})(\text{Weight})}{(72)(\text{SCr}_{ss})}$$
$$= \frac{(140 - 40 \text{ yr})(70.9 \text{ kg})}{(72)(2.3 \text{ mg/dL})}$$
$$= 42.8 \text{ mL/min}$$
$$= 42.8 \text{ mL/min} \times \frac{60 \text{ min/hr}}{1,000 \text{ mL/L}}$$
$$= 2.57 \text{ L/hr}$$

Using the estimated creatinine clearance of 2.57 L/hr as the gentamicin clearance and the volume of distribution of 38 L, the elimination rate constant (Equation 8.15) and half-life (Equation 8.10) are calculated to be approximately 0.07 hr^{-1} and approximately 10 hours, respectively:

$$K = \frac{Cl}{V}$$

$$= \frac{2.57 \, L/hr}{38 \, L}$$

$$= 0.067 \approx 0.07 \, hr^{-1}$$

$$t_{\frac{1}{2}} = \frac{0.693}{K}$$

$$= \frac{0.693}{0.07 \, hr^{-1}}$$

$$= 9.9 \approx 10 \, hr$$

Given D.H.'s half-life of approximately 10 hours and an infusion time of 0.5 hour, Equation 8.26, the steady-state bolus dose model, can be used to calculate his regimen.

$$Dose = \frac{(C_{ss1})(V)(1 - e^{-K\tau})}{(S)(F)(e^{-Kt_1})}$$

Because aminoglycoside dosing intervals are typically greater than four to five half-lives, a dosing interval of 48 hours is reasonable, given D.H.'s half-life of approximately 10 hours. Dosing interval can also be determined by rearranging Equation 8.11 to calculate the time it will take a targeted peak level, $C_0 = 10$ mg/L, to reach the targeted trough level, $C = 1$ mg/dL.

$$C = C_0 \, e^{-Kt}$$

$$t = \frac{\ln\left(\dfrac{C}{C_0}\right)}{-K} \qquad \text{(Eq. 8.28)}$$

$$= \frac{\ln\left(\dfrac{1 \, mg/L}{10 \, mg/L}\right)}{-0.07 \, hr^{-1}}$$

$$= 32.9 \, hr$$

Time difference between peak and trough levels of approximately 33 hours falls between 24- and 48-hour doing interval. Owing to impaired renal function in D.H., dosing interval of 48 hours would prevent accumulation of trough level and overexposure to gentamicin.

Making the appropriate substitution in the rearranged equation, where C_{ss1} is assumed to be 10 mg/L, t_1 is 1 hour (indicating that the peak concentration is to be obtained 1 hour after the start of the infusion), a dose of approximately 400 mg is calculated.

$$\text{Dose} = \frac{(10 \text{ mg/L})(38 \text{ L})(1 - e^{-(0.07 \text{ hr}^{-1})(48 \text{ hr})})}{(1)(1)(e^{-(0.07 \text{ hr}^{-1})(1 \text{ hr})})}$$

$$= \frac{(10 \text{ mg/L})(38 \text{ L})(0.97)}{(1)(1)(0.93)}$$

$$= 396 \text{ mg or} \approx 400 \text{ mg}$$

Although a dose of 400 mg appears to be large, this is due, in part, to the extensive third-spacing fluid and the large volume of distribution. In many cases, a somewhat lower dose might be employed; however, the peak concentration would be proportionately decreased. Also, although the dose of 400 mg seems large, D.H. is receiving this dose only every other day, and based on his adjusted IBW of 70.9 kg, this equates to approximately 3.0 mg/kg/d, which is below the lower end of the usual range (5-7 mg/kg/d). It is also important to ensure that AUC_{24} is in the desired range (70-100 mg·hr/L).

$$AUC_{24} = \frac{(\text{Dose in mg})(24 \text{ hr})/\tau \text{ in hr}}{Cl \text{ in L/hr}}$$

$$AUC_{24} = \frac{(400 \text{ mg})(24 \text{ hr})/48 \text{ hr}}{2.57 \text{ hr}}$$

$$= 77.8 \text{ mg} \cdot \text{hr/L}$$

The AUC_{24} value of approximately 78 mg·hr/L is at the lower end of the desired range (70-100 mg·hr/L), indicating that the dose could be increased if necessary depending on the severity of the infection. If the dosing interval remains 48 hours, an increase in dose will result in a proportional increase in AUC_{24} and peak concentration (see Equations 8.17 and 8.27). For example, a 30% increase in dose would result in an AUC_{24} of approximately 100 mg·hr/L and a peak concentration of 13 mg/L.

If the dosing interval of 24 hours was chosen instead, a dose of 340 mg might have achieved the target peak level of 10 mg/L, but the trough would be at a higher end of a range of 2 mg/L, resulting in overexposure to gentamicin with AUC_{24} of 132 mg·hr/L.

Question #10 *What is the significance of a changing serum creatinine in a patient receiving gentamicin?*

A rising serum creatinine level in a patient always raises the question of gentamicin-induced nephrotoxicity. In this event, the drug may be discontinued, the plasma concentration reevaluated, and/or the dose adjusted because gentamicin may accumulate substantially when renal function is impaired. Dose modification should be based on plasma gentamicin levels rather than serum creatinine levels because serum creatinine concentrations that are not at steady state can be misleading (see Creatinine Clearance [Cl_{Cr}] in Chapter "Drug Dosing in Kidney Disease and Dialysis"). This is because despite the similarity between gentamicin and creatinine clearances,[30,42] their volumes of distribution differ. Gentamicin's V of 0.25 L/kg is smaller than that of creatinine, which is 0.5 L/kg.[25,26,31,71] Because the half-life is determined by the clearance and volume of distribution (see Equation 8.10), the half-life for creatinine is approximately twice as long as that of gentamicin and the other aminoglycosides. Therefore, it will take creatinine longer to arrive at a new steady-state concentration after a change in renal function.

$$t_{\frac{1}{2}} = \frac{(0.693)(V)}{Cl}$$

When the serum creatinine is rising (ie, not at steady state), the actual renal function is worse than that predicted by the use of the serum creatinine, and any gentamicin dose calculated using the serum creatinine would be overestimated. Conversely, when the serum creatinine is falling, renal function may be better than that reflected by creatinine clearance, and the doses calculated on the basis of these levels would be underestimated.

Question #11   *D.W., a 20-year-old, 60-kg man, is receiving 120 mg of tobramycin infused IV over a 30-minute period every 12 hours. His serum creatinine has increased from 1 to 2 mg/dL over the past 24 hours. Because his renal function appears to be decreasing, three plasma samples were obtained to monitor serum tobramycin concentrations as follows: just before a dose, 1 hour after that same dose, and 12 hours after that dose (two troughs and one peak level). The serum tobramycin concentrations at these times were 3, 9, and 4 mg/L, respectively. Calculate the volume of distribution, elimination rate constant, and clearance of tobramycin for D.W.*

Because the second trough concentration of tobramycin is higher than the first, it is apparent that the drug is accumulating. Therefore, steady-state equations should not be used to calculate D.W.'s pharmacokinetic parameters. The first step that should be taken to resolve this dilemma is to calculate the elimination rate constant from the two plasma concentrations that were obtained during the elimination phase (9 and 4 mg/L). Equation 8.23 can be used to estimate the elimination rate constant; however, this K should only be used as an estimate because the two plasma concentrations were obtained less than one half-life apart.

$$K = \frac{\ln\left(\frac{C_1}{C_2}\right)}{t}$$

$$= \frac{\ln\left(\frac{9 \text{ mg/L}}{4 \text{ mg/L}}\right)}{11 \text{ hr}}$$

$$= 0.074 \text{ hr}^{-1}$$

This elimination rate constant of 0.074 hr^{-1} was calculated by assuming that the peak concentration of 9 mg/L was obtained 1 hour after the start of the tobramycin infusion and that the trough concentration was obtained just before the next dose, resulting in a time interval of 11 hours. The elimination rate constant of 0.074 hr^{-1} corresponds to a half-life of approximately 10 hours (Equation 8.10):

$$t_{1/2} = \frac{0.693}{K}$$
$$= \frac{0.693}{0.074 \ hr^{-1}}$$
$$= 9.4 \approx 10 \ hr$$

This half-life of 10 hours suggests that relatively little drug is lost during the infusion period; therefore, a bolus model is most appropriate for this situation. The volume of distribution can be estimated by assuming that the bolus dose is administered instantaneously and calculating the theoretical peak concentration using Equation 8.12. C is the measured concentration of 9 mg/L, t is the 1-hour interval between the start of the infusion and the time of sampling, and C_0 is the theoretical peak concentration for an IV bolus.

$$C_0 = \frac{C}{e^{-Kt}}$$
$$= \frac{9 \ mg/L}{e^{-(0.074 \, hr^{-1})(1 hr)}}$$
$$= \frac{9 \ mg/L}{0.93}$$
$$= 9.7 \ mg/L$$

Because the change in concentration (peak minus trough) is the result of the dose administered and the volume of distribution, V can be calculated using Equation 8.29.

$$V = \frac{Dose}{(C_{peak} - C_{min})} \qquad \text{(Eq. 8.29)}$$

$$V = \frac{120 \ mg}{(9.7 \ mg/L - 3 \ mg/L)}$$
$$= 17.9 \ L$$

This volume of distribution of 17.9 L can then be used with the elimination rate constant of 0.074 hr^{-1} in Equation 8.25 to calculate D.W.'s clearance of 1.3 L/hr or 22 mL/min:

$$Cl = (K)(V)$$
$$= (0.074 \ hr^{-1})(17.9 \ L)$$
$$= 1.3 \ L/hr \ or \ 22 \ mL/min$$

Question #12   *Using the pharmacokinetic parameters calculated for D.W. in Question 11, develop a dosing regimen that will produce reasonable peak and trough concentrations of tobramycin.*

Because D.W.'s tobramycin clearance is low (1.3 L/hr), it will be necessary to reduce his maintenance dose. There are two alternatives: (1) reduce the dose and maintain the same dosing interval or (2) adjust both the dose and the dosing interval such that the peak concentration and AUC_{24} will be approximately 10 mg/L and 70 to 100 mg·hr/L, respectively.

Reduce the dose and maintain the same dosing interval. This method is not acceptable for D.W. because the peak concentration is already near the goal with the current dose. If the dose is reduced while the dosing interval is maintained, the peak concentration will be compromised. With such a long half-life ($\approx$10 hours), even a lower dose that achieves a peak concentration of 8 mg/L will result in a trough level of approximately 3.3 mg/L if every 12-hour dosing interval is maintained.

$$C_{ss\,min} = (C_{ss\,max})(e^{-K\tau}) \hspace{3cm} \text{(Eq. 8.30)}$$

$$C_{ss\,min} = (8 \text{ mg/L})(e^{-(0.074\,hr^{-1})(12hr)})$$
$$= 3.3 \text{ mg/L}$$

This level may place D.W. at risk for tobramycin toxicity.

Adjust both the dose and dosing interval to achieve reasonable peak concentration and AUC_{24} values. The only potential limitation to this approach is that most clinicians prefer to avoid prolonged periods during which the gentamicin concentration is below the MIC of the pathogen owing to the possibility of organism regrowth. Clinical experience with dosing intervals in excess of 48 hours is limited. Nevertheless, some animal data suggest that doses that result in high peak and low trough concentrations are less likely to produce renal toxicity than the same dose administered as a continuous IV infusion (ie, the same average levels).[72] A first estimate of the dosing interval can be made by examining D.W.'s tobramycin half-life of 10 hours. If an interval of four to five half-lives is chosen, a dosing interval of 48 hours can be used. As previously stated, Equation 8.27 can be used to calculate the dose required to achieve a specific AUC_{24} (ie, 80 mg·hr/L, a value between 70 and 100 mg·hr/L). Using Equation 8.27 with the previously derived pharmacokinetic parameters and a dosing interval of 48 hours, a dose of approximately 200 mg is calculated.

$$AUC_{24} = \frac{(\text{Dose in mg})(24 \text{ hr}) / \tau \text{ in hr}}{Cl \text{ in L/hr}}$$

or

$$Dose \text{ in mg} = \frac{(AUC_{24})(Cl \text{ in L/hr})(\tau \text{ in hr})}{24 \text{ hr}}$$
$$= \frac{(80 \text{ mg} \cdot \text{hr/L})(1.3 \text{ L/hr})(48 \text{ hr})}{24 \text{ hr}}$$
$$= 208 \approx 200 \text{ mg given q48 h}$$

Because the half-life of tobramycin is long relative to the infusion time of 0.5 hour, the bolus dose model can be used to calculate the peak concentration (Equation 8.17).

A peak concentration that occurs 1 hour after the infusion has been initiated is also assumed (ie, $t_1 = 1$ hour).

$$C_{ss1} = \frac{\dfrac{(S)(F)(\text{Dose})}{V}}{(1 - e^{-K\tau})} (e^{-Kt_1})$$

$$= \frac{\dfrac{(1)(1)(200 \text{ mg})}{17.9 \text{ L}}}{(1 - e^{-(0.074 \text{hr}^{-1})(48 \text{hr})})} (e^{-(0.074 \text{hr}^{-1})(1 \text{hr})})$$

$$= \frac{11.2 \text{ mg/L}}{0.97} (0.93)$$

$$= 10.7 \text{ mg/L}$$

The trough concentration, 47 hours later, calculated using Equation 8.11, would be 0.33 mg/L.

$$C = C_0(e^{-Kt})$$
$$C = (10.7 \text{ mg/L})(e^{-(0.074 \text{hr}^{-1})(47 \text{hr})})$$
$$= 0.33 \text{ mg/L}$$

Question #13 *M.S., a 66-kg nonobese female, undergoes 4 hours of hemodialysis every 48 hours. She is functionally (not surgically) anephric, and gentamicin is to be started. Calculate a dosing regimen that achieves a peak concentration of 7 mg/L and a predialysis concentration between 3 and 5 mg/L.*

Because the gentamicin half-life for a patient who is functionally anephric is probably in excess of 30 hours, very little drug will be eliminated from the body over the 1-hour period following initiation of the infusion. Therefore, the loading dose may be calculated as though it was a bolus (Equation 8.31). Assuming S and F to be 1 and the volume of distribution to be 16.5 L (0.25 L/kg), a loading dose of approximately 120 mg would be calculated as follows:

$$\text{Loading dose} = \frac{(V)(C)}{(S)(F)} \qquad \text{(Eq. 8.31)}$$

$$= \frac{(16.5 \text{ L})(7 \text{ mg/L})}{(1)(1)}$$
$$= 115.5 \approx 120 \text{ mg}$$

The peak concentrations of 7 to 10 mg/L and a predialysis C_p of 3 to 5 mg/L for tobramycin and gentamicin (C_p of 20-30 mg/L and predialysis C_p of <10 for amikacin) have shown to be effective in eradicating infections in patients undergoing dialysis every 48 to 72 hours.[73,74] Because gentamicin elimination in M.S. will be irregular, occurring at higher rates during the dialysis, the usual maintenance dose equation cannot be used. As presented in Dialysis of Drugs in Chapter "Drug Dosing in Kidney Disease and Dialysis," there are two possible approaches to resolving this problem. One approach is to administer a daily dose such that average concentrations are maintained and then to calculate a replacement dose postdialysis. While this approach will maintain average concentrations of 4 mg/L, achieving the target peak concentration of 7 to 10 mg/L will be difficult.

A second approach is to administer the drug after dialysis only. Previously, a loading dose of 3 mg/kg and a maintenance dose of 1 to 2 mg/kg given after dialysis was able to achieve the C_p and predialysis targets, but these doses may not always achieve the target peak concentrations owing to the advanced technologies in hemodialysis treatment, including high-flux dialysis filters that are able to clear approximately 50% of aminoglycosides during hemodialysis.[73-76] Traditional postdialysis dosing regimen of 1 to 2 mg/kg is unlikely to reach the goal C_p of 7 to 10 mg/L.

Aminoglycoside dose to be given postdialysis can be calculated using Equation 8.32. The dose used is the amount of drug lost during the interdialysis and intradialysis period. In this case, the use of the patient's clearance (Cl_{pat}), dialysis clearance (Cl_{dial}), and the volume of distribution will be required. The reported clearance for aminoglycosides in functionally anephric patients is approximately 0.0043 L/kg/hr,[26,77] and aminoglycoside clearance by high-flux hemodialysis is 103 to 116 mL/min, with an average value of approximately 110 mL/min.[75,76]

Using Equation 8.32, the following are calculated: a $C_{ss\,peak}$ of 7 mg/L, a patient clearance of 0.28 L/hr (0.0043 L/hr/kg × 66 kg), and a t_1 of 44 hours (derived from a 48-hour interval between the dialyses and a dialysis time [T_d] of 4 hours), the postdialysis replacement dose is approximately 100 mg. Note that the dialysis clearance of 6.6 L/hr represents a clearance of approximately 110 mL/min and that this is the primary route of elimination during the intradialysis period.

$$\text{Postdialysis replacement dose} = (V)(C_{ss\,peak})\left(1 - \left[\left(e^{-\left(\frac{Cl_{pat}}{V}\right)(t_1)}\right)\left(e^{-\left(\frac{Cl_{pat}+Cl_{dial}}{V}\right)(T_d)}\right)\right]\right) \quad \textbf{(Eq. 8.32)}$$

$$= (16.5\ \text{L})(7\ \text{mg/L})\left(1 - \left[\left(e^{-\left(\frac{0.28\ \text{L/hr}}{16.5\ \text{L}}\right)(44\ \text{hr})}\right)\left(e^{-\left(\frac{0.28\ \text{L/hr}+6.6\ \text{L/hr}}{16.5\ \text{L}}\right)(4\ \text{hr})}\right)\right]\right)$$

$$= 115.5\ (1 - [(0.47)(0.19)])$$

$$= 105 \approx 100\ \text{mg}$$

To ensure that trough concentration just before dialysis is between 3 and 5 mg/L, the predialysis drug concentration should be calculated using Equation 8.33.

$$\text{Predialysis drug concentration} = \left[C_{ss\,peak}\right]\left[e^{-\left(\frac{Cl_{pat}}{V}\right)(t_1)}\right] \quad \textbf{(Eq. 8.33)}$$

$$= (7 \text{ mg/L}) \left[e^{\left(-\frac{0.28 \text{L/hr}}{16.5 \text{L}} (44 \text{hr}) \right)} \right]$$

$$= (7 \text{ mg/L})(0.47)$$

$$= 3.32 \text{ mg/L}$$

This predialysis concentration of approximately 3.3 mg/L is higher than usually desired in patients with normal renal function; however, because the gentamicin half-life is unusually long, it will be difficult to maintain peak levels in the range of 7 to 10 mg/L and predialysis trough concentrations of less than 2 mg/L. Unfortunately, the persistence of relatively high concentrations between dialysis periods will place M.S. at greater risk for ototoxicity.[78] One strategy to decrease the risk of ototoxicity associated with persistent high concentrations is to administer gentamicin right before dialysis. Predialysis dosing of the drug will achieve the target C_p goal, and the removal of drugs during dialysis will minimize sustained elevated serum levels. Moreover, a first predialysis C_p: MIC greater than 6 mg/L has been suggested as a predictor for decreased mortality among patients with gram-negative rod bloodstream infections, which may not be achieved with postdialysis dosing.[74]

Delayed distribution of aminoglycoside is observed in patients with renal failure; thus, the C_p level should be drawn approximately 2 hours after dose administration to avoid the distribution phase.[73,79] If postdialysis concentrations are to be measured, time should be allowed for equilibration between the plasma compartment (in which concentrations have been lowered during the dialysis period) and the extracellular fluid compartment.[80]

Question #14   *How would the abovementioned situation have differed if peritoneal dialysis rather than hemodialysis had been used?*

Peritoneal dialysis is much less effective in removing gentamicin; the usual clearance value is approximately 4 mL/min/m², with an average value of 5 to 10 mL/min for the 70-kg patient. Nonetheless, the total amount of drug removed during dialysis may be as much as 30% or more because acute intermittent peritoneal dialysis is usually continued for approximately 36 hours.[77,81]

Aminoglycosides can be administered either parenterally or intraperitoneally to achieve systemic plasma concentrations. When administered intraperitoneally, an initial loading dose of 2 to 3 mg/kg is added to the first peritoneal dialysis exchange. Then, 1.2 mg/kg/d is added to one exchange daily (usually the nighttime exchange), or a dose that produces a dialysate concentration of approximately 6 to 10 mg/L is added to each dialysate exchange. Both of these regimens result in steady-state plasma concentrations of approximately 3 mg/L with relatively little fluctuation.[82] When aminoglycoside antibiotics are placed in each peritoneal exchange, many clinicians estimate the steady-state plasma concentration to be approximately 40% of the peritoneal dialysate concentration. As an example, if 16 mg were added to each 2-L peritoneal exchange volume (8 mg/L), the steady-state plasma concentration would be 3.2 mg/L, or 40% of the 8 mg/L concentration in the dialysate exchanges.[83,84]

Question #15   *T.C. is receiving tobramycin 400 mg IV over 0.5 hour every 24 hours at 9:00 AM. Levels drawn at 11:00 AM and 9:00 PM were 17 and 1 mg/L, respectively. Calculate the peak concentration expected at 10:00 AM., or 1 hour after starting the 9:00 AM tobramycin infusion, and the AUC_{24} to determine the appropriateness of the current dosing regimen.*

The time interval between 11:00 AM and 9:00 PM is 10 hours, and Equation 8.23 can be used to determine the elimination rate constant for T.C.

$$K = \frac{\ln\left(\dfrac{C_1}{C_2}\right)}{t}$$

$$= \frac{\ln\left(\dfrac{17 \text{ mg/L}}{1 \text{ mg/L}}\right)}{10 \text{ hr}}$$

$$= \frac{2.8}{10 \text{ hr}}$$

$$= 0.28 \text{ hr}^{-1}$$

This patient-specific elimination rate constant of 0.28 hr^{-1} can be used in Equation 8.12 to calculate the expected plasma concentration at 10:00 AM (1 hour after the start of the infusion) or 1 hour before the observed peak of 17 mg/L.

$$C_0 = \frac{C}{e^{-Kt}}$$

$$= \frac{17 \text{ mg/L}}{e^{-(0.28 \text{ hr}^{-1})(1 \text{ hr})}}$$

$$= \frac{17 \text{ mg/L}}{0.76}$$

$$= 22.4 \approx 22 \text{ mg/L}$$

Because of the short $t_{\frac{1}{2}}$ ($t_{in} > \frac{1}{6} \times t_{\frac{1}{2}}$), steady-state infusion model should be used (Equation 8.21).

$$C_{ss2} = \frac{\dfrac{(S)(F)(\text{Dose}/t_{in})}{Cl}(1 - e^{-Kt_{in}})}{(1 - e^{-K\tau})}(e^{-Kt_2})$$

The equation can be rearranged to solve for clearance:

$$Cl = \frac{\dfrac{(S)(F)(\text{Dose}/t_{in})}{C_{ss2}}(1 - e^{-Kt_{in}})}{(1 - e^{-K\tau})}(e^{-Kt_2}) \qquad \textbf{(Eq. 8.34)}$$

$$Cl = \frac{\dfrac{(1)(1)(400 \text{ mg}/0.5 \text{ hr})}{1 \text{ mg/L}}(1 - e^{(0.28 \text{hr}^{-1})(0.5 \text{hr})})}{(1 - e^{-(0.28 \text{hr}^{-1})(24 \text{hr})})} \, (e^{-(0.28 \text{hr}^{-1})(11.5 \text{hr})})$$

$$= \frac{(800 \text{ L/hr})(0.13)}{(0.99)}(0.04)$$

$$= 4.2 \text{ L/hr}$$

The AUC_{24} can then be calculated using Equation 8.27.

$$AUC_{24} = \frac{(\text{Dose in mg})(24 \text{ hr})/\tau \text{ in hr}}{Cl \text{ in L/hr}}$$

$$= \frac{(400 \text{ mg})(24 \text{ hr})/24 \text{ hr}}{4.2 \text{ L/hr}}$$

$$= 95 \text{ mg} \cdot \text{hr/L}$$

This peak concentration of 22 mg/L represents a concentration that is within the target range (peak: MIC > 10) based on the breakpoint for susceptibility (2 µg/mL). The AUC_{24} is also in the target range (70-100 mg·hr/L) and suggests that T.C's tobramycin does not require dose adjustment.

Question #16   *M.R., a 5-year-old boy (height, 3 feet 11 inches [119 cm]; weight, 24 kg) with no prior medical history, is admitted for ruptured appendix. Gentamicin 80 mg IV every 8 hours, infused over 30 minutes is started after appendectomy. His serum creatinine is 0.7 mg/dL. Calculate the predicted steady-state peak concentration of gentamicin 1 hour after the infusion was started.*

Traditionally, pediatric patients are started on gentamicin and tobramycin 2.5 mg/kg every 8 hours and amikacin 15 mg/kg/d in two to three divided doses. However, variable Cl and volume of distribution in children as they grow warrant changes in aminoglycoside dosing accordingly. In general, younger children have a larger volume of distribution and Cl and require higher doses. As they get older, the volume of distribution and Cl reach adult values, and a decrease in dose is necessary. M.R's volume of distribution can be calculated using a V of 0.35 L/kg. Cl_{cr} can be calculated by adjusting GFR from Equation 8.9 by the patient's body surface area (BSA) (see Creatinine Clearance [Cl_{Cr}] in Chapter "Drug Dosing in Kidney Disease and Dialysis"). BSA values can be obtained from the appendix.

$$V = (0.35 \text{ L/kg})(24 \text{ kg})$$

$$= 8.4 \text{ L}$$

$$Cl_{Cr} \text{ for children (mL/min/1.73 m}^2) = 0.413\left(\frac{\text{Height in cm}}{(\text{SCr})}\right)$$

$$= 0.413\left(\frac{119 \text{ cm}}{(0.7 \text{ mg/dL})}\right)$$

$$= 70.2 \text{ mL/min/1.73 m}^2$$

$$Cl_{Cr} \text{ for children (mL/min)} = (Cl_{Cr} \text{ mL/min}/1.73 \text{ m}^2) \left(\frac{BSA}{1.73 \text{ m}^2} \right) \quad \text{(Eq. 8.35)}$$

$$= (70.2 \text{ mL/min}/1.73 \text{ m}^2) \left(\frac{0.89 \text{ m}^2}{1.73 \text{ m}^2} \right)$$

$$= 36.1 \text{ mL/min}$$

$$= 36.1 \text{ mL/min} \times \frac{60 \text{ min/hr}}{1,000 \text{ mL/L}}$$

$$= 2.2 \text{ L/hr}$$

The elimination rate can be calculated using the estimated creatinine clearance of 2.2 L/hr and volume of distribution of 8.4 L (Equation 8.15). Half-life can be calculated using Equation 8.10.

$$K = \frac{Cl}{V}$$

$$= \frac{2.2 \text{ L/hr}}{8.4 \text{ L}}$$

$$= 0.26 \text{ hr}^{-1}$$

$$t_{\frac{1}{2}} = \frac{0.693}{K}$$

$$= \frac{0.693}{0.26 \text{ hr}^{-1}}$$

$$= 2.67 \text{ hr}$$

The steady-state peak concentration should be calculated using Equation 8.21 for the short infusion model because $t_{in} > \frac{1}{6} \times t_{\frac{1}{2}}$

$$C_{ss2} = \frac{\dfrac{(S)(F)(Dose/t_{in})}{Cl} (1 - e^{-Kt_{in}})}{(1 - e^{-K\tau})} (e^{-Kt_2})$$

$$= \frac{\dfrac{(1)(1)(80 \text{ mg}/0.5 \text{ hr})}{2.2 \text{ L/hr}} (1 - e^{(0.26 \text{ hr}^{-1})(0.5 \text{ hr})})}{(1 - e^{-(0.26 \text{ hr}^{-1})(8 \text{ hr})})} (e^{-(0.26 \text{ hr}^{-1})(0.5 \text{ hr})})$$

$$= \frac{(72.7 \text{ mg/L})(0.12)}{(0.88)} (0.88)$$

$$= 8.7 \text{ mg/L}$$

M.R.'s total daily dose to reach the goal peak level was approximately 10 mg/kg/d, which is higher than 5 to 7 mg/kg/d typically used in adults. This is most likely due to increased V in children. If the adult V of 0.25 L/kg is used instead, the actual serum peak level measured may result in a lower value than the estimated peak, subjecting patients to the risk of subtherapeutic therapy.

Many studies support the once-daily aminoglycoside regimen in adults, and its use, although not as prevalent, is increasing in certain populations of children. The meta-analysis of once-daily regimen demonstrated a trend for better efficacy and similar low rates of nephrotoxicity and ototoxicity in children.[85] However, lack of consensus on appropriate dosing, target population, and therapeutic drug monitoring is preventing universal acceptance of once-daily dosing.[86] The difficulty in formulating once-daily dose that can be applied to all pediatric patients lies in the interpatient variability in pharmacokinetic parameters, underlying disease states, and indications for therapy. For this reason, different dosing regimens available in the literature for a specific patient population must be reviewed before applying to the general population.

Many institutions initiate pediatric patients on 7 mg/kg/d regimen for gentamicin/tobramycin and 15 to 20 mg/kg/d for amikacin.[87] However, in children less than 8 years, 7 mg/kg/d dose has shown to be inadequate to produce target peak levels of 20 to 30 mg/L.[88] In some patient populations with altered kinetics, such as critically ill patients with burn injuries or cancer, common doses used for once-daily regimen often result in less than desired C_{max} and prolonged drug-free interval. A better approach for once-daily dosing in children with cancer may be to utilize age-based dosing, followed by levels to determine patient-specific parameters.[39,89,90] The advantage of age-based dosing is that the differences in pharmacokinetics from cancer as well as from the different age groups are accounted for in the regimen. Age-based dosing recommends higher doses for younger children (10 mg/kg/d in children between 6 months and 9 years of age) and gradually lowering doses in older age groups (8 mg/kg/d in children between 9 and 12 years of age, 6 mg/kg/d in children 12 years of age).[39] Patients with burn exhibit significantly shorter $t_{1/2}$. Higher Cl and V also result from increased blood flow to the kidney and fluid resuscitation after the burn injury. Owing to these alterations, once-daily dosing is not recommended in burn patient population. Rather, increased amikacin doses of 12.5 to 20 mg/kg every 6 to 12 hours have been recommended.[91]

There is no set guideline for checking serum levels with extended-interval dosing in pediatrics. Serum level monitoring is recommended at 2 hours and 8 to 12 hours after the infusion in adult patients, but it may be prudent to check the random level earlier in children because of the larger degree of interpatient variability in aminoglycoside disposition. It is suggested to obtain an initial level at 2 hours and a second one at 6 to 8 hours later in children.[39,89] The random level, 6 to 8 hours after the start of infusion, is particularly important to ensure that the drug-free interval does not exceed 4 to 16 hours. The extended drug-free interval can be a challenge in immunocompromised patients but can be overcome with dual bacterial coverage with additional antibiotics.

In neonates, checking a 22-hour postdose level has been suggested for extended-interval dosing of 5 mg/kg to establish an appropriate interval of every 24, 36, or 48 hours.[92] A 22-hour level was chosen to confirm the appropriateness of every 24-hour dosing interval before the next dose is given. Based on the 22-hour postdose concentration, the dosing intervals can be adjusted to keep the trough level of less than 1 mg/L. A meta-analysis of aminoglycoside extended-interval dosing in neonates reported that 8% of the peak concentrations and 6% of the trough concentrations result outside the therapeutic range.[93] Body weight of neonates changes every day, and the initial aminoglycoside dose may no longer be sufficient to reach the goal C_{max} level after several days of therapy. Therefore, serum drug concentrations should be checked regularly during prolonged aminoglycoside therapy in neonatal patients with rapidly changing body weight and renal function.

When initiating extended-interval dosing in children, dosing with serum level monitoring or computer programs, such as Bayesian analysis, should be considered over nomograms because of large interpatient variability in certain disease states.[89,94]

Question #17 *J.H. is a 22-year-old female (height, 5 feet 3 inches; weight, 48 kg) with cystic fibrosis who is admitted for the treatment of an acute pulmonary exacerbation. Her serum creatinine is 0.7 mg/dL. Calculate a tobramycin regimen that will result in a peak level of 20 to 30 mg/L 0.5 hour after 0.5-hour infusion and AUC_{24} 70 to 100 mg·hr/L.*

The pharmacokinetics of a number of compounds, including aminoglycoside antibiotics, is altered in patients with cystic fibrosis. In particular, the volume of distribution appears to be larger (0.3-0.35 L/kg), and the clearance is faster than age-matched control subjects.[73] One potential explanation for the apparent difference in pharmacokinetic parameters is altered body composition. Patients with cystic fibrosis often exhibit reduced adipose mass because of malnutrition secondary to pancreatic insufficiency. When the pharmacokinetic parameters are normalized by lean body mass, the parameters are not significantly different from that of age-matched controls.[95] J.H.'s V and Cl can be calculated using a V of 0.3 L/kg, and creatinine clearance can be calculated using Equation 8.7.

$$V = (0.3 \text{ L/kg}) (48 \text{ kg})$$

$$= 14.4 \text{ L}$$

$$\text{Cl}_{cr} \text{ for females (mL/min)} = \frac{(140 - \text{Age})(\text{Weight in kg})}{(72)(\text{SCr})} (0.85)$$

$$= \frac{(140 - 22 \text{ yr})(48 \text{ kg})}{(72)(0.7 \text{ mg/dL})} (0.85)$$

$$= 95.5 \text{ mL/min}$$

$$= 95.5 \text{ mL/min} \times \frac{60 \text{ min/hr}}{1,000 \text{ mL/L}}$$

$$= 5.7 \text{ L/hr}$$

Using the estimated creatinine clearance of 5.7 L/hr as the tobramycin clearance and the volume of distribution of 14.4 L, the elimination rate constant

(Equation 8.15) and half-life (Equation 8.10) are calculated to be 0.4 hr^{-1} and 1.7 hour, respectively:

$$K = \frac{Cl}{V}$$
$$= \frac{5.7 \text{ L/hr}}{14.4 \text{ L}}$$
$$= 0.4 \text{ hr}^{-1}$$

$$t_{\frac{1}{2}} = \frac{0.693}{K}$$
$$= \frac{0.693}{0.4 \text{ hr}^{-1}}$$
$$= 1.7 \text{ hr}$$

Traditional multiple-daily dose of tobramycin will be inadequate to reach a peak concentration of 20 to 30 mg/L, and the extended-interval dosing with 24-hour interval should be utilized. Equation 8.27 can be rearranged to calculate a dose of 480 mg every 24 hours to result in AUC$_{24}$ of 85 mg·hr/L (a range between 70 and 100 mg·hr/L)

$$AUC_{24} = \frac{(\text{Dose in mg})(24 \text{ hr}) / \tau \text{ in hr}}{Cl \text{ in L/hr}}$$

$$\text{Dose in mg} = \frac{AUC_{24}(Cl \text{ in L/hr})(\tau \text{ in hr})}{(24 \text{ hr})} \qquad \text{(Eq. 8.36)}$$

$$= \frac{(85 \text{ mg} \cdot \text{hr/L})(5.7 \text{ L/hr})(24 \text{ hr})}{24 \text{ hr}}$$
$$= 484.5 \text{ mg} \approx 480 \text{ mg}$$

The steady-state peak and trough concentrations can be calculated using the *short infusion model (Equation 8.22)*:

$$C_{ss2} = \frac{\dfrac{(S)(F)(\text{Dose}/t_{in})}{Cl}(1 - e^{-Kt_{in}})}{1 - e^{-K\tau}} (e^{-Kt_2})$$

$$= \frac{(1)(1)\left(\dfrac{480 \text{ mg}}{0.5 \text{ hr}}\right)}{5.7 \text{ L/hr}} \frac{(1 - e^{-(0.4\text{hr}^{-1})(0.5\text{hr})})}{(1 - e^{-(0.4\text{hr}^{-1})(24\text{hr})})} (e^{-(0.4\text{hr}^{-1})(0.5\text{hr})})$$

$$= \frac{(168 \text{ mg/L})(0.18)}{0.99} (0.82)$$

$$= 25 \text{ mg/L}$$

The trough concentration could be calculated using the short infusion model as shown earlier or by decaying down the peak concentration using Equation 8.11, where t is the time between the two drug levels.

$$C = C_0 e^{-Kt}$$
$$= (25 \text{ mg/L})(e^{-(0.4 \text{ hr}^{-1})(23 \text{ hr})})$$
$$= 25 \text{ mg/L } (0.0001)$$
$$= 0.0025 \text{ mg/L}$$

Although the dose of tobramycin appears quite high (10 mg/kg/d), the relatively rapid clearance (when expressed per TBW) results in predicted serum concentrations that are not different than the target concentrations in other patients. In the past, the use of "once-daily" aminoglycoside regimen was not as widespread in patients with cystic fibrosis as in other patient populations. The relatively short elimination half-life raised concerns of bacterial resistance because of prolonged drug-free interval exceeding the duration of postantibiotic effect. Recent systemic reviews demonstrated that there were no differences in efficacy between multiple-daily dosing and once-daily dosing of tobramycin. No greater risk of toxicity was noted with once-daily dosing.[96] The Cystic Fibrosis Pulmonary Guideline recommends once-daily dosing of aminoglycosides over multiple-daily dosing for the treatment of acute pulmonary exacerbations.[97] The recommended dose is 10 mg/kg/d because doses exceeding that have resulted in C_{max} greater than 30 mg/L and AUC greater than 100 mg·hr/L, even in patients with cystic fibrosis with larger V and Cl.[98] For patients with cystic fibrosis, two aminoglycoside concentrations should be checked for dosage adjustment: one level 2 hours after dosing and the other 8 to 12 hours after dosing.

Question #18   *O.L., a 52-year-old man in the critical care unit with multiple organ failure, is receiving CRRT with a total output of 2 L/hr (ultrafiltration and dialysis flow rate of 1 L/hr each). His current weight is 65 kg (up from 60 kg 2 days ago), and his serum creatinine is 2.8 mg/dL. After pending cultures, he is to be started on tobramycin. Calculate a dose that will result in a peak concentration of 7 mg/L, 0.5 hour after 0.5-hour infusion, and a trough concentration of 1 mg/L 0.5 before the next dose.*

Because the patient has end-stage renal failure and is receiving CRRT, the Cockcroft and Gault equation is not a valid way to estimate renal function. Our best guess would be to use the average aminoglycoside clearance of 0.0043 L/hr/kg for functionally anephric patients. Excluding what appears to be 5 kg of excess third-space weight, the weight of 60 kg would result in a Cl_{pat} of 0.258 L/hr (0.0043 L/hr × 60 kg). Assuming that the aminoglycoside plasma binding is negligible, fu (unbound fraction) would be approximately 1 and our maximum expected Cl_{CRRT} would be 2 L/hr.

$$Cl_{CRRT} \text{ maximum} = (fu)(CRRT \text{ flow rate}) \qquad \text{(Eq. 8.37)}$$
$$= (1)(2 \text{ L/hr})$$
$$= 2 \text{ L/hr}$$

Although the initial estimate of 2 L/hr is a reasonable first approach, the literature would suggest that the actual Cl_{CRRT} is approximately 0.8 of the CRRT flow rate.[99-101] Using 0.8 as the fraction of the CRRT flow that is actually cleared, we would have a Cl_{CRRT} of 1.6 L/hr (0.8 × 2 L/hr). Now combining Cl_{CRRT} and Cl_{pat}, we estimate a total Cl of 1.86 L/hr (1.6 L/hr + 0.258 L/hr ≈ 1.86 L/hr) while the patient is receiving CRRT.

The volume of distribution would be calculated using Equation 8.4, where 60 kg represents the "Nonobese, Non–Excess Fluid Weight," 0 the "Excess Adipose Weight," and 5 kg the "Excess Third-Space Fluid Weight."

Aminoglycoside V (L) =

$$0.25\ \text{L/kg} \begin{pmatrix} \text{Nonobese,} \\ \text{Non–excess} \\ \text{fluid weight (kg)} \end{pmatrix} + 0.1 \begin{pmatrix} \text{Excess} \\ \text{adipose} \\ \text{weight (kg)} \end{pmatrix} + \begin{pmatrix} \text{Excess} \\ \text{third space} \\ \text{fluid} \\ \text{weight (kg)} \end{pmatrix}$$

$$= (0.25\ \text{L/kg} \times 60\ \text{kg}) + 0.1(0) + 1(5\ \text{kg})$$

$$= 15\ \text{L} + 0\ \text{L} + 5\ \text{L}$$

$$= 20\ \text{L}$$

Using Equations 8.15 and 8.10, we calculate a K value in hr^{-1} and a $t_{1/2}$ in hour.

$$K = \frac{Cl}{V}$$

$$= \frac{1.86\ \text{L/hr}}{20\ \text{L}}$$

$$= 0.093\ \text{hr}^{-1}$$

$$t_{1/2} = \frac{0.693}{K}$$

$$= \frac{0.693}{0.093\ \text{hr}^{-1}}$$

$$= 7.45\ \text{hr}$$

The dosing interval can be calculated using Equation 8.28 to determine the time a peak level of 7 mg/L will take to reach a trough of 1 mg/L.

$$t = \frac{\ln\left(\dfrac{C}{C_0}\right)}{-K}$$

$$t = \frac{\ln\left(\dfrac{1}{7}\right)}{-0.093}$$

$$t = 20.9\ \text{hr}$$

Given the desire to maintain dosing intervals that are easy to calculate and adhere to, an initial dosing interval of 24 hours would seem most appropriate.

Using Equation 8.26 with 7 mg/L for C_{ss1}, 20 L and 0.093 hr^{-1} for V and K, respectively, and 24 hours for τ, tobramycin dose of 140 mg can be calculated.

$$\text{Dose} = \frac{(C_{ss1})(V)(1 - e^{-K\tau})}{(S)(F)(e^{-Kt_1})}$$

$$= \frac{(7 \text{ mg/L})(20 \text{ L})(1 - e^{-(0.093\,\text{hr}^{-1})(24\,\text{hr})})}{(1)(1)(e^{-(0.093\,\text{hr}^{-1})(1\,\text{hr})})}$$

$$= \frac{(140 \text{ mg})(0.89)}{(1)(1)(0.91)}$$

$$= 137 \text{ mg} \approx 140 \text{ mg}$$

The trough concentration for the tobramycin 140 mg given IV over 0.5 hours every 24 hours can be determined using Equation 8.11

$$C = C_0 e^{-Kt}$$

where C_0 would be the steady-state peak concentration of 7 mg/L. Because the steady-state peak concentration of 7 mg/L is measured 1 hour after the start of the infusion, and the trough concentration is measured 0.5 before the next dose, t is 22.5 hours.

$$C = C_0 e^{-Kt}$$

$$= 7 \text{ mg/L} \times e^{-0.093\,\text{hr}^{-1} \times 22.5\,\text{hr}}$$

$$= 7 \text{ mg/L} \times 0.12$$

$$= 0.84 \text{ mg/L}$$

Question #19 *Using the calculated pharmacokinetic parameters, calculate extended-interval dosing regimen that will result in a peak concentration of 20 mg/L and AUC$_{24}$ 70 to 100 mg·hr/L.*

With high-dose extended-interval dosing, the dosing interval is approximately five half-lives to achieve a short drug-free interval, which is thought to reduce accumulation within the renal cortex and inner ear. Therefore, the dosing interval should be every 48 hours (5×7.45 hours $= 37.3$ hours).

Once again, the tobramycin dose can be calculated using Equation 8.26. This time, C_{ss1} is the new target peak concentration of 20 mg/L and τ is 48 hours.

$$\text{Dose} = \frac{(C_{ss1})(V)(1 - e^{-K\tau})}{(S)(F)(e^{-Kt_1})}$$

$$= \frac{(20 \text{ mg/L})(20 \text{ L})(1 - e^{-(0.093)(48\,\text{hr})})}{(1)(1)(e^{-(0.093)(1\,\text{hr})})}$$

$$= \frac{(400 \text{ mg})(0.99)}{(1)(1)(0.911)}$$

$$= 434 \text{ mg} \approx 440 \text{ mg}$$

AUC_{24} should be calculated to determine the risk for toxicity using Equation 8.27.

$$AUC_{24} = \frac{(\text{Dose in mg}) (24 \text{ hr}) / \tau \text{ in hr}}{Cl \text{ in L/hr}}$$

where a Cl of 1.86 L/hr can be calculated from Equation 8.25.

$$AUC_{24} = \frac{(440 \text{ mg})(24 \text{ hr})/48 \text{ hr}}{1.86 \text{ L/hr}}$$

$$= \frac{220 \text{ mg}}{1.86 \text{ L/hr}}$$

$$= 118 \text{ mg} \cdot \text{hr/L}$$

This value of AUC_{24} exceeds the target range of 70 to 100 mg·hr/L; therefore, the dose would need to be reduced. Considering the severity of O.L.'s infection, AUC_{24} of 85 to 100 mg·hr/L is a reasonable target to maximize the peak concentration. Equation 8.37 is a simple ratio of the AUCs that can be used to calculate the new dose.

$$\frac{AUC_{24} \text{ New}}{AUC_{24} \text{ Old}} (\text{Dose old}) = \text{New dose} \tag{Eq. 8.38}$$

$$\frac{85 \text{ mg} \cdot \text{hr/L}}{118 \text{ mg} \cdot \text{hr/L}} (440 \text{ mg}) = 316 \text{ mg} \approx 320 \text{ mg}$$

or

$$\frac{100 \text{ mg} \cdot \text{hr/L}}{118 \text{ mg} \cdot \text{hr/L}} (440 \text{ mg}) = 372 \text{ mg} \approx 380 \text{ mg}$$

The new doses with AUC_{24} of 85 and 100 mg·hr/L are 320 and 380 mg every 48 hours. Because the dose is significantly different from the dose calculated earlier, peak concentration based on these new doses should be confirmed using Equation 8.18.

$$C_{ss1} = \frac{\dfrac{(S)(F)(\text{Dose})}{V}}{(1 - e^{-K\tau})} (e^{-Kt_1})$$

$$= \frac{(1)(1)(320 \text{ mg})/20 \text{ L}}{1 - e^{-(0.093)(48hr)}} e^{-(0.093)(1hr)}$$

$$= \frac{16 \text{ mg/L}}{0.99} (0.91)$$

$$= 14.7 \text{ mg/L}$$

Similarly, the peak concentration from a dose of 380 mg every 48 hours can be calculated to be 17.5 mg/L. Because the peak concentration is directly proportional to the dose (as long as the interval is not changed), the peak concentrations could have been estimated based on a ratio of the dose and peak concentration already calculated.

Therefore, a dose between 320 and 380 mg every 48 hours would provide a steady-state peak concentration of 14.7 to 17.5 mg/L and an AUC_{24} of 85 to 100 mg·hr/L.

As indicated in Dialysis of Drugs: Continuous Renal Replacement Therapy (CRRT) in Chapter " "Drug Dosing in Kidney Disease and Dialysis," patients who are receiving CRRT are critically ill, and the CRRT procedure is often interrupted or the CRRT flow rate changed depending on the condition of the patient. For these reasons, the patient should be monitored frequently (minimally each day) to ensure that CRRT is progressing as initially planned.

REFERENCES

1. Pechere JC, Dugal R. Clinical pharmacokinetics of aminoglycoside antibiotics. *Clin Pharmacokinet.* 1979;4:170-199.

2. Craig W, Ebert SC. Killing and regrowth of bacteria in vitro: a review. *Scand J Infect Dis Suppl.* 1991;74:63-71.

3. Kapusnik JE, Hackbarth CJ, Chambers HF, Carpenter T, Sande MA. Single, large, daily dosing versus intermittent dosing of tobramycin for treating experimental pseudomonas pneumonia. *J Infect Dis.* 1988;158:7-22.

4. Leggett JE, Fantin B, Ebert S, et al. Comparative antibiotic dose–effect relations at several dosing intervals in murine pneumonitis and thigh-infection models. *J Infect Dis.* 1989;159:281-292.

5. Moore RD, Lietman PS, Smith CR. Clinical response to aminoglycoside therapy: importance of the ratio of peak concentration to minimal inhibitory concentration. *J Infect Dis.* 1987;155:93-99.

6. Craig WA, Vogelman B. The postantibiotic effect. *Ann Intern Med.* 1987;106:900-902.

7. Craig WA, Redington J, Ebert SC. Pharmacodynamics of amikacin in vitro and in mouse thigh and lung infections. *J Antimicrob Chemother.* 1991;27(suppl C):29-40.

8. Powell SH, Thompson WL, Luthe MA, et al. Once-daily vs. continuous aminoglycoside dosing: efficacy and toxicity in animal and clinical studies of gentamicin, netilmicin, and tobramycin. *J Infect Dis.* 1983;147(5):918-932.

9. Verpooten GA, Giuliano RA, Verbist L, Eestermans G, De Broe ME. Once-daily dosing decreases renal accumulation of gentamicin and netilmicin. *Clin Pharmacol Ther.* 1989;45:22-27.

10. Rybak MJ, Abate BJ, Kang SL, Ruffing MJ, Lerner SA, Drusano GL. Prospective evaluation of the effect of an aminoglycoside dosing regimen on rates of observed nephrotoxicity and ototoxicity. *Antimicrob Agents Chemother.* 1999;43:1549-1555.

11. Barza M, Ioannidis JP, Cappelleri JC, Lau J. Single or multiple daily doses of aminoglycosides: a meta-analysis. *BMJ.* 1996;312:338-345.

12. Hatala R, Dinh T, Cook DJ. Once-daily aminoglycoside dosing in immunocompetent adults: a meta-analysis. *Ann Intern Med.* 1996;124:717-725.

13. Nicolau DP, Freeman CD, Belliveau PP, Nightingale CH, Ross JW, Quintiliani R. Experience with a once-daily aminoglycoside program administered to 2,184 adult patients. *Antimicrob Agents Chemother.* 1995;39:650-655.

14. Noone P, Parsons TM, Pattison JR, Slack RC, Garfield-Davies D, Hughes K. Experience in monitoring gentamicin therapy during treatment of serious gram-negative sepsis. *Br Med J.* 1979;1:477-481.

15. McCormack JP, Jewesson PJ. A critical reevaluation of the "therapeutic range" of aminoglycosides. *Clin Infect Dis.* 1992;14:320-339.

16. Klastersky J, Daneau D, Swings G, Weerts D. Antibacterial activity in serum and urine as a therapeutic guide in bacterial infections. *J Infect Dis.* 1974;129:187-193.

17. Cox CE. Gentamicin: a new aminoglycoside antibiotic: clinical and laboratory studies in urinary tract infections. *J Infect Dis.* 1969;119:486-491.

18. Jackson GG, Arcieri G. Ototoxicity of gentamicin in man: a survey and controlled analysis of clinical experience in the United States. *J Infect Dis.* 1971;124(suppl):S130-S137.

19. Goodman EL, Van Gelber J, Holmes R, Hull AR, Sanford JP. Prospective comparative study of variable dosage and variable frequency regimens for administrations of gentamicin. *Antimicrob Agents Chemother.* 1975;8:434-438.

20. Schentag JJ, Cerra, FB, Plaut ME. Clinical and pharmacokinetic characteristics of aminoglycoside nephrotoxicity in 201 critically ill patients. *Antimicrob Agents Chemother.* 1982;21(5):721-726.

21. Wilfret JN, Burke JP, Bloomer HA, Smith CB. Renal insufficiency associated with gentamicin therapy. *J Infect Dis.* 1971;124(suppl):S148-S155.

22. Mawer GE, Ahmad R, Dobbs SM, McGough JG, Lucas SB, Tooth JA. Prescribing aids for gentamicin. *Br J Clin Pharmacol.* 1974;1:45-50.

23. Federspil P, Schätzle W, Tiesler E. Pharmacokinetics and ototoxicity of gentamicin, tobramycin, and amikacin. *J Infect Dis.* 1976;134(suppl):S200-S205.

24. Barclay ML, Duffull SB, Begg EJ, Buttimore RC. Experience of once-daily aminoglycoside dosing using a target area under the concentration-time curve. *Aust N Z J Med.* 1995;25:230-235.

25. Gyselynck AM, Forrey A, Cutler R. Pharmacokinetics of gentamicin: distribution and plasma and renal clearance. *J Infect Dis.* 1971;124(suppl):S70-S76.

26. Christopher TG, Korn D, Blair AD, Forrey AW, O'Neill MA, Cutler RE. Gentamicin pharmacokinetics during hemodialysis. *Kidney Int.* 1974;6:38-44.

27. Danish M, Schultz R, Jukso WJ. Pharmacokinetics of gentamicin and kanamycin during hemodialysis. *Antimicrob Agents Chemother.* 1974;6:841-847.

28. Barza M, Brown RB, Shen D, Gibaldi M, Weinstein L. Predictability of blood levels of gentamicin in man. *J Infect Dis.* 1975;132:165-174.

29. Sawchuk RJ, Zaske DE. Pharmacokinetics of dosing regimens which utilize multiple intravenous infusions: gentamicin in burn patients. *J Pharmacokinet Biopharm.* 1976;4:183-195.

30. Regamey C, Gordon RC, Kirby WM. Comparative pharmacokinetics of tobramycin and gentamicin. *Clin Pharmacol Ther.* 1973;14:396-403.

31. Siber GR, Echeverria P, Smith AL, Paisley JW, Smith DH. Pharmacokinetics of gentamicin in children and adults. *J Infect Dis.* 1975;132:637-651.

32. Hull J, Sarubbi FA. Gentamicin serum concentrations: pharmacokinetic predictions. *Ann Intern Med.* 1976;85:183-189.

33. Blouin RA, Mann HJ, Griffen WO Jr, Bauer LA, Record KE. Tobramycin pharmacokinetics in morbidly obese patients. *Clin Pharmacol Ther.* 1979;26:508-512.

34. Bauer LA, Blouin RA, Griffen WO Jr, Record KE, Bell RM. Amikacin pharmacokinetics in morbidly obese patients. *Am J Hosp Pharm.* 1980;37:519-522.

35. Sampliner R, Perrier D, Powell R, Finley P. Influence of ascites on tobramycin pharmacokinetics. *J Clin Pharmacol.* 1984;24:43-46.

36. Hodgman T, Dasta JF, Armstrong DK, Crist KD, Ellison C. Tobramycin disposition into ascitic fluid. *Clin Pharm.* 1984;3:203-205.

37. Kearns GL, Abdel-Rahman SM, Alander SW, Blowey DL, Leeder JS, Kauffman RE. Developmental pharmacology—drug disposition, action ad therapy in infants and children. *N Engl J Med.* 2003;349:1157-1176.

38. Esheverria P, Siber GR, Paisley J, et al. Age-dependent dose response to gentamicin. *Pediatrics.* 1975;87:805-808.

39. Dupuis LL, Sung L, Taylor T, et al. Tobramycin pharmacokinetics in children with febrile neutropenia undergoing stem cell transplantation: once-daily versus thrice-daily administration. *Pharmacotherapy.* 2004;24:564-573.

40. Shevchuk YM, Taylor DM. Aminoglycoside volume of distribution in pediatric patients. *DICP.* 1990;24:273-276.

41. Schentag JJ, Jusko WJ, Plaut ME, Cumbo TJ, Vance JW, Abrutyn E. Tissue persistence of gentamicin in man. *JAMA.* 1977;238:327-329.

42. Schentag JJ, Jusko WJ. Renal clearance and tissue accumulation of gentamicin. *Clin Pharmacol Ther.* 1977;22:364-370.

43. Mendelson J, Portnoy J, Dick V, Black M. Safety of bolus administration of gentamicin. *Antimicrob Agents Chemother.* 1976;9:633-638.

44. Lynn KL, Neale TJ, Little PJ, Bailey RR. Gentamicin by intravenous bolus injections. *N Z Med J.* 1977;80:442-443.

45. Demczar DJ, Nafziger AN, Bertino JS Jr. Pharmacokinetics of gentamicin at traditional versus higher doses: implications for once-daily aminoglycoside dosing. *Antimicrob Agents Chemother.* 1997;41:1115-1119.

46. Colburn WA, Schentag JJ, Jusko WJ, Gibaldi M. A model for the prospective identification of the pre-nephrotoxic state during gentamicin therapy. *J Pharmacokinet Biopharm.* 1978;6:179-186.

47. Evans WE, Taylor RH, Feldman S, Crom WR, Rivera G, Yee GC. A model for dosing gentamicin in children and adolescents that adjust for tissue accumulation with continuous dosing. *Clin Pharmacokinet.* 1980;5:295-306.

48. Pai MP. Estimating the glomerular filtration rate in obese adult patients for drug dosing. *Adv Chronic Kidney Dis.* 2010;17:e53-e62.

49. Dionne RE, Bauer LA, Gibson GA, Griffen WO Jr, Blouin RA. Estimating creatinine clearance in morbidly obese patients. *Am J Hosp Pharm.* 1981;38:841-844.

50. Bauer LA, Edwards WA, Dellinger EP, Simonowitz DA. Influence of weight on aminoglycoside pharmacokinetics in normal weight and morbidly obese patients. *Eur J Clin Pharmacol.* 1983;24:643-647.

51. Aronson JK. Drug therapy in kidney disease. *Br J Clin Pharmacol.* 2007;63:504-511.

52. Halacova M, Kotaska K, Kukacka J, et al. Serum cystatin c level for better assessment of glomerular filtration rate in cystic fibrosis patients treated by amikacin. *J Clin Pharm Ther.* 2008;33:409-417.

53. Šálek T, Vodička M, Gabrhelík T. Estimated glomerular filtration rate in patients overdosed with gentamicin. *J Lab Med.* 2020;44:35-39.

54. Bartelink IH, Rademaker CM, Schobben AF, van den Anker JN. Guidelines on paediatric dosing on the basis of developmental physiology and pharmacokinetic considerations. *Clin Pharamcokinet.* 2006;45:1077-1097.

55. De Cock RF, Allegaert K, Schreuder MF, et al. Maturation of the glomerular filtration rate in neonates, as reflected by amikacin clearance. *Clin Pharmacokinet.* 2012;51:105-117.

56. De Cock RF, Allegaert K, Brussee JM, et al. Simultaneous pharmacokinetic modeling of gentamicin, tobramycin and vancomycin clearance from neonates to adults: towards a semi-physiological function for maturation in glomerular filtration. *Pharm Res.* 2014;31:2643-2654.

57. Schwartz GJ, Muñoz A, Schneider MF, et al. New equations to estimate GFR in children with CKD. *J Am Soc Nephrol.* 2009;20:629-637.

58. Gao A, Cachat F, Faouzi M, et al. Comparison of the glomerular filtration rate in children by the new revised Schwartz formula and a new generalized formula. *Kidney Int.* 2013;83:524-530.

59. Holt HA, Broughall JM, McCarthy M, Reeves DS. Interactions between aminoglycoside antibiotics and carbenicillin or ticarcillin. *Infection.* 1976;4:107-109.

60. Ervin FR, Bullock WE Jr, Nuttall CE. Inactivation of gentamicin by penicillins in patients with renal failure. *Antimicrob Agents Chemother.* 1976;9:1004-1011.

61. Weibert RT, Keane WF. Carbenicillin-gentamicin interaction in acute renal failure. *Am J Hosp Pharm.* 1977;34:1137-1139.

62. Tindula RJ, Ambrose PJ, Harralson AF. Aminoglycoside inactivation by penicillins and cephalosporins and its impact on drug-level monitoring. *Drug Intell Clin Pharm.* 1983;17:906-908.

63. Lau A, Lee M, Flascha S, Prasad R, Sharifi R. Effect of piperacillin on tobramycin pharmacokinetics in patients with normal renal function. *Antimicrob Agents Chemother.* 1983;24:533-537.

64. Riff LJ, Jackson GG. Laboratory and clinical conditions for gentamicin inactivation by carbenicillin. *Arch Intern Med.* 1972;130:887-891.

65. Riff LJ, Thomason JL. Comparative aminoglycoside inactivation by beta-lactam antibiotics. Effects of a cephalosporin and six penicillins on five aminoglycosides. *J Antibiot (Tokyo).* 1982;35:850-857.

66. Konishi H, Goto M, Nakamoto Y, Yamamoto I, Yamashina H. Tobramycin inactivation by carbenicillin, ticarcillin, and piperacillin. *Antimicrob Agents Chemother.* 1983;23:653-657.

67. Pickering LK, Gerahart P. Effect of time and concentration upon interaction between gentamicin, tobramycin, netilmicin, or amikacin, and carbenicillin or ticarcillin. *Antimicrob Agents Chemother*. 1979;15:592-596.

68. Glew RH, Pavuk RA. Stability of gentamicin, tobramycin, and amikacin in combination with four beta-lactam antibiotics. *Antimicrob Agents Chemother*. 1983;24:474-477.

69. Earp CM, Barriere SL. The lack of inactivation of tobramycin by cefazolin, cefamandole, moxalactam in vitro. *Drug Intell Clin Pharm*. 1985;19:677-679.

70. Fischer JH, Hedrick PJ, Riff LJ. Pharmacokinetics and antibacterial activity of two gentamicin products given intramuscularly. *Clin Pharm*. 1984;3:411-416.

71. Blieler RE, Schedl HP. Creatinine excretion: variability and relationships to diet and body size. *J Lab Clin Med*. 1962;59:945-955.

72. Reiner N, Bloxham DD, Thompson WL. Nephrotoxicity of gentamicin and tobramycin given once daily or continuously in dogs. *Antimicrob Agents Chemother*. 1978;4(suppl A):85-101.

73. Dager WE, King JH. Aminoglycosides in intermittent hemodialysis: pharmacokinetics with individual dosing. *Ann Pharmacother*. 2006;40:9-14.

74. Heintz BH, Thompson GR III, Dager WE. Clinical experience with aminoglycosides in dialysis-dependent patients: risk factors for mortality and reassessment of current dosing practices. *Ann Pharmacother*. 2011;45:1338-1345.

75. Sowinski K, Magner SJ, Lucksiri A, Scott MK, Hamburger RJ, Mueller BA. Influence of hemodialysis on gentamicin pharmacokinetics, removal during hemodialysis, and recommended dosing. *Clin J Am Soc Nephrol*. 2008;3(2):355-361.

76. Amin NB, Padhi ID, Touchette MA, Patel RV, Dunfee TP, Anandan JV. Characterization of gentamicin pharmacokinetics in patients hemodialyzed with high-flux polysulphone membranes. *Am J Kidney Dis*. 1999;34:222-227.

77. Reguer L, Colding H, Jensen H, Kampmann JP. Pharmacokinetics of amikacin during hemodialysis and peritoneal dialysis. *Antimicrob Agents Chemother*. 1977;11:214-218.

78. Gailiunas P Jr, Dominguez-Morenzo M, Lazarus M, Lowrie EG, Gottlieb MN, Merrill JP. Vestibular toxicity of gentamicin: incidence in patients receiving long-term hemodialysis therapy. *Arch Intern Med*. 1978;138:1621-1624.

79. Halstenson CE, Berkseth RO, Mann HJ, Matzke GR. Aminoglycoside redistribution phenomenon after hemodialysis; netilmicin and tobramycin. *Int J Clin Pharmacol Ther Toxicol*. 1987;25:50-55.

80. Bauer LA. Rebound gentamicin levels after hemodialysis. *Ther Drug Monit*. 1982;4:99-101.

81. Gary NE. Peritoneal clearance and removal of gentamicin. *J Infect Dis*. 1971;124(suppl):S96-S97.

82. Lamiere N, Bogaert M, Belpaire F. Peritoneal pharmacokinetics and pharmacological manipulation of peritoneal transport. In: Gokal R, ed. *Continuous Ambulatory Peritoneal Dialysis*. Churchill Livingstone; 1986:56-93.

83. O'Brien MA, Mason NA. Systemic absorption of intraperitoneal antimicrobials in continuous ambulatory peritoneal dialysis. *Clin Pharm*. 1992;11:246-254.

84. Horton MW, Deeter RG, Sherman RA. Treatment of peritonitis in patients undergoing continuous ambulatory peritoneal dialysis. *Clin Pharm*. 1990;9:102-118.

85. Contopoulos-Ioannidis DG, Giotis ND, Baliatsa DV, Ioannidis JP. Extended-interval aminoglycoside administration for children: a meta-analysis. *Pediatrics*. 2004;114:e111-e118.

86. Knoderer CA, Everett JA, Buss WF. Clinical issues surrounding once-daily aminoglycoside dosing in children. *Pharmacotherapy*. 2003;23:44-56.

87. Jenh AM, Tamma PD, Milstone AM. Extended-interval aminoglycoside dosing in pediatrics. *Pediatr Infect Dis J*. 2011;30:338-339.

88. McDade EJ, Wagner JL, Moffett BS, Palazzi DL. Once-daily gentamicin dosing in pediatric patients without cystic fibrosis. *Pharmacotherapy*. 2010;30:248-253.

89. Newby B, Prevost D, Lotocka-Reysner H. Assessment of gentamicin 7 mg/kg once daily for pediatric patients with febrile neutropenia: a pilot project. *J Oncol Pharm Pract*. 2009;15:211-216.

90. Ho KK, Bryson SM, Thiessen JJ, Greenberg ML, Einarson TR, Leson CL. The effects of age and chemotherapy on gentamicin pharmacokinetics and dosing in pediatric oncology patients. *Pharmacotherapy*. 1995;15:754-764.

91. Yu T, Stockmann C, Healy DP, et al. Determination of optimal amikacin dosing regimens for pediatric patients with burn wound sepsis. *J Burn Care Res*. 2015;36:e244-e252.

92. Dersch-Mills D, Akierman A, Alshaikh B, Sundaram A, Yusuf K. Performance of a dosage individualization table for extended interval gentamicin in neonates beyond the first week of life. *J Matern Fetal Neonatal Med*. 2016;29:1451-1456.

93. Nestaas E, Bangstad HJ, Sandvik L, Wathne K-O. Aminoglycoside extended interval dosing in neonates is safe and effective: a meta-analysis. *Arch Dis Child Fetal Neonatal Ed*. 2005;90:F294-F300.

94. Abusham AA, Mohammed AH, Alkindi SS, Hassan MM, Al-Zakwani IS. Sub-optimal serum gentamicin concentrations in sickle cell disease patients utilizing the Hartford protocol. *J Clin Pharm Ther*. 2012;37:212-216.

95. Hennig S, Norris R, Kirkpatrick CM. Target concentration intervention is needed for tobramycin dosing in paediatric patients with cystic fibrosis—a population pharmacokinetic study. *Br J Clin Pharmacol*. 2008;65:502-510.

96. Smyth AR, Bhatt J. Once-daily versus multiple-daily dosing with intravenous aminoglycosides for cystic fibrosis. *Cochrane Database Syst Rev* 2014;(2):CD002009. doi:10.1002/14651858.CD002009.pub5.

97. Flume PA, Mogayzel PJ Jr, Robinson KA, et al; Clinical Practice Guidelines for Pulmonary Therapies Committee. Cystic fibrosis pulmonary guidelines: treatment of pulmonary exacerbations. *Am J Respir Crit Care Med*. 2009;180:802-808.

98. Prescott WA Jr, Nagel JL. Extended-interval once-daily dosing of aminoglycosides in adult and pediatric patients with cystic fibrosis. *Pharmacotherapy*. 2010;30:95-108.

99. Bickley SK. Drug dosing during continuous arteriovenous hemofiltration. *Clin Pharm*. 1988;7:198-206.

100. Golper TA. Continuous arteriovenous hemofiltration in acute renal failure. *Am J Kidney Dis*. 1985;6:373-386.

101. Pea F, Viale P, Pavan F, Furlanut M. Pharmacokinetic considerations for antimicrobial therapy in patients receiving renal replacement therapy. *Clin Pharmacokinet*. 2007;46:997-1038.

9

ANTICOAGULANTS: HEPARIN, LOW-MOLECULAR-WEIGHT HEPARIN, AND WARFARIN

Paul Wong and Toby Trujillo

Learning Objectives

By the end of the unfractionated heparin, low-molecular-weight heparins, and warfarin chapter, the learner shall be able to:

1. Describe the pharmacokinetics and pharmacodynamics of unfractionated heparin (UFH) that contribute to interpatient variability in response.
2. Identify the relevant assays used to assess the efficacy and safety of UFH, low-molecular-weight heparins (LMWHs), and warfarin.
3. Devise strategies for dosing of UFH and LMWHs for patients at the extremes of weight.
4. Review the pharmacogenetic and environmental (dietary and medication) factors that alter the pharmacokinetic and pharmacodynamic profile of warfarin.
5. Develop plans for the reversal of the anticoagulant effects of UFH, LMWHs, and warfarin.

UNFRACTIONATED HEPARIN

Heparin is a naturally occurring glycosaminoglycan possessing anticoagulant activity, useful in the treatment of numerous thrombotic conditions, such as venous thromboembolic (VTE) disease and acute coronary syndrome (ACS).[1] Notably, heparin and its derivatives possess nonanticoagulant effects, including anti-inflammatory and antineoplastic activity, though their clinical relevance has not been established.[2,3] Heparin exerts its anticoagulant activity through the formation of a complex with antithrombin (AT). Creation of the heparin-AT complex converts AT from a slow to a rapid inhibitor of the clotting factors IIa (thrombin), Xa, IXa, XIa, and XIIa, though it is most active against thrombin.[1] Multiple preparations of heparin are available, with unfractionated heparin (UFH) and low-molecular-weight heparins (LMWHs) being most used in clinical practice.[4]

UFH is available as multiple dose vials, prefilled syringes, and premixed bags of varying concentrations. In commercial preparations, UFH is a heterogeneous mixture of heparin molecules varying in size from 3,000 to 30,000 Da with a mean of 15,000 Da.[1] As a result, the drug exhibits variability with respect to its anticoagulant activity and pharmacokinetic properties in the clinical setting.

Dosing of UFH varies based on indication and route of administration. For the treatment of VTE, the American College of Chest Physicians (ACCP) Antithrombotic Therapy and Prevention of Thrombosis guidelines recommend an initial dose of intravenous (IV) UFH that is either weight based (80 units/kg IV bolus, then 18 units/kg/hr IV infusion) or fixed (5,000 units IV bolus followed by an infusion of ≥32,000 units/d).[1] When given subcutaneously (SC), it is recommended to give an initial dose, either 5,000 units IV bolus or 333 units/kg SC, followed by 250 units/kg SC twice daily (BID). When administered for ACS, a typical dose is 60 units/kg IV bolus (max 4,000 units) followed by 12 units/kg/hr IV infusion (max 1,000 units/hr).[1] Recommendations from the joint American Heart Association (AHA) and American College of Cardiology (ACC) guidelines suggest loading doses ranging from 50 to 100 units/kg depending on the severity of ACS presentation and concurrent antithrombotic therapy.[5,6] Bolus doses are important to achieve rapid anticoagulation in active thrombosis.

Therapeutic Plasma Concentrations

Direct measurements of plasma heparin concentrations are difficult to standardize, cumbersome to perform, and subject to interference from other factors.[7] Thus, indirect methods of measurement are preferred in the clinical setting. There are two preferred methods for indirectly measuring heparin plasma concentrations: (1) measuring the amount of protamine needed to neutralize the anticoagulant effect of UFH and (2) measuring the inhibition of factor Xa by heparin. Therapeutic ranges vary based on the assay used. Plasma heparin concentrations of 0.2 to 0.4 units/mL by protamine titration[8] and 0.3 to 0.7 units/mL by anti-Xa inhibition[9] are considered therapeutic.

KEY PARAMETERS: Unfractionated Heparin

THERAPEUTIC PLASMA CONCENTRATIONS	ANTI-XA ASSAY: 0.3-0.7 UNITS/ML PROTAMINE TITRATION: 0.2-0.4 UNITS/ML
F (SC)	30%
V^a	~0.07 L/kg
Cl^b	0.25-2.63 mL/min/kg
$t_{1/2}{}^c$	0.5-2 hr

[a]Unfractionated heparin binds nonspecifically to numerous plasma proteins (eg, histidine-rich glycoproteins, von Willebrand factor, platelet factor 4), endothelial cells, and macrophages.
[b]Interpatient variability and testing modality used (aPTT or anti-Xa assay) contribute to wide range of reported clearance.
[c]Half-life elimination of unfractionated heparin is dose dependent.

Historically, measurement of heparin concentrations has been difficult in the clinical setting. As such, coagulation assays, such as the activated partial thromboplastin time (aPTT) or the activated clotting time (ACT), have been used to monitor heparin's anticoagulant effects, with aPTT being the most common.[7,10] A target aPTT range of 1.5 to 2.5 times the control value was established based on a single study demonstrating a reduction in recurrent VTE when UFH therapy was titrated to maintain this aPTT.[11] Although the ratio method was used to determine the goal therapeutic range for a number of years, more recently, it has fallen out of favor.[1] This is due to the aPTT being complicated by variability in results based on the instrument and thromboplastin reagent, with over 300 instrument-reagent combinations used clinically.[10] Studies evaluating aPTT values obtained using different reagents and instruments showed poor correlation to heparin concentration measured by factor Xa inhibition, leading to the potential for routine underdosing of UFH based on aPTT values.[12-15] Therefore, each laboratory should establish an institution-specific therapeutic aPTT range that corresponds to therapeutic heparin concentrations obtained using a validated anti-Xa (0.3-0.7 units/mL) or protamine neutralization (0.2-0.4 units/mL) assay.[1] The institution's laboratory should adjust the therapeutic aPTT range whenever instruments or reagents change. Though differences in aPTT values can be partly attributed to different instrument-reagent combinations, providers should also be aware that many patient-related factors may influence aPTT, independent of the effects of UFH.[16]

The use of heparin assays to monitor UFH therapy is becoming more common, though their use can be cost-prohibitive. While protamine titration assays are cumbersome, anti-Xa assays are practical for clinical use.[7] An increase in the use of the anti-Xa assays has been spurred by studies showing an improved ability to achieve therapeutic anticoagulation more rapidly with fewer dose adjustments and fewer monitoring tests needed to maintain therapeutic levels as compared to aPTT monitoring.[16-18] This practice is supported by evidence that monitoring with aPTT and anti-Xa levels had similar rates of bleeding and thrombosis.[19-22] However, it should be noted that anti-Xa assays are subject to many of the same interferences as aPTT values.

The heparin assays have been used to determine the pharmacokinetic parameters of heparin, but issues with the test accuracy and biologic variables influencing heparin make it difficult to truly describe the pharmacokinetics of heparin.[23,24]

Bioavailability (F)

As UFH is not absorbed enterally, the preferred routes of administration are IV and SC.[1] Administration of UFH SC may result in plasma concentrations as low as 30% of that seen with an equivalent IV dose, depending on the patient and the dose.[25,26] As such, caution is warranted in the treatment of thrombotic phenomenon with SC UFH. However, low-dose UFH (5,000 units SC BID) for prophylaxis of thromboembolism is an effective regimen.[27] Intramuscular injection of UFH is not recommended owing to the risk of hematoma formation.

Volume of Distribution (V)

The usual volume of distribution (V) of UFH is approximately 0.07 L/kg, approximating the plasma volume.[23] After administration, UFH binds to multiple plasma components, including histidine-rich glycoproteins, von Willebrand factor, and platelet factor 4 (PF4).[1,28-31] In addition, UFH is known to bind to endothelial cells and macrophages.[32,33] Further complicating the distribution is evidence of greater protein binding in patients with VTE.[34] The complex protein binding contributes, in part, to the variability seen in the anticoagulant effect of heparin.

Given that the apparent V_d of UFH approximates the plasma volume, weight-based dosing regimens are recommended for the treatment of thrombotic complications. The total body weight (TBW) is recommended for dose calculations, though there is controversy over the optimal dosing weight for patients with obesity. Patients with obesity have relatively higher total plasma volumes, but adipose tissue has less vasculature compared to lean tissue.[35,36] This suggests that TBW may be less reflective of the apparent V of UFH at the upper extremes of body weight. Several studies have shown that patients with obesity require relatively lower doses of UFH in units per kilogram to achieve therapeutic aPTT or anti-Xa values compared to patients without obesity.[37-39] Thus, the use of the adjusted body weight (AdjBW) has been suggested for patients with obesity.[40-42] However, the definition of obesity varied across the studies, making it difficult to identify the optimal patient for dosing using AdjBW. As such, the use of either TBW or AdjBW for dosing calculations of UFH is appropriate, and institution-specific approaches are warranted.[10]

$$AdjBW = Ideal\ body\ weight\ (IBW) + 0.4\,(TBW - IBW)$$

where

$$IBW\ (men) = 50\ kg + 2.3\,\frac{kg}{each\ inch\ over\ 5\ ft}$$

$$IBW\ (women) = 45.5\ kg + 2.3\,\frac{kg}{each\ inch\ over\ 5\ ft}$$

Clearance (Cl)

The reported clearance (Cl) of UFH ranges between 0.25 and 2.63 mL/min/kg, with variations attributed to testing used (aPTT or anti-Xa) and interpatient differences.[34,43-45] Clearance of UFH appears to be influenced by age, the presence of active thromboembolic disease, hepatic or renal impairment, and obesity.

The clearance of UFH involves both zero-order and first-order processes.[1] The zero-order phase is a rapid, but saturable process that involves binding to endothelial cell receptors and macrophages. The first-order phase is a slower, nonsaturable process that is largely renal in nature. At therapeutic doses, the clearance is primarily driven by the rapid, saturable processes with higher doses of UFH invoking the renal clearance. This contributes to the nonlinear dose-response curve seen with UFH, leading to disproportionate increases in the intensity and duration of anticoagulant effects at higher doses.

Half-Life ($t_{1/2}$)

As the clearance of UFH shows a dose-dependent relationship (Figure 9.1), the half-life of UFH is dose dependent as well, ranging from 0.5 to 2 hours.[1,23] After administration of IV boluses of 25, 100, and 400 units/kg, the half-lives were estimated to be 30, 60, and 150 minutes, respectively.[46-48] The relatively short half-life combined with the unpredictable dose-response curve support dosing UFH as a continuous infusion with frequent monitoring in most clinical situations.

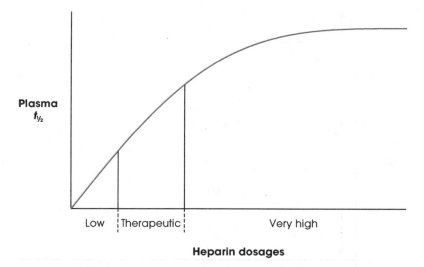

Plasma t½

Low ⋮Therapeutic⋮   Very high

Heparin dosages

FIGURE 9.1 Unfractionated heparin demonstrates dose-dependent half-life elimination. (From Garcia DA, Baglin TP, Weitz JI, Samama MM. Parenteral anticoagulants: antithrombotic therapy and prevention of thrombosis, 9th ed: American College of Chest Physicians Evidence-Based Clinical Practice Guidelines. *Chest*. 2012;141(suppl 2):e24S-e43S. doi:10.1378/chest.11-2291.)

Time to Sample

The aPTT and anti-Xa assays are most commonly used for monitoring the anticoagulant effects of UFH therapy.[1,7] Measurements of coagulation (eg, aPTT, prothrombin time [PT], and international normalized ratio [INR]) before administration of UFH are recommended to evaluate the coagulation status of the patient at baseline. When administered as a continuous IV infusion, plasma samples for coagulation tests should be obtained 4 to 8 hours after the start of the infusion or any change in the infusion rate, with sampling at 6 hours common in clinical practice. If an IV bolus dose is administered, plasma sampling after 6 to 8 hours is recommended as the bolus dose may influence the aPTT values for up to 8 hours.[49] Measurements of anticoagulant effects taken too early after a bolus dose may overestimate the degree of anticoagulation provided by the continuous infusion alone (Figure 9.2). If no IV bolus dose is administered, plasma sampling after 4 hours can be considered.

If an SC regimen is used, plasma samples should be obtained 6 hours after the dose. Once a therapeutic value has been obtained on either an IV or SC dosing regimen, plasma sampling may be spaced out to a longer duration, most typically once daily depending on the duration of therapy. When dose adjustments are made to UFH therapy, resampling after 4 to 8 hours is recommended.

Adverse Effects

Hemorrhagic complications are the main adverse effect associated with heparin therapy. Aside from bleeding, notable complications include heparin-induced thrombocytopenia (HIT) and osteoporosis.[1] HIT is an immunoglobulin G (IgG) antibody–mediated adverse drug reaction in which activated platelets target complexes of PF4 and heparin.[50] The resultant platelet aggregation can lead to thrombotic complications. Though the incidence of HIT is less than 5%, the clinical consequences are severe, and routine

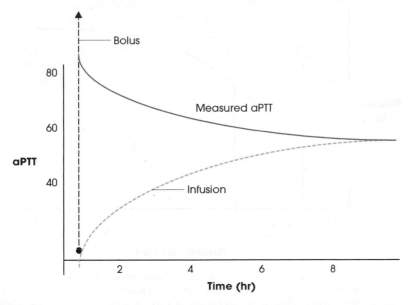

FIGURE 9.2 Timing of aPTT measurements are dependent on if a bolus dose of unfractionated heparin was used. Measurements taken too soon after a bolus dose may overestimate the degree of anticoagulation that will be achieved at steady state from the continuous infusion. aPTT, activated partial thromboplastin time. From Dager W, Gulseth M, Nutescu E, eds. *Anticoagulation Therapy: A Point-of-Care Guide.* American Society of Health-System Pharmacists; 2011.

monitoring of platelets is recommended to detect for thrombocytopenia. Osteoporosis is a long-term adverse effect of heparin therapy that results from heparin binding to osteoblasts and subsequent activation of osteoclasts.[1]

> **Question #1**   *TM is a 43-year-old man who is admitted to the hospital for the management of a right femoral deep vein thrombosis (DVT). He is 74.3 kg and 5'11". Calculate an initial UFH infusion rate for TM using pharmacokinetic modeling.*

Several methods for integrating pharmacokinetic and pharmacodynamic information into determining doses of UFH have been proposed. Chenella et al. proposed a first-order pharmacokinetic model to improve the precision and reliability of initial heparin infusion rates in achieving a therapeutic effect without excess bleeding.[51] The investigators used the following equation to determine the initial infusion rate:

$$R_0 = (C_{ss})(k_e)(V)$$

where
R_0 = initial hourly infusion rate (units/hr)
C_{ss} = desired steady-state heparin concentrations (units/mL)
k_e = elimination rate constant for heparin
V = the volume of distribution of heparin

As the heparin V approximates plasma volume, estimates of the blood volume can be used.[52]

Blood volume (men) = $(366.9 \text{ mL/mm}^3)(H^3) + (32.19 \text{ mL/kg})(\text{TBW}) + 604.1 \text{ mL}$

Blood volume (women) = $(356 \text{ mL/mm}^3)(H^3) + (33.08 \text{ mL/kg})(\text{TBW}) + 183.3 \text{ mL}$

where H = height (m)

Alternatively, the k_e and V can be estimated using population values. Using C_{ss} = 0.3 units/mL (assuming a target range of 0.2-0.4 units/mL), V = 0.07 L/kg (or 70 mL/kg), and k_e = 0.693 hour^{-1} (assuming a half-life elimination of 60 minutes), an initial infusion rate can be determined as follows:

$$R_0 = \left(0.3 \frac{\text{units}}{\text{mL}}\right)(0.693 \text{ hr}^{-1})\left(70 \frac{\text{mL}}{\text{kg}} \times 74.3 \text{ kg}\right)$$

$$R_0 = \left(0.3 \frac{\text{units}}{\text{mL}}\right)(0.693 \text{ hr}^{-1})(5,201 \text{ mL})$$

$$R_0 = 1,081 \frac{\text{units}}{\text{hr}}$$

$$R_0 = 1,100 \text{ units/hr}$$

Rounding heparin doses to the nearest 100 units/hr increment improves the ease of administration and programming of infusion pumps.

Though this equation has been used to estimate initial dosing regimens of UFH, there are two major assumptions: (1) the population values reflect a given patient's pharmacokinetic parameters and (2) heparin follows a one-compartment model. Given the interpatient variability in heparin pharmacokinetic parameters and the complex elimination of heparin, particularly at higher doses, caution is warranted in applying this method in determining initial doses. Further, the use of these models to predict heparin doses has not been shown to improve clinical outcomes over the use of weight-based dosing nomograms (described later).

Question #2 *YN is a 29-year-old man initiated on a heparin infusion for the treatment of a pulmonary embolism. He is 68.3 kg and 5'8". He was started on UFH with a 5,500 unit IV bolus followed by a 1,230 units/hr continuous IV infusion. The following data are available:*

TIME AFTER INFUSION START (HR)	APTT (SEC)	ANTI-XA (UNITS/ML)
1	58	0.49
4	46	0.36
6	39	0.24

Assuming a target aPTT of 46 to 70 seconds and an anti-Xa level of 0.3 to 0.7 units/mL, determine the dose adjustment necessary to achieve therapeutic anticoagulation.

When anti-Xa activity and aPTT can be measured concurrently, a pharmacokinetic model using non–steady-state plasma heparin concentrations can be used to adjust infusion rates to target therapeutic aPTT levels.[53,54] This method is based on equations described by Chiou et al., assuming the drug follows a linear one-compartment model and the levels are obtained at a constant drug infusion rate.[55]

$$Cl = \left(\frac{2R}{C_1 + C_2} \right) + \left(\frac{2V(C_1 - C_2)}{(C_1 + C_2)(t_2 - t_1)} \right)$$

where
Cl = apparent heparin clearance (units/hr)
R = hourly UFH infusion rate (units/hr)
C_1 = anti-Xa level obtained 1 hour after the start of UFH infusion (units/mL)
C_2 = anti-Xa level obtained 4 hours after the start of UFH infusion (units/mL)
V = volume of distribution of heparin (mL)

In this model, the following equation can be used to estimate blood volume.[56]

$$V = aH^3 + bW - c$$

where
H = height (cm)
W = weight (kg)
a = 0.000417 for men and 0.000414 for women
b = 45 mL/kg for men and 32.8 mL/kg for women
c = 30 mL

Alternatively, the V can be approximated by population data (70 mL/kg). Using the population V, the apparent clearance of heparin for YN can be determined as follows:

$$Cl = \frac{2\left(1,230 \ \frac{\text{units}}{\text{hr}} \right)}{0.49 \ \frac{\text{units}}{\text{mL}} + 0.36 \ \frac{\text{units}}{\text{mL}}} + \frac{2\left(\frac{70 \ \text{mL}}{\text{kg}} \times 68.3 \ \text{kg} \right)\left(0.49 \ \frac{\text{units}}{\text{mL}} - 0.36 \ \frac{\text{units}}{\text{mL}} \right)}{\left(0.49 \ \frac{\text{units}}{\text{mL}} + 0.36 \ \frac{\text{units}}{\text{mL}} \right)(4 \ \text{hr} - 1 \ \text{hr})}$$

$$Cl = \frac{2,460 \ \frac{\text{units}}{\text{hr}}}{0.85 \ \frac{\text{units}}{\text{mL}}} + \frac{2(4,781 \ \text{mL})\left(\frac{0.13 \ \text{units}}{\text{mL}} \right)}{\left(\frac{0.85 \ \text{units}}{\text{mL}} \right)(3 \ \text{hr})}$$

$$Cl = 2,894.12 \ \frac{\text{mL}}{\text{hr}} + \frac{1,243.06 \ \text{units}}{2.55 \ \text{units*} \frac{\text{hr}}{\text{mL}}}$$

$$Cl = 2,894.12 \, \frac{mL}{hr} + 487.47 \, \frac{mL}{hr}$$

$$Cl = 3,381.59 \, \frac{mL}{hr}$$

A new maintenance infusion rate can then be calculated using the patient-specific heparin clearance.[53,54]

$$R = Cl \times C_{ss_{des}}$$

where
R = new maintenance infusion rate (units/hr)
$C_{ss_{des}}$ = desired steady-state heparin concentration, determined by an anti-Xa assay (units/mL)

Using the patient-specific heparin clearance and a desired heparin concentration of 0.5 units/mL by anti-Xa assay (assuming a target range of 0.3-0.7 units/mL), a new maintenance infusion rate can be determined.

$$R = 3,381.59 \, \frac{mL}{hr} \times 0.5 \, \frac{units}{mL}$$

$$R = 1,690.8 \, \frac{units}{hr}$$

$$R = 1,690 \, \frac{units}{hr}$$

This pharmacokinetic model for heparin dose adjustments using heparin concentrations was better able to maintain aPTT values above 1.5 times the baseline aPTT as compared to a standard method using only aPTT values. However, obtaining multiple heparin levels may be cumbersome to healthcare providers and frequent blood sampling can be difficult on patients.

Owing to the aforementioned limitations, these models are eschewed for weight-based dosing nomograms, which are the current standard of practice. The use of dosing nomograms for UFH in clinical practice has been thoroughly evaluated.[57-67] Table 9.1 illustrates an example dosing nomogram based on aPTT values. Though this example demonstrates a recommended structure for the nomogram, care should be taken to individualize it for each specific institution and laboratory, accounting for differences in reagents and instruments used. Dosing nomograms using anti-Xa levels can be used at institutions able to perform routine anti-Xa assays (Table 9.2). These nomograms should be individualized for each institution as well.

Question #3   *MB is a 46-year-old woman who is currently receiving UFH for the treatment of an acute pulmonary embolism. Despite escalating the dose to 28 units/ kg/hr, the patient has not achieved a therapeutic aPTT value. What is the possible explanation for this phenomenon, and what can be done?*

TABLE 9.1   Example of a UFH Dosing Nomogram Using aPTT

Initial Dose	80 units/kg bolus, then 18 units/kg/hr
Subsequent Dosing Based on aPTT	
<35 sec	80 units/kg bolus and increase rate by 3 units/kg/hr
35-53 sec	40 units/kg bolus and increase rate by 2 units/kg/hr
54-96 sec	No change
96-114 sec	Decrease rate by 2 units/kg/hr
>114 sec	Hold infusion for 1 hr, then decrease rate by 3 units/kg/hr

An example dosing nomogram for UFH using aPTT values. After the initial dose is started, subsequent adjustments to therapy can be made based on the aPTT values obtained at steady state. Each laboratory should establish an institution-specific target aPTT range using their instruments and reagents. Changes to the recommended dose adjustments may be needed based on clinical practice at each institution. aPTT, activated partial thromboplastin time; UFH, unfractionated heparin.

In practice, there are cases where patients require unusually high doses of heparin to reach a therapeutic aPTT, collectively referred to as heparin resistance.[1,68] Though no standard definition of heparin resistance exists, it has been suggested that failure of 35,000 or more units/d of heparin to achieve therapeutic anticoagulation be used.[69] Among patients who require high daily doses of heparin to attain a therapeutic aPTT, switching to anti-Xa level monitoring may reduce the amount of administered heparin while maintaining clinical efficacy.[1]

The threshold of 35,000 units/d for heparin resistance may not be appropriate for every situation. In a hypothetical 81-kg patient, using the starting UFH infusion rate for the treatment of VTE of 18 units/kg/hr will reach this threshold. A weight-based dose threshold may be more appropriate (eg, >25 units/kg/hr), but no specific dose has been identified

TABLE 9.2   Example of a UFH Dosing Nomogram Using Anti-Xa Levels

Initial Dose	80 units/kg bolus, then 18 units/kg/hr
Subsequent Dosing Based on Anti-Xa Level	
<0.1 units/mL	80 units/kg bolus and increase rate by 3 units/kg/hr
0.1-0.29 units/mL	40 units/kg bolus and increase rate by 2 units/kg/hr
0.3-0.7 units/mL	No change
0.71-0.9 units/mL	Decrease rate by 2 units/kg/hr
>0.9 units/mL	Hold infusion for 1 hr, then decrease rate by 3 units/kg/hr

An example dosing nomogram for UFH using anti-Xa levels. Similar to the aPTT-based nomogram, adjustments to therapy can be made based on the anti-Xa levels obtained at steady state. Changes to the recommended dose adjustments may be needed based on clinical practice at each institution. aPTT, activated partial thromboplastin time; UFH: unfractionated heparin.

or validated. A framework that considers the weight-based dose, failure to reach therapeutic anticoagulation despite dose escalations, and the clinical consequences of failing to achieve therapeutic anticoagulation may be best to raise concern for heparin resistance.

Addressing heparin resistance involves identifying the underlying etiology. Several mechanisms for heparin resistance have been proposed, including AT deficiency, increased clearance of heparin, nonspecific binding of heparin, and elevated levels of coagulation factors.[1] In cases of AT deficiency confirmed by laboratory testing, supplementation with exogenous AT has been suggested to promote adequate anticoagulation, but experience is primarily limited to cardiac surgery and patients on extracorporeal membrane oxygenation (ECMO).[70] In addition, there is a lack of clear AT dosing guidance or goal AT activity. In cases where AT deficiency is suspected, other concurrent factors may be contributing to the lack of anticoagulant effect of UFH, rendering supplementation with AT potentially ineffective. As such, the use of alternative anticoagulants, such as the direct thrombin inhibitors, may be warranted.

Question #4   *HF is a 46-year-old woman initiated on heparin infusion for the treatment of an acute lower extremity DVT. She is 76.8 kg and 5'5". She was started on UFH with a 6,100 unit IV bolus followed by a 1,380 units/hr continuous IV infusion. Two hours after the bolus dose and the start of the infusion, she had a large, melanotic bowel movement associated with lightheadedness and a decrease in blood pressure concerning for an acute gastrointestinal bleed. Determine the most appropriate plan to neutralize the anticoagulant effect of heparin.*

When patients experience severe bleeding complications from heparin, protamine sulfate can be used to neutralize the anticoagulant effect of heparin. One milligram of protamine is estimated to neutralize approximately 100 units of heparin. As the half-life of UFH is typically 60 to 90 minutes, only the amount of heparin given within the preceding 2 to 3 hours should be considered when determining the dose of protamine required. For patient HF, the first step would be determining the total amount of heparin to be neutralized.

$$\text{Amount heparin to be neutralized} = 6,100 \text{ units} + 2 \text{ hr} \times \left(1,380 \frac{\text{units}}{\text{hr}}\right)$$

$$\text{Amount heparin to be neutralized} = 6,100 \text{ units} + 2,760 \text{ units}$$

$$\text{Amount heparin to be neutralized} = 8,860 \text{ units}$$

Using a protamine:heparin neutralization ratio of 1 mg:100 units, approximately 90 mg of protamine would be needed to neutralize this patient's heparin. However, total single doses over 50 mg are not recommended. Excessive doses of protamine may worsen bleeding complications due to protamine's intrinsic weak anticoagulant activity. High doses of protamine may also predispose patients to severe hypotension and anaphylactic or anaphylactoid reactions. These adverse effects can be mitigated by administering protamine slowly. Doses higher than 50 mg may be considered in cardiac surgery. However, as this patient is not undergoing cardiac surgery, her dose should be capped at 50 mg.

When protamine is needed to reverse the effects of heparin administered SC, a continuous infusion or repeat doses of protamine may be needed to account for continued absorption from the site of heparin administration. Measurement of aPTT can be helpful in determining the adequacy of heparin neutralization by protamine.

LOW-MOLECULAR-WEIGHT HEPARINS

LMWHs are a class of drugs derived from UFH that is subjected to either chemical or enzymatic degradation, resulting in shorter polysaccharide chains and a reduced molecular weight.[1] Though UFH and the LMWHs have a similar mechanism of anticoagulant effect, the shorter chains of the LMWHs confer comparatively greater activity against factor Xa and less activity against thrombin. The smaller size also contributes to a more advantageous pharmacokinetic and pharmacodynamic profile compared to UFH, making the LMWHs an attractive alternative. There are several commercially available LMWHs, though only dalteparin and enoxaparin are available in the United States.

KEY PARAMETERS: Low Molecular Weight Heparins

	CERTOPARIN (SANDOPARIN)[a]	DALTEPARIN (FRAGMIN)[b]	ENOXAPARIN (LOVENOX)[b]	NADROPARIN (FRAXIPARINE)[c]	REVIPARIN (CLIVARIN)[a]
Mean molecular weight (Da)	5,600	5,000	4,500	4,900	4,600
Anti-Xa: anti-IIa activity ratio	2.1:1	2.7:1	3.8:1	3.6:1	3.5:1
Therapeutic range[d]	Twice-daily dosing for treatment of VTE (anti-Xa assay): 0.6-1.0 units/mL (peak) Once-daily dosing for treatment of VTE (anti-Xa assay): 1.0-2.0 units/mL (peak)				
F (SC) (%)	90	87	90-92	98	95
V (L)	10.8	5.3	4.3	6.8	6.3
Cl (mL/min)	25	33.3	15.3	21.4	36.7
$t_{1/2}$ (hr)	4.6	3-5	4.5	3.3	3

[a]Available in Europe.
[b]Available in the United States.
[c]Available in Canada.
[d]The therapeutic ranges apply only to LMWH when dosed for the treatment of thrombotic conditions.

As with UFH, LMWHs are useful in the treatment and prevention of thrombotic phenomena. Though LMWHs are commonly referred to collectively, they each possess distinct pharmacokinetic and pharmacodynamic properties.[71-77] As such, the recommended dosing is agent and indication specific (Table 9.3). Many LMWH agents are available as prefilled injectable syringes, and weight-based doses are typically rounded to the closest available syringe size.

TABLE 9.3 FDA-Approved Dosing for Select Low-Molecular-Weight Heparins

	DALTEPARIN	ENOXAPARIN
Prophylaxis		
Abdominal surgery, postoperative	• 2,500 units SC once daily • 5,000 units SC once daily • 2,500 units SC q12h for 2 doses, then 5,000 units SC once daily	• 40 mg SC q24h, give first dose 2 hr before surgery
Knee arthroplasty, postoperative		• 30 mg SC q12h, starting 12-24 hr postoperatively
Hip arthroplasty, postoperative	• 2,500 units SC 4-8 hr after surgery, then 5,000 SC units once daily • 2,500 units SC 2 hr before surgery, then 2,500 units SC 4-8 hr after surgery, then 5,000 units SC once daily • 5,000 units SC evening before surgery, then 5,000 units 4-8 hr after surgery	• 30 mg SC q12h, starting 12-24 hr postoperatively • 40 mg SC q24h, starting 12 hr preoperatively
Hospitalized medical patients	• 5,000 units SC once daily	• 40 mg SC once daily
Treatment		
Acute ST-elevation myocardial infarction		• 30 mg IV bolus, then 1 mg/kg SC q12h (max 100 mg for first 2 doses)
Unstable angina and non–Q-wave myocardial infarction	• 120 units/kg SC twice daily (max 10,000 units)	• 1 mg/kg SC q12h
Deep vein thrombosis with or without pulmonary embolism, treatment	• 200 units/kg SC once daily • 100 units/kg SC twice daily • *Cancer associated*: 200 units/kg SC once daily for 30 d, then 150 units/kg SC once daily	• 1 mg/kg SC q24h • 1.5 mg/kg SC once daily (inpatient)

FDA, Food and Drug Administration; IV, intravenous; SC, subcutaneous.

Therapeutic Plasma Concentrations

Routine monitoring of LMWH efficacy is generally unnecessary because of a predictable anticoagulant effect.[1,78] The therapeutic range of LMWHs is wide, and usual treatment doses are expected to routinely achieve therapeutic levels. Monitoring of

LMWH therapy may be considered in certain clinical scenarios: renal impairment, obesity, and pregnancy. However, the American Society of Hematology (ASH) recommends against monitoring LMWH therapy in these patients as high-quality evidence that supports dose adjustments based on levels is lacking.[79,80] Further, the appropriate timing of levels and the therapeutic range have not been extensively validated.[78]

If monitoring of LMWH therapy is clinically warranted, the anti-Xa assay is recommended. Owing to the relatively limited effect on thrombin, aPTT measurements may not reliably reflect the degree of anticoagulant activity of LMWHs. Though the timing of levels remains controversial, consensus recommendations suggest obtaining peak levels 4 to 5 hours after a SC injection.[78] This corresponds to the peak concentration after a dose. When the LMWH is dosed BID, the target range is 0.6 to 1.0 units/mL, as opposed to a range of 1.0 to 2.0 units/mL when dosed once daily. These ranges apply only for treatment-dose LMWH.

Bioavailability (*F*)

Similar to UFH, LMWHs are minimally bioavailable via enteral administration.[81] After SC injection, LMWHs are highly bioavailable, ranging from 87% to 98%.[71-74] The onset of anticoagulant effects, as measured by anti-Xa levels, occurs 30 minutes after SC dosing and peak after 3 to 5 hours.[75] Given these favorable pharmacokinetic profiles, SC administration is the preferred route. IV administration may be considered when a more rapid anticoagulant effect is needed, such as in the treatment of ST-elevation myocardial infarctions.[6]

Bioavailability of SC administered LMWHs in critically ill patients may be reduced, particularly when patients are receiving vasoactive agents.[82,83] A number of factors, including poor peripheral blood flow and decreased cardiac output, likely contribute. However, the clinical consequences are unclear. The use of prophylactic SC LMWH at standard doses in critically ill patients appears to be effective. For critically ill patients requiring therapeutic anticoagulation, it may be reasonable to consider the use of IV UFH instead of LMWH.

Volume of Distribution (*V*)

The apparent volume of distribution of LMWHs approximates the plasma volume, ranging from 3.9 to 9.3 L.[75,76] Variations in the reported *V* of LMWHs is likely because of differences in the assays used. Compared to UFH, LMWHs have significantly decreased nonspecific protein binding, which contributes to their more favorable pharmacokinetic profile and more predictable pharmacodynamic response. Given the distribution of LMWH primarily to the plasma, weight-based dosing using TBW is recommended.

Dosing for patients at the extremes of body weight is debated. In patients with obesity (body mass index [BMI] ≥ 30 kg/m²), LMWH may not distribute well into adipose tissue.[84] Use of an AdjBW for treatment-dose LMWH has been suggested, but no trial has evaluated this strategy. Reduced weight–based treatment dosing of enoxaparin (eg, 0.7-0.8 mg/kg) has been shown to better achieve anti-Xa levels in the therapeutic range compared to standard dosing, but the impact on bleeding and thrombotic outcomes is limited.[85] Further, there is no clear correlation between supratherapeutic anti-Xa levels and bleeding outcomes.[80] Until more robust trials are conducted, it is reasonable to continue using TBW to calculate treatment-dose LMWH in patients with obesity. When used for prophylaxis, increasing the dose of LMWH by 30% may be reasonable to reduce the risk of VTE.[84] A strategy of enoxaparin 40 mg SC q12h in patients with BMI 40 kg/m^2 or more is also effective.[86]

Limited information is available on the optimal dosing for patients with low body weight. Use of TBW for treatment-dose LMWH is appropriate. Dose reductions of prophylactic LMWH in patients weighing less than 55 kg may be necessary, though clinical outcome data are lacking.[87,88]

Clearance (Cl)

Each of the LMWHs has a distinct Cl, ranging from 15.3 to 33.3 mL/min.[75,76] The LMWHs are cleared primarily through a nonsaturable renal mechanism, following first-order kinetics. Thus, unlike UFH, the Cl of LMWHs is not dose dependent, contributing to the more predictable and linear dose response seen with LMWHs.

As LMWHs are cleared primarily through the kidneys, caution is warranted in patients with renal impairment. Clearance may be reduced by as much as 44%.[84] Dose reductions are recommended for LMWHs based on the determination of creatinine clearance (Cl$_{Cr}$) using the Cockcroft-Gault method with the following equations:

$$Cl_{Cr} \text{ for males (mL/min)} = \frac{(140 - \text{Age})(\text{Weight in kg})}{(72)(\text{SCr})}$$

$$Cl_{Cr} \text{ for females (mL/min)} = (0.85)\frac{(140 - \text{Age})(\text{Weight in kg})}{(72)(\text{SCr})}$$

Note that patients with severe renal impairment (Cl$_{Cr}$ <30 mL/min) were generally excluded from the clinical trials. Pharmacodynamic studies have shown higher anti-Xa levels in patients with severe renal impairment when given treatment doses of enoxaparin.[89] There is evidence of greater rates of bleeding among patients with renal impairment treated with LMWH, though the contribution of renal insufficiency itself on bleeding outcomes must be considered.[84] Dose reductions of enoxaparin are recommended in patients with severe renal impairment, and anti-Xa level monitoring has been suggested for all LMWHs. However, current guidelines do not recommend routine monitoring of anti-Xa levels in patients with renal impairment receiving LMWHs.[80] The use of UFH instead of LMWHs may be prudent in patients with Cl$_{Cr}$ less than 20 mL/min.

Half-Life ($t_{1/2}$)

The elimination half-life for LMWHs ranges between 3 and 6 hours after SC administration.[1] The relatively longer half-lives allow for once-daily or BID dosing. As clearance is primarily renal in nature, the half-life is significantly prolonged in patients with renal impairment.[90,91] In patients with chronic renal insufficiency requiring renal replacement therapy, the half-life of LMWHs may be prolonged up to 1.9-fold compared to healthy volunteers.[92]

Time to Sample

When obtaining anti-Xa levels to monitor LMWH therapy, appropriate timing of levels is important. Anti-Xa levels should be obtained 4 to 5 hours after an SC injection.[78] The defined therapeutic range varies based on dosing frequency, with a target range of 0.6 to 1.0 units/mL for BID dosing and a target range of 1.0 to 2.0 units/mL for once-daily dosing. There is no standard for dose adjustments based on anti-Xa levels obtained while on LMWH therapy. Table 9.4 describes a potential dosing nomogram for LMWH based on anti-Xa levels.[93] However, this nomogram has only been validated in pediatric patients.

Adverse Effects

The LMWHs share an adverse effect profile with UFH, with bleeding being the major complication of therapy. Compared to UFH, the LMWHs have a lower affinity to PF4 and a 3-fold decreased incidence of HIT.[1] However, routine monitoring of platelets is warranted, and LMWHs should be avoided in patients with a history of HIT. The LMWHs also possess a lower affinity for osteoblasts and osteoclasts, leading to a reduced risk of osteoporosis compared to UFH.

TABLE 9.4   Sample Dosing Nomogram for Low-Molecular-Weight Heparins

ANTI-FACTOR XA LEVEL U/ML	HOLD NEXT DOSE?	DOSE CHANGE?	REPEAT ANTI-FACTOR XA
<0.35	No	Increase by 25%	4 hr after next dose
0.35-0.49	No	Increase by 10%	4 hr after next dose
0.5-1.0	No	No	Next day, then 1 wk later and monthly thereafter while receiving reviparin-Na treatment (at 4 hr after AM dose)
1.1-1.5	No	Decrease by 20%	Before next dose
1.6-2.0	3 hr	Decrease by 30%	Before next dose, then 4 hr after next dose
>2.0	Until anti-factor Xa 0.5 U/mL	Decrease by 40%	Before next dose, if not <0.5 unit/mL, repeat q12h

A suggested dosing nomogram for treatment-dose LMWH. Dose adjustments to LMWH therapy can be made using peak anti-Xa levels. This nomogram has only been validated in the pediatric population and may not be applicable to adults. From Monagle P, Michelson AD, Bovill E, Andrew M. Antithrombotic therapy in children. *Chest*. 2001;119(suppl 1):344S-370S. doi:10.1378/chest.119.1_suppl.344s.

Question #5   *RC is a 39-year-old man initiated enoxaparin for the treatment of an acute pulmonary embolism. He is 82.5 kg and 5'9". He was started on enoxaparin 80 mg SC q12h and discharged home. After 1 week of therapy, he developed a severe headache and was found to have a small intracranial hemorrhage. He reports adherence to his therapy, with his last dose 5 hours ago. Determine the most appropriate plan to neutralize the anticoagulant effect of enoxaparin.*

Similar to UFH, protamine can be used to neutralize the anticoagulant effects of LMWHs.[1] However, as protamine has a variable ability to neutralize the anti-Xa effects, the reversal may be incomplete. The clinical implications of this incomplete neutralization are unclear. The dose of protamine to be administered depends on the time since the last dose of LMWH. If the reversal is needed within 8 hours of the previous dose, protamine should be administered at a ratio of 1 mg/100 units (100 units = 1 mg enoxaparin). If the last dose of LMWH was between 8 and 12 hours prior, the protamine dose should be reduced to 0.5 mg/100 units. Reversal of a LMWH given greater than 12 hours prior is not necessary. The same precautions apply in giving protamine for reversal of LMWH as for UFH. The protamine dose should not exceed 50 mg and should be given slowly to reduce the risk of hypotension and anaphylactoid reactions. Assessing the efficacy of reversal using anti-Xa levels is not recommended.

Andexanet alfa, a factor Xa inhibitor reversal agent, has been investigated for use in reversing enoxaparin.[94] Though andexanet alfa has demonstrated the ability to reverse the anticoagulant effects of enoxaparin in animal models, clinical data in human trials are lacking. As such, andexanet alfa is not currently approved for the reversal of enoxaparin. This recommendation may evolve as more data emerge.

WARFARIN

Warfarin and related vitamin K antagonists (VKAs) are orally (PO) bioavailable anticoagulants used for a broad spectrum of thrombotic conditions. The VKAs inhibit the action of vitamin K epoxide reductase (VKOR), an enzyme responsible for the cyclic regeneration of vitamin K. Vitamin K is a necessary cofactor for the production of the clotting factors II, VII, IX, and X in addition to the natural anticoagulant proteins C and S.[95] Though their effectiveness has been established in clinical trials and decades of clinical experience, the use of VKAs is complicated by a narrow therapeutic window and numerous pharmacokinetic, pharmacodynamic, and genetic factors that influence the dose response. Dosing is typically individualized for each patient, with some requiring complex dosing regimens involving variable daily dosing requirements and frequent monitoring. With more convenient options in the direct oral anticoagulants (DOACs), VKAs are no longer first-line options in the management of various thromboembolic disorders. However, there are still clinical scenarios where VKAs are preferred. Of the available agents, warfarin is the most common. Warfarin is a racemic mixture of S- and R-warfarin isomers, which possess different pharmacokinetic and pharmacodynamic properties. The S-enantiomer has been reported to be 2.7 to 3.8 times more potent than the R-enantiomer.[95]

Therapeutic Plasma Concentrations

Plasma concentrations of warfarin do not predict the efficacy and safety of VKA therapy. Instead, the measurement of the PT, in seconds, describes the anticoagulant effect of VKA.[95] The PT responds to reductions in three of the four factors affected by warfarin (factors II, VII, and X). However, measurement of the PT is subject to variability in the thromboplastin responsiveness to reductions in the vitamin K–dependent clotting factors. The responsiveness of each thromboplastin reagent can be characterized by the international sensitivity index (ISI). A calibration model was developed to standardize PT measurements across different reagents and laboratories.[96] The resultant value, the INR, can be calculated using the following equation:

$$INR = \left(\frac{Patient\ PT}{Mean\ normal\ PT} \right)^{ISI}$$

It is important to note that the PT and INR can be influenced be heparin.[97] Care should be made in selecting a thromboplastin reagent that is insensitive to heparin to avoid inaccurate measurements of VKA therapy when patients are concurrently on a VKA and a heparin product.

The therapeutic INR range for VKA therapy is dependent on the indication and patient-specific factors. For many therapeutic uses, the INR goal is between 2.0 and 3.0. In patients who have undergone a mitral valve replacement with a mechanical prosthesis, an INR goal of 2.5 to 3.5 is recommended.

Bioavailability (*F*)

The PO bioavailability of warfarin is more than 90%.[98,99] After PO administration, absorption is rapid with peak plasma concentrations seen in about 90 minutes.[95] Food does not impact the bioavailability of warfarin. However, when administered with enteral nutrition via a feeding tube, plasma concentrations of warfarin may be reduced by up to 35%.[100] Adsorption to the feeding tube appears to be responsible for this effect.

Volume of Distribution (*V*)

The volume of distribution of warfarin is approximately 10 L/70 kg.[99] Warfarin is almost completely (99%) bound to plasma proteins, predominantly to serum albumin.[101] There are little to no differences in the volume of distribution and protein binding between the warfarin enantiomers.[102] As unbound warfarin is responsible for the anticoagulant effects, the response to warfarin is influenced by alterations in protein binding. In patients with chronic renal failure, plasma protein binding of warfarin may be reduced as uremic toxins compete for binding sites on albumin.[103] Unbound warfarin concentrations may be 2-fold higher in these patients. As such, dosing requirements of warfarin in patients with chronic kidney disease may be approximately 20% lower than that in patients with normal renal function.[104]

There are a number of drugs that are known to displace warfarin from protein-binding sites, including phenytoin and nonsteroidal anti-inflammatory drugs (NSAIDs).[105] However, the effect on unbound concentrations, and therefore the anticoagulant effects of warfarin, may be transient and clinically insignificant, given a corresponding increase in warfarin clearance.[106] Thus, monitoring of the patient's coagulation status without empiric dose changes is sufficient when a highly protein-bound drug is added to patient receiving warfarin.

Clearance (Cl)

Warfarin is eliminated almost entirely through hepatic metabolism and is independent of hepatic blood flow, given an extraction ratio that approaches zero.[99,102] The clearance of warfarin is approximately 0.2 L/hr/70 kg, though it is stereospecific with S-warfarin having a higher systemic clearance than R-warfarin.[99] This difference is likely due to separate metabolic pathways for the enantiomers. While both are metabolized through the cytochrome P450 system, the S-enantiomer is metabolized primarily by CYP2C9, whereas CYP1A2 and CYP3A4 are responsible for metabolizing the R-enantiomer.[95] Genetic variations in the expression of certain CYP2C9 alleles partially explain the wide interpatient variability seen in warfarin dose response.

Half-Life ($t_{1/2}$)

The racemic mixture of warfarin has a terminal half-life of approximately 35 to 45 hours, though each enantiomer has its own half-life.[95,107] As the clearance of S-warfarin is higher than R-warfarin, the half-life of the S-enantiomer is approximately 29 hours compared to 45 hours for the R-enantiomer.

Time to Sample

In patients being newly started on warfarin, daily monitoring of the INR has been recommended as changes may occur rapidly.[97] However, it is important to note that changes in the INR may not be seen for 2 to 3 days and the full antithrombotic effects for 5 to 7 days, depending on the dose administered.[95] This delay is directly related to warfarin's mechanism of anticoagulant effect. Through inhibition of the VKOR enzyme, clotting factors II, VII, IX, and X are still produced by the liver, but their level of biologic functionality is reduced. However, existing circulating clotting factors at the time of warfarin initiation continue to influence the coagulation status of the patient until they can be replaced with less functional clotting factors. Thus, the initial onset and time to the full anticoagulant effect of warfarin are dependent on the degradation of previously produced factors. An initial prolongation in the INR may be seen after 2 to 3 days due to depletion of circulating factor VII, but the full anticoagulant effect will not be seen until degradation of factors II and X (Table 9.5).

During initiation of warfarin, reduction in protein C results in a relatively hypercoagulable state.[95] Thus, in situations where rapid anticoagulation is needed and a transient hypercoagulable state could be detrimental, such as HIT, coadministration with a parenteral anticoagulant is crucial. In general, when immediate therapeutic anticoagulation is required, overlap with a parenteral anticoagulant should be continued for 5 days and until the INR is within the therapeutic range for two readings approximately 24 hours apart. In scenarios where rapid therapeutic anticoagulation is not needed, such as chronic stable atrial fibrillation, warfarin can be started without overlapping with a parenteral anticoagulant.

TABLE 9.5   Half-Lives of Vitamin K–Dependent Proteins

PROTEIN	HALF-LIFE (HR)
Factor II	42-72
Factor VII	4-6
Factor IX	21-30
Factor X	27-48
Protein C	8
Protein S	60

The half-life elimination of vitamin K–dependent proteins. Vitamin K antagonists reduce production of new clotting factors, but the onset of anticoagulant effects is delayed until actively circulating clotting factors are depleted, based on their half-life elimination.

Monitoring of the INR at least 4 to 5 times per week while determining the stable warfarin dose needed to achieve a consistent INR within the therapeutic range is recommended.[97] After the INR has been in the therapeutic range for at least two consecutive readings, the frequency of testing may be slowly spaced out to 2 to 3 times per week and then weekly if the INR continues to be therapeutic. Once a stable dose has been determined, the optimal frequency of monitoring is still up for debate. The College of American Pathologists has recommended that INR be monitored not less frequently than every 4 weeks in stable patients.[97] However, the ACCP and ASH suggest an interval of up to 12 weeks in patients on a stable dose of VKA.[80,108] The optimal interval for INR monitoring should be based on patient-specific factors. After any dose adjustments, the frequency of monitoring should be increased again until stability is redemonstrated.

Adverse Effects

As with any anticoagulant, hemorrhagic complications are the primary concern. Rare, but serious nonhemorrhagic side effects of warfarin include skin necrosis[109] and purple toe syndrome.[110] Warfarin-induced skin necrosis presents as skin lesions or petechiae, usually within 3 to 8 days of initiation. The lesions are primarily distributed to fatty tissue, caused by extensive thrombosis of the vasculature in SC fat.[95,109] This adverse effect is thought to be linked to genetic proteins C and S deficiency or rapid depletion of protein C due to high initial doses of warfarin. Purple toe syndrome typically occurs 3 to 8 weeks after initiation of warfarin, presenting as acute-onset, bilateral purple lesions on the toes and sides of the feet that are painful in nature.[110] Although these side effects are rare, clinicians should be aware of these effects because of their serious nature.

INITIAL DOSING OF WARFARIN

Initial dosing of warfarin remains controversial. Loading doses that exceed the anticipated maintenance dose were suggested in the past, but that practice is no longer recommended. The use of a loading dose does not result in more rapid attainment of anticoagulant effects and, in many instances, leads to an initial overshoot of the therapeutic range.[111] The ACCP has suggested a daily dose between 5 and 10 mg for the first 2 days of therapy for most patients, with subsequent dosing based on the INR response.[95] Caution is warranted in giving initial daily doses of 10 mg or higher as this may lead to excessive anticoagulation, precipitate a hypercoagulable state owing to the rapid decrease in protein C, and cause skin necrosis.[112] Several nomograms using initial fixed doses have been evaluated but do not fully consider individual patient factors.[113] A starting daily dose of warfarin 5 mg is reasonable for most patients, and adjustments based on the factors included in Table 9.6 should be considered.[114]

Common practice among clinicians is to instruct patients to take their warfarin doses in the evening. During appointments with their patients, clinicians may make immediate changes to a patient's warfarin regimen, such as holding a dose, based on the INR results obtained from that day.

Pharmacogenetic Considerations

There is clear evidence that pharmacogenetics plays a key role in the pharmacokinetic and pharmacodynamic disposition of warfarin, particularly when mutations occur in the genes encoding the CYP2C9 and VKOR enzymes.[95,102] Single-nucleotide polymorphisms (SNPs) in the gene coding for the CYP2C9 enzyme are responsible for decreases in enzymatic activity and impaired metabolism of warfarin. The presence of the CYP2C9*2 and CYP2C9*3 alleles has been shown to reduce the metabolism of

TABLE 9.6 Patient Factors That Influence Response to Warfarin

FACTOR	INFLUENCE ON INR RESPONSE
Advanced age	⇑
Alcohol use (acute)	⇑
Alcohol use (chronic)	⇓
Cigarette smoking	⇓
Congestive heart failure	⇑
Dietary vitamin K	⇓
Drug-drug interactions	⇑/⇓
Heart valve replacement, acute phase	⇑
Hepatic disease	⇑
Poor nutritional status	⇑
Renal disease	⇑
Thyroid disease (hyperthyroidism)	⇑
Thyroid disease (hypothyroidism)	⇓

Partial list of patient-specific factors that influence the patient response to warfarin as described by the INR.
INR, international normalized ratio.

S-warfarin by approximately 30% to 40% and approximately 80% to 90%, respectively, when compared to the wild type (CYP2C9*1).[115] As such, patients with one or two copies of this allele require lower maintenance doses to achieve a stable INR and are more susceptible to adverse bleeding outcomes. Other decrease-in-function alleles have been identified (CYP2C9*5, CYP2C9*6, CYP2C9*8, and CYP2C9*11) and contribute to interpatient dose variability. Notably, key differences in the frequency of these alleles vary by race, with individuals of European ancestry most likely to carry CYP2C9*2 and CYP2C9*3 alleles. The frequency of CYP2C9*5, CYP2C9*6, CYP2C9*8, and CYP2C9*11 alleles are highest among individuals of African ancestry.

The VKOR complex 1 (*VKORC1*) gene that results in the synthesis of the VKOR enzyme is subject to mutations as well.[95] Variants that result in a -1639G>A polymorphism lead to increased warfarin sensitivity compared to the -1639G/G homozygote and thus lower warfarin maintenance doses.[115] The U.S. Food and Drug Administration (FDA) label for warfarin now includes dosing recommendations based on pharmacogenetic factors.[116]

Integration of the CYP2C9 and VKORC1 genetic variants into warfarin dose prediction models has shown improved accuracy in identifying a stable maintenance dose compared to a clinical algorithm.[117,118] However, the use of a pharmacogenetic algorithm has not been consistently shown to improve time in the therapeutic INR range as compared to a clinical algorithm.[119-121] The 2012 ACCP guidelines recommend against the routine use of pharmacogenetic testing to determine VKA dosing.[108] When pharmacogenetic information is available, the Clinical Pharmacogenetics Implementation Consortium (CPIC) recommends using a validated published algorithm, such as the one developed by International Warfarin Pharmacogenetics Consortium.[115,117]

There continues to be evolving data on the genetic factors that influence warfarin sensitivity, including variants in CYP4F2 and rs12777823 SNP in the CYP2C cluster.[115] Inclusion of these genetic variants in warfarin dosing models appears to improve the accuracy of dose prediction, but clinical data are still needed.

Drug and Food Interactions

Warfarin is subject to numerous pharmacokinetic and pharmacodynamic drug-drug interactions.[114] These interactions can either reduce or potentiate warfarin's anticoagulant effects as evidenced by changes in the INR. Alterations in absorption, protein binding, and metabolism are responsible for these effects. Several drugs, such as cholestyramine[122] and sucralfate,[123] bind warfarin within the gastrointestinal tract and reduce warfarin absorption. Administration of the warfarin dose at least 2 to 4 hours before the binding drug can partially mitigate this interaction, but close monitoring of the INR is warranted. Though concurrent use of other highly protein-bound drugs may displace warfarin, increasing plasma concentrations, corresponding increases in warfarin clearance balance this effect, resulting in only transient and mild changes in the anticoagulant response.[124]

Addition or discontinuation of drugs that alter warfarin metabolism often necessitates significant warfarin dose adjustments with close monitoring of the INR. Concurrent use of medications that either inhibit or induce the activity of the CYP2C9 and CYP3A4 enzymes, and to a lesser extent CYP1A2, results in clinically important changes to warfarin metabolism.[125] Common CYP450 inhibitors that reliably lead to relevant drug interactions with warfarin can be remembered using the

"FAB-Four" pneumonic: fluconazole (and other azole antifungals), amiodarone, Bactrim (sulfamethoxazole-trimethoprim), and Flagyl (metronidazole).[126] Published experience with concomitant use of amiodarone and warfarin suggests an eventual 25% to 40% reduction in warfarin dose may be necessary, depending on the dose of amiodarone administered.[127,128] Similarly, coadministration of fluconazole (or other azoles), sulfamethoxazole-trimethoprim, or metronidazole with warfarin may necessitate a 25% to 40% warfarin dose reduction.[125]

Patients treated with warfarin while receiving CYP450 inducers may require substantially higher doses of warfarin. Published reports of the warfarin-rifampin interaction suggest that warfarin dose increases of up to 3 to 5 times the previous dose may be required to achieve a therapeutic INR.[129] Addition of carbamazepine to a stable warfarin regimen may require dose escalations of 50%.[130] Table 9.7 further describes

TABLE 9.7 Medications With Clinically Relevant Drug-Drug Interactions With Warfarin

POTENTIATE ANTICOAGULANT EFFECT	INHIBIT ANTICOAGULANT EFFECT	INCREASE BLEEDING RISK
Acetaminophen	Barbiturates	Aspirin
Allopurinol	Bile acid sequestrants	Direct oral anticoagulants
Amiodarone	Carbamazepine	Direct thrombin inhibitors
Anabolic steroids	Dicloxacillin	Fondaparinux
Azole antifungals	Nafcillin	GP IIb/IIIa inhibitors
Cephalosporins	Phenytoin	Heparin derivatives
Cimetidine	Rifabutin	NSAIDs
Ciprofloxacin	Rifampin	$P2Y_{12}$ Inhibitors
Danazol	St. John wort	
Disulfiram	Sucralfate	
Fibric acid derivatives	Trazodone	
Fluorouracil		
Fluvoxamine		
Isoniazid		
Levofloxacin		
Lovastatin		
Macrolide antibiotics		
Metronidazole		
Omeprazole		
Propafenone		
Sertraline		
Simvastatin		
Sulfamethoxazole		
Tetracycline antibiotics		

List of select medications that have a clinically relevant interaction with warfarin. This list is not exhaustive. NSAID, nonsteroidal anti-inflammatory drug.

medications that have a high likelihood of clinically relevant drug-drug interactions with warfarin.[131]

The onset and offset of CYP450-mediated drug interactions are dependent on the half-life of the offending agent and if the agent is an inducer or inhibitor.[132] In most cases, interactions from inhibitors can be seen within 3 to 5 days, though the effect may be delayed for interacting drugs with long half-lives. The effect of the warfarin-amiodarone interaction may be delayed for up to 2 months after initiation. The timing of offset of enzyme inhibition typically mirrors that of the onset. The onset and offset of drug interactions are also influenced by the time needed to synthesize and degrade CYP450 enzymes. Cases of warfarin-rifampin interactions persisting for weeks after rifampin discontinuation have been reported.[133]

Some clinicians employ a strategy of empiric warfarin dose adjustments when an enzyme inhibitor or inducer is added to an existing warfarin regimen. These strategies improve the time in therapeutic range but do not affect clinical outcomes.[134-136] As it is difficult to predict the degree of dose adjustment needed, preemptive changes to warfarin doses may not be an effective strategy in all patients. Close monitoring of INR, in line with the expected onset of the interaction, with corresponding dose adjustments as needed is recommended. For most drug interactions, follow-up INR monitoring within 3 to 5 days of the inhibitor or inducer initiation is appropriate.[125]

Warfarin is also susceptible to many pharmacodynamic drug interactions. Addition of antiplatelets or NSAIDs to a warfarin regimen increases the bleeding risk without changes in the INR.[114] Combining these agents with warfarin should be avoided when possible.[108] In situations where patients are indicated for treatment with both warfarin and antiplatelets, concurrent antiplatelet therapy should be minimized and continued for the shortest effective duration.[137] The use of broad-spectrum antibiotics may reduce gastrointestinal flora contributing to intrinsic vitamin K production, thereby potentiating the impact of warfarin on the INR.[138] This interaction may be particularly relevant in patients with poor nutritional status.

Food and herbal products contribute further to variability in warfarin response. High intake of foods that contain vitamin K may inhibit the anticoagulant effect of warfarin (Table 9.8).[114,139] Patients on warfarin therapy should be educated on the importance of consistency in their vitamin K intake, rather than complete avoidance. Several herbal medications have been implicated in warfarin interactions, with mechanisms ranging from influencing metabolism (eg, St. John's wort) to altering intrinsic coagulation (eg, ginseng).

The full scope of relevant drug interactions for warfarin therapy is difficult to ascertain because of evidence of varying quality.[131] Evaluation of the potential for a drug interaction should be conducted whenever warfarin is added to an existing drug regimen or a new drug is started on a patient currently taking warfarin. Where possible, avoidance of the interacting agent is recommended. If avoidance is not possible, close monitoring of the INR is necessary to minimize adverse clinical outcomes.

TABLE 9.8   Vitamin K Content of Food Products[a]

VERY HIGH (>200 µg)	HIGH (100 TO <200 µg)	LOW (<100 µg)
Collard greens	Broccoli	Asparagus
Green onions	Brussels sprouts	Avocado
Kale	Cabbage	Fruits (various)
Mustard greens	Canola oil	Olive oil
Parsley	Lettuce	
Spinach	Margarine	
Swiss chard	Mayonnaise	
Tea leaves	Salad dressing	
Turnip greens	Soybean oil	

List of select foods grouped by vitamin K content. Patients on warfarin should have a consistent intake of foods on this list to avoid variations in their INR response.
INR, international normalized ratio.
[a]Per 100 g of food product.

REVERSAL OF WARFARIN THERAPY

During treatment with warfarin, interruption or reversal of therapy may be required to address excessive anticoagulation with or without bleeding complications. A strategy of warfarin interruption is typically sufficient in patients with an elevated INR without bleeding complications.[95,108] The ACCP recommends against treating INR elevations to 4.5 to 10 if there is no clinical evidence of bleeding.[108] After holding warfarin, the INR may take greater than 96 hours to normalize when starting from 2 to 3, with longer times needed for higher INRs.[140]

In situations that warrant reversal of the anticoagulant effects of warfarin, vitamin K_1 with or without fresh-frozen plasma (FFP) or prothrombin complex concentrate (PCC) is effective. Vitamin K_1 bypasses the VKOR enzyme, allowing for the synthesis of functional clotting factors even in the presence of warfarin.[141] Vitamin K_1 may be administered PO, SC, or IV. Though the IV administration achieves a more rapid effect (reduction of INR within 4-6 hours), the magnitude of INR reduction is similar between PO and IV vitamin K_1 at 24 hours.[95] IV administration of vitamin K_1 has been reported to cause anaphylactoid reactions, though the frequency may be low at approximately 3 per 100,000 doses. Administration of the IV dose mixed in 50 mL over a minimum of 20 minutes is recommended to reduce the risk of anaphylactoid reactions. SC administration should be avoided as the effects are unpredictable and less effective.

For patients who experience INR values of greater than 10 without evidence of bleeding, warfarin should be held and PO vitamin K_1 may be administered to reverse the effect of warfarin.[108] The use of a low dose (1-5 mg) of vitamin K_1 is effective in lowering the INR in these cases.[141] Higher doses should be avoided in these cases as excess vitamin K_1 can accumulate in the liver, leading to issues in reestablishing a therapeutic INR when warfarin therapy is resumed. This resistance to warfarin may persist for up to a week after the dose.

In patients who experience major or life-threatening bleeding, administration of IV vitamin K_1 at a dose of 5-10 mg is recommended.[108] As the full effects of vitamin K_1 on the INR may take up to 24 hours to manifest, concurrent replacement of clotting factors is recommended. Where available, four-factor prothrombin complex concentrate (4F-PCC) is preferred to other PCCs or FFP.[142] The dose of 4F-PCC is dependent on the INR and the body weight: 25 units/kg (max 2,500 units) for INR 2 to less than 4, 35 units/kg (max 3,500 units) for INR 4 to 6, and 50 units/kg (max 5,000 units) for INR greater than 6. After administration of 4F-PCC, a reduction in INR should be expected within 30 minutes. If FFP is used, it should be dosed at 10 to 15 mL/kg.

For patients on warfarin who require a procedure, consideration for reversal should include assessment of the urgency of the procedure. In patients planned to undergo an elective procedure, holding warfarin with close monitoring of the INR is sufficient. If a patient requires an emergent procedure occurring in the next 6 to 8 hours, administration of 4F-PCC with IV vitamin K_1 is recommended. For procedures occurring within the next 24 to 36 hours, low-dose vitamin K_1, given either PO or IV, is appropriate.

Question #6   *OA is a 74-year-old White female being initiated on warfarin for stroke prophylaxis in atrial fibrillation. She is 5'2" and 51.2 kg. She denies a history of liver, renal, or thyroid disease. She does not drink alcohol but is a current smoker. She is currently taking metoprolol 25 mg PO BID. Genetic testing reveals she is heterozygous for the CYP2C9*2 allele. What initial warfarin dosing regimen would you recommend for OA?*

Before initiation of warfarin, a detailed review of the patient's profile should be conducted to identify any possible factors that may influence the patient's response to warfarin. In addition, the target INR should be established based on the indication. For this patient, an INR goal of 2 to 3 is appropriate. Several patient-specific factors should be considered in determining her initial dose, including her advanced age, body weight, active smoking status, and the presence of the CYP2C9*2 allele. Notably, these factors modulate the initial dose in different directions, with the advanced age, body weight, and CYP2C9*2 allele suggesting a dose reduction and her smoking status calling for dose increases. A starting dose of warfarin 5 mg daily is reasonable in most patients to minimize the risk of rapid and excessive anticoagulation. Given OA's patient-specific factors, a dose reduction is warranted, though the optimal percent decrease is difficult to characterize. Many institutions provide guidance or policies to practitioners to assist with dosing of warfarin. Online tools are another potential resource to assist clinicians. Sites such as warfarindosing.org utilize validated algorithms to predict maintenance doses, whereas nextdose.org uses Bayesian forecasting. For this patient, an initial dose of warfarin 2.5 to 4mg daily may be reasonable. Patients being newly initiated on warfarin should be assessed for the need for a parenteral anticoagulant bridge. As OA's indication for warfarin is stroke prophylaxis and not an acute thrombotic event, initiation of warfarin without a parenteral bridge is reasonable.

Key Parameters of Warfarin

Therapeutic range (INR)	Treatment of venous thromboembolism: 2.0-3.0
	Stroke prophylaxis in atrial fibrillation: 2.0-3.0
	Heart valve replacement
	• Bioprosthetic valve, aortic or mitral position: 2.0-3.0
	• Mechanical valve, aortic position: 2.0-3.0
	• Mechanical valve, mitral position: 2.5-3.5
F	>90%
V_d	10 L/70 kg
Protein binding	99%
Cl	
Racemic mixture	0.2 L/hr/70 kg
R-warfarin	0.15 L/hr/70 kg
S-warfarin	0.31 L/hr/70 kg
$t_{1/2}$ (hr)	
Racemic mixture	35-45
R-warfarin	45
S-warfarin	29

Question #7   *OA presents to her anticoagulation clinic for follow-up 1 week later. She endorses adherence to her warfarin 4 mg daily and denies any changes to her diet, cigarette smoking, or medications. Her INR at clinic is 3.2, and she denies any signs or symptoms of bleeding. She has not yet taken her warfarin dose for the day. How should her warfarin regimen be adjusted?*

When patients present to an outpatient clinic for warfarin management with an INR above the goal range, they should first be assessed for any adverse bleeding complications. Investigation into their adherence and changes in their diet or medications is pertinent to determine whether there is an outside influence on their response to warfarin. As OA denies any bleeding complications or changes that may impact her INR, a dose adjustment is warranted. Various nomograms exist to guide adjustments to warfarin therapy and may be provided by a clinician's practice site. Generally, a 5% to 20% dose adjustment should be made to the total weekly maintenance dose and the degree of change based on the degree of INR abnormality. For OA, a 5% to 10% reduction in her weekly maintenance dose of 28 mg is warranted. This would entail a weekly dose reduction to 25 to 27 mg, which does not divide evenly into a daily dose. In these cases, designing a dosing regimen with variable doses on specific days allows us to achieve this goal. A regimen of warfarin 4 mg daily, except for 1 day, when she should take warfarin 2 mg, will deliver a total weekly dose of 26 mg. The patient should be instructed to take the reduced warfarin 2 mg dose that evening to start the new weekly regimen. She should return to clinic for a follow-up within 1 week.

TABLE 9.9   Pharmacokinetics of Direct Oral Anticoagulants

	DABIGATRAN	APIXABAN	EDOXABAN	RIVAROXABAN
F (%)	6.5	50	62	80
V_d (L)	50-70	23	>300	50
Protein binding (%)	35	87	55	90
$t_{1/2}$ (hr)	12-17	9-14	10-14	5-9
Renal elimination (%)	80	25	35-50	33
Metabolic pathway	P-gp	CYP3A4, P-gp	CYP3A4, P-gp	CYP3A4, P-gp

Select pharmacokinetic parameters of the direct oral anticoagulants.
P-gp, P-glycoprotein.

Question #8   *OA returns to her anticoagulation clinic 3 months later for follow-up. Her INR has been stable on her warfarin regimen of 4 mg daily, except 2 mg on Sundays. She endorses adherence to her warfarin regimen and no dietary changes. She notes that she was recently prescribed citalopram 10 mg daily, which she started taking that morning. Today's INR is 2.7. What changes should be made to her warfarin regimen?*

Clinicians managing patients on warfarin should routinely ask if the patient has started taking new medications, including any over-the-counter medications or herbal supplements. Such assessments are important to evaluate for possible drug interactions. In this case, citalopram may potentiate the effect of warfarin, and the INR may increase as a result. Preemptive dose adjustments to therapy are not recommended as it is difficult to predict the degree of change needed to maintain the INR in the therapeutic range. OA should be instructed to follow up in clinic in 1 week to assess for changes in INR owing to the recent initiation of citalopram.

Warfarin remains a challenging medication to manage for patients and clinicians. Patients requiring anticoagulant therapy should be assessed for ability to be treated with a DOAC. In general, the DOACs offer a more favorable pharmacokinetic and pharmacodynamic profile as compared to warfarin (Table 9.9).[114] These agents do not require monitoring for efficacy and are subject to fewer environmental (drug and food interactions) and genetic influences. There remain a number of disease states where limited data exist to support the use of DOACs and warfarin remains the optimal PO anticoagulant in those patients.

REFERENCES

1. Garcia DA, Baglin TP, Weitz JI, Samama MM. Parenteral anticoagulants: antithrombotic therapy and prevention of thrombosis, 9th ed: American College of Chest Physicians Evidence-Based Clinical Practice Guidelines. *Chest*. 2012;141(suppl 2):e24S-e43S. doi:10.1378/chest.11-2291

2. Ejaz U, Akhtar F, Xue J, Wan X, Zhang T, He S. Review: inhibitory potential of low molecular weight heparin in cell adhesion; emphasis on tumor metastasis. *Eur J Pharmacol*. 2021;892:173778. doi:10.1016/j.ejphar.2020.173778

3. Paschoa AF. Heparin: 100 years of pleiotropic effects. *J Thromb Thrombolysis*. 2016;41(4):636-43. doi:10.1007/s11239-015-1261-z

4. Qiu M, Huang S, Luo C, et al. Pharmacological and clinical application of heparin progress: an essential drug for modern medicine. *Biomed Pharmacother*. 2021;139:111561. doi:10.1016/j.biopha.2021.111561

5. Amsterdam EA, Wenger NK, Brindis RG, et al; ACC/AHA Task Force Members. 2014 AHA/ACC guideline for the management of patients with non-ST-elevation acute coronary syndromes: a report of the American College of Cardiology/American Heart Association Task Force on Practice Guidelines. *Circulation*. 2014;130(25):e344-e426. doi:10.1161/cir.0000000000000134

6. O'Gara PT, Kushner FG, Ascheim DD, et al. 2013 ACCF/AHA guideline for the management of ST-elevation myocardial infarction: a report of the American College of Cardiology Foundation/ American Heart Association Task Force on Practice Guidelines. *J Am Coll Cardiol*. 2013;61(4):e78-e140. doi:10.1016/j.jacc.2012.11.019

7. Olson JD, Arkin CF, Brandt JT, et al. College of American pathologists conference XXXI on laboratory monitoring of anticoagulant therapy: laboratory monitoring of unfractionated heparin therapy. *Arch Pathol Lab Med*. 1998;122(9):782-798.

8. Chiu HM, Hirsh J, Yung WL, Regoeczi E, Gent M. Relationship between the anticoagulant and antithrombotic effects of heparin in experimental venous thrombosis. *Blood*. 1977;49(2):171-84.

9. Kearon C, Kahn SR, Agnelli G, Goldhaber S, Raskob GE, Comerota AJ. Antithrombotic therapy for venous thromboembolic disease: American College of Chest Physicians Evidence-Based Clinical Practice Guidelines (8th Edition). *Chest*. 2008;133(suppl 6):454s-545s. doi:10.1378/chest.08-0658

10. Smythe MA, Priziola J, Dobesh PP, Wirth D, Cuker A, Wittkowsky AK. Guidance for the practical management of the heparin anticoagulants in the treatment of venous thromboembolism. *J Thromb Thrombolysis*. 2016;41(1):165-186. doi:10.1007/s11239-015-1315-2

11. Basu D, Gallus A, Hirsh J, Cade J. A prospective study of the value of monitoring heparin treatment with the activated partial thromboplastin time. *N Engl J Med*. 1972;287(7):324-327. doi:10.1056/nejm197208172870703

12. Kitchen S, Preston FE. The therapeutic range for heparin therapy: relationship between six activated partial thromboplastin time reagents and two heparin assays. *Thromb Haemost*. 1996;75(5):734-739.

13. Baker BA, Adelman MD, Smith PA, Osborn JC. Inability of the activated partial thromboplastin time to predict heparin levels. Time to reassess guidelines for heparin assays. *Arch Intern Med*. 1997;157(21):2475-2479.

14. Rosborough TK. Comparison of anti-factor Xa heparin activity and activated partial thromboplastin time in 2,773 plasma samples from unfractionated heparin-treated patients. *Am J Clin Pathol*. 1997;108(6):662-668. doi:10.1093/ajcp/108.6.662

15. Koerber JM, Smythe MA, Begle RL, Mattson JC, Kershaw BP, Westley SJ. Correlation of activated clotting time and activated partial thromboplastin time to plasma heparin concentration. *Pharmacotherapy*. 1999;19(8):922-931. doi:10.1592/phco.19.11.922.31573

16. Vandiver JW, Vondracek TG. A comparative trial of anti-factor Xa levels versus the activated partial thromboplastin time for heparin monitoring. *Hosp Pract (1995)*. 2013;41(2):16-24. doi:10.3810/hp.2013.04.1022

17. Guervil DJ, Rosenberg AF, Winterstein AG, Harris NS, Johns TE, Zumberg MS. Activated partial thromboplastin time versus antifactor Xa heparin assay in monitoring unfractionated heparin by continuous intravenous infusion. *Ann Pharmacother*. 2011;45(7-8):861-868. doi:10.1345/aph.1Q161

18. Frugé KS, Lee YR. Comparison of unfractionated heparin protocols using antifactor Xa monitoring or activated partial thrombin time monitoring. *Am J Health Syst Pharm*. 2015;72(17 suppl 2):S90-S97. doi:10.2146/sp150016

19. Samuel S, Allison TA, Sharaf S, et al. Antifactor Xa levels vs. activated partial thromboplastin time for monitoring unfractionated heparin. A pilot study. *J Clin Pharm Ther*. 2016;41(5):499-502. doi:10.1111/jcpt.12415

20. Whitman-Purves E, Coons JC, Miller T, et al. Performance of anti-factor Xa versus activated partial thromboplastin time for heparin monitoring using multiple nomograms. *Clin Appl Thromb Hemost*. 2018;24(2):310-316. doi:10.1177/1076029617741363

21. Coons JC, Iasella CJ, Thornberg M, et al. Clinical outcomes with unfractionated heparin monitored by anti-factor Xa vs. activated partial thromboplastin time. *Am J Hematol.* 2019;94(9):1015-1019. doi:10.1002/ajh.25565

22. Kindelin NM, Anthes AM, Providence SM, Zhao X, Aspinall SL. Effectiveness of a calculation-free weight-based unfractionated heparin nomogram with anti-Xa level monitoring compared with activated partial thromboplastin time. *Ann Pharmacother.* 2021;55(5):575-583. doi:10.1177/1060028020961503

23. Estes JW. Clinical pharmacokinetics of heparin. *Clin Pharmacokinet.* 1980;5(3):204-220. doi:10.2165/00003088-198005030-00002

24. Hirsh J, Raschke R. Heparin and low-molecular-weight heparin: the Seventh ACCP Conference on Antithrombotic and Thrombolytic Therapy. *Chest.* 2004;126(suppl 3):188s-203s. doi:10.1378/chest.126.3_suppl.188S

25. Bara L, Billaud E, Gramond G, Kher A, Samama M. Comparative pharmacokinetics of a low molecular weight heparin (PK 10 169) and unfractionated heparin after intravenous and subcutaneous administration. *Thromb Res.* 1985;39(5):631-636. doi:10.1016/0049-3848(85)90244-0

26. Dawes J, Prowse CV, Pepper DS. Absorption of heparin, LMW heparin and SP54 after subcutaneous injection, assessed by competitive binding assay. *Thromb Res.* 1986;44(5):683-693. doi:10.1016/0049-3848(86)90169-6

27. Halkin H, Goldberg J, Modan M, Modan B. Reduction of mortality in general medical in-patients by low-dose heparin prophylaxis. *Ann Intern Med.* 1982;96(5):561-565. doi:10.7326/0003-4819-96-5-561

28. Lijnen HR, Hoylaerts M, Collen D. Heparin binding properties of human histidine-rich glycoprotein. Mechanism and role in the neutralization of heparin in plasma. *J Biol Chem.* 1983;258(6):3803-3808.

29. Rucinski B, Niewiarowski S, Strzyzewski M, Holt JC, Mayo KH. Human platelet factor 4 and its C-terminal peptides: heparin binding and clearance from the circulation. *Thromb Haemost.* 1990;63(3):493-498.

30. Young E, Prins M, Levine MN, Hirsh J. Heparin binding to plasma proteins, an important mechanism for heparin resistance. *Thromb Haemost.* 1992;67(6):639-643.

31. Manson L, Weitz JI, Podor TJ, Hirsh J, Young E. The variable anticoagulant response to unfractionated heparin in vivo reflects binding to plasma proteins rather than clearance. *J Lab Clin Med.* 1997;130(6):649-655. doi:10.1016/s0022-2143(97)90115-3

32. Bârzu T, Van Rijn JL, Petitou M, Molho P, Tobelem G, Caen JP. Endothelial binding sites for heparin. Specificity and role in heparin neutralization. *Biochem J.* 1986;238(3):847-854. doi:10.1042/bj2380847

33. Friedman Y, Arsenis C. Studies on the heparin sulphamidase activity from rat spleen. Intracellular distribution and characterization of the enzyme. *Biochem J.* 1974;139(3):699-708. doi:10.1042/bj1390699

34. Simon TL, Hyers TM, Gaston JP, Harker LA. Heparin pharmacokinetics: increased requirements in pulmonary embolism. *Br J Haematol.* 1978;39(1):111-120. doi:10.1111/j.1365-2141.1978.tb07133.x

35. Feldschuh J, Enson Y. Prediction of the normal blood volume. Relation of blood volume to body habitus. *Circulation.* 1977;56(4 Pt 1):605-612. doi:10.1161/01.cir.56.4.605

36. Lemmens HJ, Bernstein DP, Brodsky JB. Estimating blood volume in obese and morbidly obese patients. *Obes Surg.* 2006;16(6):773-776. doi:10.1381/096089206777346673

37. Riney JN, Hollands JM, Smith JR, Deal EN. Identifying optimal initial infusion rates for unfractionated heparin in morbidly obese patients. *Ann Pharmacother.* 2010;44(7-8):1141-1151. doi:10.1345/aph.1P088

38. Shin S, Harthan EF. Safety and efficacy of the use of institutional unfractionated heparin protocols for therapeutic anticoagulation in obese patients: a retrospective chart review. *Blood Coagul Fibrinolysis.* 2015;26(6):655-660. doi:10.1097/mbc.0000000000000336

39. Isherwood M, Murphy ML, Bingham AL, Siemianowski LA, Hunter K, Hollands JM. Evaluation of safety and effectiveness of standardized antifactor Xa-based unfractionated heparin protocols in obese versus non-obese patients. *J Thromb Thrombolysis.* 2017;43(4):476-483. doi:10.1007/s11239-016-1466-9

40. Myzienski AE, Lutz MF, Smythe MA. Unfractionated heparin dosing for venous thromboembolism in morbidly obese patients: case report and review of the literature. *Pharmacotherapy.* 2010;30(3):324. doi:10.1592/phco.30.3.324

41. Fan J, John B, Tesdal E. Evaluation of heparin dosing based on adjusted body weight in obese patients. *Am J Health Syst Pharm.* 2016;73(19):1512-1522. doi:10.2146/ajhp150388

42. Hosch LM, Breedlove EY, Scono LE, Knoderer CA. Evaluation of an unfractionated heparin pharmacy dosing protocol for the treatment of venous thromboembolism in nonobese, obese, and severely obese patients. *Ann Pharmacother.* 2017;51(9):768-773. doi:10.1177/1060028017709819

43. Hirsh J, van Aken WG, Gallus AS, Dollery CT, Cade JF, Yung WL. Heparin kinetics in venous thrombosis and pulmonary embolism. *Circulation.* 1976;53(4):691-695. doi:10.1161/01.cir.53.4.691

44. Beermann B, Lahnborg G. Pharmacokinetics of heparin in healthy and obese subjects and in combination with dihydroergotamine. *Thromb Haemost.* 1981;45(1):24-26.

45. Cipolle RJ, Seifert RD, Neilan BA, Zaske DE, Haus E. Heparin kinetics: variables related to disposition and dosage. *Clin Pharmacol Ther.* 1981;29(3):387-393. doi:10.1038/clpt.1981.53

46. Olsson P, Lagergren H, Ek S. The elimination from plasma of intravenous heparin. An experimental study on dogs and humans. *Acta Med Scand.* 1963;173:619-630. doi:10.1111/j.0954-6820.1963.tb17446.x

47. Bjornsson TD, Wolfram KM, Kitchell BB. Heparin kinetics determined by three assay methods. *Clin Pharmacol Ther.* 1982;31(1):104-113. doi:10.1038/clpt.1982.16

48. de Swart CA, Nijmeyer B, Roelofs JM, Sixma JJ. Kinetics of intravenously administered heparin in normal humans. *Blood.* 1982;60(6):1251-1258.

49. Dager W, Gulseth M, Nutescu E. *Anticoagulation Therapy: A Point-of-Care Guide.* American Society of Health-System Pharmacists, Inc.; 2011.

50. Cuker A, Arepally GM, Chong BH, et al. American Society of Hematology 2018 guidelines for management of venous thromboembolism: heparin-induced thrombocytopenia. *Blood Adv.* 2018;2(22):3360-3392. doi:10.1182/bloodadvances.2018024489

51. Chenella FC, Gill MA, Kern JW, Floyd RA, McGehee WG. Improved methods for estimating initial heparin infusion rates. *Am J Hosp Pharm.* 1979;36(6):782-784.

52. Joch LE, Lutomski DM, Williams DJ, Bottorff M. Accuracy of a first-order model for estimating initial heparin dosage. *Clin Pharm.* 1993;12(8):597-601.

53. Groce JB, III, Gal P, Douglas JB, Steuterman MC. Heparin dosage adjustment in patients with deep-vein thrombosis using heparin concentrations rather than activated partial thromboplastin time. *Clin Pharm.* 1987;6(3):216-222.

54. Kandrotas RJ, Gal P, Douglas JB, Groce JB, III. Rapid determination of maintenance heparin infusion rates with the use of non-steady-state heparin concentrations. *Ann Pharmacother.* 1993;27(12):1429-1433. doi:10.1177/106002809302701201

55. Chiou WL, Gadalla MA, Peng GW. Method for the rapid estimation of the total body drug clearance and adjustment of dosage regimens in patients during a constant-rate intravenous infusion. *J Pharmacokinet Biopharm.* 1978;6(2):135-151. doi:10.1007/bf01117448

56. Allen TH, Peng MT, Chen KP, Huang TF, Chang C, Fang HS. Prediction of blood volume and adiposity in man from body weight and cube of height. *Metabolism.* 1956;5(3):328-345.

57. Saya FG, Coleman LT, Martinoff JT. Pharmacist-directed heparin therapy using a standard dosing and monitoring protocol. *Am J Hosp Pharm.* 1985;42(9):1965-1969.

58. Cruickshank MK, Levine MN, Hirsh J, Roberts R, Siguenza M. A standard heparin nomogram for the management of heparin therapy. *Arch Intern Med.* 1991;151(2):333-337.

59. Hull RD, Raskob GE, Rosenbloom D, et al. Optimal therapeutic level of heparin therapy in patients with venous thrombosis. *Arch Intern Med.* 1992;152(8):1589-1595.

60. Rivey MP, Peterson JP. Pharmacy-managed, weight-based heparin protocol. *Am J Hosp Pharm.* 1993;50(2):279-284.

61. Elliott CG, Hiltunen SJ, Suchyta M, et al. Physician-guided treatment compared with a heparin protocol for deep vein thrombosis. *Arch Intern Med.* 1994;154(9):999-1004.

62. Gunnarsson PS, Sawyer WT, Montague D, Williams ML, Dupuis RE, Caiola SM. Appropriate use of heparin. Empiric vs nomogram-based dosing. *Arch Intern Med.* 1995;155(5):526-532.

63. Hollingsworth JA, Rowe BH, Brisebois FJ, Thompson PR, Fabris LM. The successful application of a heparin nomogram in a community hospital. *Arch Intern Med.* 1995;155(19):2095-2100.

64. Raschke RA, Reilly BM, Guidry JR, Fontana JR, Srinivas S. The weight-based heparin dosing nomogram compared with a "standard care" nomogram. A randomized controlled trial. *Ann Intern Med.* 1993;119(9):874-881. doi:10.7326/0003-4819-119-9-199311010-00002

65. Raschke RA, Gollihare B, Peirce JC. The effectiveness of implementing the weight-based heparin no-mogram as a practice guideline. *Arch Intern Med.* 1996;156(15):1645-1649.

66. de Groot MR, Büller HR, ten Cate JW, van Marwijk Kooy M. Use of a heparin nomogram for treatment of patients with venous thromboembolism in a community hospital. *Thromb Haemost.* 1998;80(1):70-73.

67. Bernardi E, Piccioli A, Oliboni G, Zuin R, Girolami A, Prandoni P. Nomograms for the administration of unfractionated heparin in the initial treatment of acute thromboembolism—an overview. *Thromb Haemost.* 2000;84(1):22-26.

68. Levy JH, Connors JM. Heparin resistance–clinical perspectives and management strategies. *N Engl J Med.* 2021;385(9):826-832. doi:10.1056/NEJMra2104091

69. Levine MN, Hirsh J, Gent M, et al. A randomized trial comparing activated thromboplastin time with heparin assay in patients with acute venous thromboembolism requiring large daily doses of heparin. *Arch Intern Med.* 1994;154(1):49-56.

70. Spiess BD. Treating heparin resistance with antithrombin or fresh frozen plasma. *Ann Thorac Surg.* 2008;85(6):2153-2160. doi:10.1016/j.athoracsur.2008.02.037

71. Hirsh J, Levine MN. Low molecular weight heparin. *Blood.* 1992;79(1):1-17.

72. McCart GM, Kayser SR. Therapeutic equivalency of low-molecular-weight heparins. *Ann Pharmaco-ther.* 2002;36(6):1042-1057. doi:10.1345/aph.10264

73. Gray E, Mulloy B, Barrowcliffe TW. Heparin and low-molecular-weight heparin. *Thromb Haemost.* 2008;99(5):807-818. doi:10.1160/th08-01-0032

74. Jeske W, Wolf H, Ahsan A, Fareed J. Pharmacologic profile of certoparin. *Expert Opin Investig Drugs.* 1999;8(3):315-327. doi:10.1517/13543784.8.3.315

75. Frydman A. Low-molecular-weight heparins: an overview of their pharmacodynamics, pharmacoki-netics and metabolism in humans. *Haemostasis.* 1996;26(suppl 2):24-38. doi:10.1159/000217270

76. Samama MM, Gerotziafas GT. Comparative pharmacokinetics of LMWHs. *Semin Thromb Hemost.* 2000;26(suppl 1):31-38. doi:10.1055/s-2000-9497

77. Andrassy K, Eschenfelder V, Koderisch J, Weber E. Pharmacokinetics of clivarin a new low mo-lecular weight heparin in healthy volunteers. *Thromb Res.* 1994;73(2):95-108. doi:10.1016/0049-3848(94)90084-1

78. Laposata M, Green D, Van Cott EM, Barrowcliffe TW, Goodnight SH, Sosolik RC. College of Ameri-can Pathologists Conference XXXI on laboratory monitoring of anticoagulant therapy: the clinical use and laboratory monitoring of low-molecular-weight heparin, danaparoid, hirudin and related com-pounds, and argatroban. *Arch Pathol Lab Med.* 1998;122(9):799-807.

79. Bates SM, Rajasekhar A, Middeldorp S, et al. American Society of Hematology 2018 guidelines for management of venous thromboembolism: venous thromboembolism in the context of pregnancy. *Blood Adv.* 2018;2(22):3317-3359. doi:10.1182/bloodadvances.2018024802

80. Witt DM, Nieuwlaat R, Clark NP, et al. American Society of Hematology 2018 guidelines for man-agement of venous thromboembolism: optimal management of anticoagulation therapy. *Blood Adv.* 2018;2(22):3257-3291. doi:10.1182/bloodadvances.2018024893

81. Dryjski M, Schneider DE, Mojaverian P, Kuo BS, Bjornsson TD. Investigations on plasma activity of low molecular weight heparin after intravenous and oral administrations. *Br J Clin Pharmacol.* 1989;28(2):188-192. doi:10.1111/j.1365-2125.1989.tb05415.x

82. Priglinger U, Delle Karth G, Geppert A, et al. Prophylactic anticoagulation with enoxaparin: is the sub-cutaneous route appropriate in the critically ill? *Crit Care Med.* 2003;31(5):1405-1409. doi:10.1097/01.Ccm.0000059725.60509.A0

83. Dörffler-Melly J, de Jonge E, Pont AC, et al. Bioavailability of subcutaneous low-molecular-weight hep-arin to patients on vasopressors. *Lancet.* 2002;359(9309):849-850. doi:10.1016/s0140-6736(02)07920-5

84. Nutescu EA, Spinler SA, Wittkowsky A, Dager WE. Low-molecular-weight heparins in renal impair-ment and obesity: available evidence and clinical practice recommendations across medical and surgi-cal settings. *Ann Pharmacother.* 2009;43(6):1064-1083. doi:10.1345/aph.1L194

85. Sebaaly J, Covert K. Enoxaparin dosing at extremes of weight: literature review and dosing recommen-dations. *Ann Pharmacother.* 2018;52(9):898-909. doi:10.1177/1060028018768449

86. Wang TF, Milligan PE, Wong CA, Deal EN, Thoelke MS, Gage BF. Efficacy and safety of high-dose thromboprophylaxis in morbidly obese inpatients. *Thromb Haemost.* 2014;111(1):88-93. doi:10.1160/th13-01-0042

87. Rojas L, Aizman A, Ernst D, et al. Anti-Xa activity after enoxaparin prophylaxis in hospitalized patients weighing less than fifty-five kilograms. *Thromb Res.* 2013;132(6):761-764. doi:10.1016/j.thromres.2013.10.005

88. Yam L, Bahjri K, Geslani V, Cotton A, Hong L. Enoxaparin thromboprophylaxis dosing and anti-factor Xa levels in low-weight patients. *Pharmacotherapy.* 2019;39(7):749-755. doi:10.1002/phar.2295

89. Becker RC, Spencer FA, Gibson M, et al. Influence of patient characteristics and renal function on factor Xa inhibition pharmacokinetics and pharmacodynamics after enoxaparin administration in non-ST-segment elevation acute coronary syndromes. *Am Heart J.* 2002;143(5):753-759. doi:10.1067/mhj.2002.120774

90. Brophy DF, Wazny LD, Gehr TW, Comstock TJ, Venitz J. The pharmacokinetics of subcutaneous enoxaparin in end-stage renal disease. *Pharmacotherapy.* 2001;21(2):169-174. doi:10.1592/phco.21.2.169.34113

91. Sanderink GJ, Guimart CG, Ozoux ML, Jariwala NU, Shukla UA, Boutouyrie BX. Pharmacokinetics and pharmacodynamics of the prophylactic dose of enoxaparin once daily over 4 days in patients with renal impairment. *Thromb Res.* 2002;105(3):225-231. doi:10.1016/s0049-3848(02)00031-2

92. Goudable C, Ton That H, Damani A, et al. Low molecular weight heparin half life is prolonged in haemodialysed patients. *Thromb Res.* 1986;43(1):1-5. doi:10.1016/0049-3848(86)90039-3

93. Monagle P, Michelson AD, Bovill E, Andrew M. Antithrombotic therapy in children. *Chest.* 2001;119(suppl 1):344S-370S. doi:10.1378/chest.119.1_suppl.344s

94. Powell J, Taylor J, Garland SG. Andexanet alfa: a novel factor Xa inhibitor reversal agent. *Ann Pharmacother.* 2019;53(9):940-946. doi:10.1177/1060028019835209

95. Ageno W, Gallus AS, Wittkowsky A, Crowther M, Hylek EM, Palareti G. Oral anticoagulant therapy: antithrombotic therapy and prevention of thrombosis, 9th ed: American College of Chest Physicians Evidence-Based Clinical Practice Guidelines. *Chest.* 2012;141(suppl 2):e44S-e88S. doi:10.1378/chest.11-2292

96. Kirkwood TB. Calibration of reference thromboplastins and standardisation of the prothrombin time ratio. *Thromb Haemost.* 1983;49(3):238-244.

97. Fairweather RB, Ansell J, van den Besselaar AM, et al. College of American Pathologists Conference XXXI on laboratory monitoring of anticoagulant therapy: laboratory monitoring of oral anticoagulant therapy. *Arch Pathol Lab Med.* 1998;122(9):768-781.

98. Breckenridge A, Orme M, Wesseling H, Lewis RJ, Gibbons R. Pharmacokinetics and pharmacodynamics of the enantiomers of warfarin in man. *Clin Pharmacol Ther.* 1974;15(4):424-430. doi:10.1002/cpt1974154424

99. Holford NH. Clinical pharmacokinetics and pharmacodynamics of warfarin. Understanding the dose-effect relationship. *Clin Pharmacokinet.* 1986;11(6):483-504. doi:10.2165/00003088-198611060-00005

100. Klang M, Graham D, McLymont V. Warfarin bioavailability with feeding tubes and enteral formula. *JPEN J Parenter Enteral Nutr.* 2010;34(3):300-304. doi:10.1177/0148607109337257

101. Chan E, McLachlan AJ, Pegg M, MacKay AD, Cole RB, Rowland M. Disposition of warfarin enantiomers and metabolites in patients during multiple dosing with rac-warfarin. *Br J Clin Pharmacol.* 1994;37(6):563-569. doi:10.1111/j.1365-2125.1994.tb04305.x

102. Takahashi H, Echizen H. Pharmacogenetics of warfarin elimination and its clinical implications. *Clin Pharmacokinet.* 2001;40(8):587-603. doi:10.2165/00003088-200140080-00003

103. Gulyassy PF, Depner TA. Impaired binding of drugs and endogenous ligands in renal diseases. *Am J Kidney Dis.* 1983;2(6):578-601. doi:10.1016/s0272-6386(83)80038-9

104. Sakaan SA, Hudson JQ, Oliphant CS, et al. Evaluation of warfarin dose requirements in patients with chronic kidney disease and end-stage renal disease. *Pharmacotherapy.* 2014;34(7):695-702. doi:10.1002/phar.1445

105. MacLeod SM, Sellers EM. Pharmacodynamic and pharmacokinetic drug interactions with coumarin anticoagulants. *Drugs.* 1976;11(6):461-470. doi:10.2165/00003495-197611060-00006

106. Sands CD, Chan ES, Welty TE. Revisiting the significance of warfarin protein-binding displacement interactions. *Ann Pharmacother.* 2002;36(10):1642-1644. doi:10.1345/aph.1A208

107. Kelly JG, O'Malley K. Clinical pharmacokinetics of oral anticoagulants. *Clin Pharmacokinet.* 1979;4(1):1-15. doi:10.2165/00003088-197904010-00001

108. Holbrook A, Schulman S, Witt DM, et al. Evidence-based management of anticoagulant therapy: antithrombotic therapy and prevention of thrombosis, 9th ed: American College of Chest Physicians Evidence-Based Clinical Practice Guidelines. *Chest.* 2012;141(suppl 2):e152S-e184S. doi:10.1378/chest.11-2295

109. Nazarian RM, Van Cott EM, Zembowicz A, Duncan LM. Warfarin-induced skin necrosis. *J Am Acad Dermatol.* 2009;61(2):325-332. doi:10.1016/j.jaad.2008.12.039

110. Talmadge DB, Spyropoulos AC. Purple toes syndrome associated with warfarin therapy in a patient with antiphospholipid syndrome. *Pharmacotherapy.* 2003;23(5):674-677. doi:10.1592/phco.23.5.674.32200

111. O'Reilly RA, Aggeler PM. Studies on coumarin anticoagulant drugs. Initiation of warfarin therapy without a loading dose. *Circulation.* 1968;38(1):169-177. doi:10.1161/01.cir.38.1.169

112. Harrison L, Johnston M, Massicotte MP, Crowther M, Moffat K, Hirsh J. Comparison of 5-mg and 10-mg loading doses in initiation of warfarin therapy. *Ann Intern Med.* 1997;126(2):133-136. doi:10.7326/0003-4819-126-2-199701150-00006

113. Dager WE. Initiating warfarin therapy. *Ann Pharmacother.* 2003;37(6):905-908. doi:10.1345/aph.1D038

114. Nutescu EA, Burnett A, Fanikos J, Spinler S, Wittkowsky A. Pharmacology of anticoagulants used in the treatment of venous thromboembolism. *J Thromb Thrombolysis.* 2016;41(1):15-31. doi:10.1007/s11239-015-1314-3

115. Johnson JA, Caudle KE, Gong L, et al. Clinical Pharmacogenetics Implementation Consortium (CPIC) guideline for pharmacogenetics-guided warfarin dosing: 2017 update. *Clin Pharmacol Ther.* 2017;102(3):397-404. doi:10.1002/cpt.668

116. *Coumadin (warfarin)* [package insert]. Princeton, NJ: Bristol-Myers Squibb Company. https://www.accessdata.fda.gov/drugsatfda_docs/label/2011/009218s107lbl.pdf. October 2011. Accessed June 3, 2023.

117. Klein TE, Altman RB, Eriksson N, et al. Estimation of the warfarin dose with clinical and pharmacogenetic data. *N Engl J Med.* 2009;360(8):753-764. doi:10.1056/NEJMoa0809329

118. Gage BF, Eby C, Johnson JA, et al. Use of pharmacogenetic and clinical factors to predict the therapeutic dose of warfarin. *Clin Pharmacol Ther.* 2008;84(3):326-331. doi:10.1038/clpt.2008.10

119. Kimmel SE, French B, Kasner SE, et al. A pharmacogenetic versus a clinical algorithm for warfarin dosing. *N Engl J Med.* 2013;369(24):2283-2293. doi:10.1056/NEJMoa1310669

120. Verhoef TI, Ragia G, de Boer A, et al. A randomized trial of genotype-guided dosing of acenocoumarol and phenprocoumon. *N Engl J Med.* 2013;369(24):2304-2312. doi:10.1056/NEJMoa1311388

121. Pirmohamed M, Burnside G, Eriksson N, et al. A randomized trial of genotype-guided dosing of warfarin. *N Engl J Med.* 2013;369(24):2294-2303. doi:10.1056/NEJMoa1311386

122. Jähnchen E, Meinertz T, Gilfrich HJ, Kersting F, Groth U. Enhanced elimination of warfarin during treatment with cholestyramine. *Br J Clin Pharmacol.* 1978;5(5):437-440. doi:10.1111/j.1365-2125.1978.tb01651.x

123. Mungall D, Talbert RL, Phillips C, Jaffe D, Ludden TM. Sucralfate and warfarin. *Ann Intern Med.* 1983;98(4):557. doi:10.7326/0003-4819-98-4-557_2

124. Benet LZ, Hoener BA. Changes in plasma protein binding have little clinical relevance. *Clin Pharmacol Ther.* 2002;71(3):115-121. doi:10.1067/mcp.2002.121829

125. Vazquez SR. Drug-drug interactions in an era of multiple anticoagulants: a focus on clinically relevant drug interactions. *Blood.* 2018;132(21):2230-2239. doi:10.1182/blood-2018-06-848747

126. Thi L, Shaw D, Bird J. Warfarin potentiation: a review of the "FAB-4" significant drug interactions. *Consult Pharm.* 2009;24(3):227-230. doi:10.4140/tcp.n.2009.227

127. Sanoski CA, Bauman JL. Clinical observations with the amiodarone/warfarin interaction: dosing relationships with long-term therapy. *Chest.* 2002;121(1):19-23. doi:10.1378/chest.121.1.19

128. Holm J, Lindh JD, Andersson ML, Mannheimer B. The effect of amiodarone on warfarin anticoagulation: a register-based nationwide cohort study involving the Swedish population. *J Thromb Haemost.* 2017;15(3):446-453. doi:10.1111/jth.13614

129. MacDougall C, Canonica T, Keh C, BA PP, Louie J. Systematic review of drug-drug interactions between rifamycins and anticoagulant and antiplatelet agents and considerations for management. *Pharmacotherapy.* 2022;42(4):343-361. doi:10.1002/phar.2672

130. Mannheimer B, Andersson ML, Järnbert-Pettersson H, Lindh JD. The effect of carbamazepine on warfarin anticoagulation: a register-based nationwide cohort study involving the Swedish population. *J Thromb Haemost.* 2016;14(4):765-771. doi:10.1111/jth.13268

131. Holbrook AM, Pereira JA, Labiris R, et al. Systematic overview of warfarin and its drug and food interactions. *Arch Intern Med.* 2005;165(10):1095-1106. doi:10.1001/archinte.165.10.1095

132. Michalets EL. Update: clinically significant cytochrome P-450 drug interactions. *Pharmacotherapy.* 1998;18(1):84-112.

133. Krajewski KC. Inability to achieve a therapeutic INR value while on concurrent warfarin and rifampin. *J Clin Pharmacol.* 2010;50(6):710-713. doi:10.1177/0091270009353030

134. Ahmed A, Stephens JC, Kaus CA, Fay WP. Impact of preemptive warfarin dose reduction on anticoagulation after initiation of trimethoprim-sulfamethoxazole or levofloxacin. *J Thromb Thrombolysis.* 2008;26(1):44-48. doi:10.1007/s11239-007-0164-z

135. Holt RK, Anderson EA, Cantrell MA, Shaw RF, Egge JA. Preemptive dose reduction of warfarin in patients initiating metronidazole. *Drug Metabol Drug Interact.* 2010;25(1-4):35-39. doi:10.1515/dmdi.2010.002

136. Powers A, Loesch EB, Weiland A, Fioravanti N, Lucius D. Preemptive warfarin dose reduction after initiation of sulfamethoxazole-trimethoprim or metronidazole. *J Thromb Thrombolysis.* 2017;44(1):88-93. doi:10.1007/s11239-017-1497-x

137. Kumbhani DJ, Cannon CP, Beavers CJ, et al. 2020 ACC expert consensus decision pathway for anticoagulant and antiplatelet therapy in patients with atrial fibrillation or venous thromboembolism undergoing percutaneous coronary intervention or with atherosclerotic cardiovascular disease: a report of the american college of cardiology solution set oversight committee. *J Am Coll Cardiol.* 2021;77(5):629-658. doi:10.1016/j.jacc.2020.09.011

138. Greenblatt DJ, von Moltke LL. Interaction of warfarin with drugs, natural substances, and foods. *J Clin Pharmacol.* 2005;45(2):127-132. doi:10.1177/0091270004271404

139. U.S. Department of Agriculture, Agricultural Research Service. FoodData Central. https://fdc.nal .usda.gov/. Accessed 2022.

140. White RH, McKittrick T, Hutchinson R, Twitchell J. Temporary discontinuation of warfarin therapy: changes in the international normalized ratio. *Ann Intern Med.* 1995;122(1):40-42. doi:10.7326/0003-4819-122-1-199501010-00006

141. Hirsh J, Fuster V, Ansell J, Halperin JL. American Heart Association/American College of Cardiology Foundation guide to warfarin therapy. *J Am Coll Cardiol.* 2003;41(9):1633-1652. doi:10.1016/s0735-1097(03)00416-9

142. Tomaselli GF, Mahaffey KW, Cuker A, et al. 2020 ACC expert consensus decision pathway on management of bleeding in patients on oral anticoagulants: a report of the American College of Cardiology Solution Set Oversight Committee. *J Am Coll Cardiol.* 2020;76(5):594-622. doi:10.1016/j.jacc.2020.04.053

10

ANTIFUNGAL AGENTS: TRIAZOLES

Russell E. Lewis

Learning Objectives

By the end of the antifungal agents: triazoles chapter, the learner shall be able to:

1. Compare and contrast the main causes of pharmacokinetic (PK) variability among triazole antifungals that could jeopardize the efficacy and/or safety of treatment.
2. Identify specific factors for each triazole antifungal and formulation that may predispose patients to PK interactions.
3. Describe strategies of how triazole antifungal dosing can be optimized when inadequate drug exposures are identified by therapeutic drug monitoring.

Invasive fungal diseases are a major cause of morbidity and mortality in the immunocompromised patients, causing an estimated 1.5 million deaths per year—a figure that surpasses the number of deaths as a result of either tuberculosis or malaria.[1] Although diagnostic advances and new antifungal agents have improved outcomes in recent years, mortality rates still approach 25% to 50% for the most commonly encountered invasive fungal infections and result in prolonged hospitalization or delays in life-saving chemotherapy or transplantation for malignancy or organ failure.

For over 40 years, amphotericin B deoxycholate was the only reliable antifungal treatment for invasive yeast and mold infections. Its effectiveness is compromised by frequent infusion-related reactions and nephrotoxicity that may require interruption of treatment. During the 1990s, amphotericin B was reformulated into lipid or liposomal carriers to improve the drug's tolerability profile, but nephrotoxicity is still encountered with prolonged therapy, in patients with preexisting renal disease, or those patients receiving multiple concomitant nephrotoxic therapies.

The introduction of triazoles antifungals provided the first possibility of treating serious fungal infections without dose-limiting nephrotoxicity. Triazole antifungals were also the first class of antifungals approved for use in both oral and intravenous

(IV) formulations, thus allowing patients to continue their treatment outside the hospital without a central venous catheter (Table 10.1).

As a result, triazoles are now the most widely prescribed class of antifungal agents despite some limitations. First, all triazole antifungals arrest fungal cell growth by inhibiting a key fungal cytochrome (CY) P450 enzyme (14α-demethylase) that converts lanosterol to the fungal cell membrane sterol ergosterol. This mechanism is not entirely selective for fungi, because all triazoles also inhibit, to varying degrees human CYP450 enzymes involved in the metabolism of thousands of endogenous and exogenous chemicals.[2] Consequently, triazole therapy places patients at risk for many pharmacokinetic (PK) drug-drug interactions.

A second limitation of triazole pharmacology is that binding affinity to 14α-demethylase depends on the lipophilic nature of the molecule. Chemical modifications designed to broaden the spectrum of triazole antifungals produce molecules with large volume of distribution, complex biotransformation (metabolism) profiles, and poorer bioavailability.

Collectively, these characteristics and potential for drug interactions mean that triazole PKs can be unpredictable in patients, even if dosing is standardized to body weight. In some cases, this PK variability has been shown to jeopardize the effectiveness

TABLE 10.1   Systemic Antifungals Timeline of Introduction

SITE OF ACTION IN FUNGI	MECHANISM	DRUG (YEAR INTRODUCED)

Cell membrane	Ergosterol binding	Polyene antifungals
		  Amphotericin B (1958)
		  Amphotericin B lipid complex (1995)
		  Liposomal amphotericin B (1996)

	Ergosterol synthesis inhibition (14α-demethylase)	Imidazoles Ketoconazole (1981)

		Triazoles
		  Fluconazole (1990)
		  Itraconazole (1992)
		  Voriconazole (2002)
		  Posaconazole (2006)
		  Isavuconazole (2015)

Cell wall	β-Glucan synthesis inhibition (β-1,3-D-Glucan synthase)	Echinocandins
		  Caspofungin (2001)
		  Micafungin (2005)
		  Anidulafungin (2007)
		  Ibrexafungerp (2021)
		  Rezafungin

Intracellular	Pyrimidine analogs/ thymidylate synthase inhibitor	Flucytosine (1971)

and safety of treatment for invasive fungal diseases, suggesting that some patients could benefit from therapeutic drug monitoring (TDM).[3] This chapter focuses on the PK characteristics of triazole antifungals with particular emphasis on agents that potentially require TDM in patients at risk or documented to have invasive fungal disease.

Fluconazole

Fluconazole was the first triazole antifungal developed for clinical use. It is a relatively small (molecular weight 306 g/mol) hydrophilic molecule (log P 0.58) that is a reversible inhibitor of fungal 14α-demethylase. Fluconazole is the narrowest-spectrum triazole antifungal with activity primarily against yeast (*Candida* and *Cryptococcus* spp.), some activity against endemic (dimorphic) fungi, including *Coccidioides immitis*, *Coccidioides posadasii*, and *Blastomyces dermatitidis*, but no clinically useful activity against molds such as *Aspergillus* spp., *Fusarium* spp., or Mucorales. Fluconazole is used for the treatment of mucocutaneous *Candida* infections, *Candida* urinary tract infections, or as a step-down (second-line) regimen for invasive candidiasis after initial echinocandin treatment if susceptibility of the isolate is confirmed.[4] Fluconazole is also administered as prophylaxis for mucocutaneous and invasive candidiasis in some high-risk immunocompromised populations.

THERAPEUTIC RANGE OF FLUCONAZOLE

Fluconazole exhibits concentration- and time-dependent antifungal activity with a prolonged postantifungal effect. The ratio of free drug area under the concentration-time curve from 0 to 24 hours to minimum inhibitory concentration ($fAUC_{0-24hr}/MIC$) is considered the PK/pharmacodynamic (PD) index predictive of antifungal activity.[5] An AUC_{0-24hr}/MIC of 50 is associated with fungistatic activity, with optimal outcomes in immunocompromised or critically ill patients reported as $fAUC_{0-24hr}/MIC$ approaches 100.[6] Based on current susceptibility breakpoints for *Candida* spp., an AUC 400 mg·hr/L (equivalent to a C_{min} >10-15 mg/L) is recommended. Currently, there are insufficient data linking target serum fluconazole concentrations to the development of toxicities.

BIOAVAILABILITY (F)

Fluconazole is available in both IV and oral formulations (tablet and suspensions). The oral bioavailability of fluconazole is excellent (>90%) and not appreciably affected by food or gastric pH. Fluconazole achieves peak concentrations in the serum within 1 to 2 hours after oral administration.

VOLUME OF DISTRIBUTION (V)

Fluconazole is widely distributed throughout the body with a volume of distribution of approximately 0.7 L/kg and good penetration into the cerebrospinal fluid (50%-90% of serum levels depending on meningeal inflammation), eye, peritoneal fluid, sputum, skin, and urine.[7]

CLEARANCE (Cl)

Fluconazole is largely excreted unchanged (>80%) through the kidneys but undergoes partial metabolism (11%) through CYP3A4 to an inactive N-oxide and glucuronide metabolites that are excreted in the urine. Fluconazole has predictable dose-proportional linear PKs with a nearly 1:1 relationship between the daily dose of fluconazole (in mg) and the observed serum AUC in patients with normal renal function and average body habitus. As a result, fluconazole dose/MIC is occasionally used as a surrogate for AUC/MIC in PD calculations.

The typical total body clearance rate of fluconazole in adult patients is 0.23 mL/min/kg. Fluconazole clearance in pediatric patients is more rapid (0.4-0.6 mL/min/kg), resulting in a shorter half-life. Using the following standard PK equation (Equation 10.1), the predicted half-life is approximately 35 hours in adults and 16 to 20 hours in children.[8]

$$t_{1/2} = \frac{0.693 \times V_d}{Cl} \qquad \text{(Eq. 10.1)}$$

Fluconazole doses are adjusted in patients with renal dysfunction. In patients with estimated glomerular filtration rate (GFR) of 50 to 80 mL/min, normal doses are recommended. If the GFR is 10 to 50 mL/min or less than 10 mL/min, then 50% of the daily dose is administered. The clearance of fluconazole (Equation 10.3) can be predicted in patients with renal impairment in relation to the estimated (Equation 10.2) or measured (Equation 10.4) creatinine clearance using the following equations:

$$\frac{G \times (140 - Age) \times Weight\ (kg)}{Serum\ creatinine\ (mg/dL) \times 72} \quad G = 1(male),\ 0.85(female) \qquad \text{(Eq. 10.2)}$$

$$Cl/F\ (mL/min/kg) = 0.064 + 0.003 \times Cockcroft\ and\ Gault\ Cl_{Cr}\ (mL/min) \qquad \text{(Eq. 10.3)}$$

$$Cl/F\ (mL/min/kg) = 0.129 + 0.002 \times Measured\ Cl_{Cr}\ (mL/min) \qquad \text{(Eq. 10.4)}$$

Fluconazole is removed by dialysis, but the dosing recommendations vary depending on the type of dialysis. In patients receiving intermitted hemodialysis, 100% of a daily dose is administered after hemodialysis, or 50% of the dose is administered every 24 hours after the dialysis session. Similarly, for peritoneal dialysis, 50% of the fluconazole dose is administered daily. In patients undergoing hemofiltration, 200 to 400 mg of fluconazole is recommended once daily for patients undergoing continuous venovenous hemofiltration (CVVH). In patients undergoing continuous venovenous hemodialysis (CVVHD) or continuous venovenous hemodiafiltration (CVVHDF), 400 to 800 mg/d of fluconazole is recommended; however, higher doses may be required depending on the dialysis flow rate.

KEY PARAMETERS: Fluconazole[a]

THERAPEUTIC CONCENTRATIONS	C_{min} >10-15 mg/L
F[b]	90%
V_d[c]	0.6-0.8 L/kg
Cl	0.97 L/hr
AUC_{0-24hr}[d]	350 mg·hr/L
$t_{1/2}$ in adults	35 hr
fu (fraction unbound)	89%

[a]Pharmacokinetic parameters may vary depending on patient characteristics and renal function.
[b]Bioavailability not affected by gastric pH or food.
[c]Widely distributed throughout body tissues and fluids such as the kidney, skin, saliva, sputum, nail, blister fluid, and prostate. Cerebrospinal fluid penetration is 50%-94% of concurrent serum concentrations.
[d]400 mg daily dose.

Depending on the treatment indication, doses of fluconazole typically range from 400 to 800 mg daily for invasive fungal diseases. The recommended dose for patients with invasive candidiasis is a 12 mg/kg loading dose on day 1, followed by 6 mg/kg once daily. Administration of weight-based loading and maintenance doses is recommended for bloodstream candidiasis because the infection can progress to sepsis with marked changes in patient volume of distribution, resulting in subtherapeutic fluconazole exposures. Indeed, PK point-prevalence studies of intensive care unit patients in Europe have reported that one-third of patients do not achieve therapeutic fluconazole exposures largely because fixed 200 or 400 mg daily doses are administered without loading doses, irrespective of patient weight.[9] The excellent bioavailability of the tablet and suspension formulations of fluconazole allows easy IV to oral switching when patients are clinically stable. Fluconazole is a recommended "step-down" narrowest-spectrum therapy of choice for patients who were previously receiving an echinocandin for the treatment of invasive candidiasis, provided the susceptibility of the infecting isolate to fluconazole is confirmed.[4]

PHARMACOKINETIC DRUG INTERACTIONS

Fluconazole is a potent inhibitor of CYP2C9 and CYP2C19 and a moderate inhibitor of CYP3A4. Inhibiting effects may persist for 4 to 5 days after discontinuation owing to the long half-life of fluconazole.[2] Fluconazole is also a substrate of CYP3A4. Strong inducers of CYP3A4 (ie, rifampin) will increase the nonrenal clearance of fluconazole, potentially resulting in subtherapeutic exposures.[10] Drug-drug interactions are often dose dependent, with stronger effects observed at higher fluconazole doses.[2] Fluconazole must be used with caution when other drugs are metabolized via CYP450 enzymes.

ADVERSE EFFECTS

Fluconazole is generally well tolerated, even at high doses. Patients occasionally develop problems of gastrointestinal (GI) intolerance or rash. Reversible alopecia has been reported in patients receiving more than 400 mg/d owing to inhibition of endogenous retinoic acid metabolism.[11] Elevation of serum transaminases can also occur and, in rare case, hepatitis. However, in general, these toxicities are idiosyncratic and do not correlate with fluconazole serum concentrations. Similar to other triazoles, fluconazole therapy may be associated with prolongation of the QTc interval. Some experts have recommended monitoring serum levels in patients at high risk for QTc prolongation, especially in the setting the renal dysfunction.[3]

TIME TO SAMPLE

TDM is not typically recommended for patients receiving fluconazole because of the drug's relatively predictable linear PKs and excellent tolerability profile.[3] However, special circumstances may warrant monitoring of serum drug levels, for example, patients on CVVHD with severe infections, patients infected with *Candida* spp. with a high MIC (eg, 2-4 mg/L), *Candida* infections of the central nervous system (CNS), and, possibly, pediatric patients.[8] In most cases, the most practical sampling approach is to measure serum C_{min} immediately before the next dose. A serum C_{min} of 10 to 15 mg/L would be indicative of a free drug AUC/MIC greater than 100 for *Candida* spp. with MICs up to 2 mg/L. Patients can be sampled immediately after the first maintenance dose if a loading dose is administered; otherwise, the first C_{min} sample should be drawn between 3 and 5 days of therapy.

CLINICAL APPLICATION OF FLUCONAZOLE PHARMACOKINETICS

A relatively straightforward approach can be used to evaluate fluconazole PKs. If fluconazole C_{min} is low, the dose (mg/d) can be increased in a proportional manner to achieve serum concentration exposures of 10 to 15 mg/L. C_{min} above this target range does not require dose reduction if the patient is tolerating the therapy.

Question #1 *S. V. is a 52-year-old, 68-kg female with a recent history of necrotizing pancreatitis that was complicated by sepsis, acute renal injury during sepsis, and candidemia. She was originally treated with caspofungin but has increasing transaminase levels, and the plan is to switch to IV fluconazole. There is concern about the patient having excessive fluconazole serum levels because she is receiving other medications that prolong the QTc interval. The Candida albicans isolated from the blood was found to be susceptible to fluconazole MIC (1 mg/L). Her current serum creatinine is 2.1 mg/dL. You are asked to recommend an IV dosing regimen for this patient that would ideally maintain plasma concentrations above 10 mg/L, but not produce excessive exposures that could place her at higher risk for QTc prolongation.*

The clearance of fluconazole can be estimated using an estimate of the Cl_{Cr} and Equation 10.2.

$$Cl_{Cr}(mL/min) = \frac{(0.85)(140 - 52)(68\,kg)}{(2.1\,mg/dL)(72)}$$

$$= 33.6\,mL/min$$

Cl/F (mL/min/kg) = 0.064 + 0.003 × 34 (mL/min) or 0.17 mL/min/kg, resulting in an estimate of 11.3 mL/min or 0.68 L/hr for this patient.

V can be estimated using the population value of 0.7 L/kg.

$$V = 0.7\,L/kg\,(68\,kg)$$

$$= 47.6\,L$$

The elimination rate constant can be calculated based on the Cl and V.

$$K = \frac{Cl}{V}$$

$$= \frac{0.68\,L/hr}{47.6\,L}$$

$$= 0.014\,hr^{-1}$$

The half-life is then calculated using Equation 10.1. In the case of this patient, the expected half-life would be $t_{\frac{1}{2}}$ = (0.693 × 47.6 L)/0.68 L/hr or 49.5 hours.

The patient should be administered a standard 12 mg/kg loading dose of fluconazole (~800 mg administered as a bolus injection). Loading doses are not adjusted on the basis of renal function. An 800-mg loading dose in this patient would result in an expected C_{max} of 16.8 mg/L, assuming a V_d of 0.7 L/kg using the following equation:

$$C_{max} = \frac{Dose}{V_d} \qquad \text{(Eq. 10.5)}$$

$$C_{max} = \frac{800\,mg}{47.6\,L} = 16.8\,mg/L$$

The expected trough 24 hours after the loading dose in this patient can be estimated using the following equation:

$$C_{min} = C_0 \times e^{-K_e(t)} \qquad \text{(Eq. 10.6)}$$

$$C_{min} = 16.8\,mg/L \times e^{-(0.014\,hr^{-1})(24\,hr)}$$

$$= 12.0\,mg/L$$

Hence, the patient has only eliminated approximately 28% of the dose after 24 hours, with 72% of the drug remaining. The cumulative impact of slower fluconazole clearance could be estimated, for example, if the patient was administered a standard 400 mg daily maintenance dose. At day 5 of therapy, the fluconazole trough concentrations would be predicted using the non–steady-state equation:

$$C_{min} = \left(\frac{\frac{Dose}{V_d}}{(1 - e^{-K_e(\tau)})} \right)(1 - e^{-K_e(N)(\tau)})(e^{-K_e\tau_2}) \tag{Eq. 10.7}$$

$$C_{min} = \left(\frac{\frac{400}{47.6\ L}}{(1 - e^{-(0.014\ hr^{-1})(24\ hr)})} \right)(1 - e^{-(0.014\ hr^{-1})(5)(24\ hr)})(e^{-(0.014\ hr^{-1})(24\ hr)})$$

$$= 17.1\ mg/L$$

where τ is the dosing interval of 1, N the number of doses administered,[5] and t_2 the time elapsed from the last dose until the time of the C_{min} (1 day). The predicted C_{min} is approximately 17 mg/L by day 5—nearly double the trough concentration that is required. Figure 10.1 shows how this accumulation would look over time. By reducing the administered dose by 50% to 200 mg every 24 hours, the patient could be maintained at therapeutic exposures of fluconazole (>10 mg/L) while reducing excessive peak concentrations that may be a concern in the setting of this patient's risk for QTc prolongation.

$$C_{min} = \left(\frac{\frac{Dose}{V_d}}{(1 - e^{-K_e(\tau)})} \right)(e^{-K_e\tau_2}) \tag{Eq. 10.8}$$

$$= \left(\frac{\frac{200\ mg}{47.6\ L}}{(1 - e^{-(0.014\ hr^{-1})(24\ hr)})} \right)(e^{-(0.014\ hr^{-1})(24\ hr)})$$

$$= 10.6\ mg/L$$

Itraconazole

Itraconazole was the second triazole approved for the treatment of superficial and invasive fungal diseases. It is a larger (molecular weight 705 g/mol) more lipophilic (log P 5.48) molecule compared to fluconazole that is an irreversible inhibitor of fungal 14α-demethylase. The spectrum of itraconazole is also broader than fluconazole, including yeast (*Candida* and *Cryptococcus* spp.) and endemic dimorphic fungi

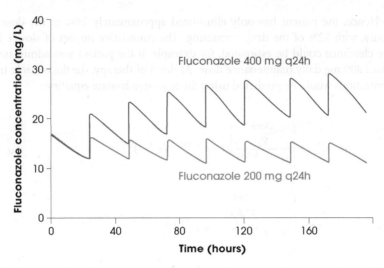

FIGURE 10.1 Predicted fluconazole serum concentrations over time in a patient with renal dysfunction.

(*C. immitis, C. posadasii, B. dermatitidis, Histoplasma capsulatum*) as well as common molds such as *Aspergillus* spp. Use of itraconazole has been largely supplanted by newer, better tolerated broad-spectrum triazoles, but it remains an important drug for the treatment of endemic mycoses, including histoplasmosis, blastomycosis, and coccidioidomycosis.

THERAPEUTIC RANGE OF ITRACONAZOLE

When corrected for protein binding, itraconazole is similar to fluconazole in that the fAUC/MIC is the PK/PD threshold associated with treatment efficacy. Several studies and a meta-analysis of 3,957 patients have examined the relationship between itraconazole serum C_{min} and risk for breakthrough invasive fungal diseases in patients with hematologic malignancies taking itraconazole as antifungal prophylaxis.[12-15] Breakthrough fungal infections were more common among patients with serum itraconazole C_{min} less than 0.25 to 0.5 mg/L measured by a high-performance liquid chromatography (HPLC) assay. Therefore, a C_{min} above 0.5 mg/L is recommended to ensure adequate protection during itraconazole prophylaxis. In a clinical study examining the use of itraconazole capsules for the treatment of invasive aspergillosis, improved outcomes were observed when itraconazole serum concentrations surpassed 8 mg/L (measured by bioassay; equivalent to >1 mg/mL measured by HPLC).[14] Therefore, C_{min} concentrations of itraconazole greater than 1 mg/L are advocated in patients with active fungal disease.

One study performed in patients with chronic obstructive pulmonary aspergillosis reported significantly higher rates of toxicity (GI adverse effects and fluid retention) when itraconazole serum levels measured by bioassay exceeded 17 mg/L.[16,17] This bioassay concentration is roughly equivalent to an itraconazole C_{min} greater than 4 mg/L (measured by HPLC).

BIOAVAILABILITY

Itraconazole is typically administered as 200 to 400 mg daily as a divided dose. In patients with severe fungal disease, a loading dose of 200 mg 3 times daily for the first 3 days of therapy is recommended. Itraconazole bioavailability depends on the formulation administered (see Key Parameters: Itraconazole). The capsule formulation (100 mg) consists of drug-coated microspheres to enhance the surface area for dissolution of the drug in the stomach. In healthy volunteers with normal gastric acidity, the bioavailability of the capsules is 55% when taken with food. The time to peak serum concentrations ranges between 1 and 4 hours. However, dissolution of the drug is reduced in patients with GI dysfunction or increased gastric pH (eg, on acid suppression therapy), resulting in less absorbable drug delivered to the duodenum and significantly lower bioavailability. To overcome this problem, a cyclodextrin oral solution formulation of itraconazole was developed that can be taken without food and does not require low gastric pH. The bioavailability of the oral solution is approximately 60% but has, for many patients, an unpalatable taste and higher rates of GI adverse effects. This is because of the fact that the cyclodextrin vehicle is not absorbed from the GI tract and acts as an osmotic agent to retain water in the intestine. An IV form of itraconazole (administered in cyclodextrin) is available in Europe and Asia but is no longer available in the United States.

More recently, a new oral formulation of itraconazole was approved (SUper-BioAvailable-Itraconazole [SUBA-itraconazole], Tolsura), which consists of a solid dispersion of itraconazole particles in a pH-sensitive drug-polymer matrix delivered as a 65-mg capsule. When the capsule is ingested, itraconazole is retained in polymer until the capsule reaches higher pH (pH ~6), in the duodenum where itraconazole is released at concentrations optimized for maximal absorption. By bypassing the need for slow dissolution in the stomach, SUBA-itraconazole avoids many of the factors that contribute to erratic bioavailability of itraconazole capsules in a more convenient and palatable formulation.

The relative bioavailability of SUBA-itraconazole was 173% higher than the capsule formulation with 21% less variability between subjects.[18] This translated to an absolute bioavailability of 90% for SUBA-itraconazole versus 55% for the capsules. Thus, the SUBA-itraconazole formulation reintroduces a possibility of using oral itraconazole in a wider range of patients where other formulations were unreliable or not well tolerated.

VOLUME OF DISTRIBUTION (V)

Itraconazole has a very large volume of distribution (10.7 L/kg) that includes penetration into the skin, liver, bone, adipose tissue, nail, and bronchial fluids.[7] However, high molecular weight and extensive protein binding (90%-99%) limit its penetration into the vitreous fluid of the eye and cerebrospinal fluid (concentrations often undetectable), even though successful treatment of cerebral fungal infections and cryptococcal meningitis are reported. Little active drug is present in urine.

CLEARANCE (Cl)

Itraconazole displays a saturable, nonlinear pattern of elimination with increasing doses. The PKs are more complex than fluconazole, with serum concentrations best predicted with a two-compartment model with oral absorption described by four-transit compartments. Itraconazole is extensively metabolized in the liver by predominantly CYP3A4 to an active (hydroxyl-itraconazole) and inactive metabolites. The ratio of metabolites depends, in part, on the synthesis of itraconazole, which is compared of four *cis*-isomers with varying affinity for CYP3A4. The active hydroxyl-itraconazole metabolite can be detected in concentrations of 1 to 1.6 times higher than the parent compound.[19] The presence of the active metabolite will influence how serum concentrations are reported; most reference laboratories will report both the metabolite and parent compound concentrations. If itraconazole concentrations are analyzed using a (microbial) bioassay methodology, the reported concentrations will be roughly 5-fold higher.

Approximately 55% of the itraconazole dose is excreted via biliary elimination, and 35% excreted as active and inactive metabolites through the kidney. At steady state, the clearance rate is approximately 3.8 mL/min/kg. Using Equation 10.1, this results in an estimated half-life of 32 hours.

KEY PARAMETERS: Itraconazole[a]

THERAPEUTIC CONCENTRATIONS	C_{min} 0.5-4 mg/L (MEASURED BY HPLC)
F	55% capsules (with food; solution 30% higher when administered without food)
	90% SUBA-itraconazole
V_d	10.7 L/kg
Cl[b]	16 L/hr
AUC_{0-24hr}[c]	15.4 mg·hr/L
$t_{1/2}$	35 hr
fu (fraction unbound)	<5%

[a]Pharmacokinetic parameters may vary depending on patient characteristics and liver dysfunction; administered as a 200-mg dose.
[b]Mean body clearance.
[c]200 mg twice daily dose.

Itraconazole doses do not need to be reduced in patients with renal dysfunction. However, patients with moderate-to-severe liver dysfunction are likely to have reduced rates of clearance. Patients should be carefully monitored for evidence of toxicity and consideration given to performing TDM for itraconazole.

PHARMACOKINETIC DRUG INTERACTIONS

Itraconazole is a substrate and inhibitor of CYP3A4 and P-glycoprotein (P-gp) and is associated with the potential for many drug-drug interactions. Patients should have their medication profiles carefully reviewed whenever starting or stopping itraconazole therapy. Strong inducers of CYP3A4 (ie, rifampin, phenytoin, carbamazepine) will result in low or undetectable itraconazole concentrations and are contraindicated. Similarly, the use of itraconazole with other medications metabolized through CYP3A4 pathways that increase QTc interval is contraindicated. Itraconazole will reduce the clearance of many cardiovascular, anesthesia, immunosuppressant, and chemotherapy agents. Careful dosage adjustment of the second drug or avoidance of itraconazole may be required because some of these interactions are potentially life-threatening.

In addition to CYP3A4-associated interactions, drugs that increase gastric pH (antacids, H_2 antagonists, and protein-pump inhibitors) reduce the bioavailability of itraconazole capsules. Cola drinks have been shown to increase the absorption of the capsules in patients with achlorhydria or those taking H_2-receptor antagonists or other gastric acid suppressors. Grapefruit/grapefruit juice may increase itraconazole serum levels because of the inhibition of intestinal P-gp.

ADVERSE EFFECTS

Although itraconazole is tolerated by many patients, it is associated with higher rates of GI intolerance and hepatic toxicity compared to fluconazole. Hypokalemia, cardiotoxicity with a negative inotropic effect that can lead to new to or exacerbations of congestive heart failure, neuropathies, adrenal insufficiencies (more common with longer term, higher dose therapy), gynecomastia, leg edema, tremor, and hearing loss are also observed more frequently with itraconazole than fluconazole. Itraconazole carries a risk of QTc prolongation and interacts with many other agents that also prolong QTc. Therefore, concomitant use should be avoided.

TIME TO SAMPLE

Without a loading dose, itraconazole concentrations reach steady state after 2 weeks. If a loading dose is administered, the first C_{min} sample can be collected on days 5 to 7 of therapy or soon thereafter. Owing to the long half-life of the drug, samples drawn for TDM in the middle of the dosing interval will not differ substantially from the actual C_{min} concentration.

CLINICAL APPLICATION OF ITRACONAZOLE PHARMACOKINETICS

TDM is recommended for all patients receiving itraconazole to ensure adequate exposures. If the C_{min} concentration of itraconazole is low (<0.5 mg/L) on days 5 to 7 of therapy, then the patient should be carefully assessed for factors to improve the drug bioavailability (ie, administer with cola beverage if taking capsules, stop protein-pump inhibitors), or switch to the oral solution or new SUBA capsule formulation. If the patient is going to continue taking conventional itraconazole capsules, the dose should be increased by 100 mg twice daily and recheck a serum concentration. Patients with elevated C_{min} concentrations (>4 mg/L) can be continued on the same dose without changes if they are tolerating itraconazole, but dose reduction (100 mg twice daily) should be considered if they are experiencing adverse effects and cannot be switched to an alternative antifungal agent.

> **Question #2**   A.J. is a 34-year-old male patient (height 5 feet 6 inches, weight 55 kg) with cystic fibrosis who is to be initiated on itraconazole 200 mg capsules orally every 12 hours for the treatment of allergic bronchopulmonary aspergillosis. What is the predicted steady-state C_{min} on this regimen?

Because the frequency of drug administration (eg, 12 hours) is approximately one-third of the half-life (eg, 35 hours), the continuous infusion model (Equation 10.9) can be used to predict the average steady-state concentration.

$$C_{ss} = \frac{(S)(F)(\text{Dose})}{(\text{Cl})(\tau)} \qquad \text{(Eq. 10.9)}$$

$$C_{ss} = \frac{(1)(0.55)(200 \text{ mg})}{(16.7 \text{ L/hr})(12 \text{ hr})}$$

$$= 0.55 \text{ mg/L}$$

The concentration of 0.55 mg/L is within the desired therapeutic range for the trough concentration, indicating that this regimen is appropriate. A measured concentration should be obtained in 2 weeks to confirm the achievement of a therapeutic concentration and to assess clinical response. Patients with cystic fibrosis typically receive acid suppressor therapy for the treatment of acid reflux or to enhance the activity of pancreatic enzyme supplements; therefore, the dose of itraconazole often needs to be increased in this population to achieve therapeutic concentrations.

Voriconazole

Voriconazole is structurally similar to fluconazole (349 g/mol) but is a more lipophilic (log P 1.82) and irreversibly binds to fungal 14α-demethylase, resulting in a broader spectrum of activity that covers yeast and *Aspergillus*, some *Fusarium* spp., and black molds, but not Mucorales. Along with isavuconazole, voriconazole is considered a first-line choice for the treatment of invasive aspergillosis in patients who have not received prior triazole therapy.[20]

THERAPEUTIC RANGE OF VORICONAZOLE

Voriconazole exposure-response relationships have been investigated in a number of studies and are similar to other triazoles in that the fAUC/MIC best predicts outcome.[17] Specifically, serum C_{min} concentrations are predictive of the patient's AUC. A C_{min} of greater than 1 mg/L has been identified in several studies as a threshold voriconazole exposure associated with a higher probability of successful clinical outcome in patients with invasive aspergillosis.[21-23] In an analysis of phase 2/3 studies of voriconazole treatment for invasive aspergillosis and invasive candidiasis, C_{min}-to-MIC ratios of 2 to 5 were associated with a higher probability of successful clinical outcome.[24]

Voriconazole C_{min} greater than 5.5 to 6 mg/L are associated with a higher probability of CNS adverse effects (encephalopathy) and visual hallucinations. In one prospective study investigating voriconazole TDM, patients who were randomized to undergo routine TDM monitoring during voriconazole therapy experienced fewer adverse effects and were less likely to have treatment interruptions compared to those who did not undergo routine TDM.[25]

Although voriconazole C_{min} is often elevated in patients with liver dysfunction, there is inconclusive evidence of a "cutoff" concentration of voriconazole that can be used to predict hepatotoxic events.[26]

BIOAVAILABILITY (F)

Voriconazole is typically administered IV as 6 mg/kg loading dose for two doses and then 4 mg/kg twice daily as a maintenance dose. An oral tablet and suspension formulations are available. Oral tablet doses are lower (fixed 200 mg dose twice daily), but many experts still recommend continued weight-based dosing (4 mg/kg twice daily), even with the tablet formulation. Time to peak serum levels is approximately 1 hour. Dosing for patients less than 40 kg is lower (100 mg twice daily), whereas pediatric patients require higher doses (discussed below). Voriconazole tablets are well absorbed without food (86% bioavailability) when taken 1 hour before or 2 hours after meals. Absorption is independent of gastric pH but is reduced by 24% if tablets are taken with food. Some population PK models in neutropenic patients have suggested that bioavailability is lower (60%-65%) in patients with chemotherapy-associated mucositis,[19] or in pediatric patients.[27-30]

The IV formulation of voriconazole is solubilized in a sulfobutyl ether-cyclodextrin (SBECD) vehicle. In patients with renal dysfunction, and in animal models, accumulation of the SBECD has been associated with reversible changes in the renal and bladder epithelium, but the clinical significance of these changes in humans is unknown. The manufacturer does not recommend using the IV formulation in patients with impaired renal function (GFR < 50 mL/min), and SBECD is only moderately removed by dialysis. However, several case series have described successful use of IV voriconazole in critically ill patients with renal dysfunction or on dialysis without problems.[31-33]

VOLUME OF DISTRIBUTION (V)

Voriconazole is widely distributed in tissues, including the CNS and vitreous fluid of the eye. Cerebral spinal fluid concentrations are approximately 50% of serum concentration.[7] The volume of distribution differs between children and adults. In children, a biphasic V_d has been described, with a V_d (central) compartment of 0.81 L/kg and V_d (peripheral) compartment of 2.2 L/kg. In adults, the V_d is 4.6 L/kg. Little active drug is present in urine.

CLEARANCE

Clearance rates of voriconazole are dose dependent, saturable at higher doses (non-linear Michaelis Menten pharmacokinetics), and can vary tremendously from one patient owing to a number of factors. Voriconazole is metabolized predominantly by CYP2C19 and, to a lesser extent, CYP2C9 and CYP3A4 to inactive metabolite (N-oxide voriconazole), which is excreted in the urine. CYP2C19 exhibits genetic polymorphism (15%-20% Asians may be poor metabolizers of voriconazole; 3%-5% Caucasians and African Americans may be poor metabolizers).

Pediatric patients have much higher clearance rates of voriconazole compared to adults because of a 3- to 5-fold greater rate of CYP2C19 metabolism and enhanced activity of flavin-containing monooxygenase 3.[27-29,34] Clearance of voriconazole in adolescents (age 12-14 years) depends on weight with children greater than 50 kg exhibiting PK characteristics similar to adults. Currently, recommended doses for children aged 2 to 12 years less than 50 kg are an IV dose of 9 mg/kg twice daily on day 1, then 8 mg/kg twice daily thereafter. Oral dosing is 9 mg/kg twice daily and then followed by 9 mg/kg every 12 hours.[28] However, PKs are extremely variable, and TDM is often needed to guide dosing. Occasionally, infants and younger children may require every 8-hour dosing of voriconazole to achieve therapeutic concentrations.

Voriconazole clearance is not affected by renal function. However, avoidance of IV voriconazole is recommended by the manufacturer if patients have an estimated GFR of less than 50 mL/min owing to the risk of accumulation of cyclodextrin vehicle. Lower doses of voriconazole should be considered in patients with hepatic insufficiency. For mild-to-moderate hepatic insufficiency (Child-Pugh Classes A and B): 6 mg/kg every 12 hours × 2 doses (load), then 2 mg/kg IV every 12 hours with serum concentration monitoring is recommended.

KEY PARAMETERS: Voriconazole[a]

THERAPEUTIC CONCENTRATIONS	C_{min}: 1-6 mg/L
F	86% capsules without food (adults)
	50%-65% (pediatrics)
V_d	4.6 L/kg
Cl^b	2.07 mg/L (adults)
K_m^c	5.16 mg/L (pediatrics)
V_{max}^d	1.7 mg/kg/d (pediatrics)
	0.54 mg/kg/d (adults)
AUC_{0-12hr}^e	17.99 mg·hr/L
$t_{1/2}$	6 hr, variable and dose dependent
fu (fraction unbound)	40%

[a]Pharmacokinetic parameters may vary depending on patient characteristics and liver dysfunction; administered as a 200-mg dose.
[b]Voriconazole exhibits Michaelis-Menten (nonlinear) pharmacokinetics in some patients, meaning that dosage escalation may lead to a disproportionate increase in systemic drug exposures (AUC) because of saturable metabolism. Conversely, accurate estimation of voriconazole exposure (clearance) is not always possible as the maximal rate of voriconazole clearance (V_{max}) often changes as therapeutically achieved concentrations.[30] This saturable metabolism appears to occur at lower doses (mg/kg) in adults than children owing to a greater than 2-fold higher concentration required to saturate metabolic capacity (K_m).
[c]K_m concentration in central compartment where clearance is half-maximal. Median calculated value from population pharmacokinetic studies, subject to wide interpatient variability.
[d]V_{max} is the maximal rate of enzymatic inactivation of voriconazole. Median calculated value from population pharmacokinetic studies, subject to wide interpatient variability.
[e]6 mg/kg loading dose, then 4 mg/kg twice daily.

PHARMACOKINETIC DRUG INTERACTIONS

Voriconazole is a substrate of CYP2C19 and a potent inhibitor of CYP3A4.[2] Patients should have their medication profiles carefully reviewed with starting or stopping voriconazole therapy. Strong inducers of CYP3A4 (ie, rifampin, phenytoin, carbamazepine, efavirenz) generally result in low or undetectable voriconazole concentrations and are contraindicated. Similarly, the use of voriconazole with other medications metabolized through CYP3A4 pathways that increase QTc interval is not recommended. Voriconazole will reduce the clearance of many cardiovascular, anesthesia, immunosuppressant, and chemotherapy agents. Careful dosage adjustment of the victim drug or avoidance of voriconazole may be required, because some of these interactions are potentially life-threatening.

Medications that are inhibitors of CYP2C19 (ie, omeprazole) have been used in some case series to "boost" voriconazole serum concentrations but can result in an increased risk of CNS side effects.[35,36]

ADVERSE EFFECTS

The most common adverse effect during voriconazole therapy is transient photopsia (abnormal vision described as blurriness, color changes, and enhanced vision) due to selective and reversible inhibition of retinal ON-bipolar cells in both rod and cone pathways. The visual adverse effects are seen in 20.6% of patients, but fewer than 1% require treatment discontinuation. The duration of visual abnormalities usually lasts less than 30 minutes, typically starting 30 minutes after dosing. Patients may also develop increased transaminases (13%) and alkaline phosphatase with therapy discontinuation required in 4% to 8% of cases. Other less common adverse effects include rash and hallucinations.

Encephalopathy is an adverse effect of voriconazole that is associated with C_{min} concentrations of greater than 5.5 mg/L.[21,22] Other rare adverse effects seen with long-term therapy include phototoxicity that can evolve into squamous cell carcinoma, alopecia with skin and nail changes, and periostitis and/or skeletal fluorosis.

TIME TO SAMPLE

Voriconazole concentrations reach steady state by 5 days, but a C_{min} sample on days 2 to 5 after the loading dose is acceptable for early TDM assessment. Many experts recommend repeating a C_{min} sample during the second week of therapy to confirm the patient is within the therapeutic range. Autoinduction of voriconazole metabolism has been reported to occur at higher-than-usual doses, resulting in decreased C_{min} over time, which may require further dose modification to maintain therapeutic concentrations.

CLINICAL APPLICATION OF VORICONAZOLE PHARMACOKINETICS

TDM is recommended in patients receiving voriconazole for the treatment of invasive aspergillosis and is considered essential for effective dosing of pediatric patient[28] Similar to other triazole antifungals, C_{min} is reasonable predictive of AUC and is used to monitor therapy. The first C_{min} sample for voriconazole can be drawn after 3 to 5 days (after the fifth dose, including the loading doses) to confirm serum concentrations fall between 1 and 6 mg/L.

Patients who have changes in their voriconazole dose, are switched from IV to oral therapy, or have a change in their clinical condition (eg, suspected breakthrough infections or toxicity) should have voriconazole serum concentrations checked. TDM may also be helpful in patients who have additional medications with possible PK interactions with voriconazole started or stopped.

If the voriconazole C_{min} is low (<1 mg/L), it is important to ensure that the voriconazole dose (including loading dose) was administered appropriately. If the patient was recently switched from IV to a fixed oral dose, the oral dose could be increased to the same weight-based (mg/kg) dose that was administered IV. If the C_{min} is very low (<0.5 mg/L), the patient should be switched to IV if on oral, and the daily dose should be increased by 50% with follow-up monitoring 2 to 5 days later. Careful screening for clinical scenarios that alter voriconazole PKs (eg, drug interactions, compliance) is critical.

If the predose voriconazole C_{min} concentrations are high (>6 mg/L), the patient should be carefully screened for clinical factors that may be influencing voriconazole PKs and ensure that the C_{min} sample was appropriately drawn. Dose reduction may not be needed if the patient is tolerating voriconazole without CNS adverse effects; however, close monitoring is recommended. In one prospective randomized study of voriconazole TDM, patients with C_{min} greater than 10 mg/L had the next voriconazole dose held, and subsequent doses were reduced by 50% until concentrations fell within the therapeutic range.

Question #3 *F.P. is a 9-year-old, 35-kg male who received a matched related allogeneic hematopoietic stem cell transplant for acute lymphoblastic leukemia 70 days ago that has been complicated by acute graft versus host disease. He is receiving oral trimethoprim-sulfamethoxazole, valacyclovir, and fluconazole as prophylaxis. His current immunosuppression regimen is tacrolimus 0.03 mg/kg/d, and his last level was 10.2 ng/mL. His renal and liver function are within normal limits. In the last 72 hours, F.P. has developed a fever (38.5 °C) that has not responded to broad-spectrum antibiotics, and a computed tomography scan of the chest reveals lesions suspicious for invasive aspergillosis. F.P. was started on IV voriconazole 250 mg (7 mg/kg) twice daily, and, on day 5 of therapy, a C_{min} serum level is 0.5 mg/L. How should F.P.'s voriconazole dosing be managed to achieve a C_{min} above 1.0 mg/L?*

Because F.P. is pediatric patient, he is expected to have much higher clearance of voriconazole than adults; 7 mg/kg twice daily may still not be sufficient. Although the PKs of voriconazole are complex and difficult to predict because of wide interpatient variations in metabolism, the Km value reported in most pediatric PK studies is higher than in adults (see Key Parameters: Voriconazole) and surpasses average voriconazole concentrations expected in this patient. This can be demonstrated by using a formula relating C_{min} (μg/mL) concentrations to voriconazole AUC (mg·hr/L) reported in pediatric population PK studies (Figure 10.2).

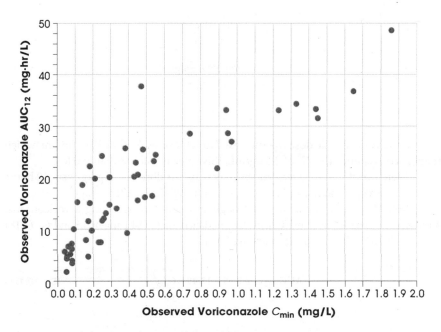

FIGURE 10.2   Observed voriconazole AUC_{0-12hr} versus C_{min} at steady state in children receiving 7 mg/kg intravenous every 12 hours and 200 mg orally every 12 hours with a $C_{min} < 2$ µg/mL. (From Driscoll TA, Yu LC, Frangoul H, et al. Comparison of pharmacokinetics and safety of voriconazole intravenous-to-oral switch in immunocompromised children and healthy adults. *Antimicrob Agents Chemother.* 2011;55(12):5770-5779.)

$$AUC_{0-12\ hr} = 11.45 + 14.97 \times C_{min} \qquad \textbf{(Eq. 10.10)}$$

Using this equation, a patient with a trough of 0.5 µg/mL would have an expected AUC of 18.9 mg·h/L.

$$AUC_{0-12\ hr} = 11.45 + 14.97 \times 0.5\ mg/L$$

$$= 18.9\ mg·hr/L$$

The clearance can be calculated from the AUC using Equation 10.11 as follows:

$$Cl\,(L/kg · hr) = \frac{(S)(F)(Dose)}{AUC} \qquad \textbf{(Eq. 10.11)}$$

$$= \frac{(1)(1)(7\ mg/kg)}{18.9\ mg/L · hr}$$

$$= 0.37\ L/kg·hr$$

Using Equation 10.9, we can estimate the average steady-state concentration, C_{ss} of 1.58 µg/mL, which is well below the typical medial K_m reported in population PK studies (5.16 µg/mL).

$$C_{ss} = \frac{(S)(F)(\text{Dose})}{(\text{Cl})(\tau)}$$

$$= \frac{(1)(1)(7 \text{ mg/kg})}{0.37 \text{ L/kg} \cdot \text{hr}}$$

$$= 1.58 \text{ mg/L}$$

If the voriconazole dose was increased to achieve an AUC of 30 µg/mL·hr, which roughly corresponds to a C_{ss} of 2.5 µg/mL, this value is still less than the K_m.

Therefore, it would be reasonable to increase the dose by 2 mg/kg every 12 hours to 9 mg/kg every 12 hours, and recheck serum trough levels after 3 days.

Note that for an adult with a trough of 0.5 µg/mL receiving a voriconazole 4 mg/kg maintenance dose twice daily, the predicted AUC (14.1 mg·hr/L) and C_{ss} (1.18) is modestly lower based on the following formula:

$$\text{AUC}_{0-12 \text{ hr}} = 7.39 + 13.49 \times C_{min} \qquad \text{(Eq. 10.12)}$$

$$= 7.39 + 13.49 \ (0.5 \text{ mg/L})$$

$$= 14.1 \text{ mg·hr/L}$$

However, the C_{ss} (1.18) is much closer to reported K_m values (2.07 µg/mL), suggesting adult patients will approach saturable (nonlinear) drug elimination at lower mg/kg doses. Therefore, if an adult patient has a trough of 0.5 µg/mL, a more modest dose increase of 1 to 5 mg/kg every 12 hours may be more reasonable with a recheck of the serum trough levels after 3 days.

Question #4   *How should tacrolimus dosing be changed in light of the PK drug interaction with voriconazole?*

When starting voriconazole in patients already receiving tacrolimus, it is recommended that the tacrolimus dose be reduced to one-third of the original dose and followed with frequent monitoring of the tacrolimus blood levels (therapeutic range 10-15 ng/mL). When voriconazole is discontinued, tacrolimus levels should be carefully monitored and the dose increased as necessary.

Posaconazole

Posaconazole is a large molecular weight (700 g/mol) highly lipophilic (log P 5.50) triazole structurally similar to itraconazole. Posaconazole is one of the two broadest-spectrum triazoles, with activity against yeast (*Candida* spp. and *Cryptococcus* spp.), molds (*Aspergillus*, *Fusarium* spp., and black molds, including some Mucorales), and endemic dimorphic fungi (*C. immitis*, *C. posadasii*, and *B. dermatitidis*). Similar to itraconazole capsules, the suspension formulation of posaconazole requires food and low gastric pH for absorption.

THERAPEUTIC RANGE OF POSACONAZOLE

Posaconazole has similar PD characteristics as other triazoles. Exposure-response relationships for posaconazole are primarily derived from phase III studies that evaluated posaconazole prophylaxis in patients with hematologic malignancies[37] or acute graft versus host disease after allogeneic hematopoietic stem cell transplantation.[38] Additional exposure-response data were also available from an open-label salvage study in patients with probable or proven invasive aspergillosis.[39] In prophylaxis studies, higher rates of breakthrough fungal infection or treatment discontinuation were observed in patients with random serum or C_{min} less than 0.7 mg/L.[40] In the open-label salvage study of patients with invasive fungal disease, the highest response rates were observed in patients with random serum levels or C_{min} greater than 1.25 mg/L.[39]

To date, serum concentrations of posaconazole have not been shown to be predictive of toxicity during posaconazole treatment, although there is a relationship between serum posaconazole concentrations and risk of grade II/IV liver injury[41] or pseudohyperaldosteronism.[42,43]

BIOAVAILABILITY (*F*)

The bioavailability of posaconazole suspension when administered at 600 to 800 mg/d in divided doses (3-4 times daily) with a high-fat meal is approximately 50%. Without food or divided doses, or in the setting of increased gastric pH, the bioavailability decreases by more than 30%. Similar to itraconazole, acidic beverages increase the bioavailability of posaconazole. The need for 3 to 4 times daily dosing with posaconazole is not related to the half-life of the drug, rather divided dosing improves the dissolution of the solid dosage form in the stomach. Doses higher than 800 mg/d of the suspension will not improve blood levels because of limited additional dissolution.

Because frequent administration of posaconazole with high-fat meals is problematic in target population who would most benefit from posaconazole prophylaxis (ie, hematologic malignancy patients receiving chemotherapy), a delayed-release tablet formulation was introduced that releases the drug in the small intestine. As a result, absorption of the tablet does not require food or low gastric pH to achieve 60% bioavailability. However, bioavailability is still further improved if the tablet is administered with food. Dosing for the delayed-release tablet differs from the suspension: 300 mg orally twice daily for day 1, then 300 mg once daily.

An IV formulation of posaconazole solubilized in cyclodextrin was also introduced and is useful for patients who cannot take the gastro-resistant tablet. IV dosing is similar to the tablet: 300 mg IV twice daily for 1 day, then 300 mg IV once daily.

VOLUME OF DISTRIBUTION (*V*)

Similar to itraconazole, posaconazole is widely distributed in tissues with a V_d of approximately 7 L/kg.[7] Posaconazole is highly protein bound (>98%) and, like itraconazole, has limited penetration into the vitreous fluid of the eye and low concentrations in the cerebrospinal fluid, even though successful treatment of cerebral fungal infections has been reported.[7] The terminal elimination half-life is approximately 35 hours (steady-state attained at 7-10 days). Little active drug is present in urine.

CLEARANCE (Cl)

Posaconazole is primarily metabolized in the liver, where it undergoes glucuronidation, and is transformed into inactive metabolites. Posaconazole is predominantly eliminated in feces (71%). Renal clearance is a minor elimination pathway (13%).

Posaconazole dosing should not be adjusted in patients with renal dysfunction. Limited data are available on dosing posaconazole in patients with liver disease; standard dosing is recommended with caution.

KEY PARAMETERS: Posaconazole[a]

THERAPEUTIC CONCENTRATIONS	C_{min}: > 0.7 mg/L
F	50% suspension with food and divided dosing; 54% tablets without food and single daily dose
V_d	7 L/kg
Cl	11 L/hr
AUC_{0-24hr}	15.9 mg·hr/L
$t_{1/2}$	35 hr
fu (fraction unbound)	2%

[a]Pharmacokinetic parameters may vary depending on patient characteristics and formulation administered.

PHARMACOKINETIC DRUG INTERACTIONS

Posaconazole is metabolized via uridine diphosphate (UDP) glucuronidation (phase II enzymes). It is a substrate of P-gp efflux and an inhibitor of CYP3A4. As a result, the clearance of drugs is metabolized, although CYP3A4 will be affected by posaconazole.[2] Similar precautions are recommended as with other triazoles that inhibit CYP3A4. Posaconazole serum concentrations may be decreased with the coadministration of UDP glucuronidation or P-gp inducers.

ADVERSE EFFECTS

Posaconazole is generally well tolerated with a side-effect profile similar to fluconazole. The most common adverse effects are nausea, vomiting, and abdominal pain. Increases in serum aminotransferases or hyperbilirubinemia are occasionally reported. No recommendations are currently available with respect to posaconazole serum concentration monitoring to reduce the risk of toxicity.

TIME TO SAMPLE

Without a loading dose or when using the suspension formulation, posaconazole concentrations reach steady state after 7 to 10 days. Typically, the first C_{min} sample can be collected on days 5 to 7 of therapy or soon thereafter. For tablets or IV formulation, serum levels of C_{min} can be initially samples on days 3 to 5. Owing to the long half-life of the posaconazole, samples drawn for TDM in the middle of the dosing interval will not differ substantially from the actual C_{min} concentration.

CLINICAL APPLICATION OF POSACONAZOLE PHARMACOKINETICS

TDM is recommended for most patients receiving posaconazole suspension, especially during the treatment of suspected or documented fungal infections. The need for routine TDM with the gastro-resistant tablet or IV formulation is less well defined but could be considered in situations of suspected clinical failure or drug interactions. Typically, a C_{min} concentration of posaconazole is checked after the first 3 to 5 days of therapy with the tablet or IV formulation to ensure that the levels are above 0.7 mg/L. A serum C_{min} greater than 0.35 mg/L sample on days 2 to 3 with the suspension will likely surpass 0.7 mg/L at steady state.[44]

If predose C_{min} concentration is low (<0.7 mg/L prophylaxis or <1 mg/L treatment), the patients should be assessed for clinical scenarios affecting bioavailability and compliance. Patients receiving the suspension formulations can be switched to the gastro-resistant tablet or IV formulation. If the patient requires suspension formulation, the daily dose should be increased from 600 to 800 mg administered in four divided doses with food or acidic beverage, stop acid suppression therapy if feasible. C_{min} concentrations can be rechecked after 5 to 7 days. The safety and PKs of higher maintenance doses of gastro-resistant tablets of IV formulations above 300 mg/d are not well defined.

Question #5   *R.T. is a 54-year-old, 80-kg male undergoing remission-induction chemotherapy for acute myelogenous leukemia. As part of his prophylaxis regimen, he was prescribed posaconazole gastro-resistant tablet (three 100 mg tablets daily), but now has difficulties swallowing as a result of mucositis and has been switched to the oral suspension formulation of posaconazole (200 mg 3 times daily). A trough serum level was checked after switching and returned as undetectable. How should R.T.'s posaconazole be managed to achieve a C_{min} above 0.7 mg/L?*

Although posaconazole tablets are now the preferred formulation of posaconazole, in many centers, they may be challenging to swallow in patients with poor oral intake and mucositis. Unfortunately, poor appetite or difficulty swallowing may also limit the absorption of the suspension formulation, which requires low gastric pH, food (preferably a high-fat meal), and divided dosing to maximize absorption. Strategies for maximizing the absorption of posaconazole may include increasing the dose of the suspension formulation to 800 mg/d given in four divided doses, administering each dose with Ensure or some other enteral nutrition product, or taking posaconazole suspension with an acidic cola beverage. Acid suppression therapy such as proton-pump inhibitors or H_2 antagonists should be stopped if possible.

Ultimately, it may be necessary to switch the patient to IV posaconazole, and re-check serum C_{min}, to ensure that adequate concentrations are then considered switch-ing back to oral therapy once mucositis and oral intake improve.

Question #6   *If the patient is switched to the IV formulation but not adminis-tered a loading dose, what would be the predicted trough after the first IV dose (only given 300 mg daily)?*

The population estimate of V can be used.

$$V = 7 \text{ L/kg (80 kg)}$$

$$= 560 \text{ L}$$

The elimination rate constant can be calculated based on the Cl and V.

$$K = \frac{Cl}{V}$$

$$= \frac{11 \text{ L/hr}}{560 \text{ L}}$$

$$= 0.0196 \text{ hr}^{-1}$$

Using Equation 10.5, the initial concentration after the dose is estimated as follows:

$$C_0 = \frac{(S)(F)(\text{Dose})}{V}$$

$$= \frac{(1)(1)(300 \text{ mg})}{560 \text{ L}} = 0.54 \text{ mg/L}$$

$$= 0.54 \text{ mg/L}$$

The trough concentration can then be estimated using Equation 10.6:

$$C_{min} = C_0 \times e^{-K_e \tau}$$

$$= 0.54 \text{ mg/L} \times e^{-(0.0196 \text{ hr}^{-1})(24 \text{ hr})}$$

$$= 0.34 \text{ mg/L}$$

Question #7   *How long would it take for the patient to achieve a trough concen-tration above 0.7 mg/L?*

Using the non–steady-state Equation 10.7, we can calculate the predicted troughs on days 2, 3, and 4.

$$C_{min} = \left(\frac{\dfrac{Dose}{V_d}}{(1 - e^{-K_e \tau})} \right) (1 - e^{-K_e (N)(\tau)})(e^{-K_e \tau})$$

$$C_{min\,(2nd\ dose)} = \left(\frac{\dfrac{300\ mg}{560\ L}}{(1 - e^{(-0.02\ hr^{-1}) \times 24\ hr})} \right) (1 - e^{(-0.02\ hr^{-1})(2) \times (24\ hr)})(e^{-0.02 \times 24\ hr})$$

With each successive dose, N is changed to 3, 4, 5, and so on.

The results are 0.55 mg/L on day 2, 0.68 mg/L on day 3, and 0.72 mg/L on day 4.

Question #8   *If the patient is administered a loading dose (300 mg twice daily on day 1), what is the predicted trough before the dose on day 2 (24 hours after loading dose started)?*

Using Equation 10.7, we can calculate the predicted trough 24 hours after the loading dose was started.

$$C_{min} = \left(\frac{\dfrac{Dose}{V_d}}{(1 - e^{-K_e (\tau)})} \right) (1 - e^{-K_e (N)(\tau)})(e^{-K_e \tau})$$

$$= \left(\frac{\dfrac{300\ mg}{560\ L}}{(1 - e^{(-0.02\ hr^{-1}) \times (12\ hr)})} \right)$$

$$= 0.75\ mg/L$$

Isavuconazole

Isavuconazole is a smaller (molecular weight 437 g/mol) lipophilic (log P 3.9) triazole with a similar spectrum of activity to posaconazole. Isavuconazole is unique, however, in that it is formulated as a water-soluble prodrug (isavuconazonium sulfate) that is rapidly cleaved by serum esterases to the active moiety (isavuconazole). As a result, both the oral tablet and IV formulation avoid the need for cyclodextrin. Isavuconazole is as effective for the treatment of invasive aspergillosis as voriconazole but is associated with fewer visual, CNS and hepatic toxicities, and less variable PKs.[45] Isavuconazole is primarily used as a first-line treatment for invasive aspergillosis but may also be an effective alternative to amphotericin B for patients with mucormycosis.[46]

THERAPEUTIC RANGE OF ISAVUCONAZOLE

Although isavuconazole exhibits similar PK/PD characteristics as other triazole antifungals, no relationship between serum drug levels and treatment outcome was reported in phase II/III clinical studies.[47,48] A provisional C_{min} target of greater than 1 mg/L has been proposed based on the isolate susceptibility of PK/PD simulations.[49] To date, serum concentrations of isavuconazole have not been shown to be predictive of toxicity during isavuconazole treatment, although troughs greater than 5.15 have been reported to be associated with higher rates of GI toxicity.[50]

BIOAVAILABILITY (F)

The typical IV or oral dose of isavuconazole is 372 mg isavuconazonium (equivalent to 200 mg isavuconazole) 3 times daily for the first 2 days as a loading dose and then 372 mg once daily. The loading dose is required to ensure serum drug concentrations exceed 1 mg/L in the first 24 to 48 hours of therapy.[41] Isavuconazole exhibits linear and dose-proportional PKs up to 600 mg/d. Bioavailability of oral tablets is estimated at 98%. Maximal serum concentrations are reached 2 to 3 hours after either single or multiple dosing. Absorption of isavuconazonium tablets is not markedly affected by food or gastric pH.

VOLUME OF DISTRIBUTION (V)

Isavuconazole is widely distributed into tissues with a V_d of approximately 6 to 7 L/kg at steady state. Isavuconazole is highly protein bound (99%) and achieves low concentrations in the cerebrospinal fluid but penetrates the brain parenchyma. Little active drug is present in urine.

CLEARANCE (Cl)

Following IV administration, prodrug is not found in serum 1.25 hours after a 1-hour infusion. Isavuconazonium is rapidly hydrolyzed to isavuconazole by esterases along with some minor, inactive metabolites. Isavuconazole is a substrate of cytochrome P450 3A4 and 3A5 and undergoes extensive hepatic metabolism with fecal excretion. Renal excretion accounts for less than 1% of the administered dose. Isavuconazole is unique among the triazoles because of the extended elimination half-life (100 hours). Clearance of isavuconazole is not impacted by renal impairment. The clearance of isavuconazole in patients with mild-to-moderate hepatic impairment (Child-Pugh Classes A and B) is reduced, but no dosage adjustment is recommended. There are no data for patients who have Child-Pugh Class C liver disease.

Isavuconazole clearance may be affected by race. Chinese subjects were found to have a lower clearance of isavuconazole (2.6 L/hr vs 1.6 L/hr) compared to Caucasian subjects and a 50% higher AUC. However, no dosage adjustment has been recommended based on race. No PK studies of isavuconazole have been reported in children.

PHARMACOKINETIC DRUG INTERACTIONS

Isavuconazole is a substrate and a moderate inhibitor of CYP3A4. Isavuconazole is also a mild inhibitor of P-gp and organic cation transporter 2. Similar to itraconazole, voriconazole, and posaconazole, concomitant use of isavuconazole is contraindicated with strong CYP3A4 inducers (eg, rifampin). Medications that are metabolized through CYP3A4 should be used with caution in combination with isavuconazole and may require dosage adjustment with careful TDM (eg, tacrolimus, sirolimus, cyclosporine). Similar concurrent use of isavuconazole with strong CYP3A4 inducers (eg, rifampin) should be avoided because they will result in subtherapeutic exposures of isavuconazole.

KEY PARAMETERS: Isavuconazole[a]

THERAPEUTIC CONCENTRATIONS (PROVISIONAL)	C_{min}: >1 mg/L
F	98%
V_d	>7 L/kg
Cl	2-3 L/hr
AUC_{0-24hr}	97.9 mg·hr/L
$t_{1/2}$	100 hr
fu (fraction unbound)	1%

[a]Pharmacokinetic parameters may vary depending on patient characteristics and formulation administered.

ADVERSE EFFECTS

Isavuconazole was well tolerated in clinical trials, patients who received isavuconazole experienced fewer adverse effects (visual disturbances, liver function test abnormalities) compared to voriconazole. The most common reactions are headache, GI complaints, and mild elevation in serum transaminases. Isavuconazole is uniquely associated with QTc shortening (instead of QTc prolongation observed with other triazoles) and is contraindicated in patients with familial short QTc syndrome.

TIME TO SAMPLE

Following a loading dose, steady-state concentrations of isavuconazole are achieved after 5 to 7 days. A C_{min} sample is recommended immediately before the next dose after this time. Owing to the long half-life of the drug, samples drawn for TDM in the middle of the dosing interval will not differ substantially from the actual C_{min} concentration.

CLINICAL APPLICATION OF ISAVUCONAZOLE PHARMACOKINETICS

Currently, there are limited data supporting the need for routine TDM for isavuconazole. However, TDM may be warranted in patients with suspected clinical failure or progression of the infection on treatment, infection with a resistant pathogen, or PK drug interactions. A C_{min} concentration of greater than 1 mg/L (but ideally 2-4 mg/L) would suggest adequate drug exposures. After ruling out drug interactions or other possible causes of inadequate exposures, switching to IV therapy (if on oral) or dosage escalation up to 600 mg/d could be considered in select patient with low isavuconazole blood levels.

REFERENCES

1. Brown GD, Denning DW, Gow NAR, Levitz SM, Netea MG, White TC. Hidden killers: human fungal infections. *Sci Transl Med.* 2012;4(165):165rv13.

2. Brüggemann RJM, Alffenaar JWC, Blijlevens NMA, et al. Clinical relevance of the pharmacokinetic interactions of azole antifungal drugs with other coadministered agents. *Clin Infect Dis.* 2009;48(10):1441-1458.

3. Ashbee HR, Barnes RA, Johnson EM, Richardson MD, Gorton R, Hope WW. Therapeutic drug monitoring (TDM) of antifungal agents: guidelines from the British Society for Medical Mycology. *J Antimicrob Chemother.* 2014;69(5):1162-1176.

4. Pappas PG, Kauffman CA, Andes DR, et al. Clinical practice guideline for the management of candidiasis: 2016 update by the infectious diseases society of America. *Clin Infect Dis.* 2016;62(4): e1-50.

5. Johnson MD. Antifungals in clinical use and the pipeline. *Infect Dis Clin North Am.* 2021;35(2):341-371.

6. Rodríguez-Tudela JL, Almirante B, Rodríguez-Pardo D, et al. Correlation of the MIC and dose/MIC ratio of fluconazole to the therapeutic response of patients with mucosal candidiasis and candidemia. *Antimicrob Agents Chemother.* 2007;51(10):3599-3604.

7. Felton T, Troke PF, Hope WW. Tissue penetration of antifungal agents. *Clin Microbiol Rev.* 2014; 27(1):68-88.

8. van der Elst KCM, Pereboom M, van den Heuvel ER, Kosterink JGW, Schölvinck EH, Alffenaar JWC. Insufficient fluconazole exposure in pediatric cancer patients and the need for therapeutic drug monitoring in critically ill children. *Clin Infect Dis.* 2014;59(11):1527-1533.

9. Sinnollareddy MG, Roberts JA, Lipman J, et al; DALI Study authors. Pharmacokinetic variability and exposures of fluconazole, anidulafungin, and caspofungin in intensive care unit patients: data from multinational Defining Antibiotic Levels in Intensive care unit (DALI) patients Study. *Crit Care.* 2015;19(1):33.

10. Nicolau DP, Crowe HM, Nightingale CH, Quintiliani R. Rifampin-fluconazole interaction in critically ill patients. *Ann Pharmacother.* 1995;29(10):994-996.

11. Thompson GR III, Krois CR, Affolter VK, et al. Examination of fluconazole-induced alopecia in an animal model and human cohort. *Antimicrob Agents Chemother.* 2019;63(2):e01384-18. doi:10.1128/AAC.01384-18

12. Glasmacher A, Molitor E, Hahn C, et al. Antifungal prophylaxis with itraconazole in neutropenic patients with acute leukaemia. *Leukemia.* 1998;12(9):1338-1343.

13. Glasmacher A, Prentice A, Gorschlüter M, et al. Itraconazole prevents invasive fungal infections in neutropenic patients treated for hematologic malignancies: evidence from a meta-analysis of 3,597 patients. *J Clin Oncol.* 2003;21(24):4615-4626.

14. Glasmacher A, Hahn C, Molitor E, Marklein G, Sauerbruch T, Schmidt-Wolf I. Itraconazole trough concentrations in antifungal prophylaxis with six different dosing regimens using hydroxypropyl-beta-cyclodextrin oral solution or coated-pellet capsules. *Mycoses.* 1999;42(11-12):591-600.

15. Glasmacher A, Hahn C, Leutner C, et al. Breakthrough invasive fungal infections in neutropenic patients after prophylaxis with itraconazole. *Mycoses.* 1999;42(7-8):443-451.

16. Lestner JM, Roberts SA, Moore CB, Howard SJ, Denning DW, Hope WW. Toxicodynamics of itraconazole: implications for therapeutic drug monitoring. *Clin Infect Dis.* 2009;49(6):928-930.

17. Lepak AJ, Andes DR. Antifungal pharmacokinetics and pharmacodynamics. *Cold Spring Harb Perspect Med.* 2014;5(5):a019653.

18. Abuhelwa AY, Foster DJR, Mudge S, Hayes D, Upton RN. Population pharmacokinetic modeling of itraconazole and hydroxyitraconazole for oral SUBA-itraconazole and sporanox capsule formulations in healthy subjects in fed and fasted states. *Antimicrob Agents Chemother.* 2015;59(9):5681-5696.

19. Wiederhold NP, Pennick GJ, Dorsey SA, et al. A reference laboratory experience of clinically achievable voriconazole, posaconazole, and itraconazole concentrations within the bloodstream and cerebral spinal fluid. *Antimicrob Agents Chemother.* 2014;58(1):424-431.

20. Patterson TF, Thompson GR III, Denning DW, et al. Practice guidelines for the diagnosis and management of aspergillosis: 2016 update by the Infectious Diseases Society of America. *Clin Infect Dis.* 2016;63(4):e1-e60.

21. Pascual A, Csajka C, Buclin T, et al. Challenging recommended oral and intravenous voriconazole doses for improved efficacy and safety: population pharmacokinetics-based analysis of adult patients with invasive fungal infections. *Clin Infect Dis*. 2012;55(3):381-390.

22. Pascual A, Calandra T, Bolay S, Buclin T, Bille J, Marchetti O. Voriconazole therapeutic drug monitoring in patients with invasive mycoses improves efficacy and safety outcomes. *Clin Infect Dis*. 2008;46(2):201-211.

23. Dolton MJ, Ray JE, Chen SCA, Ng K, Pont LG, McLachlan AJ. Multicenter study of voriconazole pharmacokinetics and therapeutic drug monitoring. *Antimicrob Agents Chemother*. 2012;56(9):4793-4799.

24. Troke PF, Hockey HP, Hope WW. Observational study of the clinical efficacy of voriconazole and its relationship to plasma concentrations in patients. *Antimicrob Agents Chemother*. 2011;55(10):4782-4788.

25. Park WB, Kim NH, Kim KH, et al. The effect of therapeutic drug monitoring on safety and efficacy of voriconazole in invasive fungal infections: a randomized controlled trial. *Clin Infect Dis*. 2012;55(8):1080-1087.

26. Tan K, Brayshaw N, Tomaszewski K, Troke P, Wood N. Investigation of the potential relationships between plasma voriconazole concentrations and visual adverse events or liver function test abnormalities. *J Clin Pharmacol*. 2006;46(2):235-243.

27. Neely M, Rushing T, Kovacs A, Jelliffe R, Hoffman J. Voriconazole pharmacokinetics and pharmacodynamics in children. *Clin Infect Dis*. 2010;50(1):27-36.

28. Groll AH, Castagnola E, Cesaro S, Dalle JH. Fourth European Conference on Infections in Leukaemia (ECIL-4): guidelines for diagnosis, prevention, and treatment of invasive fungal diseases in paediatric patients with cancer or allogeneic haemopoietic stem-cell transplantation. *Lancet Oncol*. 2014;15(8):e327-e340. http://www.sciencedirect.com/science/article/pii/S1470204514700178

29. Friberg LE, Ravva P, Karlsson MO, Liu P. Integrated population pharmacokinetic analysis of voriconazole in children, adolescents, and adults. *Antimicrob Agents Chemother*. 2012;56(6):3032-3042.

30. Hope W, Johnstone G, Cicconi S, et al. Software for dosage individualization of voriconazole: a prospective clinical study. *Antimicrob Agents Chemother*. 2019;63(4):e02353-18. doi:10.1128/AAC.02353-18

31. Abel S, Allan R, Gandelman K, Tomaszewski K, Webb DJ, Wood ND. Pharmacokinetics, safety and tolerance of voriconazole in renally impaired subjects: two prospective, multicentre, open-label, parallel-group volunteer studies. *Clin Drug Investig*. 2008;28(7):409-420.

32. Burkhardt O, Thon S, Burhenne J, Welte T, Kielstein JT. Sulphobutylether-beta-cyclodextrin accumulation in critically ill patients with acute kidney injury treated with intravenous voriconazole under extended daily dialysis. *Int J Antimicrob Agents*. 2010;36(1):93-94.

33. Turner RB, Martello JL, Malhotra A. Worsening renal function in patients with baseline renal impairment treated with intravenous voriconazole: a systematic review. *Int J Antimicrob Agents*. 2015;46(4):362-366.

34. Driscoll TA, Yu LC, Frangoul H, et al. Comparison of pharmacokinetics and safety of voriconazole intravenous-to-oral switch in immunocompromised children and healthy adults. *Antimicrob Agents Chemother*. 2011;55(12):5770-5779.

35. Boyd NK, Zoellner CL, Swancutt MA, Bhavan KP. Utilization of omeprazole to augment subtherapeutic voriconazole concentrations for treatment of Aspergillus infections. *Antimicrob Agents Chemother*. 2012;56(11):6001-6002.

36. Wood N, Tan K, Purkins L, Layton G. Effect of omeprazole on the steady-state pharmacokinetics of voriconazole. *Br J Clin Pharmacol*. 2003;56(suppl 1):56-61. http://onlinelibrary.wiley.com/doi/10.1046/j.1365-2125.2003.02000.x/full

37. Cornely OA, Maertens J, Winston DJ, et al. Posaconazole vs. fluconazole or itraconazole prophylaxis in patients with neutropenia. *N Engl J Med*. 2007;356(4):348-359.

38. Ullmann AJ, Lipton JH, Vesole DH, et al. Posaconazole or fluconazole for prophylaxis in severe graft-versus-host disease. *N Engl J Med*. 2007;356(4):335-347.

39. Walsh TJ, Raad I, Patterson TF, et al. Treatment of invasive aspergillosis with posaconazole in patients who are refractory to or intolerant of conventional therapy: an externally controlled trial. *Clin Infect Dis*. 2007;44(1):2-12.

40. Jang SH, Colangelo PM, Gobburu JVS. Exposure-response of posaconazole used for prophylaxis against invasive fungal infections: evaluating the need to adjust doses based on drug concentrations in plasma. *Clin Pharmacol Ther*. 2010;88(1):115-119.

41. Tverdek FP, Heo ST, Aitken SL, Granwehr B, Kontoyiannis DP. Real-life assessment of the safety and effectiveness of the new tablet and intravenous formulations of posaconazole in the prophylaxis of invasive fungal

infections via analysis of 343 courses. *Antimicrob Agents Chemother.* 2017;61(8):e00188-17. doi:10.1128/AAC.00188-17

42. Davis MR, Nguyen MVH, Gintjee TJ, Odermatt A, Young BY, Thompson GR. Management of posaconazole-induced pseudohyperaldosteronism. *J Antimicrob Chemother.* 2020;75(12):3688-3693.

43. Nguyen MVH, Davis MR, Wittenberg R, et al. Posaconazole serum drug levels associated with pseudohyperaldosteronism. *Clin Infect Dis.* 2020;70(12):2593-2598.

44. Suh HJ, Kim I, Cho JY, et al. Early therapeutic drug monitoring of posaconazole oral suspension in patients with hematologic malignancies. *Ther Drug Monit.* 2018;40(1):115-119.

45. Maertens JA, Raad II, Marr KA, et al. Isavuconazole versus voriconazole for primary treatment of invasive mould disease caused by Aspergillus and other filamentous fungi (SECURE): a phase 3, randomised-controlled, non-inferiority trial. *Lancet.* 2016;387(10020):760-769.

46. Marty FM, Ostrosky-Zeichner L, Cornely OA, et al; VITAL and FungiScope Mucormycosis Investigators. Isavuconazole treatment for mucormycosis: a single-arm open-label trial and case-control analysis. *Lancet Infect Dis.* 2016;16(7):828-837.

47. Kaindl T, Andes D, Engelhardt M, Saulay M, Larger P, Groll AH. Variability and exposure-response relationships of isavuconazole plasma concentrations in the Phase 3 SECURE trial of patients with invasive mould diseases. *J Antimicrob Chemother.* 2019;74(3):761-767.

48. Andes DR, Ghannoum MA, Mukherjee PK, et al. Outcomes by MIC values for patients treated with isavuconazole or voriconazole for invasive aspergillosis in the phase 3 SECURE and VITAL trials. *Antimicrob Agents Chemother.* 2019;63(1):e01634-18. doi:10.1128/AAC.01634-18

49. Arendrup MC, Meletiadis J, Mouton JW, et al; Subcommittee on Antifungal Susceptibility Testing (AFST) of the ESCMID European Committee for Antimicrobial Susceptibility Testing (EUCAST). EUCAST technical note on isavuconazole breakpoints for Aspergillus, itraconazole breakpoints for Candida and updates for the antifungal susceptibility testing method documents. *Clin Microbiol Infect.* 2016;22(6):571.e1-571.e4.

50. Furfaro E, Signori A, Di Grazia C, et al. Serial monitoring of isavuconazole blood levels during prolonged antifungal therapy. *J Antimicrob Chemother.* 2019;74(8):2341-2346.

11

CARBAMAZEPINE

Laura F. Ruekert and Jeanne H. VanTyle[†]

Learning Objectives

By the end of the carbamazepine chapter, the learner shall be able to:

1. Estimate the initial dosage for a patient on carbamazepine (CBZ), including the population estimates for V_d and clearance.
2. Explain why loading doses of CBZ are not recommended.
3. List and perform the pharmacokinetic calculations necessary for initial adjustments in the maintenance dose of CBZ.
4. Describe the metabolism and clearance of CBZ and anticipate possible drug interactions or adverse reactions related to clearance.
5. Understand and explain the role of pharmacogenetics with pharmacokinetics and pharmacodynamics of CBZ and its adverse drug reaction profile.

Carbamazepine (CBZ) is an anticonvulsant compound that is structurally similar to the tricyclic antidepressant agents. It blocks voltage-dependent sodium channels and is the drug of choice for the treatment of trigeminal neuralgia (tic douloureux, glossopharyngeal neuralgia syndrome) and is used in the treatment of a variety of seizure disorders. It has the Food and Drug Administration (FDA) approval for generalized tonic-clonic (grand mal) and partial (psychomotor, temporal lobe) seizures, bipolar disorders, and in acute mania and mixed episodes. It is used off-label in a variety of other conditions, including pain syndromes, migraine headaches, and other neurologic disorders. CBZ is most frequently prescribed for those patients who have failed to respond to other anticonvulsant therapy or for those who have developed significant side effects from other anticonvulsant agents.[1,2]

CBZ is available in many dosage forms, including oral suspension, chewable tablets, oral tablets, extended-release tablets, and extended-release capsules. High-fat meals will increase the rate, but not the extent, of absorption. The contents of the capsule cannot be altered by chewing but may be sprinkled on applesauce if required.[3]

[†]Deceased.

CBZ is available generically from several manufacturers. It is labeled for use in children through adulthood. The most commonly used dose for children less than 6 years is 10 to 20 mg/kg/d initially but, at steady state, is likely to be 20 to 30 mg/kg/d orally divided twice daily. Effective doses for adults with seizure disorders are in the range of 15 to 25 mg/kg/d (or 800-1,200 mg/d) at steady state. Migraine prophylaxis doses are usually in the range of 10 to 20 mg/kg/d given twice daily with extended-release products.

KEY PARAMETERS: Carbamazepine

Therapeutic plasma concentrations	4-12 mg/L
F	80% tablets
S	1.0
V^a	1.1 L/kg
$Cl^{a,b}$ (L/kg/hr)	
Monotherapy	0.064
Polytherapy	0.10
Children (monotherapy)	0.11
Free fraction	0.2-0.3
$t_{1/2}$ (hr)	
Adult monotherapy	15
Adult polytherapy[b]	10

[a]The values for volume of distribution and clearance are approximations based upon oral administration data and an estimate of bioavailability.
[b]The clearance and half-life values represent adult values after induction has taken place. Polytherapy represents a patient receiving other enzyme-inducing anticonvulsants (eg, phenobarbital, phenytoin).

CBZ is metabolized by CYP3A4 and CYP3A5, producing a carbamazepine-10, 11-epoxide, metabolite responsible for both therapeutic and adverse effects. The half-life of 10,11-epoxide is approximately 34 hours. The carbamazepine-10,11-epoxide to CBZ ratios are higher in infants and preschool children. Children have been shown to have increased CYP3A4 activity as compared to adults. Less than 2% of CBZ is excreted unchanged in the urine. CBZ is approximately 75% bound to plasma albumin and α_1-acid glycoprotein. Usual half-life of CBZ, 24 to 30 hours, as monotherapy would suggest achievement of steady state within a week. However, the time to achieve steady state is highly variable, with reports of 4 to 15 days owing to autoinduction.

THERAPEUTIC AND TOXIC PLASMA CONCENTRATIONS

The range of therapeutic serum concentrations for CBZ is reported to be 4 to 12 mg/L (SI: 17-51 µmol/L). The conversion of mass units to SI units is 1 µg/mL = 4.23 µmol/L. Many patients will develop symptoms of toxicity, including cardiovascular toxicity, such as second- and third-degree heart block, when plasma concentrations exceed 10 mg/L. For this reason, many clinicians prefer to use a therapeutic range of approximately 4 to 8 mg/L, especially in patients on other anticonvulsants. Adverse reactions such as neuromuscular disturbances can be difficult to tolerate, and some clinicians prefer a lower therapeutic range. The clinician should be aware of conditions that can increase the formation of 10,11-epoxide,[4–6] such as simultaneous administration of quetiapine,[7] phenytoin, and valproate sodium.[8] In most patients, the CBZ to its major metabolite (10,11-epoxide) ratio is relatively constant,[9,10] with serum concentrations of the epoxide metabolite ranging from 15% to 40% of CBZ.[4,7] In some patients, such as in overdose situations when protein binding is saturated, it might be useful to monitor total CBZ and the 10,11-epoxide metabolite because serum concentrations will significantly increase to 50% to 80% of the CBZ concentration.[4,11]

ADVERSE EFFECTS

CBZ is associated with numerous adverse drug reactions. The most common adverse effects associated with CBZ involve the central nervous system (CNS) and include dizziness, nystagmus, ataxia, blurred vision, diplopia, dry mouth, nausea, vomiting, drowsiness, and suicidality. Cardiovascular, renal, and hepatic effects vary in severity and include tachycardia, hyponatremia, hepatic porphyria, and hepatotoxicity. Idiosyncratic dermatologic and hematologic reactions associated with CBZ include agranulocytosis, aplastic anemia, mild maculopapular eruption and drug hypersensitivity syndrome or drug reaction with eosinophilia and systemic symptoms (DRESS), Stevens-Johnson syndrome (SJS),[12] and toxic epidermal necrolysis (TEN).[13]

The appropriateness of pharmacogenomics testing should be evaluated when considering the initiation of CBZ or when there is a diagnosis of SJS, TEN, DRESS, or other cutaneous reaction such as mild maculopapular eruption potentially secondary to CBZ, owing to the significant associated morbidity and mortality. The presence of either the HLA-A*31:01 or HLA-B*15:02 allele has been associated with the development of these cutaneous reactions, with reported odds ratios (ORs) of 9 and 113 in all populations.[14,15] Clinical Pharmacogenetics Implementations Consortium guidelines and the FDA recommended patients with ancestry in at-risk populations should be screened for the presence of HLA-B*1502 allele before starting CBZ.[16-18] Studies confirm highest at-risk individuals include those of Han Chinese descent, followed by Vietnam, Cambodia, the Reunion Islands, Thailand, India, Malaysia, and Hong Kong.[14,15] Any individual with at least one copy of HLA-B15:02 allele should avoid CBZ unless the benefits outweigh the risks *and* the patient has taken the drug for 3 months or more without any development of cutaneous adverse reactions.[18] Whereas HLA-B*15:02 is more strongly associated with SJS/TEN, particularly in Han Chinese (OR 1,357),[18,19] HLA-A*31:01 is associated with all phenotypes of CBZ-induced cutaneous reactions in Japanese, Korean, European, and mixed ancestries (OR 9).[15,16,20] It is noteworthy that some patients without copies of the allele have experienced SJS/TEN, regardless of ancestry.

CBZ, pregnancy class D, is teratogenic and has been associated with neural tube defects by antagonizing enzymes in folate metabolism and interfering with folate absorption.[21,22] Polymorphism in genes associated with folate metabolism, including methylenetetrahydrofolate reductase, methionine synthase reductase, and methylenetetrahydrofolate dehydrogenase, may lead to difference in the susceptibility of individuals to folate antagonists.[23] CBZ and 10,11-epoxide both pass into the breast milk, and clinicians should take into consideration the importance of the drug to the mother while balancing the risks to the nursing infant.

Many antiepileptic drugs, including CBZ, appear to increase the risk of suicidal thoughts or behavior. Patients should be monitored for worsening of depression, suicidal thoughts, and/or any changes in mood or behavior. In one study of 827 suicidal acts in

297,620 treatment episodes, oxcarbazepine, tiagabine, lamotrigine, valproate, and pheno-barbital had rates greater than CBZ.[24] Unlike the risk of suicidality associated with anti-depressants, the risk of suicidality associated with antiepileptics shows no relationship to age and may persist for the duration of treatment. To minimize the risk of CBZ adverse effects, a baseline comprehensive history and physical examination along with baseline and periodic complete blood count, comprehensive metabolic panel, liver function tests, drug levels, and electrocardiogram are recommended monitoring parameters.

PHARMACOKINETICS

Bioavailability (*F*)

CBZ is a lipid-soluble compound that is slowly and variably absorbed from the gastro-intestinal tract. Peak plasma concentrations following immediate-release products oc-cur at approximately 6 hours (range 2-24 hours) after oral ingestion. Grapefruit juice increases the bioavailability of CBZ by inhibiting CYP3A4 in the gut wall and liver. There is evidence that CYP induction/inhibition modulates drug transporter expres-sion of P-glycoprotein, MRP2 (multidrug resistance protein 2), and MRP3 (multidrug resistance protein 3). A high-fat meal has been shown to increase the rate of absorp-tion and elevate the peak concentration while not changing the extent as measured by the area under the curve. Following administration of an intravenous product, bioavailability is shown to be 0.78.[25,26] Because CBZ is slowly absorbed, changes in gastrointestinal function, especially those associated with rapid transit, could decrease its bioavailability and result in variable plasma concentrations of CBZ. For clinical purposes, the authors assume the bioavailability factor (*F*) to be approximately 0.8 for CBZ when administered as an oral tablet, chewable tablet, or suspension.

Volume of Distribution (*V*)

On average, the volume of distribution for CBZ is approximately 1.1 L/kg.[27] CBZ, a neutral compound, is primarily bound to albumin and α_1-acid glycoprotein and has a free fraction (α) of approximately 0.2 to 0.3. In uremic patients, increases in free CBZ concentrations may be observed. Although CBZ is bound to plasma proteins, there are very few clinical studies exploring alterations in plasma-binding characteristics. This may be because CBZ is bound to multiple plasma proteins and, with a free fraction of 0.2 to 0.3, a fairly large change in plasma binding would be required for the change in binding to become clinically significant. CBZ daily dose should be based on ideal body weight, but not on total body weight.[28] Loading doses of CBZ are not commonly uti-lized because time must be allowed for concentrations to rise to steady state, because autoinduction alters the pharmacokinetics of CBZ.

Clearance (Cl)

CBZ is eliminated almost exclusively by metabolism, with less than 2% of an oral dose being excreted remain unchanged in the urine. CBZ is metabolized in the liver by CYP3A4/5 isoenzymes and induces CYP1A2 (strong), CYP2B6 (moderate), CYP2C8/9 (strong), CYP2C19 (strong), and CYP3A4 (strong) to accelerate the he-patic metabolism of other drugs (see Figure 11.1). The average clearance value appears

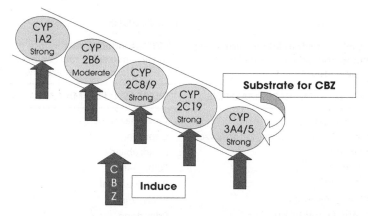

FIGURE 11.1   The metabolism of carbamazepine is via CYP3A4. Carbamazepine is capable of inducing CYP1A2, CYP2B6, CYP2C8/9, CYP2C19, and CYP3A4/5. The induction of the same system as is used for "autoinduction." This leads to unique pharmacokinetic difficulties until steady-state conditions are reached. Carbamazepine also induces P-gp production and uses UGT1A1 and UGT2B7. CBZ, carbamazepine; P-gp, P-glycoprotein.

to be approximately 0.064 L/kg/hr in adult patients who have received the drug chronically. Data indicate gender and racial differences account for variability in CBZ clearance.[29] Studies indicate that absolute clearance (L/hr/kg) was significantly lower in men as compared to women (0.039 vs 0.049, $P = .007$) and in African Americans as compared to Caucasians (0.039 vs 0.048, $P = .019$).[25] A majority of studies show that apparent CYP3A4 activity is higher in women (and children) than in men.[30]

In patients who are taking other enzyme-inducing antiepileptic drugs concurrently (polytherapy), the clearance is increased to approximately 0.1 L/kg/hr. Single-dose studies suggest a clearance that is one-half to one-third of the values observed in patients on chronic therapy. The increase in clearance associated with chronic therapy is apparently owing to autoinduction of its metabolic enzymes.

Drug Interactions

CBZ has many drug interactions resulting from both CYP inhibition and induction that alter observed concentrations. CBZ has been shown to induce the metabolism of warfarin through CYP2C9. CBZ greatly reduces the serum concentrations of atorvastatin and rosuvastatin, probably by inducing the metabolism.[31] Because pravastatin is not metabolized by CYP3A4, it is not associated with this interaction.[32] In addition, CBZ induces the phase II metabolism isoenzymes UGT1A9 and UGT2B7 found in the liver, kidneys, and lower gastrointestinal tract. UGT1A9 and UGT2B7 play a major role in conjugation.[33] Table 11.1 lists selected drug interactions via CYP3A4.

CBZ induces its own metabolism through time- and dose-dependent autoinduction, resulting in the curvilinear relationship between the CBZ dose and the epoxide metabolite. Therefore, the use of clearance values from single-dose studies is impractical in the calculation of a maintenance dose and may lead to errors. The autoinduction of CBZ metabolism has many clinical implications. It is important to initiate patients on relatively low doses to avoid side effects early in therapy. The maintenance dose can be increased at 1- to 2-week intervals by 200 mg/d. The autoinduction phenomenon

TABLE 11.1   Carbamazepine Drug Interactions

CYP3A4 **inhibitors** that inhibit carbamazepine metabolism and increase plasma carbamazepine include	CYP3A4 **inducers** that induce the rate of carbamazepine metabolism and decrease plasma carbamazepine include
INCREASED PLASMA CARBAMAZEPINE	**DECREASED PLASMA CARBAMAZEPINE**
Azole antifungals	Carbamazepine[b]
Fluconazole, itraconazole, ketoconazole, voriconazole	Cisplatin
	Doxorubicin
Cimetidine	Felbamate
Clarithromycin[a]	Phenobarbital
Chloroquine, mefloquine	Phenytoin
Dalfopristin/Quinupristin	Primidone
Diltiazem	Rifampin
Erythromycin[a]	Theophylline
Fluoxetine	
Fluvoxamine	
Grapefruit juice	
Isoniazid	
Lithium	
Loratadine	
Loxapine	
Niacinamide	
Protease inhibitors	
Indinavir, nelfinavir, ritonavir	
Quetiapine	
Quinine	
Ranolazine	
Troleandomycin	
Valproate[a]	
Verapamil	
Zileuton	

Partial list of drugs known to affect serum concentrations of carbamazepine.
[a]Inhibit epoxide hydrolase, resulting in increased concentrations of carbamazepine 10,11-epoxide.
[b]Autoinduction.

also limits pharmacokinetic study and manipulation of CBZ dosing. For example, it is uncertain whether induction is an all-or-none or a graded process that is dose related. Induction should be complete within 5 to 7 days but may take up to a few weeks. Finally, autoinduction of metabolism commonly causes changes in steady-state CBZ levels that are less than proportional to an increase in the maintenance dose.

As with many of the anticonvulsant agents, CBZ has been associated with cross-induction of other anticonvulsants. For this reason, whenever CBZ is added to an anticonvulsant regimen or other agents are added to a CBZ regimen, additional plasma level monitoring may be appropriate to ensure that the maintenance regimen continues to result in plasma levels that are optimal for therapeutic control.

Table 11.2 provides examples of monitoring recommendations for selected drug interactions. Under certain conditions, as with valproate, erythromycin, and clarithromycin, the CBZ concentration is reduced, and the 10,11-epoxide concentration is increased.[33] This may explain the observation of CNS side effects in some patients with relatively low CBZ plasma concentrations and may warrant checking the epoxide metabolite level in addition to the CBZ drug concentration.

Patients treated with a combination of antiretroviral agents and CBZ are at increased risk of interactions.[34] CBZ use is common in the treatment of HIV-infected patients because approximately 10% of patients have seizures secondary to neurologic manifestations of HIV and opportunistic CNS infections. CBZ can reduce concentrations of antiretroviral agents and, importantly, be implicated in the loss of virologic response. In particular, the well-established efficacy of recommended first-line integrase strand transfer inhibitor regimens containing dolutegravir for HIV can be compromised and warrants dolutegravir dosing increases from once daily to twice daily when given concomitantly with CBZ.[34,35] Various protease inhibitors, nucleoside reverse transcription inhibitors (NRTIs), non-nucleoside reverse transcriptase inhibitors (NNRTIs), and their associated combination products interact with CBZ and should be carefully evaluated to optimize treatment response.

TABLE 11.2 Effects of Carbamazepine on Other Select Drugs

DRUG(S)	MECHANISM	EFFECT	RECOMMENDATION
Efavirenz/ other NNRTIs	Induction of CYP3A4 by carbamazepine	Reduction in plasma concentration of NNRTI and loss of virologic response	Monitor carbamazepine concentrations and adjust. Consider alternative AED agent
Lithium	Pharmacodynamic effect	Neurotoxic effects	A reduced lithium dose may be needed
Oral contraceptives	Induction of CYP3A4 by carbamazepine	Enhanced metabolism of EE and norethindrone resulting in contraceptive failure	Backup method of contraception required; barrier or IUD
Phenytoin Primidone	Hepatic metabolism induced	Combination may alter levels of both drugs; may increase CNS depression	Monitor serum concentrations of phenytoin and carbamazepine
Warfarin	Induction of CYP1A2 and CYP3A4	Decreased anticoagulant effect	Increased monitoring and change in dose may be required. Consider alternative anticoagulant

AED, antiepileptic drug; CNS, central nervous system; EE, ethinylestradiol; IUD, intrauterine device; NNRTIs, non-nucleoside reverse transcriptase inhibitors.

Estradiol is metabolized by CYP1A2, and CYP1A2 is induced by CBZ. Studies have shown lowered sex hormone levels secondary to enzyme-induced accelerated metabolism and higher sex hormone–binding globulin that reduces the free concentrations of the hormones.[36] Induced metabolism of sex steroid hormones by CBZ increases the risk of contraceptive failure and may result in pregnancy.[37] This is especially true for women on low-dose contraceptive hormones.[37-40]

Half-Life ($t_{1/2}$)

Single-dose studies predict a CBZ half-life of approximately 30 to 35 hours. However, steady-state data suggest a half-life of approximately 15 hours in adult patients receiving CBZ monotherapy and approximately 10 hours in patients receiving other enzyme-inducing antiepileptic drugs (eg, phenytoin, phenobarbital) concurrently. Children metabolize CBZ more rapidly than adults do, with reported steady-state half-lives of 4 to 12 hours.

Time to Sample

Obtaining CBZ plasma samples within the first few weeks of therapy may be useful to establish a relationship between CBZ concentration and a patient's clinical response. However, these data should be interpreted cautiously if one is attempting to predict the long-term relationship between a CBZ dosing regimen and plasma levels. Once steady state has been achieved, the time of sampling within a dosing interval is somewhat arbitrary, given the long half-life and relatively short dosing interval for CBZ. It is important to establish a fixed relationship between drug intake and blood sampling. The most sensible time to take routine samples is in the early morning (trough) before the first dose of medication is administered, or later in the day, before the next dose. Such samples will reflect the trough concentration and are comparable from day to day. In addition, the clinician can monitor plasma drug levels without concern for artifactual errors, including the influence of diet and food intake on absorption of the drug from the gastrointestinal tract. Nevertheless, it is reasonable to obtain CBZ plasma samples at a consistent time within the dosing interval. As a rule, samples should be obtained just before a dose (trough) unless this is markedly inconvenient for the patient. Inconvenience is most likely to be encountered in ambulatory patients who may be taking the drug on a schedule that is not consistent with their clinic appointments.

PHARMACOGENETICS

It has been suggested that single-nucleotide polymorphisms (SNPs) within the CBZ pathway contribute to the variability seen with its pharmacokinetics and thus response or even resistance. SCN1A gene belongs to a family of genes that provide instructions for making sodium channels. Overall, 25 SNPs have been identified and may account for the variability in CBZ pharmacokinetics. For example, SNPs associated with CYP3A, EPHX1 (epoxide hydrolase 1), UGT2B7, and drug transporters (ABCB1 and ABCB2) may alter clearance, volume of distribution, serum drug levels, and the CBZ to the epoxide metabolite ratio and, subsequently, may be implicated in the setting of drug interactions, adverse reactions, suboptimal treatment response.[41]

Oxcarbazepine (Trileptal)

CBZ has a number of limitations, including autoinduction, many drug interactions, toxicities, and teratogenicity. Oxcarbazepine (Trileptal) was developed as chemically similar to CBZ with an improved safety profile. Oxcarbazepine has a chemical structure similar to CBZ but with different metabolism. Oxcarbazepine is a prodrug of 10-monohydroxycarbazepine (MHD), the active metabolite that is responsible for the majority of drug actions. Oxcarbazepine is completely absorbed and converted to MHD. The volume of distribution is approximately 0.7 L/kg in adults. MHD has a half-life of about 9 hours, is taken 2 times a day, steady state is reached in 2 to 3 days, and about 40% is protein bound primarily to albumin. Oxcarbazepine biotransformation does not involve epoxide metabolite formation. The lack of an epoxide may contribute to the better tolerability of oxcarbazepine. More than 95% appears in the urine as metabolites, with less than 1% as unchanged drug. No dose adjustment is required for liver dysfunction but is for creatinine clearance of less than 30 mL/min. It is in pregnancy category C. Oxcarbazepine can inhibit CYP2C19 and induce CYP3A4/5. with potentially important effects on plasma concentrations of other drugs. The inhibition of CYP2C19 by oxcarbazepine and MHD can cause increased plasma concentrations of drugs that are substrates of CYP2C19. No autoinduction has been observed with oxcarbazepine. Coadministration of oxcarbazepine with an oral contraceptive has been shown to decrease the plasma concentrations of the two hormonal components, ethinylestradiol and levonorgestrel.[42]

Eslicarbazepine (Aptiom)

Eslicarbazepine is the newest member of this antiepileptic drug group. Eslicarbazepine is approved for both adjunctive and monotherapy of partial-onset seizures in adults and children (6-17 years).[43] It is used off-label for bipolar disorder and trigeminal neuralgia. It is structurally different from CBZ and oxcarbazepine. Eslicarbazepine has a linear pharmacokinetic profile, low binding to plasma proteins (<40%), and a half-life of 20 to 24 hours and is mainly excreted by the kidneys in an unchanged form or as glucuronide conjugates. It has a low potential for drug interactions.[42,44,45] Like oxcarbazepine, it is not metabolized to an epoxide. A common concern of the three agents is hyponatremia that has been reported with all. The hyponatremia appears to be caused by syndrome of inappropriate antidiuretic hormone secretion and is dose related. It also induces oral contraceptives and may cause oral contraceptives to be less effective by lowering concentrations of ethinylestradiol and levonorgestrel. Oxcarbazepine and eslicarbazepine do not have black-box warnings for HLA-B*1502, aplastic anemia, or agranulocytosis.[43,45,46]

> **Question #1** *N.S., a 36-year-old, 60-kg female, is to be started on CBZ as an anticonvulsant agent. How would you initiate therapy? Explain your rationale. Estimate the amount needed at steady state and then propose how to start the patient on therapy. Calculate a daily dose that will produce an average steady-state plasma concentration of approximately 6 mg/L.*

Do not give a loading dose of CBZ because of autoinduction. To calculate an average steady-state plasma concentration, the maintenance dose equation is used with an assumed bioavailability of 0.8 and an average clearance value of 3.84 L/hr (0.064 L/kg/hr × 60 kg). The fraction of the administered dose that is active drug (S) is 1.0.

$$Cl_{monotherapy} = 0.064 \text{ L/kg} \times 60 \text{ kg} = 3.84 \text{ L/hr} \qquad \text{(Eq. 11.1)}$$

$$\text{Maintenance dose} = \frac{(Cl)(C_{ss\,ave})(\tau)}{(S)(F)}$$

$$= \frac{(3.84 \text{ L/hr})(6 \text{ mg/L})(24 \text{ hr/1 day})}{(1)(0.8)}$$

$$= 691.2 \text{ mg/d}$$

This dose (~700 mg/d) is that which would be required to achieve the steady-state level of 6 mg/L after autoinduction of CBZ metabolism had taken place. For this reason, N.S. should be started on a lower daily dose initially and increased at 1- to 2-week intervals based on her clinical response. The usual initial daily dose for adult patients is 200 by mouth twice daily, with increases of approximately 200 mg/d every 7 to 14 days. When discontinuing treatment, reduce the dose gradually to avoid the risk of seizure.

Question #2   *After 2 months, the CBZ dose of N.S. has been increased to 300 mg orally 2 times a day. On this regimen, she has had some reduction in seizure frequency; however, seizure control is still considered unsatisfactory. The steady-state CBZ level at this time is reported to be 4 mg/L. What are possible explanations for this observed plasma level? What dose would be required to achieve a new steady-state CBZ level of 6 mg/L?*

Using the steady-state continuous infusion equation and a clearance of 3.84 L/hr, the anticipated CBZ level in N.S. for a dose of 600 mg/d would be approximately 5 mg/L. One should also consider whether to use literature values or patient observations when you have patient data that allow you to calculate clearance for the patient. Using the literature information:

$$C_{ss\,ave} = \frac{(S)(F)(\text{Dose}/\tau)}{(Cl)} \qquad \text{(Eq. 11.2)}$$

$$= \frac{(1)(0.8)(300 \text{ mg/12 hr})}{3.84 \text{ L/hr}}$$

$$= 5.2 \text{ mg/L}$$

The observed level of 4.0 mg/L is within the predicted range, considering the fact that both bioavailability and clearance values derived from average literature values may not be correct for N.S. At this point, it would be difficult to establish whether a slightly lower-than-expected bioavailability or a higher-than-average clearance was responsible for the observed level of 4.0 mg/L.

Because of CBZ's relatively slow absorption characteristics and long half-life, it is probable that the measured concentration of 4 mg/L represents an average steady-state value. At steady state, the average plasma concentration should be proportional to the daily dose. Therefore, to increase the plasma concentration from 4 to 6 mg/L, one would simply increase the CBZ dose by 50% (ie, from 600 to 900 mg/d).

$$\text{New maintenance dose} = \left(\frac{C_{ss\ ave\ new}}{C_{ss\ ave\ old}} \right) \text{Old maintenance dose} \qquad \textbf{(Eq. 11.3)}$$

$$= \left(\frac{C_{ss\ ave\ new}}{C_{ss\ ave\ old}} \right) 600\ mg/d$$

$$= 900\ mg/d$$

Another approach might be to calculate the apparent CBZ clearance for patient N.S. using a rearrangement of the maintenance dose Equation 11.1, the current maintenance dose of 300 mg/12 hr, and an assumed bioavailability of 0.8. In this case, patient observations are used rather than literature clearance:

$$Cl = \frac{(S)(F)(Dose/\tau)}{C_{ss\ ave}} \qquad \textbf{(Eq. 11.4)}$$

$$= \frac{(1)(0.8)(300\ mg/12\ hr)}{4\ mg/L}$$

$$= 5\ L/hr$$

This clearance value could then be used in the maintenance dose equation to calculate the maintenance dose as illustrated. However, this time, the clearance value that has been derived from the patient's specific data is used rather than an average value from the literature:

$$\text{Maintenance dose} = \frac{(Cl)(C_{ss\ ave})(\tau)}{(S)(F)}$$

$$= \frac{(5\ L/hr)(6\ mg/L)(24\ hr/d)}{(1)(0.8)}$$

$$= 900\ mg/d$$

If N.S. was receiving other anticonvulsant agents, it would be appropriate to monitor their concentrations as well, because CBZ could induce their metabolism, thereby reducing their steady-state concentrations.

Question #3 *The decision is made to add valproic acid to attempt better control of the seizures. N.S. returns 2 weeks later to the clinic. The patient complains that recently, she is sleepy and "feels funny." A CBZ concentration is drawn and reported to be 9 µg/mL. What is your explanation?*

Owing to the addition of valproic acid, a CYP3A4 enzyme inhibitor, the metabolism of CBZ is decreased, which, in turn, increases CBZ serum concentrations as well as the carbamazepine-10,11-epoxide, which also has some activity. This leads to increased serum concentration, and because the epoxide has activity, it can cause further sedation than was seen on the lower dose of CBZ. After serum levels have stabilized, the body may adjust to the higher level and her sleepiness will become less of a noticeable side effect.

In addition, valproic acid can inhibit the metabolism of CBZ via CYP3A4 and can displace CBZ from protein-binding sites, thus increasing the free fraction of CBZ. Valproic acid can increase the formation of the epoxide metabolite, which may also be picked up by the assay (about 7%) for CBZ. These factors can lead to an increase in CBZ's serum concentration, which could result in side effects such as drowsiness.

Question #4 *A.B. is a 60-year-old male (65 kg) currently receiving the following:*

MEDICATION	STEADY-STATE CONCENTRATION (µg/mL)
CBZ 200 mg 3 times a day	7
Phenytoin extended 300 mg orally at bedtime	11

Despite these agents, seizures persist, and the decision is made to add valproic acid of 250 mg orally 3 times a day. One month following the addition of valproic acid, A.B. complains of drowsiness. Drug concentrations are drawn, and the levels obtained are CBZ 7.6 µg/mL, phenytoin 8 µg/mL, and valproic acid 50 µg/mL. The serum albumin level reported is 4.2 g/dL. What is your explanation for the patient complaints?

Figure 11.2 depicts the effects valproic acid may have on CBZ and phenytoin levels. CBZ level is slightly increased because of the concurrent use of valproic acid, a CYP3A4 enzyme inhibitor, which decreases the metabolism of the CBZ. A possibility that the increase is only modest is because of the use of phenytoin, a CYP3A4 enzyme inducer, which may also be affecting the amount of CBZ being metabolized. Phenytoin levels are likely decreased owing to the increased CBZ level with additional increase in CBZ epoxide levels. From these increases, an increase in CYP3A4 induction occurs,

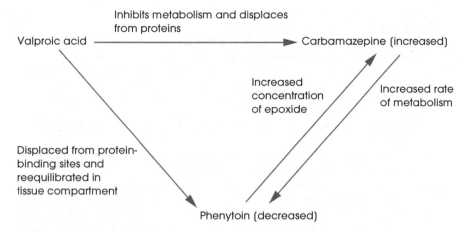

FIGURE 11.2   Complex interaction between carbamazepine, valproic acid, and phenytoin.

which causes an increase in phenytoin metabolism and a decrease in phenytoin serum levels. Valproic acid levels are within the therapeutic range but would potentially be higher if it was used as monotherapy and was not being influenced by the enzyme induction of phenytoin and CBZ.

REFERENCES

1. Johannessen-Landmark C, Johannessen SI. Pharmacological management of epilepsy: recent advances and future prospects. *Drugs*. 2008;68:1925-1939.

2. Glauser T, Ben-Menachem E, Bourgeois B, et al. ILAE treatment guidelines: evidence-based analysis of antiepileptic drug efficacy and effectiveness as initial monotherapy for epileptic seizures and syndromes. *Epilepsia*. 2006;47:1094-1120.

3. Equetro. Package insert. Validus Pharmaceuticals; 2012.

4. Russell JL, Spiller HA, Baker DD. Markedly elevated carbamazepine-10,11-epoxide/carbamazepine ratio in a fatal carbamazepine ingestion. *Case Rep Med*. 2015;2015:369707.

5. Burianová I, Bořecká K. Routine monitoring of the active metaboite of carbamazepine: is it really necessary? *Clin Biochem*. 2015;48(13-14):866-869.

6. Potter JM, Donnelly A. Carbamazepine-10,11-epoxide in therapeutic drug monitoring. *Ther Drug Monitor*. 1998;20(6):652-657.

7. Fitzgerald BJ, Okos AJ. Elevation of carbamazepine-10,11-epoxide by quetiapine. *Pharmacotherapy*. 2002;22(11):1500-1503.

8. Bernus I, Dickinson RG, Hooper WD, Eadie MJ. The mechanism of the carbamazepine-valproate interaction in humans. *Br J Clin Pharmacol*. 1997;44:21-27.

9. Tutor-Crespo MJ, Hermida J, Tutor JC. Relative proportions of serum carbamazepine and its pharmacological active 10,11-epoxy derivative: effect of polytherapy and renal insufficiency. *Ups J Med Sci*. 2008;113(2):171-180.

10. Ma CL, Jiao Z, Wu XY, Hong Z, Wu ZY, Zhong MK. Association between PK/PD-involved gene polymorphisms and carbamazepine-individualized therapy. *Pharmacogenonomics*. 2015;16(13):1499-1512.

11. Sol EL, Ruggles KH, Cascino GD, Ahmann PA, Weatherford KW. Seizure exacerbation and status epilepticus related to carbamazepine-10,11-epoxide. *Ann Neurol*. 1994;35(6):743-746.

12. Ferrell PB, McLeod HL. Carbamazepine, HLA-B* 1502 and the risk of Stevens-Johnson syndrome and toxic epidermal necrolysis: US FDA recommendations. *Pharmacogenomics*. 2008;9:1543-1546.

13. Anderson GD. Pharmacokinetics, pharmacodynamic, and pharmacogenetic targeted therapy of antiepileptic drugs. *Ther Drug Monit*. 2008;30:173-180.

14. Whirl-Carrillo M, McDonagh EM, Hebert JM, et al. Pharmacogenomics knowledge for personalized medicine. *Clin Pharmacol Ther*. 2012;92(4):414-417.

15. Leckband SG, Kelsoe JR, Dunnenberger HM, et al; Clinical Pharmacogenetics Implementation Consortium. Clinical Pharmacogenetics Implementation Consortium (CPIC) guidelines for HLA-B genotype and carbamazepine dosing. *Clin Pharmacol Ther*. 2013;94(3):324-328.

16. Genin E, Chen D-P, Hung S-I, et al. HLA-A*31:01 and different types of carbamazepine-induced severe cutaneous adverse reactions: an international study and meta-analysis. *Pharmacogenomics J*. 2014;14:281-288.

17. Hung S-I, Chung W-H, Jee S-H, et al. Genetic susceptibility to carbamazepine-induced cutaneous adverse drug reactions. *Pharmacogenet Genomics*. 2006;16:297-306.

18. Tangamornsuksan W, Chaiyakinapurk N, Somkrua R, Lohitnavy M, Tassaneeyakul W. Relationship between the HLA-B*1502 allele and carbamazepine-induced Stevens-Johnson syndrome and toxic epidermal necrolysis: a systematic review and meta-analysis. *JAMA Dermatol*. 2013;149(9):1025-1032.

19. Man CB, Kwan P, Baum L, et al. Association between HLA-B*1502 allele and antiepileptic drug-induced cutaneous reactions in Han Chinese. *Epilepsia*. 2007;48:1015-1018.

20. Amstutz U, Shear NH, Rieder MJ, et al; CPNDS Clinical Recommendation Group. Recommendations for HLA-B*15:02 and HLA-A*31:01 genetic testing to reduce the risk of carbamazepine-induced hypersensitivity reactions. *Epilepsia*. 2014;55(4):496-506.

21. Tomson T, Xu WH, Battino D. Major congenital malformations in children of women with epilepsy. *Seizure*. 2015;28:46-50.

22. Arpino C, Brescianini S, Robert E, et al. Teratogenic effects of antiepileptic drugs: use of an International Database on Malformations and Drug Exposure (MADRE). *Epilepsia*. 2000;41:1436-1443.

23. van Gelder MM, van Rooij IA, Miller RK, Zielhuis GA, de Jong-van den Berg LT, Roeleveld N. Teratogenic mechanisms of medical drugs. *Hum Reprod Update*. 2010;16(4):378-394.

24. Patorno E, Bohn RL, Wahl PM, et al. Anticonvulsant medications and the risk of suicide, attempted suicide, or violent death. *JAMA*. 2010;303(14):1401-1409.

25. Marino SE, Birnbaum AK, Leppil IE, et al. Steady-state carbamazepine pharmacokinetics following oral and stable-labeled intravenous administration in epilepsy patients: effects of race and sex. *Clin Pharmacol Ther*. 2012;91(3):483-488.

26. Tolbert D, Cloyd J, Biton V, et al. Bioequivalence of oral and intravenous carbamazepine formulations in adult patients with epilepsy. *Epilepsia*. 2015;56(6):915-923.

27. Landmark CJ, Johannessen SI, Tomson T. Host factors affecting antiepileptic drug delivery-pharmacokinetic variability. *Adv Drug Deliv Rev*. 2012;64:896-910.

28. Caraco Y, Zylber-Katz E, Berry EM, Levy M. Carbamazepine pharmacokinetics in obese and lean subjects. *Ann Pharmacother*. 1995;29:843-847.

29. Puranik YG, Birnbaum AK, Marino SE, et al. Association of carbamazepine major metabolism and transport pathway gene polymorphisms and pharmacokinetics in patients with epilepsy. *Pharmacogenomics*. 2013;14(1):35-45.

30. Harris RZ, Benet LZ, Schwartz JB. Gender effects in pharmacokinetic and pharmacodynamics. *Drugs*. 1995;50(2):222-239.

31. Parrish RH, Pazdur DE, O'Donnell PJ. Effect of carbamazepine initiation and discontinuation on antithrombotic control in a patient receiving warfarin: case report and review of the literature. *Pharmacotherapy*. 2006;26:1650-1653.

32. Bellosta S, Paoletti R, Corsini A. Safety of statins: focus on clinical pharmacokinetics and drug interactions. *Circulation*. 2004;109(23 suppl 1):III50-III57.

33. Caruso A, Bellia C, Pivetti A, et al. Effects of EPHX1 and CYP3A4 polymorphisms on carbamazepine metabolism in epileptic patients. *Pharmgenomics Pers Med*. 2014;7:117-120.

34. Günthard HF, Saag MS, Benson CA, et al. Antiretroviral drugs for treatment and prevention of HIV infection in adults. 2016 recommendations of the International Antiviral Society-USA panel. *JAMA*. 2016;316(2):191-210.

35. Song I, Weller S, Patel J, et al. Effect of carbamazepine on dolutegravir pharmacokinetics and dosing recommendation. *Eur J Clin Pharmacol*. 2016;72(6):665-670.

36. Brodie MJ, Mintzer S, Pack AM, Gidal BE, Vecht CJ, Schmidt D. Enzyme induction with antiepileptic drugs: cause for concern? *Epilepsia*. 2013;54(1):11-27.

37. Davis AR, Westhoff CL, Stanczyk FZ. Carbamazepine coadministration with an oral contraceptive: effects on steroid pharmacokinetics, ovulation, and bleeding. *Epilepsia*. 2011;52(2):243-247.

38. Lagana AS, Triolo O, D'Amico V, et al. Management of women with epilepsy: from preconception to post-partum. *Arch Gynecol Obstet*. 2016;293(3):493-503.

39. Bhajta J, Bainbridge J, Borgelt L. Teratogenic medications and concurrent contraceptive use in women of childbearing ability with epilepsy. *Epilepsy Behav*. 2015;52(Pt A):212-217.

40. Verrotti A, Mencaroni E, Castagnini M, Zaccara G. Foetal safety of old and new antiepileptic drugs. *Expert Opin Drug Saf*. 2015;14(10):1563-1571.

41. Daci A, Beretta G, Vllasaliu D, et al. Polymorphic variants of SCN1A and EPHX1 influence plasma carbamazepine concentration, metabolism, and pharmacoresistance in a population of Kosovar Albanian Epileptic Patients. *PLoS ONE*. 2015;10(11):1-17.

42. Zaccara G, Perucca E. Interactions between antiepileptic drugs, and between antiepileptic drugs and other drugs. *Epileptic Disord*. 2014;16(4):409-431.

43. Gierbolini J, Giarratano M, Benbadis SR. Carbamazepine-related antiepileptic drugs for the treatment of epilepsy—a comparative review. *Expert Opin Pharmacother*. 2016;17(7):885-888.

44. Tambucci R, Basti C, Maresca M, Coppola G, Verrotti A. Update on the role of eslicarbazepine acetate in the treatment of partial-onset epilepsy. *Neuropsychiatr Dis Treat*. 2016;12:1251-1260.

45. Zelano J, Ben-Menachem E. Eslicarbazepine acetate for the treatment of partial epilepsy. *Expert Opin Pharmacother*. 2016;17(8):1165-1169.

46. Zaccara G, Giovannelli F, Cincotta M, Carelli A, Verrotti A. Clinical utility of eslicarbazepine: current evidence. *Drug Des Devel Ther*. 2015;9:781-789.

12

PRECISION ONCOLOGY: PHARMACOKINETICS AND GENOMICS TO GUIDE CANCER THERAPY

James Kevin Hicks

Learning Objectives

By the end of the precision oncology: pharmacokinetics and genomics to guide cancer therapy chapter, the learner shall be able to:

1. Discuss how pharmacokinetics and genomics can be integrated into oncology practice to guide drug selection and mitigate toxicities.
2. Describe the methotrexate plasma concentrations and time course that would
   a. Identify patients at risk for methotrexate toxicity.
   b. Identify patients who would be most likely to have therapeutic benefit from methotrexate.
3. Convert methotrexate concentrations from mg/L to μM (10^{-6} M) and μM to mg/L.
4. Outline the usual dosing strategy for leucovorin rescue and conditions under which (concentration and time) the leucovorin rescue dose should be increased.
5. Describe the apparent two-compartment modeling of methotrexate and what would be the most appropriate volume of distribution to use when a loading dose is administered over a relatively short time period.
6. Identify patients who would be at risk for methotrexate toxicity considering the following:
   a. Renal function.
   b. Significant third spacing of fluid.
   c. Receiving drugs that are known to, or would be expected to, decrease methotrexate clearance.

7. Discuss the biphasic elimination of methotrexate and why the biphasic elimination is important to the timing of the methotrexate plasma samples and projection of when rescue will be achieved.

8. Do the following if a patient history and a methotrexate infusion dose over 36 hours are given:
   a. Calculate the patients' expected methotrexate clearance.
   b. Calculate the expected methotrexate C_{ss} ave at 36 hours.
   c. Calculate the expected methotrexate concentration 48 and 60 hours after starting the methotrexate regimen.

9. Calculate the recommended starting dose of busulfan in a patient who is:
   a. Less than 25% above their ideal body weight (IBD).
   b. More than 25% above their IBD.

10. Convert busulfan concentrations from µg/L to µM and from µM to µg/L.

11. Convert busulfan area under the curve (AUC) in units of µM·min to busulfan C_{ss} in units of µg/L and C_{ss} in µg/L to AUC in units of µM·min.

12. Describe the busulfan plasma AUC or C_{ss} that is associated with the following after hematopoietic stem cell transplant:
   a. An increased risk of developing hepatic veno-occlusive disease.
   b. An increased risk of disease relapse or failure to engraft.

13. Identify the appropriate blood sample collection schedule for the determination of busulfan AUC or C_{ss}.

14. Given a set of busulfan concentration-versus-time data, determine the following:
   a. The busulfan plasma AUC using the rule of linear trapezoids.
   b. The busulfan plasma C_{ss} using the rule of linear trapezoids.
   c. The busulfan AUC using the model-derived parameters obtained from a compartmental model fit of the data.
   d. The busulfan C_{ss} using the model-derived parameters.

15. Calculate the recommended adjusted dose of busulfan that will give the targeted AUC or C_{ss}.

16. Describe how pharmacogenetic test results can preemptively identify individuals at risk of drug-induced toxicities.
   a. Identify appropriate mercaptopurine dose adjustments based on *TPMT* genetic test results.

17. Describe how genetic testing of the cancer genome can inform drug selection.

The utilization of unique patient characteristics to individualize anticancer therapy for the purpose of optimizing response and mitigating adverse events has evolved greatly over the past few decades. It has long been recognized that body weight along with renal and liver function partially explains interindividual differences in drug exposure, and for certain anticancer drugs, these patient characteristics can be used to individualize dosage. For cytotoxic agents such as methotrexate and busulfan, real-time monitoring of drug concentrations, referred to as *therapeutic drug monitoring* (TDM), can also be used to optimize anticancer therapy. More recently, genetic testing of the inherited (ie, germline) genome and cancer (ie, somatic) genome have been integrated into oncology practice to assist with drug selection and dosage.[1] The term *precision pharmacotherapy* has been coined to refer to the use of weight, liver and renal function, TDM, genetics, environmental exposures, and other unique patient or disease characteristics to guide drug selection and dosage.[2] For patients with cancer, the term *precision oncology* is often used with an emphasis on genetic testing to identify opportunities for targeted therapy. This chapter provides specific examples of using pharmacokinetics and genetics to individualize drug therapy in the oncology setting.

PHARMACOKINETICS

The principle of treating patients with maximal safe doses of cytotoxic chemotherapy is reflected in the way that these drugs are developed for clinical use. During the early stages of clinical testing, doses of cytotoxic drugs are escalated in small cohorts of patients until unacceptable or dose-limiting toxicity is observed. Once toxicity is encountered, the dosage in subsequent patients is reduced to a level where an "acceptable" proportion of patients experience unacceptable toxicity (typically defined as <33%). The resulting "maximum tolerated dose" becomes the recommended starting dose for future clinical use. Moreover, cytotoxic agents typically display steep dose-response curves and narrow therapeutic windows. Optimal cytotoxic drug therapy is complicated by the contribution of both pharmacokinetic and pharmacodynamic variability. Although little is known about the causes and extent of pharmacodynamic variability, a great deal of effort has been spent determining the magnitude and potential sources of the wide patient-to-patient variations seen in the pharmacokinetics of most cytotoxic drugs. As a result of the many factors that contribute to differences in pharmacokinetics, the clearances of most of the commonly used cytotoxic drugs vary over a 3- to 10-fold range. The wide ranges in the rates of elimination result in correspondingly large variations in total drug exposures (eg, area under the concentration-time curve [AUC] and steady-state drug concentration [C_{ss}]) in patients treated with equivalent doses. As a result, individuals given identical doses of cytotoxic agents can have up to 10-fold differences in measured drug exposures. For drugs with steep dose-response curves and narrow therapeutic windows, the implication of such pharmacokinetic variability is significant and leads to unpredictability in antitumor response and toxicity. Therefore, several methods are used in an attempt to minimize the wide intersubject and intrasubject pharmacokinetic variability.[3]

DOSING BASED ON BODY SURFACE AREA

One of the earliest approaches to normalizing cytotoxic drug exposures was the use of body surface area (BSA) to correct for differences in individual patient size.[4] During the initial stages of clinical drug development, BSA is used to guide dosage escalation up to the point of a definition of the maximum tolerated dose. The recommended doses of drugs that are developed in this way are ultimately assigned on the basis of a BSA-based dosing algorithm. As a result, it has become common practice in clinical oncology to dose anticancer drugs on the basis of a patient's BSA with the aim of reducing interindividual variability in drug exposure caused by factors related to patient size.

DOSING BASED ON RENAL FUNCTION

The pharmacokinetics of anticancer agents are often associated with the functional indices of the major drug-clearing organs, the liver and kidneys. Depending on the major route of elimination for a particular drug, it can be reliably predicted that significant changes in either hepatic or renal function will result in corresponding changes in drug clearance. Carboplatin is associated with an increased risk of severe toxicity in patients with creatinine clearances of less than 60 mL/min because of decreased drug clearance and greater total drug exposure.[5] Calvert and colleagues[6] first demonstrated that carboplatin AUC could be accurately predicted using an equation that takes into account the patient's pretreatment glomerular filtration rate (GFR):

$$\text{Carboplatin dose (mg)} = \text{AUC (mg/mL·min)} \times (\text{GFR} + 25)(\text{mL/min})$$

This a priori method for carboplatin dosing has led to a substantial reduction in pharmacokinetic variability, and carboplatin is one the few drugs of any class that is routinely dosed to achieve a target systemic exposure. The original Calvert formula was developed using an accurate measurement of GFR based on urinary ^{51}Cr-ethylenediaminetetraacetic acid clearance. The method of choice for current clinical practice uses either a measured or a calculated creatinine clearance (Cl_{Cr}) instead of the measured GFR. Although the accepted formulas for calculating Cl_{Cr} typically lead to biased estimates of GFR, they are more suited to routine clinical use. An important caveat is that because of the change in the methodology for measuring serum creatinine, lower values are being reported, leading to much higher estimates of Cl_{Cr}. Therefore, the Food and Drug Administration currently recommends that when using established formulas to calculate carboplatin doses in patients with normal kidney function, the estimate of GFR should be capped at 125 mL/min to avoid overdosing.

DOSING BASED ON HEPATIC FUNCTION

The rationale for reducing the dose of cytotoxic drugs in the presence of hepatic impairment is well documented for agents such as etoposide, doxorubicin, vincristine, docetaxel, and paclitaxel. However, unlike Cl_{Cr} and kidney function, there is no single laboratory test that can be used to accurately predict pharmacokinetics. In patients with hepatic impairment, the recommended guidelines for dose adjustment are based on clinical measures of liver function, such as bilirubin (eg, doxorubicin and vincristine), serum glutamic-oxaloacetic transaminase (eg, paclitaxel and docetaxel), alkaline phosphatase (eg, docetaxel), or albumin (eg, etoposide). More recently, the Childs-Pugh classification has been proposed as an alternative to single laboratory measures of hepatic capacity.

THERAPEUTIC DRUG MONITORING

Evans et al reported the first-ever large prospective randomized trial comparing individualized doses of cytotoxic chemotherapy versus standard doses.[7] In this trial, children with acute lymphoblastic leukemia were randomized to receive either conventional doses of methotrexate, cytarabine, and teniposide or individualized doses based on real-time pharmacokinetic determinations. Patients who were randomized to receive individualized chemotherapy doses had a significantly better disease-free survival than those patients who received fixed doses. Although this study established the clinical utility of TDM in cytotoxic chemotherapy, it also illustrated the difficulty of such an approach. The ability to perform real-time pharmacokinetic monitoring of even a single cytotoxic agent requires dedicated laboratory personnel and resources typically only available at major medical centers. Therefore, despite a high degree of pharmacokinetic variability, steep dose-response relationships, and narrow therapeutic windows, there are currently only two cytotoxic agents for which TDM plays an accepted role in the management of patients.[3,8,9]

Methotrexate

Methotrexate is a folic acid antimetabolite that competitively inhibits dihydrofolate reductase, the enzyme responsible for converting folic acid to reduced or active folate cofactors. Methotrexate is used to treat a number of neoplasms, including leukemia, osteogenic sarcoma, breast cancer, and non-Hodgkin lymphoma. Methotrexate is administered by the parenteral route when doses exceed 30 mg/m^2 because oral absorption is limited.[10] Current dosing regimens range from as low as 2.5 mg to as high as 12 g/m^2 or more. High-dose methotrexate is administered over a period as short as 3 to 6 hours to as long as 40 hours.[11,12]

Approximately 50% of methotrexate is bound to plasma proteins.[10,11] Methotrexate is primarily renally cleared. It is a weak acid with a pK_a of 5.4. At low pH, the drug has limited solubility and may precipitate in the urine, causing renal damage. Therefore, a patient receiving high-dose methotrexate should receive hydration, and the urine pH should be maintained above 7. Methotrexate has some minor metabolites with weak activity, the most important of which is 7-hydroxy-methotrexate. The concentration of this metabolite may become significant with high doses of methotrexate. Although 7-hydroxy-methotrexate has only about 1/200 of the clinical activity of methotrexate, it is one-third to one-fifth as soluble. As a result, it may precipitate in the renal tubules, causing acute nephrotoxicity.[13] This solubility problem is an additional reason why patients receiving high doses of methotrexate should be adequately hydrated and have their urine alkalinized.[11,12]

UNITS

Methotrexate is generally administered in milligram or gram doses, and the plasma concentrations are reported in units of mg/L, μg/mL, and molar (M) or micromolar (μM) units. When methotrexate concentrations are reported in molar units, they usually range from values of 10^{-8} to 10^{-2} M. In addition, they are commonly reported in micromolar (or 10^{-6} M) units. To interpret methotrexate concentrations accurately, it is important to establish which units are being reported and how those units correspond to the generally accepted therapeutic or toxic values. Methotrexate has a molecular weight of 454 g/mol; therefore, a value of 0.454 mg/L is equal to 1×10^{-6} M or 1 μM.

To convert methotrexate concentrations in units of mg/L to molar concentrations, Equation 12.1 can be used:

$$\text{Methotrexate concentration in } 10^{-6} \text{ M} = \frac{\text{Methotrexate concentration in mg/L}}{0.454} \qquad \text{(Eq. 12.1)}$$

TOXIC PLASMA CONCENTRATIONS

The primary goal of methotrexate plasma monitoring is to ensure that patients receive adequate doses of the rescue agent to prevent serious toxicity. Because most high-dose rescue regimens are designed to "save" the average patient, the vast majority of methotrexate plasma levels that are obtained for monitoring will be routine and are unlikely to require intervention. Nevertheless, plasma concentration monitoring can be used to identify patients with unusual methotrexate disposition that could result in serious toxicity. The therapeutic and toxic effects of methotrexate are closely linked to its plasma concentrations. Plasma concentrations exceeding 1×10^{-7} M for 48 hours or more are associated with methotrexate toxicity.[14] The most common toxic effects of methotrexate include myelosuppression, oral and gastrointestinal mucositis, and acute hepatic dysfunction.[10,12,14]

Leucovorin Rescue

To ensure that methotrexate toxicities do not occur in moderate- and high-dose treatment regimens, leucovorin is administered every 4 to 6 hours in doses that range from 10 to 100 mg/m². The usual course of rescue therapy is from 12 to 72 hours, or until the plasma concentration of methotrexate falls below the critical value of 1×10^{-7} M. In some rescue protocols, concentrations of 5×10^{-8} (0.05 µM) are considered to be the value indicating the rescue is complete.[11]

Methotrexate concentrations in excess of 1×10^{-6} M (1 µM) at 48 hours are associated with an increased incidence of methotrexate toxicity, even in the face of leucovorin rescue doses of 10 mg/m². When the methotrexate concentration exceeds 1×10^{-6} M at 48 hours, increasing the leucovorin rescue dose to 50 to 100 mg/m² or more reduces methotrexate toxicity.[14] Presumably, this increased dose enables leucovorin factor to compete successfully with methotrexate for intracellular transport and to thereby rescue host tissues.

Although rescue regimens vary considerably, most employ a leucovorin dosing regimen of approximately 10 mg/m² administered every 6 hours for 72 hours. If the methotrexate concentration falls below 1×10^{-7} M (0.1 µM) or 5×10^{-8} M (0.05 µM) before the completion of the 72-hour rescue period, then the rescue factor can be discontinued. If the methotrexate concentrations are still greater than 1×10^{-7} but less than 1×10^{-6} at 48 hours, then rescue with leucovorin is continued at doses of approximately 10 mg/m² every 6 hours until the methotrexate concentration falls below the rescue value of 1×10^{-7} M (0.1 µM) or 5×10^{-8} M (0.05 µM). If methotrexate concentrations are greater than 1×10^{-6} at 48 hours, leucovorin doses should be increased to 100 mg/m² intravenous (IV) every 3 hours and continued at that dose until levels are below 1×10^{-6}, at which point leucovorin can be decreased to approximately 10 mg/m^2 every 6 hours until the methotrexate concentration falls below the rescue value of 1×10^{-7} M (0.1 µM) or 5×10^{-8} M (0.05 µM).

KEY PARAMETERS: Methotrexate

THERAPEUTIC PLASMA CONCENTRATION	VARIABLE
Toxic concentration	
Plasma	$>1 \times 10^{-7}$ M for >48 hr
CNS	$>1 \times 10^{-6}$ M at >48 hr requires increased leucovorin rescue doses
	Continuous CNS methotrexate concentrations $>10^{-8}$ M
F	100%
Dose < 30 mg/m^2	Variable
Dose < 30 mg/m^2	
V_i (initial) (L/kg)	0.2
V AUC (L/kg)	0.7
Cl	$[1.6][Cl_{Cr}]$
$t_{1/2}$ (hr)	
α^a	3
β^b	10
fu (fraction unbound in plasma)	0.5

$^a t_{1/2}$ of 3 hours generally employed with methotrexate plasma concentrations greater than 5×10^{-7} M.
$^b t_{1/2}$ of 10 hours generally employed with methotrexate plasma concentrations of less than 5×10^{-7} M.
CNS, central nervous system.

VOLUME OF DISTRIBUTION (V)

The relationship between methotrexate plasma concentrations and volume of distribution is complex. The drug displays at least a biexponential elimination curve, indicating that there is an initial plasma volume of distribution of about 0.2 L/kg and a second larger volume of distribution of 0.5 to 1 L/kg following complete distribution.[15,16] The evaluation of the apparent volume of distribution for methotrexate is further complicated by the fact that it appears to increase at higher plasma concentrations.[15] This phenomenon may reflect an active transport system that becomes saturated at high plasma concentrations and reverts to passive intracellular diffusion of methotrexate. The multi-compartmental modeling as well as the variable relationship between the plasma concentration and apparent volume of distribution of methotrexate makes the calculation of methotrexate loading doses somewhat speculative. Nevertheless, when loading doses are required, a volume of distribution of 0.2 to 0.5 L/kg is usually employed.

The presence of third-space fluids such as ascites, edema, or pleural effusions can also influence the volume of distribution of methotrexate.[17] Although pleural effusions do not substantially increase the volume of distribution, the high concentrations of methotrexate that accumulate in these spaces can be important because equilibration with plasma is delayed. In patients with pleural effusions, the initial elimination half-life appears to be normal; however, the second elimination phase is prolonged.[18] Prolongation of this terminal elimination phase is significant because the time required for patients to achieve a methotrexate plasma concentration of less than 1×10^{-7} can be extended. In this situation, additional doses and/or higher doses of leucovorin rescue factor may have to be administered beyond the usual rescue period (see Figure 12.1, Half-Life $[t_{1/2}]$, and Question 2).

CLEARANCE (Cl)

The vast majority of methotrexate is eliminated by the renal route.[18] Methotrexate clearance ranges from 1 to as much as 2 times the creatinine clearance.[12,13,15] Methotrexate clearance by an active transport mechanism that may be saturable results in a renal clearance value that varies (relative to creatinine clearance) with methotrexate plasma concentrations.[13] There are emerging data suggesting that genetic variants in the *SLCO1B1* gene, which encodes for a drug transporter mostly found in the liver, may also influence methotrexate clearance.[19] However, individualizing methotrexate dose based on *SLCO1B1* genetic test results has not been fully elucidated.

The renal clearance of methotrexate is also influenced by a number of compounds (eg, probenecid and salicylates influence weak acid secretion). In addition, sulfisoxazole and other weak acids have been reported to diminish the renal transport of methotrexate.[13,20] Proton-pump inhibitors such as omeprazole have also been associated with delays in methotrexate clearance and prolonged methotrexate half-life.[21] Because methotrexate renal clearance may be inhibited, all drugs should be added cautiously to the regimen of a patient receiving methotrexate therapy. Although early reports attributed salicylate-induced methotrexate toxicity to plasma protein displacement of methotrexate, the most likely mechanism is an alteration in renal clearance. An alteration in plasma binding is an unlikely explanation because methotrexate is only 50% bound to plasma proteins.[13,18]

Changes in renal function are important when designing and monitoring methotrexate therapy. Therefore, all patients receiving moderate- and high-dose methotrexate therapy should have their plasma level of methotrexate and their renal function monitored. Although the therapeutic dose of methotrexate may range over several grams, serious toxicity and death have been attributed to doses as low as 10 mg of methotrexate when administered to a patient with inadequate renal function.[22,23]

Concomitant administration of the prostaglandin inhibitors indomethacin and ketoprofen with methotrexate has been associated with an acute decrease in renal function and a greatly prolonged exposure to high methotrexate concentrations.[24,25] This interaction presumably results from the combined renal effects of the nonsteroidal anti-inflammatory agent with methotrexate. Although this interaction has not been described for all nonsteroidal anti-inflammatory agents, these agents should be avoided in patients receiving methotrexate therapy.

A relatively small percentage of methotrexate is metabolized; nevertheless, significant amounts of methotrexate metabolites can be found in the urine when large doses are administered. This is especially true during the late phase of methotrexate elimination when the majority of the parent compound has been eliminated. The most extensively studied metabolite is the 7-hydroxy-methotrexate compound, which is considered to be potentially nephrotoxic because of its low water solubility.[13]

HALF-LIFE ($t_{1/2}$)

The relationship between methotrexate's volume of distribution and clearance is complex. Because of the potential for capacity-limited intracellular transport and capacity-limited renal clearance, the apparent half-lives for methotrexate are determined by both a changing volume of distribution and a changing clearance. Consequently, the elimination of methotrexate is not accurately described by linear pharmacokinetic modeling. Given these problems, a relatively simple two-compartment model with an initial α half-life of 2 to 3 hours and a β or terminal half-life of approximately 10 hours appears to represent the elimination phase reasonably well.[16,18] The terminal or β half-life of approximately 10 hours often does not become apparent until plasma concentrations decline into the range of 5×10^{-7} M (0.5×10^{-6} or 0.5 μM). Because the terminal phase is also independent of the dose administered, it probably reflects a change in the distribution and elimination of methotrexate.

Whereas the apparent terminal half-life of methotrexate is somewhat variable, it does not appear to increase with increasing doses. Unlike most other two-compartmental drugs, significant methotrexate is eliminated during the α phase. In fact, a very large percentage of the total methotrexate dose may be eliminated during the α phase. Nevertheless, the terminal phase is also important because retention of even a very small amount of the administered dose can be potentially toxic to the patient.[16,17]

Pleural effusions or other third-space fluid collections can significantly prolong the terminal half-life of methotrexate, and leucovorin rescue regimens may need to be extended over a longer period in these situations. Some patients may unexpectedly develop acute changes in renal function or prolonged elimination characteristics that are unpredictable and independent of renal function. For this reason, continued monitoring of methotrexate is essential, even if early plasma level monitoring indicates that an adjustment of the methotrexate dose or leucovorin regimen is unnecessary.

Question #1 *P.J., a 61-year-old, 69-kg man ($S_{Cr} = 1.1$ mg/dL), is to receive a course of methotrexate therapy for acute lymphoblastic leukemia. His regimen will consist of a 400-mg methotrexate loading dose to be administered over 15 minutes, followed by an IV infusion of 50 mg/hr for the next 36 hours. He will then receive a 100 mg ($=50$ mg/m^2) dose of leucovorin every 6 hours IV for the first 4 doses, followed by 8 doses orally of 20 mg ($=10$ mg/m^2) at 6-hour intervals or until the methotrexate concentration is less than 0.5×10^{-7} M. The leucovorin regimen will begin immediately after the 36-hour methotrexate infusion has been discontinued and is scheduled to continue for the next 72 hours, with the last dose given 102 hours after initiation of the methotrexate therapy. Methotrexate levels are scheduled to be obtained 24 hours after the beginning of the 50-mg/hr infusion, at 48 hours (12 hours after the end of the 36-hour infusion), and at 60 hours (24 hours after the end of the methotrexate infusion). Calculate the anticipated methotrexate concentrations at the scheduled sampling times.*

Before the anticipated methotrexate concentrations can be calculated, it is first necessary to determine P.J.'s creatinine clearance, using Equation 12.2:

$$Cl_{Cr} \text{ for males}(mL/min) = \frac{(140-Age)(Weight)}{(72)\,(S_{Crss})} \qquad \textbf{(Eq. 12.2)}$$

$$= \frac{(140-61)(69)}{(72)(1.1)}$$

$$= 68.8 \text{ mL/min}$$

The creatinine clearance of 68.8 mL/min can be converted to 4.13 L/hr:

$$Cl_{Cr}(L/hr) = [Cl_{Cr}(mL/min)]\left[\frac{60 \text{ min/hr}}{1{,}000 \text{ mL/L}}\right]$$

$$= [68.8\,mL/min]\left[\frac{60 \text{ min/hr}}{1{,}000 \text{ mL/L}}\right]$$

$$= 4.13 \text{ L/hr}$$

This creatinine clearance of 4.13 L/hr can then be placed into Equation 12.3 to calculate a methotrexate clearance (Cl_{MTX}) of 6.6 L/hr.

$$Cl_{MTX} = (1.6)(Cl_{Cr}) \qquad \textbf{(Eq. 12.3)}$$

$$= [1.6][4.13\,L/hr]$$

$$= 6.6 \text{ L/hr}$$

The 24-hour concentration represents an average steady-state level. The steady-state level of methotrexate in mg/L can then be calculated by using the equation for steady-state concentration (Equation 12.4):

$$C_{ss\,ave} = \frac{(S)(F)(Dose/\tau)}{Cl} \qquad \textbf{(Eq. 12.4)}$$

$$= \frac{(1)(1)(50\,mg/1\,hr)}{6.6\,L/hr}$$

$$= 7.6 \text{ mg/L}$$

The values of S and F were assumed to be 1, and this methotrexate concentration in mg/L can be converted to a concentration in the units of micromoles or 10^{-6} M using Equation 12.1.

$$\text{Methotrexate concentration in } 10^{-6} \text{ M} = \frac{\text{Methotrexate concentration in mg/L}}{0.454}$$

$$= \frac{7.6 \text{ mg/L}}{0.454}$$

$$= 16.7 \times 10^{-6} \text{ M or } 1.67 \times 10^{-5} \text{ M}$$

The resultant methotrexate concentration of approximately 16.7×10^{-6} or 1.67×10^{-5} M assumes that steady state has been achieved 24 hours after the infusion rate of 50 mg/hr has been initiated. Steady state is assumed to have been achieved because the methotrexate plasma concentrations are relatively high. At concentrations greater than 10^{-7} M, a half-life of 2 to 3 hours appears to determine the elimination and accumulation of most of the methotrexate in the body. As noted earlier, this model is not consistent with the traditional view of a two-compartment model in which the terminal half-life plays an important role in the accumulation toward steady state. Although there is the possibility of some continued accumulation, this generally appears to be minor, and the use of the shorter, 2- to 3-hour, methotrexate half-life in evaluating initial methotrexate loss or accumulation is satisfactory in most cases.

Assuming the plasma concentration at the end of the 36-hour infusion is 16.7×10^{-6} M, a plasma concentration of 1.04×10^{-6} M (10.4×10^{-7} M) at 48 hours (or 12 hours after the infusion has been discontinued) can be calculated using Equation 12.5.

$$C_2 = C_1(e^{-Kt}) \qquad \text{(Eq. 12.5)}$$

C_1 is the methotrexate plasma concentration at the end of the infusion, and t is the 12-hour time interval spanning from the end of the 36-hour infusion to the time of sampling at 48 hours. K is the elimination rate constant calculated from a rearrangement of the equation for $t_{1/2}$ (Equation 12.6) and using the shorter elimination half-life of 3 hours.

$$t_{1/2} = \frac{0.693}{K} \qquad \text{(Eq. 12.6)}$$

$$K = \frac{0.693}{t_{1/2}} \qquad \text{(Eq. 12.7)}$$

$$K = \frac{0.693}{t_{1/2}}$$

$$= \frac{0.693}{3 \text{ hr}}$$

$$= 0.231 \text{ hr}^{-1}$$

$$C_2 = C_1(e^{-Kt})$$

$$C_2 = (16.7 \times 10^{-6} \text{M})(e^{-(0.231 \text{ hr}^{-1})(12 \text{ hr})})$$

$$= (16.7 \times 10^{-6} \text{M})(0.0625)$$

$$= 1.04 \times 10^{-6} \text{M or } 10.4 \times 10^{-7} \text{M}$$

Because this methotrexate concentration is 1×10^{-6} M 48 hours after starting the methotrexate therapy, the leucovorin rescue dose does not have to be increased. The planned leucovorin rescue schedule should be continued until the concentration falls to 0.5×10^{-7}.

Calculation of the methotrexate concentration 60 hours after the infusion has been initiated (24 hours after the infusion has been concluded) is more problematic. The half-life for methotrexate tends to increase as the methotrexate concentration approaches 0.2 to 0.7×10^{-6} M (2 to 7×10^{-7} M). Therefore, the use of a traditional two-compartment model for this drug is inappropriate because the more prolonged terminal half-life correlates more closely with a specific concentration range than with a specific time interval following discontinuation of the infusion. This unusual phenomenon may be related to a change in the active transport system that is influenced by plasma concentration.

One technique that is used to predict methotrexate concentrations several hours after the infusion has been discontinued is to decay the methotrexate concentration to a range of 0.2 to 0.7×10^{-6} M using a half-life of 3 hours. The longer or β half-life of 10 hours is then used to predict subsequent decay. If a plasma concentration of 0.5×10^{-6} is arbitrarily selected as the cutoff concentration for using a half-life of 3 hours, the time required for the initial decay can be calculated using Equation 12.8:

$$t = \frac{\ln\left(\dfrac{C_1}{C_2}\right)}{K} \qquad \textbf{(Eq. 12.8)}$$

C_1 represents the initial plasma concentration of 16.7×10^{-6} M, C_2 the arbitrary cutoff plasma concentration of 0.5×10^{-6} M, and K the elimination rate constant corresponding to the initial half-life of 3 hours (0.231 hr^{-1}). Using Equation 12.8, the time (t) required for the methotrexate concentration to fall to 0.5×10^{-6} M would be 15.2 hours after the end of the infusion or 51.2 hours after the methotrexate regimen is begun:

$$t = \frac{\ln\left(\dfrac{16.7 \times 10^{-6} \text{ M}}{0.5 \times 10^{-6} \text{ M}}\right)}{0.231 \text{ hr}^{-1}}$$

$$= \frac{3.5}{0.231 \ hr^{-1}}$$

$$= 15.2 \ hr$$

To calculate the plasma concentration at 60 hours, the plasma level at 51.2 hours (36-hour infusion + 15.2-hour decay) would have to be decayed for an additional 8.8 hours. In this case, however, the elimination rate constant that corresponds to the terminal elimination half-life of 10 hours would be used (Equation 12.7).

$$K = \frac{0.693}{t_{\frac{1}{2}}}$$

$$= \frac{0.693}{10 \ hr}$$

$$= 0.0693 \ hr^{-1}$$

Using these values and the equation for first-order elimination of a drug from the body (Equation 12.5), a methotrexate concentration of 2.7×10^{-7} M at 60 hours can be calculated.

$$C_2 = C_1(e^{-Kt})$$
$$= (0.5 \times 10^{-6} \ M)(e^{-(0.0693 \ hr^{-1})(8.8 \ hr)})$$
$$= 0.27 \times 10^{-6} \ M \ \text{or} \ 2.7 \times 10^{-7} \ M$$

These calculations suggest that an additional 24 hours will be required to decay the concentration to 0.5×10^{-7} M:

$$t = \frac{\ln\left(\dfrac{0.27 \times 10^{-6} \ M}{0.05 \times 10^{-6} \ M}\right)}{0.6931 \ hr^{-1}}$$

$$= \frac{1.68}{0.0693 \ hr^{-1}}$$

$$= 24 \ hr$$

Because this concentration will decay to a concentration below 0.5×10^{-7} (0.05 µM) (the rescue value) in a little more than two half lives, it would appear from our calculations that P.J. will have been rescued by leucovorin successfully.

Therefore, the rescue concentration will be achieved before leucovorin is scheduled to be discontinued. Nevertheless, these predicted concentrations are only approximations and cannot replace the measured methotrexate concentrations. A graphic representation of the expected methotrexate concentrations (filled triangle) is plotted in Figure 12.1. Unless there is a dramatic increase in the methotrexate half-life, the concentration will be well below 1×10^{-7} M long before the leucovorin is scheduled to be discontinued.

> **Question #2** *P.J.'s methotrexate levels were reported as 13.5×10^{-6} M at 24 hours, 0.83×10^{-6} M (8.3×10^{-7} M) at 48 hours, and 0.44×10^{-6} M (4.4×10^{-7} M) at 60 hours. How would one interpret each of these methotrexate values? What would be an appropriate course of action regarding P.J.'s rescue therapy?*

The initial plasma concentration of 13.5×10^{-6} is lower than the predicted concentration calculated in Question 1 (16.7×10^{-6} M). The lower-than-predicted concentration suggests that P.J.'s methotrexate clearance is greater than expected; however, the difference between the predicted and actual concentrations is well within the expected variation.

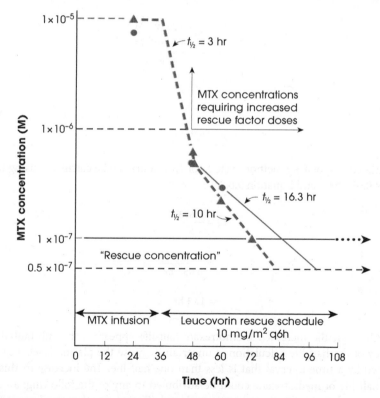

FIGURE 12.1 Methotrexate (MTX). This figure represents a semilog plot of the expected (*filled triangle*) and measured (*filled circle*) MTX plasma concentrations during and following a 36-hour infusion. Levels were obtained at 24, 48, and 60 hours after the start of the infusion. Note that leucovorin rescue should be continued as long as the MTX concentration is greater than the rescue value, represented here as either 1×10^{-7} M (0.1 µM) or 0.5×10^{-7} M (0.05 µM) and that the rescue dose should be increased for MTX levels greater than 1×10^{-6} M at 48 hours and beyond.

The plasma level of 8.3×10^{-7} M at 48 hours (12 hours after the end of the infusion) suggests that P.J. is progressing as expected during the initial elimination phase. The difference between the expected (10.4×10^{-7} M) and observed concentrations is minimal, considering the fact that the initial plasma level was slightly lower than predicted (see Figure 12.1). Because the observed plasma level is below 1×10^{-6} M at 48 hours, it is unnecessary to increase the leucovorin dose.

The measured methotrexate concentration of 4.4×10^{-7} M (0.44 µM) at 60 hours is greater than the predicted concentration of 2.7×10^{-7} M (0.27 µM). Although the differences are not remarkable, it is of some concern that P.J.'s half-life is longer than anticipated. P.J.'s elimination rate constant of 0.053 hr^{-1} can be calculated using these two methotrexate concentrations, the time interval between the concentrations, and rearranging Equation 9.8 to form Equation 12.9.

$$K = \frac{\ln\left(\dfrac{C_1}{C_2}\right)}{t} \qquad \text{(Eq. 12.9)}$$

$$t = \frac{\ln\left(\dfrac{8.3 \times 10^{-7}\ M}{4.4 \times 10^{-7}\ M}\right)}{12\,hr}$$

$$= \frac{0.63}{12\ hr}$$

$$= 0.053\ hr^{-1}$$

P.J.'s corresponding methotrexate $t_{1/2}$ of 13.1 hours can be calculated using the K value of 0.053 hr^{-1} and Equation 9.6.

$$t_{1/2} = \frac{0.693}{K}$$

$$= \frac{0.693}{0.053\ hr^{-1}}$$

$$= 13.1\ hr$$

Although the increased methotrexate half-life appears to be substantial, the accuracy of the half-life calculation is uncertain because the plasma levels used are separated by a time interval that is less than one half-life. The increase in this terminal half-life of methotrexate could be attributed to any of the following: an assay error, accumulation of methotrexate in a pleural effusion or other third-space fluid, a drug-induced reduction in the renal clearance of methotrexate (eg, salicylates), or a normal variance in methotrexate elimination. If this is the result of pleural effusion or third-space fluids, one would expect slower elimination, without a significant decrease in levels. Often in the case of pleural effusion, levels may fluctuate because of the redistribution of the methotrexate between the third-space fluid and intravascular circulation. One would need to continue to give leucovorin rescue and monitor levels until methotrexate levels drop below 0.05 µM. In addition, there may be times when methotrexate will cause an increase in serum creatinine. This may delay methotrexate clearance. Again, one would continue leucovorin rescue and monitor levels until methotrexate levels drop below 0.05 µM.

Regardless of the cause, it is important to determine whether P.J. will achieve a plasma concentration of less than 0.5×10^{-7} M by the time the leucovorin rescue is scheduled to be discontinued. Using the patient-specific or revised elimination rate constant of 0.053 hr^{-1} and Equation 9.8, it appears as though P.J.'s methotrexate concentration will fall to 0.5×10^{-7} M after another 41 hours (101 hours after starting the methotrexate therapy). This is just at the time scheduled for the last dose of leucovorin (102 hours after starting the methotrexate infusion).

$$t_{1/2} = \frac{\ln\left(\dfrac{C_1}{C_2}\right)}{K}$$

$$= \frac{\ln\left(\dfrac{4.4 \times 10^{-7}\ M}{0.5 \times 10^{-7}\ M}\right)}{0.053\ hr^{-1}}$$

$$= \frac{2.17}{0.053\ hr^{-1}}$$

$$= 41\ hr^{-1}$$

This calculation should not be used as the sole criterion for evaluating the success of rescue therapy because the elimination rate constant calculation is uncertain, and the methotrexate terminal half-life may become more prolonged as the plasma concentration declines. In this particular case, additional methotrexate plasma levels should be obtained to ensure that the actual plasma concentration is below the critical value of 0.5×10^{-7} before leucovorin rescue is discontinued. If this critical value has not been achieved by 102 hours, then additional doses of leucovorin will have to be administered until P.J. has achieved a plasma level below 0.5×10^{-7} M (see Figure 12.1). Note that the observed methotrexate levels suggest that P.J. has a more prolonged terminal half-life.

BUSULFAN

Busulfan is a bifunctional alkylating agent that kills dividing cells by forming DNA cross-links. When the resulting DNA damage cannot be repaired, cells undergo programmed cell death or apoptosis. Busulfan is especially toxic to hematopoietic cells in the bone marrow and was originally introduced as a treatment for patients with chronic myelogenous leukemia.[26] Owing to its potent myelosuppressive effects, busulfan is commonly used in bone marrow ablative regimens given before hematopoietic stem cell transplantation (HSCT). Busulfan is typically used in combination with other marrow ablative agents, such as radiation, cyclophosphamide, melphalan, or fludarabine. Busulfan was originally only available as an oral tablet, and the parental formulation did not come on the market until long after its role in HSCT conditioning had been established. The dosage of busulfan most often used in adults undergoing HSCT is 0.8 mg/kg IV or 1 mg/kg orally given every 6 hours for 4 days (12 or 16 mg/kg total dose). IV busulfan is also given on a once-daily schedule at a dose of 3.2 mg/kg/d. IV administration is now the preferred route because of the high incidence of emesis that occurs with oral dosing, often requiring error-prone estimation and replacement of the vomited tablets. Variability in busulfan systemic exposure and identification of a strong correlation between drug concentrations and both toxicity and therapeutic outcome in patients undergoing HSCT have led to the routine use of TDM.

UNITS

Busulfan is administered in milligram doses, and the plasma concentrations are typically reported in units of µg/L or µM. To interpret busulfan concentrations accurately, it is critically important to know which units are being reported and how those units correspond to the therapeutic ranges being targeted. Busulfan has a molecular weight of 246 g/mol. Therefore, a value of 246 µg/L is equal to 1×10^{-6} M or 1 µM. To convert busulfan concentrations in units of µg/L to µM concentrations, the following equation can be used:

$$\text{Busulfan conc. (µM)} = \text{Busulfan conc. (µg/L)}/246 \text{ µg/µmol} \qquad \textbf{(Eq. 12.10)}$$

TARGET PLASMA CONCENTRATIONS

Hepatic veno-occlusive disease (VOD) is a common life-threatening complication resulting from the chemoablative regimens used in HSCT, occurring in 20% to 40% of patients.[27,28] VOD results from injury to small veins and sinusoids of the liver, followed by deposition of protein aggregates that progressively block venous outflow, leading to intrahepatic hypertension. Clinically, VOD is characterized by jaundice, weight gain, ascites, and painful swelling of the liver. Mortality rates as a result of VOD range from 20% to 50%. A first-dose busulfan AUC greater than 1,500 µmol/L·min has been linked to an increased risk of VOD.[27] Others using the average busulfan plasma concentration (C_{ave}) as a measure of drug exposure have demonstrated that a C_{ave} of greater than 900 µg/L also results in an increased risk of VOD.[29] To convert the busulfan AUC to C_{ave}, one must first convert the AUC value to units of µg/L·hr and then divide the AUC by the dosing interval (τ) using Equation 12.11.

$$\text{Busulfan } C_{ave} \text{ (µg/L)} = \text{Busulfan AUC (µg/L·hr)}/\tau \qquad \textbf{(Eq. 12.11)}$$

In addition to the relationship between higher exposures and toxicity, it has been demonstrated that lower busulfan exposures are associated with poorer outcomes following HSCT. Patients with busulfan AUC of less than 800 μmol/L·min or C_{ave} of less than 600 μg/L have a higher rate of disease relapse and engraftment failure.[29,30] Therefore, the accepted therapeutic window for busulfan when given every 6 hours for 16 doses is a first dose AUC of 900 to 1,500 μM·min or a C_{ave} of 600 to 900 μg/L. Although the optimal therapeutic window for once-daily busulfan has yet to be determined, most transplant centers are using an AUC range of 900 to 1,500 μM·min, which is equivalent to 4 times the AUC range on an every 6-hour dosing schedule.[31]

TIME TO SAMPLE

For the determination of the busulfan plasma AUC, the timing for collection of samples depends on the route of administration. Following an oral dose, blood samples are collected at 15 and 30 minutes, 1, 1.5, 2, 3, 4, 5, and 6 hours following administration. Following an IV dose, samples are collected immediately before the end of the 2-hour infusion and then 15 and 30 minutes, 3, 4, 5, and 6 hours after the end of the infusion. Additional samples are required with oral dosing because of the unpredictability of oral absorption and the importance of collecting samples around the C_{max} for accurate determination of the AUC. Approaches utilizing as few as two timed blood samples have been suggested for patients receiving IV busulfan; however, these limited samples strategies have not yet been validated in prospective clinical trials. Plasma is separated from whole blood, and the complete set of samples is sent to the lab for analysis. Although some transplant centers have the capability for on-site testing, many do not. There can be a 12- to 24-hour delay between the time that the samples are collected and the time the results are available. As a result, an additional two to four doses of busulfan must be given before an adjustment can be made. Because of this, some transplant centers prefer to use a test dose strategy whereby a low, subtherapeutic dose of busulfan is given before the start of the full-dose regimen for prediction of busulfan pharmacokinetics.[32,33]

BUSULFAN ASSAYS

Analysis of busulfan in plasma is commonly performed using gas chromatography-mass spectrometric detection (GC-MS). GC methods require that busulfan in plasma be derivatized so that it becomes volatile enough to enter the gas phase and fly through the capillary column. Electrochemical detection is also an option but requires longer run times owing to the less selective nature of the detection method. More recently, liquid chromatography combined with tandem mass spectrometry (LC-MS/MS) has been used to measure busulfan. LC-MS/MS analysis does not require derivatization and is significantly more sensitive than GC-based methods. The major disadvantage is that LC-MS/MS instruments are significantly more expensive to purchase and maintain.

METHODS FOR ESTIMATING BUSULFAN AREA UNDER CURVE

Both noncompartmental and model-derived methods are used for the determination of busulfan AUC.[34] Noncompartmental data analysis relies on the rule of linear trapezoids and does not require special curve-fitting software. Programs that are available on almost every computer, such as Excel, can be used to calculate the AUC. Furthermore, noncompartmental analysis is the preferred approach in cases where the plasma concentration-versus-time data are erratic, for example, when the oral absorption is unpredictable. Because the target therapeutic ranges are based on the AUC extrapolated to infinity, the portion of the AUC after the last measured time point must also be calculated using the terminal elimination rate constant derived from the last two to three sample measurements. The equation (12.12) for calculating the AUC of busulfan using the trapezoidal rule is as follows:

$$AUC_{trapezoidal} = \sum_{i=0}^{n-1} \frac{(t_i + 1 - t_i)(C_i + 1 + C_i)}{2} + \frac{C_{last}}{\lambda} \qquad \text{(Eq. 12.12)}$$

where t_i and C_i are the times and concentrations at the ith time point. The terminal elimination rate constant for extrapolating to infinity is calculated using Equation 12.13:

$$\lambda = \frac{\ln\,(C_{last} - 1) - \ln(C_{last})}{t(last) - t(last - 1)} \qquad \text{(Eq. 12.13)}$$

Model-derived approaches depend on software packages, such as ADAPT and WinNonlin. Busulfan disposition is best described by a one-compartment first-order elimination model. Figure 12.2 shows a concentration-versus-time data set from a patient receiving IV busulfan. The actual data points are depicted by the open triangles, and the smooth curve was generated using ADAPT.

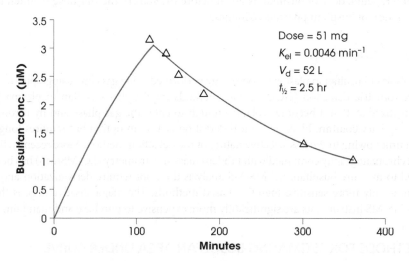

FIGURE 12.2 Busulfan. This figure is a typical busulfan plasma concentration-versus-time curve following an intravenous dose of 0.8 mg/kg infused over 120 minutes. The symbols (*open triangle*) indicate the measured plasma concentration at 115, 135, 150, 180, 300, and 360 minutes, and the line represents the best-fit curve generated using the ADAPT software.

BIOAVAILABILITY (*F*)

The availability of an IV busulfan formulation has made it possible to determine its absolute bioavailability, which has been reported to be 80%.[29,35,36] Busulfan is rapidly absorbed with peak plasma drug concentrations occurring between 1.5 and 2.5 hours after an oral dose, with more rapid absorption after the administration of crushed tablets. There are no known food-drug interactions for busulfan, although patients are advised not to eat or drink anything 1 hour before and 1 hour after each oral dose. Approximately 25% of patients experience delayed absorption or prolonged elimination of oral busulfan. In some cases, plasma concentrations can continue to increase throughout the entire 6-hour dosing interval, making it impossible to determine a terminal elimination rate constant. In such cases, the mean population terminal elimination rate constant is used to extrapolate the AUC to infinity.

KEY PARAMETERS: Busulfan

Therapeutic plasma concentrations	
q6h dosing	$AUC_{0-\infty}$ = 900 − 1,500 µM·min
q24h dosing[a]	or C_{ave} = 600 – 900 µg/L
	$AUC_{0-\infty}$ = 3,600 – 6,000 µM·min
F (%)	80
V/F (L/kg)	
Adults and children >4 yr	0.6-1.0
Children <4 yr	1.4-1.6
Cl/F (mL/min/kg)	
Adults and children >4 yr	2.5-4.5
Children <4 yr	6.8-8.4
$t_{1/2}$ (hr)	
Adults and children >4 yr	2.5-3.0
Children <4 yr	1.5-2.0
fu (fraction unbound in plasma)	0.6-0.7

[a]The optimal range for once-daily dosing has not yet been determined. A range of 3,600 to 6,000 µM·min has been proposed because it is equivalent to 4 times the range established for the every 6-hour dosing schedule.

VOLUME OF DISTRIBUTION

The mean volume of distribution (*V*) after administration of an IV dose of busulfan is 0.8 L/kg in adults and 1.5 L/kg in very young children.[29,35,36] There is no difference in the V_d of busulfan in older children versus adults. Age-related differences in busulfan disposition are possibly because of the larger liver volume normalized to body weight in younger children, which could explain the need for higher doses of drugs that are primarily cleared by the liver, such as busulfan, when they are dosed on a milligram per kilogram basis in very young children.

When calculating the dose of busulfan in a patient with obesity, it is recommended that the dose be based on an adjusted ideal body weight (IBW) calculated using the ABW25 equation[37]:

$$\text{Adjusted IBW} = \text{IBW} + (0.25 \times [\text{ABW} - \text{IBW}]) \qquad \textbf{(Eq. 12.14)}$$

Approximately 30% of the drug is irreversibly bound to plasma proteins. The erythrocyte-to-plasma ratio of busulfan is 1.05. Busulfan freely distributes into the cerebrospinal fluid (CSF), with CSF concentrations approximating those in the plasma, accounting for why some patients experience seizures after high doses.[38]

CLEARANCE (Cl)

There are also age-related differences in busulfan Cl between very young children versus older children and adults. The Cl of busulfan in children older than 4 years and adults is in the range of 2.5 to 4.5 mL/min/kg, whereas Cl in children less than 4 years ranges from 6.8 to 8.4 mL/min/kg.[29,35,36] Cl is independent of dose up to a daily IV dose of 3.2 mg/kg. Excretion of unchanged busulfan in the urine is very low (1%-2%), and the majority of busulfan is eliminated through hepatic metabolism via glutathione conjugation predominantly via GSTA1, with minor contributions from GSTM1 and GSTP1.[39] Children have been shown to conjugate busulfan more efficiently than adults, which likely explains the larger apparent V_d/F and faster clearance in very young children compared to older children and adults.

HALF-LIFE ($t_{1/2}$)

The elimination half-life of busulfan in adults and older children ranges from 2.5 to 3.0 hours. In children less than 4 years, the range is between 1.5 and 2.0 hours.[29,35,36]

Question #3 *R.C., a 43-year-old, 82-kg woman (IBW = 58 kg), is receiving a course of busulfan and cyclophosphamide as her pretransplant conditioning regimen for acute myelogenous leukemia. The regimen includes 0.8 mg/kg of IV busulfan given every 6 hours for a total of 16 doses. Each busulfan dose is administered over 120 minutes, and serial blood samples are collected around the first dose for the determination of the busulfan AUC. Calculate the correct starting dose for R.C.*

Because R.C. is obese, it is recommended that her starting busulfan dose be calculated on the basis of an adjusted IBW using the ABW25 Equation 12.14:

$$\text{Adjusted IBW} = \text{IBW} + (0.25 \times [\text{ABW} - \text{IBW}])$$

$$= 58 + (0.25[82 - 58 \text{ kg}])$$

$$= 64 \text{ kg}$$

According to the ABW25 equation, R.C.'s adjusted IBW is 64 kg. Therefore, the correct starting dose for R.C. would be 0.8 mg/kg × 64 kg or 51 mg.

Question #4 *The results of the analysis of her busulfan levels came back from the lab and are shown in the following table. First, calculate the busulfan AUC using the rule of linear trapezoids; then using the pharmacokinetic parameters from Figure 12.2, calculate the model-derived AUC.*

TIME (MIN)	BUSULFAN (µM)
115	3.18
135	2.93
150	2.56
180	2.22
300	1.34
360	1.04

The busulfan AUC can be calculated using the rule of linear trapezoids (Equation 12.12):

$$AUC_{trapezoidal} = \sum_{i=0}^{n-1} \frac{(t_i + 1 - t_i)(C_i + 1 + C_i)}{2} + \frac{C_{last}}{\lambda}$$

Based on the first term in the equation, the AUC from time zero to the time of the last busulfan measurement is 642 µM·min.

$$AUC_{0-360min} = \frac{(0 + 3.18\,\mu M)(115.18 \text{ ns})}{2} + \frac{(2.93 + 3.18\,\mu M)(1,353 + 3.18 \text{ ns})}{2}$$
$$+ \frac{(2.56 + 2.93\,\mu M)(1,506 + 2.93 \text{ ns})}{2} + \frac{(2.22 + 2.56\,\mu M)(1,802 + 2.56 \text{ ns})}{2}$$
$$+ \frac{(1.34 + 2.22\,\mu M)(3,004 + 2.22 \text{ ns})}{2} + \frac{(1.04 + 1.34\,\mu M)(3,604 + 1.34 \text{ ns})}{2}$$

$$= (182.9 + 61.1 + 41.2 + 71.7 + 213.6 + 71.4)$$

$$= 642\ \mu M \cdot min$$

To extrapolate the AUC to infinity, the terminal elimination rate constant is calculated according to Equation 12.13:

$$\lambda = \frac{\ln(C_{last} - 1) - \ln(C_{last})}{t(last) - t(last - 1)}$$

$$\lambda = \frac{ln(1.34\,\mu M) - \ln(1.04\,\mu M)}{360 - 300 \text{ min}}$$

The calculated λ for R.C. is 0.0042 min^{-1}. When the last measured busulfan concentration is divided by λ and added to the first term in the trapezoidal rule, the AUC equation results in a final AUC$_{trapezoidal}$ estimate extrapolated to infinity of 890 μM·min.

$$AUC_{360-\infty} = \frac{C_{last}}{\lambda}$$

$$= \frac{1.04\,\mu M}{0.0042\ min^{-1}}$$

$$= 248\ \mu M/min$$

$$AUC_{0-\infty} = 642 + 248 = 890\ \mu M/min$$

The busulfan AUC$_{0-\infty}$ can also be calculated using the model-derived parameters provided in Figure 12.2 according to the following equations:

$$AUC_{0-\infty} = \frac{Dose}{Cl}$$

$$Cl = V_d \times \lambda$$

To be consistent with the AUC$_{trapezoidal}$, the busulfan dose of 51 mg must first be converted to units of micromoles by multiplying by 1,000 μg/mg and dividing by the busulfan molecular weight of 246 μg/μmol. This conversion results in a busulfan dose of 207.3 μmol.

$$Busulfan\ dose\ (\mu M) = \frac{(Dose\ in\ mg)(1{,}000\ \mu g/mg)}{246\ \mu g/\mu mol}$$

$$= \frac{(51\ mg)(1{,}000\ \mu g/mg)}{246\ \mu g/\mu mol}$$

$$= 207.3\ \mu mol$$

Using the busulfan dose in μmol and substituting $V \times K_{el}$ in Figure 12.2 for Cl, the model-derived AUC$_{0-\infty}$ estimate for R.C. is 867 μM·min.

$$AUC_{0-\infty} = \frac{Dose\ (\mu mol)}{(K)(V)}$$

$$= \frac{207.3\ \mu mol}{(0.0046\ min^{-1})(52\,L)}$$

$$= 867\ \mu M \cdot min$$

Question #5 *R.C.'s hematologist wants to target an AUC of 1,200 μM·min. What dose would you recommend? The hematologist is also considering targeting an average plasma concentration (C_{ave}) of 750 μg/L instead of AUC. What is R.C.'s first-dose busulfan C_{ave}, and what would be the expected C_{ss} if you were to change the dose as calculated earlier?*

Using the $AUC_{trapezoidal}$ of 890 μM·min measured following a dose of 51 mg, one can calculate the dose expected to result in an AUC of 1,200 μM·min by using the following equation (Equation 12.15):

$$\text{Adjusted dose (mg)} = \text{First dose (mg)} \times \frac{\text{AUC (Target)}}{\text{AUC (First dose)}} \qquad \textbf{(Eq. 12.15)}$$

$$= 51\,\text{mg}\left(\frac{1,200\,\mu\text{m}\cdot\text{min}}{890\,\mu\text{m}\cdot\text{min}}\right)$$

This results in a recommended adjusted busulfan dose of 69 mg.

To determine the first-dose busulfan C_{ss}, one must first convert the $AUC_{trapezoidal}$ in units of μM·min to units of μg/L·hr by multiplying 890 μmol/L·min by 246 μg/μmol and dividing by 60 min/hr, which results in a $AUC_{trapezoidal}$ of 3,649 μg/L·hr.

$$AUC_{trapezoidal}(\mu\text{g}/\text{L}\cdot\text{hr}) = \frac{AUC_{trapezoidal}(\mu\text{M}\cdot\text{min})(246\,\mu\text{g}/\mu\text{mol})}{60\,\text{min}/\text{hr}}$$

$$= \frac{\left(890\,\mu\text{M}\cdot\text{min}\right)\left(246\,\mu\text{g}/\mu\text{mol}\right)}{60\,\text{min}/\text{hr}}$$

$$= 3,649\,\mu\text{g}/\text{L}\cdot\text{hr}$$

The C_{ss} can then be calculated using Equation 12.11, where the dosing interval τ is equal to 6 hours:

$$\text{Busulfan } C_{ss}\,(\mu\text{g}/\text{L}) = \text{Busulfan AUC }(\mu\text{g}/\text{L}\cdot\text{hr})/\tau$$

$$= \frac{3,649\,\mu\text{g}/\text{L}\cdot\text{hr}}{6\,\text{hr}}$$

$$= 608\,\mu\text{g}/\text{L}$$

resulting in a first-dose busulfan C_{ss} estimate of 608 μg/L. Increasing the busulfan dose to 69 mg, one would expect a new C_{ss} of 608 μg/L × (69 mg/51 mg), or 823 μg/L. If the hematologist truly wants to target a busulfan C_{ss} of 750 μg/L instead of an AUC of 1,200 μM·min, an adjusted busulfan dose of 51 mg $\times \dfrac{750\,\mu g/L}{608\,\mu g/L}$, or 63 mg would be more appropriate.

PHARMACOGENETICS

Research dating back to at least the 1940s[40,41] introduced the concept that inherited genetic variants (ie, germline variations) can influence drug response, with Friedrich Vogel coining the term *pharmacogenetics* in 1959.[42] Much of the early work in the field of pharmacogenetics focused on determining if genetic variants in genes encoding for drug-metabolizing enzymes or transporters influenced drug exposure or response. Similar to renal and liver function assays, initial studies showed that pharmacogenetic testing could assist in predicting drug elimination. Strong clinical evidence emerged demonstrating that pharmacogenetic testing could identify patients at an elevated risk of a drug toxicity or nonresponse, thus allowing clinicians to preemptively select a different dose or drug before an adverse event occurred. However, genotyping assays were expensive and had slow turnaround times, making large-scale clinical applications impracticable. It was not until the early 2010s that pharmacogenetic testing was more widely integrated into clinical practice, bolstered by the Human Genome Project that led the way for cheaper DNA genotyping and sequencing technologies that had faster turnaround times.[2]

The majority of pharmacogenetic assays currently used in the oncology setting test for genetic variants that influence drug metabolism. Dependent on the pharmacogenetic test results, individuals can be assigned a drug-metabolizing phenotype as follows: ultrarapid, rapid, normal, intermediate, or poor metabolizer.[43] Ultrarapid and rapid metabolizers are predicted to eliminate certain drugs more quickly, thus having lower drug exposure and an elevated risk of nonresponse. Intermediate and poor metabolizers are predicted to eliminate certain drugs more slowly, thus having greater drug exposure and an elevated risk of toxicity. The reverse is true for prodrugs, where ultrarapid and rapid metabolizers bioactive the prodrug faster, leading to greater exposure to the active compound. Intermediate and poor metabolizers have slower bioactivation of the prodrug, resulting in lower exposure to the active compound.

Numerous gene-drug pairs are applicable to oncology practice, including *CYP2D6*-tamoxifen, *DPYD*-fluoropyrimidines, *TPMT*-thiopurines, *UGT1A1*-belinostat, and *UGT1A1*-irinotecan. In addition, several supportive care medications used in the oncology setting are influenced by pharmacogenetic variants, including *CYP2C19*-voriconazole, *CYP2D6*-antiemetics, *CYP2D6*-opioids, and *G6PD*-rasburicase. Table 12.1 briefly discusses the importance of these gene-drug pairs. The Clinical Pharmacogenetics Implementation Consortium (CPIC; www.cpicpgx.org) was established to provide evidence-based guidelines for utilizing pharmacogenetic test results to optimize drug therapy.[44] The CPIC guidelines can help clinicians to interpret pharmacogenetic test results and provide specific recommendations (eg, dose adjustments) for optimizing drug therapy. There are CPIC guidelines for over 50 gene-drug pairs.

In addition to pharmacogenes that influence drug metabolism, there are a growing number of germline variants that have implications for both cancer susceptibility and pharmacotherapy. Breast cancer 1 (*BRCA1*) and breast cancer 2 (*BRCA2*) gene

TABLE 12.1 Example Pharmacogenetic Gene-Drug Pairs Applicable to Oncology

GENE-DRUG PAIR	CLINICAL SIGNIFICANCE
CYP2D6-tamoxifen	CYP2D6 metabolizes tamoxifen to the more potent anti-estrogen endoxifen that is used to treat hormone receptor–positive breast cancer. Intermediate and poor metabolizers have lower endoxifen exposure that may elevate the risk of breast cancer recurrence.
DPYD-fluoropyrimidines	DPYD intermediate and poor metabolizers have greater exposure to the chemotherapy drugs 5-fluorouracil and capecitabine that elevates the risk of serious and life-threatening toxicities.
NUDT15-thiopurines	Thiopurines such as mercaptopurine are used to treat certain hematologic malignancies. NUDT15 intermediate and poor metabolizers have greater exposure to active thiopurine metabolites that can elevate the risk of serious and life-threatening toxicities.
TPMT-thiopurines	Thiopurines such as mercaptopurine are used to treat certain hematologic malignancies. TPMT intermediate and poor metabolizers have greater exposure to active thiopurine metabolites that can elevate the risk of serious and life-threatening toxicities.
UGT1A1-belinostat	UGT1A1 poor metabolizers have greater exposure to the anticancer drug belinostat that elevates the risk of serious toxicities.
UGT1A1-irinotecan	UGT1A1 poor metabolizers have greater exposure to the activate metabolite (SN-38) of the anticancer drug irinotecan that elevates the risk of serious toxicities.
CYP2C19-voriconazole	CYP2C19 ultrarapid or rapid metabolizers are predicted to have low plasma concentrations of the antifungal voriconazole that may potentiate breakthrough fungal infections in neutropenic patients with cancer.
CYP2D6-ondansetron	CYP2D6 ultrarapid metabolizers are predicted to have lower exposure to the antiemetic ondansetron that may result in uncontrolled chemotherapy-induced nausea and vomiting.
CYP2D6-opioids	CYP2D6 bioactivates certain pain medications such as codeine and tramadol into more active metabolites. Ultrarapid metabolizers are at an elevated risk of toxicity and poor metabolizers are at an elevated risk of nonresponse.
*G6PD-rasburicase	G6DP deficiency increases the risk of rasburicase-induced hemolytic anemia. Rasburicase is a recombinant urate oxidase enzyme that is used to treat hyperuricemia caused by tumor lysis syndrome.

*G6PD (glucose-6-phosphate dehydrogenase) is an example of a pharmacogene that is not involved in drug metabolism. G6PD has a role in protecting erythrocytes from oxidative stress that can be caused by drugs.

mutations, as the name implies, were initially discovered as risk factors for the development of breast cancer. Mutations in BRCA1 or BRCA2 disrupt the DNA damage response pathway, which can be targeted by anticancer drugs such as PARP (poly [ADP-ribose] polymerase) inhibitors.[45,46] Genetic testing for mutations in DNA damage repair genes such as BRCA1 or BRCA2 to identify opportunities for targeted therapy is becoming part of routine clinical care for certain cancer types, including breast, ovarian, pancreatic, and prostate cancers.

TPMT-THIOPURINES

Thiopurines consist of the drugs azathioprine, mercaptopurine, and thioguanine. Azathioprine and mercaptopurine are used to treat autoimmune and inflammatory diseases. Mercaptopurine is also used as part of chemotherapy regimens to treat certain types of hematologic malignancies such as acute lymphoblastic leukemia (ALL). Thioguanine is rarely used in the clinical setting.

TPMT genotyping to guide thiopurine dose selection was one of the first pharmacogenetic tests to be used in the oncology setting. Thiopurines can be catabolized to compounds with less pharmacologic activity by thiopurine methyltransferase (TPMT) or converted to thioguanine nucleotides. The active thioguanine nucleotides are incorporated into the DNA of leukocytes, resulting in cell death and myelosuppression. TPMT genetic variants can impact enzyme function.[47] Those with reduced TPMT activity have more parent drug available that can be converted to thioguanine nucleotides, thus increasing the risk of severe myelosuppression.

Each individual has two gene copies, one copy inherited maternally and one copy inherited paternally. Pharmacogenetics uses the star-allele nomenclature system to summarize genetic variants inherited on each gene copy.[48] Four TPMT alleles account for approximately 90% of the genetic polymorphisms that result in loss of TPMT function: TPMT*2, TPMT*3A, TPMT*3B, and TPMT*3C. The wild-type or normal function allele is TPMT*1. Individuals who have one copy of a normal function allele and one copy of a no-function allele (eg, TPMT*1/*2) are predicted to be intermediate metabolizers, and individuals with two copies of a no-function allele (eg, TPMT*3A/*3C) are predicted to be poor metabolizers. Those with two copies of a normal function allele (eg, TPMT*1/*1) are predicted to be normal metabolizers.

The CPIC guidelines provide recommendations for thiopurine dosing based on the TPMT genotype.[49] TPMT normal metabolizers prescribed mercaptopurine to treat hematologic malignancies are recommended to receive the normal starting dose (eg, 75 mg/m^2/d). When compared to normal metabolizers, TPMT intermediate metabolizers are predicted to have high concentrations of thioguanine nucleotides that can increase the risk of toxicities, such as myelosuppression. TPMT intermediate metabolizers are recommended to start with a 30% to 80% dose reduction (eg, 60 mg/m^2/d) of mercaptopurine to prevent toxicities. TPMT poor metabolizers are predicted to have extremely high concentrations of thioguanine nucleotides when compared to normal metabolizers. To prevent severe toxicities, TPMT poor metabolizers are recommended to start with an approximately 10-fold dose reduction of mercaptopurine (eg, 10 mg/m^2) and reduce the frequency of administration from daily to thrice weekly. The CPIC guidelines also provide thiopurine dosing recommendations based on the *NUDT15* genotype, which also influences exposure to thioguanine nucleotides. Recommendations for *NUDT15* are similar to those for *TPMT*.

> **Question #6**   *J.K., who is an 8-year-old female, was recently diagnosed with ALL. As part of her chemotherapy regimen, she is planning to receive mercaptopurine. A TPMT pharmacogenetic test that was performed to guide mercaptopurine dosing reported TPMT*2/*3C. What are the predicted TPMT metabolizer status and recommended dose reduction?*

J.K. has two copies of no-function allele. She is predicted to be a TPMT poor metabolizer.

Per the CPIC guidelines, TPMT poor metabolizers are recommended to start with an approximately 10-fold reduction of the normal mercaptopurine dose and reduce the frequency of administration to 3 times per week instead of daily.[49]

CANCER GENETICS

One of the first examples of testing a tumor for molecular alterations to personalize drug therapy occurred in the late 1990s when trastuzumab was approved to target human epidermal growth factor receptor 2 (HER2)-positive breast cancer. A few years later, the tyrosine kinase inhibitor imatinib was approved to treat hematologic cancers harboring the BCR-ABL tyrosine kinase fusion protein. Similar to pharmacogenetic testing, it was not until the 2010s that sequencing of the cancer genome (ie, somatic genome) was more widely integrated into clinical practice due, in part, to the Human Genome Project developing cheaper and more efficient sequencing technologies. Also contributing to the uptake of cancer genomic sequencing in clinical practice was the exponential growth of commercially available drugs that target specific genetic alterations. Studies have suggested that over 50% of cancers harbor mutations that are amendable to targeted therapy.[50] As new targeted therapies are developed, the percent of cancers that can be treated with genomics-driven therapy is expected to increase. Sequencing the cancer genome to guide therapeutic decision-making is now part of routine clinical practice for numerous cancer types.

Lung cancer is an exemplary example of how targeted therapies drastically changed treatment strategies. Up until the early 2000s, patients with metastatic lung cancer received cytotoxic chemotherapy agents with poor survival outcomes. Then in 2004, the epidermal growth factor receptor (EGFR) tyrosine kinase inhibitor erlotinib was approved for lung cancer treatment based on research showing EGFR had a role in lung cancer tumorigenesis and clinical trials demonstrating improved responses with erlotinib.[51] Subsequent studies revealed that tumors harboring gain-of-function *EGFR* mutations (eg, *EGFR* exon 19 deletions, EGFR[L858R]) had better responses to erlotinib, thus promoting the integration of *EGFR* genotyping into patient care. There are now over 20 drugs that target specific genetic mutations in lung cancer summarized in Table 12.2.

There is an ongoing paradigm shift in cancer treatment where an increasing number of patients are receiving oral kinase inhibitors or other types of targeted

TABLE 12.2   Examples of Targeted Therapy in Lung Cancer

SOMATIC MUTATION	TARGETED THERAPY
ALK gene rearrangements	Alectinib, brigatinib, ceritinib, crizotinib, lorlatinib
BRAF^{V600E}	Dabrafenib combined with trametinib
EGFR exon 19 deletion, EGFR^{L858R}	Afatinib, dacomitinib, erlotinib, gefitinib, osimertinib
EGFR$^{S768I, L861Q, G719X}$	Afatinib, osimertinib
EGFR^{T790M}	Osimertinib
EGFR exon 20 insertion	Amivantamab, mobocertinib
ERBB2-activating mutations	Ado-trastuzumab emtansine, fam-trastuzumab deruxtecan-nxki
KRAS^{G12C}	Sotorasib
MET exon 14 skipping	Capmatinib, tepotinib
NTRK gene rearrangements	Entrectinib, larotrectinib
RET gene rearrangements	Pralsetinib, selpercatinib
ROS1 gene rearrangements	Entrectinib

therapy based on somatic sequencing results, instead of cytotoxic chemotherapy. In the not-too-distant future, certain types of cancer may be managed as a chronic disease where patients take oral kinase inhibitors targeting specific genetic alterations for years or even decades. This may lead to new opportunities for TDM in oncology practice by using drug concentrations to optimize oral kinase inhibitor therapy.[52]

ACKNOWLEDGMENT

The important work of Courtney Yuen and Timothy W. Synold in previous versions of this chapter is acknowledged.

REFERENCES

1. Hicks JK, Howard R, Reisman P, et al. Integrating somatic and germline next-generation sequencing into routine clinical oncology practice. *JCO Precis Oncol.* 2021;5:PO.20.00513.
2. Hicks JK, Aquilante CL, Dunnenberger HM, et al. Precision pharmacotherapy: integrating pharmacogenomics into clinical pharmacy practice. *J Am Coll Clin Pharm.* 2019;2(3):303-313.
3. Masson E, Zamboni WC. Pharmacokinetic optimisation of cancer chemotherapy. Effect on outcomes. *Clin Pharmacokinet.* 1997;32:324-343.
4. Du Bois D, Du Bois EF. A formula to estimate the approximate surface area if height and weight be known. 1916. *Nutrition.* 1989;5:303-311.

5. Egorin MJ, Van Echo DA, Olman EA, Whitacre MY, Forrest A, Aisner J. Prospective validation of a pharmacologically based dosing scheme for the cis-diamminedichloroplatinum(II) analogue diammi-necyclobutanedicarboxylatoplatinum. *Cancer Res.* 1985;45:6502-6506.

6. Calvert AH, Newell DR, Gumbrell LA, et al. Carboplatin dosage: prospective evaluation of a simple formula based on renal function. *J Clin Oncol.* 1989;7:1748-1756.

7. Evans WE, Relling MV, Rodman JH, Crom WR, Boyett JM, Pui CH. Conventional compared with indi-vidualized chemotherapy for childhood acute lymphoblastic leukemia. *N Engl J Med.* 1998;338:499-505.

8. van den Bongard HJ, Mathot RA, Beijnen JH, Schellens JH. Pharmacokinetically guided administra-tion of chemotherapeutic agents. *Clin Pharmacokinet.* 2000;39:345-367.

9. Paci A, Veal G, Bardin C, et al. Review of therapeutic drug monitoring of anticancer drugs part 1–cytotoxics. *Eur J Cancer.* 2014;50:2010-2019.

10. Wan SH, Huffman DH, Azarnoff DL, Stephens R, Hoogstraten B. Effect of route of administration and effusions on methotrexate pharmacokinetics. *Cancer Res.* 1974;34:3487-3491.

11. Bleyer WA. Methotrexate: clinical pharmacology, current status and therapeutic guidelines. *Cancer Treat Rev.* 1977;4:87-101.

12. Bleyer WA. The clinical pharmacology of methotrexate: new applications of an old drug. *Cancer.* 1978;41:36-51.

13. Shen DD, Azarnoff DL. Clinical pharmacokinetics of methotrexate. *Clin Pharmacokinet.* 1978;3:1-13.

14. Stoller RG, Hande KR, Jacobs SA, Rosenberg SA, Chabner BA. Use of plasma pharmacokinetics to predict and prevent methotrexate toxicity. *N Engl J Med.* 1977;297:630-634.

15. Leme PR, Creaven PJ, Allen LM, Berman M. Kinetic model for the disposition and metabolism of moderate and high-dose methotrexate (NSC-740) in man. *Cancer Chemother Rep.* 1975;59:811-817.

16. Pratt CB, Howarth C, Ransom JL, et al. High-dose methotrexate used alone and in combination for measurable primary or metastatic osteosarcoma. *Cancer Treat Rep.* 1980;64:11-20.

17. Evans WE, Pratt CB. Effect of pleural effusion on high-dose methotrexate kinetics. *Clin Pharmacol Ther.* 1978;23:68-72.

18. Isacoff WH, Morrison PF, Aroesty J, et al. Pharmacokinetics of high-dose methotrexate with citrovo-rum factor rescue. *Cancer Treat Rep.* 1977;61:1665-1674.

19. Taylor ZL, Vang J, Lopez-Lopez E, Oosterom N, Mikkelsen T, Ramsey LB. Systematic review of phar-macogenetic factors that influence high-dose methotrexate pharmacokinetics in pediatric malignan-cies. *Cancers (Basel).* 2021;13(11):2837.

20. Liegler DG, Henderson ES, Hahn MA, Oliverio VT. The effect of organic acids on renal clearance of methotrexate in man. *Clin Pharmacol Ther.* 1969;10:849-857.

21. Beorlegui B, Aldaz A, Ortega A, Aquerreta I, Sierrasesúmega L, Giráldez J. Potential interaction be-tween methotrexate and omeprazole. *Ann Pharmacother.* 2000;34:1024-1027.

22. Cadman EC, Lundberg WB, Bertino JR. Systemic methotrexate toxicity: a pharmacological study of its oc-currence after intrathecal administration in a patient with renal failure. *Arch Intern Med.* 1976;136:1321-1322.

23. Ahmad S, Shen FH, Bleyer WA. Methotrexate-induced renal failure and ineffectiveness of peritoneal dialysis. *Arch Intern Med.* 1978;138:1146-1147.

24. Ellison NM, Servi RJ. Acute renal failure and death following sequential intermediate-dose metho-trexate and 5-FU: a possible adverse effect due to concomitant indomethacin administration. *Cancer Treat Rep.* 1985;69:342-343.

25. Thyss A, Milano G, Kubar J, Namer M, Schneider M. Clinical and pharmacokinetic evidence of a life-threatening interaction between methotrexate and ketoprofen. *Lancet.* 1986;1:256-258.

26. Jones RJ, Grochow LB. Pharmacology of bone marrow transplantation conditioning regimens. *Ann N Y Acad Sci.* 1995;770:237-241.

27. Grochow LB, Jones RJ, Brundrett RB, et al. Pharmacokinetics of busulfan: correlation with veno-occlusive disease in patients undergoing bone marrow transplantation. *Cancer Chemother Phar-macol.* 1989;25:55-61.

28. Vassal G, Koscielny S, Challine D, et al. Busulfan disposition and hepatic veno-occlusive disease in children undergoing bone marrow transplantation. *Cancer Chemother Pharmacol.* 1996;37:247-253.

29. McCune JS, Gibbs JP, Slattery JT. Plasma concentration monitoring of busulfan: does it improve clinical outcome? *Clin Pharmacokinet.* 2000;39:155-165.

30. McCune JS, Gooley T, Gibbs JP, et al. Busulfan concentration and graft rejection in pediatric patients undergoing hematopoietic stem cell transplantation. *Bone Marrow Transplant.* 2002;30:167-173.

31. Madden T, de Lima M, Thapar N, et al. Pharmacokinetics of once-daily IV busulfan as part of pre-transplantation preparative regimens: a comparison with an every 6-hour dosing schedule. *Biol Blood Marrow Transplant.* 2007;13:56-64.

32. Takamatsu Y, Sasaki N, Eto T, et al. Individual dose adjustment of oral busulfan using a test dose in hematopoietic stem cell transplantation. *Int J Hematol.* 2007;86:261-268.

33. Kangarloo SB, Naveed F, Ng ESM, et al. Development and validation of a test dose strategy for once-daily i.v. busulfan: importance of fixed infusion rate dosing. *Biol Blood Marrow Transplant.* 2012;18:295-301.

34. Olson MT, Lombardi L, Clarke W. Clinical consequences of analytical variance and calculation strategy in oral busulfan pharmacokinetics. *Clin Chim Acta.* 2011;412:2316-2321.

35. Hassan M, Ljungman P, Bolme P, et al. Busulfan bioavailability. *Blood.* 1994;84:2144-2150.

36. Hassan M. The role of busulfan in bone marrow transplantation. *Med Oncol.* 1999;16:166-176.

37. Bubalo J, Carpenter PA, Majhail N, et al; American Society for Blood and Marrow Transplantation practice guideline committee. Conditioning chemotherapy dose adjustment in obese patients: a review and position statement by the American Society for Blood and Marrow Transplantation practice guideline committee. *Biol Blood Marrow Transplant.* 2014;20:600-616.

38. Caselli D, Rosati A, Faraci M, et al; Bone Marrow Transplantation Working Group of the Associazione Italiana Ematologia Oncologia Pediatrica. Risk of seizures in children receiving busulphan-containing regimens for stem cell transplantation. *Biol Blood Marrow Transplant.* 2014;20:282-285.

39. Czerwinski M, Gibbs JP, Slattery JT. Busulfan conjugation by glutathione S-transferases alpha, mu, and pi. *Drug Metab Dispos.* 1996;24:1015-1019.

40. Lederberg J. J. B. S. Haldane (1949) on infectious disease and evolution. *Genetics.* 1999;153(1):1-3.

41. Sawin PB, Glick D. Atropinesterase, a genetically determined enzyme in the rabbit. *Proc Natl Acad Sci U S A.* 1943;29(2):55-59.

42. Vogel F. Moderne problem der humangenetik. *Ergeb Inn Med U Kinderheik.* 1959;12:52-125.

43. Caudle KE, Dunnenberger HM, Freimuth RR, et al. Standardizing terms for clinical pharmacogenetic test results: consensus terms from the Clinical Pharmacogenetics Implementation Consortium (CPIC). *Genet Med.* 2017;19(2):215-223.

44. Relling MV, Klein TE. CPIC: Clinical Pharmacogenetics Implementation Consortium of the Pharmacogenomics Research Network. *Clin Pharmacol Ther.* 2011;89(3):464-467.

45. Mateo J, Carreira S, Sandhu S, et al. DNA-repair defects and olaparib in metastatic prostate cancer. *N Engl J Med.* 2015;373(18):1697-1708.

46. Golan T, Hammel P, Reni M, et al. Maintenance olaparib for germline BRCA-mutated metastatic pancreatic cancer. *N Engl J Med.* 2019;381(4):317-327.

47. Evans WE. Pharmacogenetics of thiopurine S-methyltransferase and thiopurine therapy. *Ther Drug Monit.* 2004;26(2):186-191.

48. Kalman LV, Agúndez J, Appell ML, et al. Pharmacogenetic allele nomenclature: International workgroup recommendations for test result reporting. *Clin Pharmacol Ther.* 2016;99(2):172-185.

49. Relling MV, Schwab M, Whirl-Carrillo M, et al. Clinical pharmacogenetics implementation consortium guideline for thiopurine dosing based on TPMT and NUDT15 genotypes: 2018 update. *Clin Pharmacol Ther.* 2019;105(5):1095-1105.

50. Sadaps M, Funchain P, Mahdi H, et al. Precision oncology in solid tumors: a longitudinal tertiary care center experience. *JCO Precis Oncol.* 2018;2:1-11.

51. Shepherd FA, Rodrigues Pereira J, Ciuleanu T, et al; National Cancer Institute of Canada Clinical Trials Group. Erlotinib in previously treated non-small-cell lung cancer. *N Engl J Med.* 2005;353(2):123-132.

52. Mueller-Schoell A, Groenland SL, Scherf-Clavel O, et al. Therapeutic drug monitoring of oral targeted antineoplastic drugs. *Eur J Clin Pharmacol.* 2021;77(4):441-464.

13

IMMUNOSUPPRESSANTS (MAINTENANCE THERAPY)

Tony K. L. Kiang and Mary H. H. Ensom

Learning Objectives

By the end of the immunosuppressants chapter, the learner shall be able to:

1. Know the therapeutic range of the immunosuppressive drugs discussed in this chapter (ie, cyclosporine, tacrolimus, sirolimus, and mycophenolate). The learner shall also be able to explain the consequences of subtherapeutic concentrations and the toxicities associated with supratherapeutic concentrations.
2. Identify drugs that can significantly alter the pharmacokinetics of cyclosporine, tacrolimus, sirolimus, and mycophenolate. The learner shall also be able to propose dosing strategies to increase or decrease cyclosporine, tacrolimus, sirolimus, or mycophenolate concentrations using principles of therapeutic drug monitoring (TDM) for each agent.
3. Describe alternative approaches to TDM (ie, dried blood spot, concentration variability) for tacrolimus and mycophenolate.
4. Understand the differences in the pharmacokinetics between the original cyclosporine formulation and the cyclosporine-modified formulation.
5. Convert between intravenous and oral formulations for cyclosporine modified or tacrolimus.
6. Explain, using the criteria outlined in Chapter "Drug Dosing in Kidney Disease and Dialysis," why dialysis is not likely to remove significant amounts of cyclosporine, tacrolimus, sirolimus, and mycophenolate.
7. Describe the evidence supporting the implementation of clinical pharmacogenomics of cyclosporine, tacrolimus, sirolimus, and mycophenolate.

Immunosuppression plays a vital role in preventing and treating allograft rejection in the transplant recipient and in the management of various autoimmune disorders.

Many of the immunosuppressive drugs have a narrow therapeutic window and exhibit pharmacokinetic variability. There can be large fluctuations in the observed blood/plasma concentrations between patients receiving the same dose normalized to weight (interpatient variability) and within the same patient receiving the same dose (intrapatient variability). Subtherapeutic concentrations and wide fluctuations in drug concentrations are risk factors for allograft rejection, whereas supratherapeutic concentrations increase the likelihood of developing adverse effects. Therapeutic drug monitoring (TDM) is essential in optimizing the patient's immunosuppressive drug regimen to minimize the risk of allograft rejection and concentration-related adverse effects.

Immunosuppressive drug therapy is usually individualized to the patient and tailored to the specific organ(s) transplanted, time after transplant, indication for transplantation, and transplant center–specific immunosuppression protocols. Although many antirejection drugs are available, this chapter focuses on the four drugs used in the maintenance immunosuppression setting that commonly undergo TDM: cyclosporine, tacrolimus, sirolimus, and mycophenolic acid (hereafter designated as mycophenolate). The clinical pharmacokinetics, pharmacodynamics, pharmacogenomics, and current methods for clinical pharmacokinetic monitoring for each immunosuppressant pertaining to adult subjects (ie, >18 years of age) are presented.

Cyclosporine

Cyclosporine is a cyclical peptide used in clinical practice in combination with other immunosuppressants for the prevention of allograft rejection in solid organ (ie, heart, liver, kidney) transplant recipients, for the treatment or prevention of graft-versus-host disease in bone marrow transplant recipients (as off-label usage), and for the management of various autoimmune disorders (as off-label usage).[1,2] The primary immunosuppressive effects of cyclosporine are to reduce the production of interleukin-2 (IL-2) and other inflammatory chemokines by inhibiting the calcineurin enzyme. IL-2 plays a vital role in the cellular rejection process by signaling for cytotoxic T-lymphocyte activation and proliferation.[3,4] Cyclosporine is not considered the first-line calcineurin inhibitor in solid organ transplant patients because of the improved efficacy of tacrolimus.[5] Cyclosporine is usually given in combination with a corticosteroid and an antiproliferative agent, such as mycophenolate.[3]

KEY PARAMETERS: Cyclosporine[a,2,6]

Therapeutic concentrations	See text for discussions
F^b	Original formulation: average ~30%, range 2%-90% (ie, highly variable)
	Modified formulation: generally higher than the original formulation (not well characterized)
V^c	4-6 L/kg (reduced in cardiac transplant recipients)

KEY PARAMETERS: Cyclosporine[a,2,6] (continued)

Cl[d]	5-7 mL/min/kg
$t_{1/2}$	Original formulation: average ~19 hr Modified formulation: average ~8 hr
fu[e] (fraction unbound)	2%-10%

[a]Pharmacokinetic parameters are based on population averages and may vary from patient to patient.
[b]Bioavailability depends on the formulation and type of transplant.
[c]Cyclosporine is distributed into multiple tissue and fluid compartments.
[d]Clearance value obtained from the intravenous formulation. Primarily cleared via intestinal/hepatic intrinsic clearance with little renal clearance.
[e]Cyclosporine is extensively bound (ie, >90%) to lipoproteins. Binding is saturable at higher concentrations.

Cyclosporine is available in several formulations in various brands/generics; the reader should refer to Table 13.1 for the discussed immunosuppressive drug formulations in Canada and the United States. The original formulation of cyclosporine, Sandimmune, exhibits relatively poor and erratic absorption and is, therefore, not commonly used anymore. Today, the majority of patients prescribed de novo cyclosporine are started with the modified formulation. The modified cyclosporine is a microemulsion formulation with improved absorption characteristics and hence improved bioavailability.[2,6] The modified cyclosporine formulations are absorbed faster (ie, shorter time-to-maximal concentration, t_{max}) to a greater extent (higher area under the concentration-time curve [AUC] and higher maximum concentration, C_{max}), with reduced variability compared to the original formulation.[7] Figure 13.1 illustrates

TABLE 13.1 Immunosuppressive Drug Formulations[2,6,8-13]

DRUG	FORMULATIONS
Cyclosporine Sandimmune	25 and 100 mg capsules 100 mg/mL oral solution 50 mg/mL ampules for intermittent intravenous infusion
Cyclosporine modified Neoral, Gengraf, and others	25, 50, and 100 mg capsules 100 mg/mL oral solution
Tacrolimus Prograf (or generic) Astagraf XL or Advagraf Envarsus XR/PA	0.5, 1, and 5 mg capsules 5 mg/mL ampules for intravenous infusion 0.5, 1, 3, and 5 mg extended-release capsules 0.75, 1, and 4 mg extended-release tablets
Sirolimus Rapamune (or generic)	0.5, 1, and 2 mg tablets 1 mg/mL oral solution
Mycophenolate mofetil Mycophenolate sodium Mycophenolate mofetil hydrochloride	250 mg capsule, 500 mg tablet, 200 mg/mL oral solution 180 and 360 mg delayed-release tablets 500 mg vial for injection

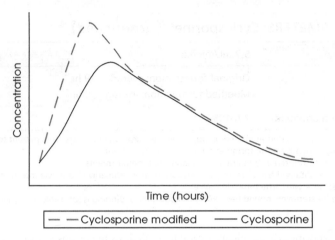

FIGURE 13.1 Representative average concentration-time profiles of the original cyclosporine and cyclosporine modified after respective oral doses.

the average concentration-time profiles of the original cyclosporine and cyclosporine modified after respective oral (PO) doses. As the original cyclosporine and cyclosporine modified exhibit different pharmacokinetic characteristics, they are not considered interchangeable therapeutically.

The typical starting PO dose of cyclosporine-modified maintenance therapy (in combination with corticosteroids and antimetabolites) to prevent allograft rejection is approximately 2 to 6 mg/kg q12h.[2] Renal and hepatic transplant recipients are usually given a higher starting dose compared to heart patients.[2] If patients are unable to tolerate PO formulations, an intravenous (IV) original (ie, nonmodified) formulation may be considered and is typically dosed at one-third of the PO dose as an intermittent infusion over 2 to 6 hours.[2] Doses should be further tailored to the individual patient utilizing target cyclosporine blood concentrations (see later in this chapter).

Cyclosporine original and cyclosporine modified are available in PO liquid formulations for those unable to swallow the capsules (see Table 13.1). The graduated PO syringe enclosed with the solution packages should be used to measure the liquid dose to ensure accuracy.[2,6] To improve the taste, the cyclosporine-modified solution can be diluted with orange juice or apple juice, and the original formulation diluted with milk products, at room temperature using a glass container.[2,6] Prepared solutions should be ingested immediately owing to the lack of stability data. The glass container should be rinsed, and the diluent consumed to ensure the complete dose is given.[2,6] Grapefruit or its juice is contraindicated as a diluent with all formulations of cyclosporine owing to its inhibitory effects toward cytochrome P450 3A4 (CYP3A4) and P-glycoprotein transporter enzymes, which are responsible for the metabolism and efflux of cyclosporine.[14-16]

Cyclosporine has a narrow therapeutic window. The concentration range between subtherapeutic concentrations, at which patients are at increased risk of acute rejection, and toxic concentrations, where the patient is at increased risk of experiencing adverse effects, is relatively narrow. Routine TDM or clinical pharmacokinetic monitoring is conducted as a part of the post-transplant protocol in most transplant centers. TDM is essential for maintaining cyclosporine concentrations within a target blood concentration range to maximize immunosuppression and minimize dose-related adverse effects. The therapeutic target usually depends on the time post-transplant (ie, typically decreases rapidly over the initial post-transplant year) and the type of graft and is specific to each transplant center tailored to the patient receiving care.

THERAPEUTIC AND TOXIC CONCENTRATIONS (BLOOD)

Cyclosporine is lipid soluble and distributed into granulocytes (up to 12%) and erythrocytes (up to 58%), and up to 47% remains in the plasma where it is highly bound to lipoproteins.[6] Thus, whole blood is the ideal TDM matrix.[17,18] Liquid chromatography tandem mass spectrometry (LC-MS/MS) is commonly used today for the quantification of cyclosporine concentrations. Owing to their specificity for cyclosporine, LC-MS/MS assays can generate concentrations lower than the traditional immune-based assays,[19] which may also detect cyclosporine metabolites in addition to the parent compound. Clinicians should be aware of the assay method used at their institution to ensure appropriate interpretation of cyclosporine concentrations. The target concentration range can vary based on the type of transplant (ie, kidney vs liver), the timing of the sample (ie, trough concentration, or C_0 vs cyclosporine concentration at 2 hours postdosing, or C_2), and the time post-transplant. In general, the target range is typically the highest immediately post-transplant and is gradually reduced over several months. For example, when concentrations in whole blood are measured using the LC/MS/MS, the typical concentration range based on an institutional target for adult kidney transplant patients are less than 1 month post-transplant (300-350 ng/mL for C_0 or 1,300 ng/mL for C_2), 1 to 2 months (250-300 ng/mL for C_0 or 1,100 ng/mL for C_2), 3 to 6 months (150-250 ng/mL for C_0 or 800-900 ng/mL for C_2), 7 to 12 months (125-200 ng/mL for C_0 or 700 ng/mL for C_2), and greater than 12 months (75-125 ng/mL for C_0 or 450-600 ng/mL for C_2).[19] These targets will differ based on the institution. More importantly, clinicians should treat the patient rather than a therapeutic concentration target.

ADVERSE EFFECTS[2,3,6]

The most common adverse effects associated with cyclosporine are hypertension, headache, hand tremors, hypertrichosis/hirsutism, elevated triglycerides, nausea, gum hyperplasia, various types of infections, and renal dysfunction (elevated serum creatinine), which can improve when the dose is decreased or the drug is discontinued. Hypertension is likely the most common adverse reaction to cyclosporine, and some patients may benefit from antihypertensive pharmacotherapy. Although the mechanism for nephrotoxicity is unclear, it may be related to cyclosporine-induced renal vasoconstriction. Pharmacists can reduce the incidence of cyclosporine-induced nephrotoxicity by carefully managing the patient's coadministered medications, avoiding the usage of concurrent nephrotoxic drugs (eg, nonsteroidal anti-inflammatory drugs [NSAIDs], vancomycin, aminoglycosides) and ensuring the blood concentration is within the therapeutic target.

BIOAVAILABILITY (F)[2,3,6]

Cyclosporine is a lipophilic drug with limited and highly variable bioavailability. Cyclosporine undergoes first-pass metabolism via intestinal and hepatic CYP3A4/5. In addition, cyclosporine is a substrate for P-glycoprotein, an efflux transporter. These factors contribute in part to cyclosporine's incomplete and variable absorption. Low or variable bioavailability is a risk factor for allograft rejection.[20,21] Peak concentrations occur in about 2 to 6 hours for the original cyclosporine formulation and 1 to 2 hours for the modified formulations.[2] Rapid gastrointestinal transit may also reduce bioavailability and should be considered in patients with diarrhea who are receiving PO cyclosporine.[22] The bioavailability of modified cyclosporine is generally higher and is probably more consistently absorbed than the original formulation.[2]

VOLUME OF DISTRIBUTION (V)[2,6]

The volume of distribution of cyclosporine is approximately 4 to 6 L/kg. This relatively large V is consistent with the observation that cyclosporine is significantly bound to components in plasma and blood, that the unbound portion in the plasma is usually less than 10%, and that cyclosporine is probably extensively bound to organ tissues outside the vascular space.[23-25] The V is reduced in heart transplant recipients and patients with end-stage renal disease.[2] The large interindividual variability associated with cyclosporine's V is unlikely to affect clinical dosing because loading doses are not administered and TDM is commonly practiced to ensure precision dosing (see Clinical Application of Cyclosporine Pharmacokinetics).

CLEARANCE (Cl)

Cyclosporine undergoes extensive first-pass metabolism via CYP3A4/5 in enterocytes and hepatocytes in the formation of multiple metabolites.[2,6] These metabolites are generally thought to be less active than cyclosporine itself.[6] The whole blood clearance of cyclosporine is approximately 5 to 7 mL/kg/min in adult patients,[6] suggesting that it exhibits a low extraction ratio when administered IV or PO. Therefore, the total clearance of cyclosporine is more likely to be influenced by the unbound cyclosporine fraction and hepatic/intestinal intrinsic clearance but is independent of hepatic blood flow. As such, drug interactions that result in protein-binding displacement (ie, altered free fraction), modulation of hepatic metabolism (ie, induction or inhibition of CYP3A4/5), or loss-of-function genetic polymorphisms associated with binding and metabolism enzymes may lead to differential effects on total and free cyclosporine concentrations. With respect to altered intrinsic clearance, numerous drugs have been reported to influence the metabolism of cyclosporine via CYP3A4 or P-glycoprotein induction or inhibition (Table 13.2).

HALF-LIFE (t½)

The average half-life calculated from the values indicated in the preceding sections and Equation 13.1 would suggest a value of approximately 7 hours.

TABLE 13.2   Immunosuppressive Drug-Drug Interactions Associated With Cyclosporine, Sirolimus, and Tacrolimus[2,19]

EXAMPLES OF DRUGS THAT MAY INHIBIT CYTOCHROME P450 (CYP3A4) AND P-GLYCOPROTEIN[a] (AND POTENTIALLY INCREASE CYCLOSPORINE/SIROLIMUS/TACROLIMUS CONCENTRATIONS)

Nondihydropyridine calcium channel blockers	Azole antifungals
Diltiazem	Fluconazole
Nicardipine	Itraconazole
Verapamil	Ketoconazole
Macrolide antibiotics	Posaconazole
Clarithromycin	Voriconazole
Erythromycin	Antidepressants
Azithromycin	Fluoxetine
HIV protease inhibitors	Fluvoxamine
Indinavir	Sertraline
Ritonavir	Paroxetine
Gastrointestinal prokinetic agents	Venlafaxine
Metoclopramide	Mirtazapine
	Others
	Amiodarone
	Cimetidine
	Danazol
	Ethinyl estradiol
	Grapefruit juice
	Nefazodone

EXAMPLES OF DRUGS THAT MAY INDUCE CYTOCHROME P450 (CYP3A4/5) AND P-GLYCOPROTEIN[a] (AND POTENTIALLY DECREASE CYCLOSPORINE/SIROLIMUS/TACROLIMUS CONCENTRATIONS)

Antibiotics	Anticonvulsants
Caspofungin	Carbamazepine
Nafcillin	Phenobarbital
Rifabutin	Phenytoin
Rifampin	Primidone
Others	
St. John wort (*Hypericum perforatum*)	

[a]This is not an exhaustive list of drugs that can interact with cyclosporine, sirolimus, or tacrolimus.

$$t_{1/2} = \frac{(0.693)(V)}{Cl} \qquad \text{(Eq. 13.1)}$$

$$= \frac{(0.693)(4.5\ \text{L/kg})}{(7.5\ \text{mL/kg/min})\left(\dfrac{60\ \text{min/hr}}{1,000\ \text{mL/L}}\right)}$$

$$= 6.93\ \text{hr}$$

The half-life of cyclosporine also exhibits a wide range because of variability associated with the volume of distribution and clearance estimates for cyclosporine. The multicompartmental nature of cyclosporine may also lead to an underestimation of the terminal half-life and the associated pharmacokinetic parameters. The most commonly reported values for cyclosporine half-life are in the range of 10 to 27 hours for the original cyclosporine formulation and 5 to 18 hours for the modified formulations.[2]

TIME TO SAMPLE

Although there are several ways to monitor cyclosporine therapy, the most widely used methods are to sample the trough (ie, just before the dose) or 2-hour postdose (C_2) concentrations.[19] Cyclosporine blood exposure as represented by the area under the concentration-time curve (AUC) is the most accurate method for predicting clinical outcomes because it directly reflects drug exposure. However, the AUC approach is rarely used in the clinic because multiple blood samples over the 12-hour dosing interval are necessary. The cyclosporine concentration at 2 hours after administration of modified formulations (eg, C_2) is the most accurate time marker for AUC_{0-4}[26] (an AUC marker predictive of acute graft rejection), but the C_2 sample should be taken on time in order to maintain the correlation. The precise timing of the sample dictates that this method of monitoring should be performed in a controlled environment, such as a hospital or transplant clinic. Furthermore, abbreviated AUC (or limited sampling strategy [LSS]) algorithms utilize a limited number of sampling points and multiple regression or population pharmacokinetic-based equations to estimate the cyclosporine AUC.[27,28] However, these LSSs should be validated and used only in patients who have similar characteristics compared to the subjects/conditions in which the equations were originally developed and validated. Despite improved accuracy and/or predictive performance of the AUC or LSS approaches, their requirement for multiple sampling means that the trough and C_2 concentrations are still the most commonly used methods to monitor cyclosporine therapy today.

CLINICAL PHARMACOGENOMICS OF CYCLOSPORINE

Currently (June 2022), there are insufficient data to support a pharmacogenomics-guided dosing for cyclosporine, with inconsistent data linking genetic polymorphisms to pharmacokinetics[29-37] (see Pharmacogenomic Applications).

Clinical Application of Cyclosporine Pharmacokinetics

When the cyclosporine concentration is low, the dose is increased; when the concentration is high, the dose is decreased. If the cyclosporine concentration is low, the pharmacist should evaluate patient adherence to the prescribed regimen and determine whether drugs have been added that might decrease cyclosporine absorption, increase efflux transport, or increase metabolism. If there are no easily correctable problems, most clinicians would increase the dose *modestly* (the extent of dose change typically is limited to within 25% of the original dose, although individual transplant centers might follow their own protocols), recognizing that the change in concentration should be approximately proportional to the change in the maintenance dose.

If the cyclosporine concentration is high, it is important to determine whether the sample has been obtained at the appropriate time (ie, trough or C_2). In addition, patient adherence should be assessed and the potential for any drug-drug interactions (ie, CYP3A4 inhibition) that might account for the increased cyclosporine concentration should be determined. If the sample is valid, many clinicians will hold a dose and then restart on a proportionally lower maintenance dose, or simply lower the dose to bring the cyclosporine concentration into the desired therapeutic target range. The steady-state (ie, after ~5 half-lives) cyclosporine concentration should be verified to ensure the patient has achieved therapeutic concentrations. Occasionally, patients have an isolated elevated or decreased cyclosporine concentration for which no logical explanation can be found. In these scenarios, the patient should be assessed to determine whether they are clinically stable, and the clinician should then recheck the cyclosporine concentration as soon as reasonably possible.

Question #1 *R.I., a 39-year-old, 51-kg woman, received a living-unrelated renal transplant over a decade ago. Her serum creatinine had been stable in the range of 1.4 to 1.7 mg/dL. She has been receiving cyclosporine modified PO, 125 mg 2 times (BID). Cyclosporine concentrations have been 85 to 110 µg/L (whole blood). Her last clinic appointment was 3 weeks ago. Other immunosuppressive medications included prednisone 10 mg/d and mycophenolate mofetil 1,000 mg BID. She returned to the clinic yesterday complaining of increasing fatigue since her last clinic appointment. Blood and urine cultures were taken, and she was admitted to the hospital with a serum creatinine of 2.8 mg/dL. How would you adjust R.I.'s cyclosporine-modified dose to increase the cyclosporine concentration to approximately 200 µg/L?*

First, it is important to determine whether the rise in serum creatinine is caused by graft rejection or cyclosporine toxicity. If the increase in serum creatinine is presumed to be a sign of allograft rejection (ie, after confirmatory investigations with renal ultrasound and/or biopsy), the patient should also receive additional acute immunosuppressant therapy, including methylprednisolone and/or antithymocyte globulin. Using approach number three as outlined in Interpretation of Plasma Drug Concentrations; Choosing a Model to Revise or Estimate a Patient's Clearance at Steady State in Chapter "Selecting the Appropriate Equation and Interpretation of Measured Drug Concentrations," a revised set of pharmacokinetic parameters can be calculated.

First, we would start by estimating a revised elimination rate constant.

$$K_{revised} = \frac{\ln\left(\dfrac{C_{ss\,min} + \dfrac{(S)(F)(Dose)}{V}}{C_{ss\,min}}\right)}{\tau}$$

(Eq. 13.2)

The average cyclosporine concentration of approximately 100 µg/L would be used as the $C_{ss\,min}$, F would be 0.3 (average value), and the dose would be expressed as 125,000 μg. The V would have to be estimated (4.5 L/kg), and τ would be 12 hours. Using these values, the revised elimination rate constant is approximately 0.0807 hr^{-1}.

$$= \frac{\ln\left(\dfrac{100\ \mu g/L> + \dfrac{(1)(0.3)(125{,}000\ \mu g)}{(4.5\ L/kg)\ (51\ kg)}}{100\ \mu g/L}\right)}{12\ hr}$$

$$= \frac{\ln\left(\dfrac{263.4\ \mu g/L}{100\ \mu g/L}\right)}{12}$$

$$= 0.0807\ hr^{-1}$$

This $K_{revised}$ would correspond to a clearance of 18.5 L/hr:

$$Cl = (K_{revised})(V) \qquad \text{(Eq. 13.3)}$$

$$= (0.0807\ hr^{-1})(4.5\ L/kg)(51\ kg)$$

$$= (0.0807\ hr^{-1})(229.5\ L)$$

$$= 18.5\ L/hr$$

and a half-life of approximately 8 or 9 hours.

$$t_{\frac{1}{2}} = \frac{0.693}{K} \qquad \text{(Eq. 13.4)}$$

$$= \frac{0.693}{0.0807\ hr^{-1}}$$

$$= 8.6\ hr$$

Using the revised pharmacokinetic parameters, a new dose can be calculated by rearranging Equation 13.5.

$$C_{ss\ min} = \frac{\dfrac{(S)(F)(Dose)}{V}}{(1 - e^{-K\tau})}(e^{-K\tau}) \qquad \text{(Eq. 13.5)}$$

$$\text{Dose} = \frac{(C_{ss\,min})(V)(1-e^{-K\tau})}{(S)(F)(e^{-K\tau})} \qquad \text{(Eq. 13.6)}$$

Making the appropriate substitutions for $C_{ss\,min}$, V, S, F, K, and τ, a dose of approximately 250 mg can be calculated.

$$= \frac{(200\ \mu g/L)(4.5\ L/kg)(51\ kg)(1 - e^{-(0.0807)(12)})}{(1)(0.3)(e^{-(0.0807)(12)})}$$

$$= \frac{(200\ \mu g/L)(229.5\ L)(1 - 0.38)}{(1)(0.3)(0.38)}$$

$$= 249.631\ \mu g\ \text{or} \approx 250\ mg\ q12h$$

Note that this dose adjustment to 250 mg q12h is double the original dose of 125 mg q2h and should result in a proportional change in the steady-state trough concentration. This method of using the desired change in the plasma concentration as the same ratio change for maintenance dose is useful as long as the dosing interval is not altered. Because the dosing interval remains the same, this is the most common method of adjusting the cyclosporine dose. *Most clinicians do not calculate the elimination rate constant or clearance values associated with steady-state cyclosporine trough concentrations. They simply make a proportional or clinically reasonable change and determine the steady-state concentrations of cyclosporine after making the dose change.* In this case, the steady-state cyclosporine (trough or C_2) concentration should be ordered 2 days after dose change, which corresponds to greater than five half-lives as determined for this patient.

Question #2 *E.R., a 48-year-old, 59-kg male patient, received a living-related renal transplant many years ago. He is currently receiving Neoral 300 mg PO as the solution BID and, in addition, prednisone 5 mg/d and mycophenolate mofetil 1,000 mg BID. E.R.'s current serum creatinine is 2.1 mg/dL, and his steady-state cyclosporine trough concentration is 590 μg/L. The physician has ruled out the possibility of rejection and believes that the recent rise in serum creatinine is because of cyclosporine toxicity. What questions would one ask E.R., and how would one adjust his cyclosporine regimen to achieve a new steady-state cyclosporine concentration of approximately 200 μg/L?*

First, confirm that E.R. has been taking his Neoral 300 mg BID as prescribed and determine whether any new medications have been added to his regimen or if he has consumed grapefruit or grapefruit juice. In addition, verify the time of sampling relative to when he took his last dose to ensure that the concentration is in fact a trough concentration. The pharmacist should also conduct a physical assessment to determine whether E.R. is experiencing any symptoms of cyclosporine-related adverse effects. If there are no easily correctable reasons for the elevated cyclosporine concentration, at least one cyclosporine dose should be held and then E.R. should be restarted on a new regimen. The dose decrease should approximate the proportionate decrease in cyclosporine concentration that is desired:

$$\text{Desired dose} = \frac{C_{ss\ desired}}{C_{ss\ current}} \times \text{Current dose} \qquad \text{(Eq. 13.7)}$$

Using the current steady-state cyclosporine concentration of 590 µg/L and the new target concentration of 200 µg/L, the new cyclosporine dose is approximately 100 mg.

$$\text{Desired dose} = \frac{200\ \mu g/L}{590\ \mu g/L} \times 300\ mg$$

$$= 0.339 \times 300\ mg$$

$$= 101.7\ mg\ or \approx 100\ mg$$

This new dose assumes that the bioavailability remains the same, that E.R.'s hepatic function remains the same, and that the drug will be administered at the same interval of 12 hours. It is unclear why E.R. requires a lower-than-average cyclosporine dose (200 mg/d or ≈3.4 mg/kg/d). He may be absorbing more than the typical population, his hepatic metabolism may be unusually low, or he may be affected by a combination of both factors. The steady-state (ie, >5 half-lives) trough cyclosporine concentration should be determined after the dose change to ensure that E.R.'s concentration is within the therapeutic target.

> **Question #3**   M.J., a new 78-kg liver transplant patient, is receiving 200 mg/d of cyclosporine as an intermittent IV infusion (the patient was intolerant to tacrolimus). Currently, his hepatic function tests appear to be stable, and for the past 3 days, he has been improving clinically with steady-state cyclosporine concentrations of approximately 220 µg/L. What would be an appropriate PO cyclosporine dose for M.J.? The hepatologist is also asking whether genotyping would help guide dosing for this patient. Which genes would you target, and why?

Because the usual bioavailability for cyclosporine is approximately 30%, most clinicians give a PO dose that is 3 times the parenteral dose. In this case, it would be approximately 600 mg/d, or 300 mg q12h. Some clinicians prefer dividing the dose to reduce the volume of cyclosporine liquid or the number of capsules per dose. Dividing the daily dose would maintain the same steady-state average concentration but increase the trough and decrease the peak concentrations. This is because when the same rate of drug administration is given as smaller doses more often, a continuous IV infusion model is more closely approximated, and the peak and trough concentrations are moving toward the steady-state average (see Interpretation of Plasma Drug Concentrations; Revising Pharmacokinetic Parameters; Clearance in Figure 2.11 of Chapter "Selecting the Appropriate Equation and Interpretation of Measured Drug Concentrations"). Again, pharmacokinetic calculations could have been performed; however, the outcome would have been essentially the same as adjusting the dose in proportion to the desired change in steady-state plasma concentration.

In this case, we have the additional factor of a change in route and, therefore, bioavailability to consider:

$$\text{New dose} = \frac{C_{ss\ desired}}{C_{ss\ current}} \times \frac{F_{current}}{F_{new\ dosage\ form}} \times \text{Current dose} \qquad \text{(Eq. 13.8)}$$

Assuming the reported cyclosporine concentration of 220 µg/L is acceptable, the new dose will be approximately 600 mg/d.

$$= \frac{220\ \mu g/L}{220\ \mu g/L} \times \frac{1.0}{0.3} \times 200\ mg$$

$$= 1 \times 3.33 \times 200\ mg$$

$$= 666\ mg \approx 600\ mg$$

If the dose is divided and given as 300 mg q12h, trough concentrations will be somewhat higher than those produced by single-daily doses. However, the bioavailability will probably be a more important influence on the trough cyclosporine concentration. The clinician should obtain a steady-state blood concentration in 2 to 3 days to confirm that switching the formulation has not affected the steady-state concentrations. Currently, there is insufficient evidence to support genotype-guided dosing of cyclosporine. Select polymorphisms (eg, CYP3A4*1B, CYP3A4*18B) may be of interest, but further systematic studies are needed to establish the utility of genotyping (see Pharmacogenomic Applications). Conventional TDM via blood concentration measurement is still the best means to achieve precision dosing of cyclosporine today.

Tacrolimus

Tacrolimus is a macrolide antibiotic with immunosuppressive effects. Whereas tacrolimus has a chemical structure similar to sirolimus, its mechanism of action is similar to that of cyclosporine. Tacrolimus, like cyclosporine, inhibits the activity of calcineurin, leading to a decrease in the production and release of IL-2. Tacrolimus is used as part of a combination immunosuppressive drug regimen to prevent allograft rejection.[8,9]

Tacrolimus is available as 0.5, 1, and 5 mg immediate-release capsules (Prograf and various generic brands); 0.5, 1, and 5 mg extended-release capsules (Astagraf XL or Advagraf); 0.75, 1, and 4 mg extended-release tablets (Envarsus); and a 5 mg/mL solution for IV administration.[8] The recommended initial PO dose of tacrolimus is approximately 0.2 mg/kg/d for the immediate-release formulations (in combination with other immunosuppressants) in kidney transplant recipients, 0.075 mg/kg/d immediate-release formulation in heart transplant recipients, and 0.1 to 0.15 mg/kg/d in liver transplant recipients.[8] Immediate-release formulations (rather than extended-release) are typically started in de novo transplant patients because of more flexibility in dose adjustment and are typically administered q12h. The IV formulation (0.01-0.05 mg/kg/d, based on the indication) is usually given as a continuous infusion.[8] IV tacrolimus is not commonly used because most patients can take tacrolimus PO immediately after transplant. Tacrolimus has a narrow therapeutic window and exhibits variability in its pharmacokinetic parameters.[38] Similar to cyclosporine and sirolimus, tacrolimus is a substrate for CYP3A4/5 and P-glycoprotein.[39] Table 13.2 lists commonly used drugs that can interact with tacrolimus. Similar to cyclosporine, TDM of tacrolimus is essential in optimizing immunosuppression and minimizing dose-related toxicity.[38]

KEY PARAMETERS: Tacrolimus[8,9]

Therapeutic concentration[a]	5-20 µg/L
F	~25% (range: 7%-32%, depending on the type of transplant)
V[b]	Range: 0.85-1.4 L/kg, in kidney and liver transplants
Cl[b]	Mean ~30 mL/min/kg
$t_{1/2}$[c]	Immediate release: 2-36 hr
	Extended release: 35-41 hr
fu (fraction unbound in plasma[d])	0.01

[a]Whole blood trough concentration. Target concentrations will vary with the organ(s) transplanted, transplant center–specific immunosuppression protocols, and the patient's clinical status.
[b]Based on blood concentrations.
[c]$t_{1/2}$ may be prolonged in individuals with liver dysfunction.
[d]Extensive partitioning into blood cells. Tacrolimus is bound mainly to albumin and α_1-acid glycoprotein.

THERAPEUTIC AND TOXIC CONCENTRATIONS (BLOOD)[19,38,39]

The therapeutic range of tacrolimus is approximately 5 to 20 µg/L (ng/mL), but the exact target is center specific. Subtherapeutic tacrolimus concentrations are associated with an increased risk for allograft rejection, and concentrations above the therapeutic range are associated with increased risk for toxic effects (eg, renal dysfunction, neurotoxicity, and hypertension).[40] Owing to the narrow therapeutic range and the wide interindividual variability in tacrolimus pharmacokinetics, patients may experience rejection and/or exhibit signs of toxicity, even within the therapeutic range. The target blood concentrations of tacrolimus will vary according to the organ(s) transplanted, time after transplant, transplant center–specific immunosuppression protocols, and the patient's clinical status.

ADVERSE EFFECTS[3,8,9]

Tacrolimus is associated with a wide range of adverse effects. The most common dose-related adverse effects include nephrotoxicity, post-transplant diabetes mellitus (dose dependency is still being investigated), neurotoxicity (headache, fine hand tremor, paresthesia, and seizure), hypertriglyceridemia, diarrhea, and hypertension. Other adverse effects include hyperkalemia, hypomagnesemia, nausea, diarrhea, myocardial hypertrophy, alopecia, opportunistic infections, and malignancies. The IV formulation contains castor oil, which, on very rare occasions, can cause anaphylactic reactions.

BIOAVAILABILITY (F)

The PO bioavailability of tacrolimus is relatively poor. The bioavailability ranges from 7% to 32%, suggesting large variability between patients.[8,39,41] The low bioavailability may be the result of extensive first-pass metabolism in the intestinal wall by CYP3A4/5 and the drug efflux pump, P-glycoprotein.[39,42,43] Tacrolimus is a lipophilic compound whose absorption may be affected by gut motility and significantly increased by diarrhea, the exact mechanisms to which remain unknown.[39] Food, especially those with high-fat content, can also decrease tacrolimus PO absorption.[8,44] To minimize the variability of absorption, tacrolimus should be taken consistently with or without food. Tacrolimus is rapidly absorbed, albeit with large intraindividual variability, with peak concentrations being reached in approximately 0.5 to 6 hours in most patients.[8,9,39]

VOLUME OF DISTRIBUTION (V)[39,41]

The volume of distribution of tacrolimus is greater than 20 L/kg when based on plasma concentration.[39,41] This indicates extensive distribution outside the plasma compartment. The blood-to-plasma ratio of 15 (range: 4-114) is consistent with extensive distribution into the blood component,[39] therefore warranting TDM to be conducted in the blood matrix. The volume of distribution is approximately 1 L/kg using blood concentrations.[39] The plasma protein binding of tacrolimus is approximately 99%.[39] Tacrolimus is bound mainly to albumin and α_1-acid glycoprotein.[39]

CLEARANCE (Cl)[39]

Tacrolimus undergoes extensive metabolism in the enterocytes and hepatocytes via CYP3A4/5 to several hydroxylated and demethylated metabolites. Several of the metabolites have immunosuppressive activity.[45] The presence of metabolites should be taken into consideration when using immune-based tacrolimus assays (not the standard of practice in major transplant centers today) that can potentially react with both the parent compound and its metabolites, falsely inflating the concentration of tacrolimus. The extensive distribution of tacrolimus into red blood cells limits its clearance from the blood, with systemic clearance values ranging from 7 to 103 mL/kg/min.[8] Clearance decreases as hepatic function progressively declines.[39] With respect to intrinsic clearance, numerous drugs have been reported to influence the metabolism and transport of tacrolimus via CYP3A4 or P-glycoprotein (Table 13.2).

HALF-LIFE ($t_{1/2}$)

The elimination half-life of tacrolimus is approximately 2 to 36 hours in transplant recipients. The half-life may be prolonged in subjects with impaired hepatic function.[8,9]

TIME TO SAMPLE

The measurement of AUC is the ideal, but not the practical, approach for the TDM of tacrolimus. Therefore, in the majority of transplant centers, tacrolimus blood concentrations are usually drawn just before the dose (trough) for clinical pharmacokinetic monitoring, with therapeutic targets varying by the time post-transplant, the type of graft, and center-specific clinical guidelines.[19,38] Given the elimination half-life of about 2 to 36 hours, it is reasonable to wait 2 to 3 days after initiating or altering therapy before checking tacrolimus blood concentrations to ensure steady-state conditions.[8,39] In addition to trough concentration monitoring, emerging data are available, suggesting the potential benefits of utilizing the trough concentration:AUC ratio or within-subject variability of the trough concentration for the purpose of TDM.[38] Moreover, instead of monitoring tacrolimus concentrations in blood, alternative matrices such as capillary dried blood spotting or intracellular concentrations have gained significant research interest.[38,46]

CLINICAL PHARMACOGENOMICS OF TACROLIMUS

If the patient's CYP3A5 genotype status is already known, it may be appropriate to adjust the starting dose of tacrolimus based on their phenotype.[47] For example, intermediate and extensive metabolizers of CYP3A5 (those who carry one and two fully functional alleles, respectively) can be advised to have their starting tacrolimus dose increased by 1.5 to 2 times (while not exceeding a dose of 0.3 mg/kg/d),[47] whereas those who carry two copies of the loss-of-function CYP3A4 allele (ie, poor metabolizers) can utilize the conventional starting dose per drug label.[47] It is worthwhile noting that a recent meta-analysis indicated that genotype-guided dosing of tacrolimus can improve therapeutic target concentration attainment but does not improve clinical outcomes, such as delayed graft function, acute graft rejection, or overall graft survival[48] (see Pharmacogenomic Applications).

> **Question #5**   *C.F. is a 55-year-old man who just received a liver transplant. His current immunosuppression regimen is IV methylprednisolone 160 mg/d and mycophenolate mofetil 1,000 mg PO BID. His weight is 80 kg, and his serum creatinine is 1.1 mg/dL. The liver donor had previously been determined to have the CYP3A5*1/*1 (extensive metabolizer) genotype. What dose (immediate-release vs extended-release) of tacrolimus would you recommend?*

The recommended starting dose for the immediate-release formulations is approximately 0.1 mg/kg/d given as 0.05 mg/kg q12h. Clinicians typically initiate tacrolimus therapy using the immediate-release formulation because it allows them more flexibility in dosing. Only in settings of noncompliance or greater-than-normal variabilities (as determined in tacrolimus TDM) would patients be switched to the extended-release (ie, once-daily) formulations.

$$\text{Daily dose} = 80 \text{ kg} \times 0.1 \text{ mg/kg/d} = 8 \text{ mg/d}$$

$$\text{Administered dose} = 4 \text{ mg PO q12h}$$

In the absence of genetic (ie, CYP3A5) information, many clinicians can elect to initiate therapy at lower doses and increase the dose over the next few days to determine whether the patient will tolerate tacrolimus. Typical starting doses range from 1 to 2 mg PO q12h and would be increased over the next few days to a target dose of 4 mg PO q12h if tolerated. Alternatively, some clinicians would just empirically start the patient at the target dose (ie, 4 mg PO q12h) and monitor concentrations after attaining steady state.

However, because prior genetic information is available for this patient, genomic-guided dosing should be considered following the Clinical Pharmacogenetics Implementation Consortium (CPIC) published clinical guideline (see Pharmacogenomic Applications). Because this patient now carries the donor liver with the CYP3A5*1/*1 genotype, he would be classified as an "extensive metabolizer" and should be started on a higher tacrolimus dose (ie, 1.5-2 times the labeled dose, which would be 6-8 mg PO q12h). Although pharmacogenomic-guided dosing has been proven to attain therapeutic tacrolimus concentrations more efficiently, these strategies have yet been associated with improved tacrolimus pharmacodynamics (ie, reduced toxicity and graft loss). As such, standard TDM is still required per routine practice in this setting.

It is necessary to wait approximately five half-lives to reach steady state after initiating or altering therapy. Given the elimination half-life of approximately 2 to 36 hours, it would be reasonable to wait 2 days before checking tacrolimus blood concentrations. Tacrolimus concentrations are usually drawn as trough concentrations (just before the dose).

Clinically, tacrolimus blood concentrations are monitored on a twice-weekly basis during the immediate post-transplant period. The frequency of tacrolimus concentration monitoring decreases over time as the patient's graft becomes more stable.

Question #6   *C.F. continues to improve clinically 4 days after the liver transplant. Owing to his CYP3A5 genotype (CYP3A5*1/*1), the team had started him on a higher tacrolimus dose of 6 mg PO BID (on day 1 post-transplant). Trough tacrolimus concentrations have been obtained serially daily in the morning (day 2: 8 µg/L; day 3: 10 µg/L; and day 4: 12 µg/L). The transplant physician would like the patient to have a higher therapeutic target of tacrolimus because of elevated risk of organ rejection in this immediate post-transplant period. The team would like you to adjust the tacrolimus dose to achieve a trough concentration of 18 µg/L. Show your approach.*

The pharmacokinetics of tacrolimus is highly variable within an individual patient and between patients. A linear proportionality between dose and exposure may be assumed for the purpose of dose adjustments. Assuming nothing else has changed (ie, renal function, hepatic function, and coadministered drugs) and doses have been administered on time (ie, based on the medication administration record), in this case, it is reasonable to increase the tacrolimus dose to 9 mg PO BID using Equation 13.7. After attaining a steady state (~5 half-lives, usually 2-3 days), one should verify the trough concentration to ensure that the desired target has been obtained.

$$\text{Desired dose} = \frac{C_{ss \text{ desired}}}{C_{ss \text{ current}}} \times \text{Current dose}$$

$$= \frac{18 \text{ μg/mL}}{12 \text{ μg/mL}} \times 12 \text{ mg/d}$$

$$= 18 \text{ mg/d or 9 mg q12h}$$

Question #7   *L.J. is a 45-year-old woman who had a liver transplant. She is receiving a stable regimen of tacrolimus 4 mg PO q12h and prednisone 5 mg PO daily. Two weeks ago, her tacrolimus concentration on this regimen was 12 μg/L. She was prescribed diltiazem XR 300 mg PO daily for hypertension 1 week ago and now presents with headaches and tremors. Her serum creatinine is 1.4 mg/dL (baseline 1.1 mg/dL), and her current tacrolimus concentration is 26 μg/L. How can you account for the elevated tacrolimus concentration? How would you manage her tacrolimus dose to achieve a tacrolimus concentration of 10 to 15 μg/L? What alternative antihypertensive agents would you recommend to minimize the interaction?*

L.J. is likely experiencing adverse effects as a result of elevated tacrolimus blood concentrations. Nephrotoxicity and neurotoxicity may be related to elevated tacrolimus concentrations. In assessing the elevated tacrolimus concentration, one should determine whether the tacrolimus blood concentration was drawn at the appropriate time relative to when the last dose was taken. Concentrations drawn too early or too late (ie, after dose given) may not represent trough concentrations. In addition, patient adherence should be assessed, and one should determine whether the patient is taking any additional medications or foods that may interact with tacrolimus or is having episodes of diarrhea which may also increase blood concentrations.

Tacrolimus is primarily metabolized by CYP3A4/5 in the liver and the gut, which accounts for significant first-pass metabolism. In addition to being a substrate for CYP3A4/5, tacrolimus is also a substrate for P-glycoprotein, the drug efflux pump in the gut. P-glycoprotein is a membrane-localized drug transporter found on the luminal face of enterocytes that pumps drug from the cells back into the lumen of the gut. Diltiazem is an inhibitor of both CYP3A4 and P-glycoprotein. The net effect is increased absorption (from decreased gut wall metabolism) with decreased drug efflux and decreased first-pass hepatic metabolism. L.J. can be managed by either discontinuing diltiazem and choosing another antihypertensive agent that does not inhibit CYP3A4 (eg, the use of dihydropyridine calcium channel blockers such as amlodipine that does not interact with CYP3A4 or P-glycoprotein enzymes) or decreasing the dose of tacrolimus. The pharmacokinetics of tacrolimus is highly variable within an individual patient and between patients. After attaining a steady state, it is reasonable to decrease the tacrolimus dose by one-half and to target a tacrolimus concentration range of 10 to 15 μg/L using Equation 13.7.

$$\text{Desired dose} = \frac{\text{Exposure desired}}{\text{Exposure current}} \times \text{Current dose}$$

$$= \left(\frac{12 \ \mu g/mL}{26 \ \mu g/mL} \right) 8 \ mg/d$$

$$= (0.461) \ 8 \ mg/d$$

$$= 3.7 \ mg/d \approx 4 \ mg/d$$

or

2 mg q12h

Question #8 *D.J. is a 55-year-old male who received a kidney transplant 3 months ago. He presents with a 2-day history of fever and cough. A chest radiograph reveals a cavitary lesion consistent with pulmonary aspergillosis. D.J. is started on antifungal therapy with IV micafungin. After 2 weeks of therapy, D.J. has responded well to IV micafungin and is to be transitioned to PO voriconazole. His immunosuppression regimen consists of tacrolimus 6 mg PO BID, prednisone 5 mg PO daily, and mycophenolic acid enteric-coated 720 mg PO BID. The most recent tacrolimus concentration was 8.5 µg/L. Are there any dosage modifications to D.J.'s immunosuppressive regimen that should be considered before starting voriconazole? How should tacrolimus concentrations be monitored?*

Voriconazole is a potent inhibitor of cytochrome CYP3A4/5 and P-glycoprotein. Concomitant administration of voriconazole can potentially increase the exposure (AUC_r) of tacrolimus by approximately 3-fold.[8] The clinician might consider to empirically decrease the dose of tacrolimus to approximately one-third of the original dose to prevent the development of potentially toxic blood concentrations. For D.J., the dose of tacrolimus can be empirically decreased to 2 mg PO BID when voriconazole is started. Tacrolimus concentrations should be monitored closely and appropriate dosage adjustments made to maintain tacrolimus within the desired therapeutic range, when both drugs have reached their respective steady states. The inhibitory effects of voriconazole will be fully apparent when it has reached steady state; thus, the timing of the tacrolimus concentration should correspond to this variable (ie, voriconazole's half-life) as well. More importantly, the patient's renal function should be monitored closely. The dose of mycophenolate and prednisone may not need to be adjusted in the setting of stable graft function.

Question #9 *L.A., a 62-kg liver transplant recipient, is receiving tacrolimus 4 mg PO BID, mycophenolate mofetil 1,000 mg PO BID, and prednisone 10 mg PO daily. Currently, his hepatic function tests appear to be stable, with a recent tacrolimus concentration of 11 µg/L. He underwent surgery for a small bowel obstruction and will not be able to take medications PO for a few days. What would be an appropriate IV tacrolimus dose for L.A.?*

Because the usual bioavailability of tacrolimus is approximately 25%, most clinicians give an IV dose of approximately one-fourth to one-third of the PO dose. In this case, it would be approximately 2 mg/d. Although pharmacokinetic calculations could have been performed, the outcome would be the same as adjusting the dose in proportion to the desired change in steady-state concentration. In this situation, we also have the additional factor of a change in route and, therefore, bioavailability to consider:

$$\text{New dose} = \frac{C_{ss\ desired}}{C_{ss\ current}} \times \frac{F_{current}}{F_{new\ dosage\ form}} \times \text{Current dose}$$

Assuming the reported tacrolimus concentration of 11 µg/L is reasonable, the IV dose will be 2 mg/d (0.032 mg/kg/d). This is consistent with an IV dosing of approximately 0.03 to 0.05 mg/kg/d for liver or kidney transplant recipients. The recommended IV dose for heart transplant recipients is 0.01 mg/kg/d.

$$= \frac{11\ \mu g/L}{11\ \mu g/L} \times \frac{0.25}{1.0} \times 8\ mg$$

$$= 1 \times 0.25 \times 8\ mg$$

$$= 2\ mg$$

IV tacrolimus is usually given as a continuous infusion, but intermittent (ie, 4 hours) infusion protocols are also available in some transplant centers. The method of administration is usually dictated by institutional guidelines. In general, IV tacrolimus is not given unless the patient cannot tolerate PO medications. Most patients are able to tolerate medications by the PO route following transplantation.

Question #10 *P.S. is a 57-year-old male who received a kidney transplant 3 years ago. He reports decreased urine output and gaining approximately 5 pounds over the past week. His creatinine is now 3.7 mg/dL (was 1.3 mg/dL 6 weeks ago). His immunosuppression regimen consists of tacrolimus 6 mg PO BID and prednisone 5 mg PO daily. Other medications include metoprolol 25 mg PO BID, dapsone 100 mg PO daily, glipizide 5 mg PO BID, and naproxen 500 mg PO BID as needed for knee pain (started about 2 weeks ago). How would you assess P.S.'s renal function?*

Allograft rejection of the kidney and calcineurin inhibitor (tacrolimus or cyclosporine) toxicity can have a similar presentation (decreased urine output and rising serum creatinine). A tacrolimus concentration should be obtained to determine whether it is within the therapeutic range. A kidney ultrasound and biopsy will aid in determining whether allograft rejection is a cause of P.S.'s renal failure. Compliance with P.S.'s medication regimen should be assessed. The current immunosuppression regimen should be reassessed (eg, the reason for not using an additional agent such as mycophenolate, azathioprine, or sirolimus should be clarified). In addition, P.S.'s medication list should be reviewed to determine whether any nephrotoxic drugs were recently started. Naproxen, like other NSAIDs, can potentiate the nephrotoxic effects of calcineurin inhibitors such as tacrolimus and should be substituted with a non-nephrotoxic analgesic such as acetaminophen.

> **Question #11** *P.S. states that he has been taking his immunosuppressive medications as ordered. A tacrolimus concentration of 10.3 µg/L and a clinical course consistent with NSAID-induced nephrotoxicity make acute rejection less likely. Despite stopping the naproxen, P.S.'s renal function continues to deteriorate. It is decided that hemodialysis will be performed. Does the dose of tacrolimus need to be adjusted for hemodialysis?*

Tacrolimus is a large lipophilic molecule with a molecular weight of 822 (g/mol), is highly protein bound (99%), and extensively partitions into whole blood. The large volume of distribution for tacrolimus suggests extravascular uptake. Tacrolimus is metabolized in the liver and gastrointestinal tract primarily by CYP3A4/5, with less than 1% of the administered dose excreted unchanged in the urine. Because tacrolimus is highly lipid soluble, almost completely metabolized, has a large volume of distribution, is extensively protein bound, and partitions into blood, it is not removed efficiently by hemodialysis or continuous hemofiltration.[49,50] A top-up dose of tacrolimus is also not recommended. Cyclosporine and sirolimus have similar physiochemical properties and, as such, are not removed by hemodialysis either. Even though tacrolimus does not accumulate in the setting of renal dysfunction nor is it removed by hemodialysis, many clinicians in this setting will target blood concentrations in the lower range in an effort to minimize any adverse effects on renal function.

Sirolimus

Sirolimus is a macrolide compound that has a chemical structure similar to tacrolimus. Although sirolimus and tacrolimus are structurally related, they have different mechanisms of action. Tacrolimus blocks the production of IL-2 by inhibiting calcineurin, whereas sirolimus prevents the IL-2–driven cell cycle progression.[10,11] Sirolimus is usually given, not as first-line therapy, in combination with a reduced dose of calcineurin inhibitor or a calcineurin inhibitor–free regimens (with mycophenolate and prednisone) to prevent graft rejection.[3,19,51] Sirolimus, rarely used in liver, lung, and cardiac transplants, is primarily used in kidney (or kidney-pancreas) transplant recipients who have developed severe toxicities to calcineurin inhibitors or acquired BK virus–associated nephropathy during calcineurin inhibitor therapy.[3,19] Sirolimus may have a specific place of therapy for patients with skin cancer or renal carcinoma due to its antiproliferative effects.[3,19]

Sirolimus, like cyclosporine and tacrolimus, has a narrow therapeutic window and exhibits variability in its pharmacokinetic parameters. Sirolimus is also a substrate for CYP3A4/5 and P-glycoprotein.[10] Many drugs are known to affect the intrinsic clearance and transport of sirolimus. Table 13.2 lists commonly used drugs that can interact with sirolimus.

Dosing depends on the immunologic risks of the patient: For subjects with low immunologic risk, a weight-based regimen is typically used where patients weighing less than 40 kg would receive a loading dose of 3 mg/m^2, then 1 mg/m^2 as maintenance; patients greater than 40 kg should receive a loading dose of 6 mg, followed by 2 mg/d of maintenance.[10] In subjects classified as high immunologic risk, the suggested loading and maintenance doses are 15 mg and 5 mg/d, respectively.[10,11]

Sirolimus is available as 0.5-, 1-, and 2-mg tablets (Rapamune and various generics) and PO solution (1 mg/mL).[10] The solution should be mixed with at least 60 to 120 mL (2-4 ounces) of water or orange juice in a glass or plastic container. Owing to limited information on the stability of the diluted solution, other diluent liquids should be avoided, and the solution should be consumed immediately after mixing. After drinking the mixture, the container should be rinsed with a similar volume of water or orange juice and the diluent consumed to maximize the delivery of the dose.[10,11,19]

THERAPEUTIC AND TOXIC CONCENTRATIONS (BLOOD)

The therapeutic range of sirolimus is 5 to 15 µg/L. Concentrations less than 5 µg/L are associated with an increased risk of rejection, and concentrations greater than 15 µg/L are associated with an increased risk of adverse effects. The target concentration will vary according to the organ(s) transplanted, concurrent immunosuppression (ie, lower target if given concurrently with calcineurin inhibitors and mycophenolate vs higher target if sirolimus is used alone), and transplant center-specific immunosuppression protocols.[19] Results from assays may differ depending on methodology. Chromatographic methods such as high-performance liquid chromatography (HPLC) with tandem MS detection (ie, the most common today) will be generate lower concentrations than immunoassay techniques for whole blood concentrations.[52] Adjustments for the target concentrations should be made based on the assay used.

ADVERSE EFFECTS

The most common adverse effects associated with sirolimus are dose-dependent hypertension, headache, acne, hypertriglyceridemia, hypercholesterolemia, constipation, anemia, thrombocytopenia, and leukopenia. Other adverse effects include hypokalemia, impaired wound healing (therefore sirolimus is never started in de novo patients right after the transplant surgery), formation of lymphoceles, rash, and increased risk of hepatic artery thrombosis in liver transplant recipients (therefore sirolimus is not the first-line agent). Although sirolimus has a chemical structure similar to tacrolimus, it is not associated with the nephrotoxic effects commonly seen with tacrolimus; however, proteinuria and delayed recovery of renal function have been reported.[10,11,19,53-55]

KEY PARAMETERS: Sirolimus[10,56]

Therapeutic concentration[a]	5-15 µg/L
F^b	
Liquid formulation	14%
Tablet formulation	18%
V^c	Mean 12 L/kg (4-20 L/kg)
Cl^d	208 ± 95 mL/kg/hr
$t_{1/2}^{e}$	Mean 62 hr (46-78 hr)
fu (fraction unbound in plasma[f])	0.02-0.08

[a]Trough blood concentration. Target concentrations may vary with the organ(s) transplanted, concurrent immunosuppression regimens, and transplant center–specific immunosuppression protocols.
[b]Liquid and tablet formulations are not considered bioequivalent.
[c]Volume of distribution and clearance are calculated as V/F and Cl/F, respectively. Therefore, true values are lower than those reported (see Sirolimus; Volume of Distribution and Clearance).
[d]Sirolimus is extensively metabolized in the liver and intestines and is a substrate of CYP3A4/5 and P-glycoprotein.
[e]Half-life can be drastically increased in extensive liver impairment.
[f]Primarily binds to serum albumin.

BIOAVAILABILITY (F)

Sirolimus is a lipophilic compound with relatively limited PO absorption. The systemic bioavailability of the liquid formulation is approximately 14%. When sirolimus is given with a high-fat meal, the AUC is increased by approximately up to 35% (but with a reduced C_{max}).[10] To minimize variability in absorption, sirolimus should be taken consistently with or without food. The bioavailability of the tablets is about 27% higher than the solution[10]; that is, the tablets are approximately 18% absorbed ($F \approx 0.18$). Whereas the tablets are not bioequivalent to the liquid formulation, the 2-mg dose may be considered clinically equivalent,[10,11] and TDM is recommended when switching between formulations.

VOLUME OF DISTRIBUTION (V)

The volume of distribution of sirolimus is approximately 12 L/kg.[10,11] This large volume of distribution was calculated from PO dosing. The reported value is V/F, indicating that the actual volume of distribution is in the range of one-tenth (assuming a PO bioavailability of 10%) to one-fifth (assuming a PO bioavailability of 20%) of the reported value. Sirolimus extensively distributes in tissues. The blood-to-plasma ratio of sirolimus is relatively high (~38 in kidney transplant patients), indicating that sirolimus partitions extensively into blood cells. Sirolimus in the plasma is also extensively protein bound (~92%) to albumin, α_1-acid glycoprotein, and lipoproteins.[10,56] Although sirolimus bioavailability is low, peak concentrations occur approximately 1 to 6 hours after a PO dose.[10]

CLEARANCE (Cl)

Sirolimus undergoes extensive liver and gut metabolism.[10,11] The apparent PO clearance of sirolimus is approximately 208 ± 95 mL/kg/hr.[56] Sirolimus, like cyclosporine and tacrolimus, is a substrate for CYP3A4/5 and P-glycoprotein. Drugs that inhibit CYP3A4/5, such as fluconazole, erythromycin, and diltiazem, can decrease the intrinsic clearance of sirolimus and result in increased blood concentrations. Similar to cyclosporine and tacrolimus, grapefruit and grapefruit juice can also inhibit CYP3A4 and P-glycoprotein and should be avoided. On the other hand, drugs that increase the intrinsic clearance (eg, rifampin) of sirolimus can result in decreased sirolimus concentrations (Table 13.2).[10,19]

HALF-LIFE ($t_{1/2}$)

The elimination half-life of sirolimus is approximately 62 hours and may be increased in subjects with severe hepatic dysfunction.[10,19,56]

TIME TO SAMPLE

Because sirolimus has a relatively long half-life (~62 hours), it is reasonable to wait at least 2 to 3 weeks (or five half-lives to achieve steady state) when obtaining a whole blood concentration after initiating or changing therapy. Trough concentrations are most commonly used when monitoring sirolimus drug concentrations.[10,11,19]

CLINICAL PHARMACOGENOMICS OF SIROLIMUS

Currently (June 2022), there are insufficient, inconsistent data to support a pharmacogenomics-guided dosing for sirolimus[29,57-60] (see Pharmacogenomic Applications).

Question #12 *A.B. just received a cadaveric renal transplant. It is determined that A.B. (60 kg) will receive an immunosuppression regimen that utilizes sirolimus, cyclosporine modified, and prednisone. What dose of sirolimus should A.B. receive, assuming A.B. is not considered at high immunologic risk based on pretransplant assessment? Is genetic-guided dosing of sirolimus warranted in this case?*

Because sirolimus has a relatively long half-life, a loading dose is commonly used to achieve therapeutic concentrations in a timely manner. The usual daily maintenance dose of sirolimus is 2 mg (although this depends on the nature of the transplant, eg, immunologic risk, and patient's weight). The loading dose is typically 3 times the maintenance dose; in this case, 6 mg. A.B. should receive 6 mg of sirolimus as a loading dose immediately and then begin a maintenance dose of 2 mg/d starting the next day. The current literature does not support pharmacogenomics-guided dosing of sirolimus. Conventional TDM (ie, trough sirolimus concentrations) is recommended.

Question #13 *A.B. is to begin an immunosuppression regimen consisting of cyclosporine modified 300 mg PO BID, sirolimus 2 mg PO daily, and prednisone taper. Does it matter when A.B. takes his sirolimus?*

Sirolimus is typically given in combination with other immunosuppressive drugs (eg, cyclosporine and prednisone). When sirolimus is administered simultaneously with cyclosporine-modified capsules, the C_{max} and AUC of sirolimus are increased.[10,11,19] It is recommended by the manufacturer to administer sirolimus 4 hours after cyclosporine is modified to minimize the interaction. To further mitigate this interaction, patients are advised to consistently take their medications at the same time of the day to minimize variations.[56,61]

Question #14   *A.B. is being given sirolimus in a liquid formulation during his hospital stay. He mixes his daily dose with orange juice but does not like the taste. Can A.B. be switched to the tablet formulation?*

Sirolimus is available in both liquid and tablet formulations. The liquid formulation must be mixed with water or orange juice and consumed immediately. Other liquids for dilution should not be used because of the lack of stability data and potential drug interactions (ie, grapefruit juice). The tablet formulation may be more convenient in an outpatient setting because it does not need to be refrigerated or diluted before administration. A.B. can be switched from the liquid to the tablet formulation at the same dose of 2 mg/d. However, doses other than 2 mg may not be considered interchangeable. TDM is recommended after the formulation has been changed.

Question #15   *C.G. was taking a stable regimen of cyclosporine modified 200 mg PO BID, sirolimus 2 mg PO daily, and prednisone 10 mg PO daily. Her steady-state cyclosporine concentration was 200 µg/L and steady-state sirolimus concentration was 9 µg/L on this regimen. C.G. was started on fluconazole 200 mg PO daily to treat a fungal infection. Two weeks later, her platelet count decreased from 200 to 75 K, and her white blood cells decreased from 7 to 2.5 K. Her latest cyclosporine blood concentration was 470 µg/L and sirolimus concentration was 22 µg/L. What could account for her thrombocytopenia and leukopenia and elevated cyclosporine and sirolimus concentrations? How would you manage this interaction?*

Patient adherence should always be assessed. The timing of the drug concentrations should be verified. In addition, it should be determined whether there have been any changes to C.G.'s medication regimens and how C.G. takes her sirolimus. It appears that C.G. was on a stable immunosuppression regimen, with therapeutic, steady-state cyclosporine and sirolimus blood concentrations. She was recently started on fluconazole, which is a known inhibitor of CYP3A4 and P-glycoprotein. Like cyclosporine, sirolimus is a substrate for both CYP3A4 and P-glycoprotein. Fluconazole can decrease the metabolism of sirolimus and cyclosporine and result in increased blood concentrations, and the elevated blood concentrations of sirolimus could account for her thrombocytopenia and leukopenia. Because C.G. is showing signs of toxicity (leukopenia, thrombocytopenia) from a supratherapeutic concentration of sirolimus, a lower dose of sirolimus would be warranted. Similar to the management of tacrolimus or cyclosporine, the blood concentration of sirolimus is dose proportional over a wide range. If her dose of sirolimus was lowered to 1 mg/d, her sirolimus concentration would be estimated to be approximately 11 µg/L. Given the long half-life of sirolimus, a repeat trough concentration is warranted in 2 to 3 weeks after dose adjustment, in addition to repeat complete blood count. Alternatively, she could be given another appropriate antifungal regimen that does not inhibit CYP3A4 (eg, micafungin) and be maintained on her current immunosuppression regimen. In this scenario, a steady-state trough concentration measurement (after 2-3 weeks of stopping fluconazole) is still warranted to ensure that the sirolimus concentration is within therapeutic targets.

Mycophenolate[12,13,62-66]

Mycophenolate suppresses the proliferation of B and T lymphocytes by inhibiting inosine monophosphate dehydrogenase.[12,13,62-66] It is primarily used in kidney, liver, heart, and lung transplantations, although off-label usage in other conditions, such as autoimmune hepatitis, lupus, and psoriasis, is also practiced.[12] Similar to the other immunosuppressants discussed in this chapter, mycophenolate is almost always used as part of a combined immunosuppressive regimen (eg, in conjunction with calcineurin inhibitors with or without corticosteroids). Mycophenolate can be administered as a prodrug (mycophenolate mofetil, CellCept, and generics) or as the sodium salt of mycophenolic acid (Myfortic or various generics). The prodrug formulation is inert but, once in the vasculature, undergoes rapid and complete activation (via hydrolysis) to form mycophenolic acid. On the other hand, the sodium formulation does not require bioactivation and is formulated only as a PO enteric-coated product for the purpose of minimizing gastrointestinal irritation.

Owing to the different pharmacokinetic characteristics, the PO dosage forms (CellCept and Myfortic, or various generics) are not considered interchangeable.[12,13,62-66] Mycophenolate mofetil is available as 250- or 500-mg capsules/tablets and a 200 mg/mL suspension. The enteric-coated mycophenolate sodium is available as 180- and 360-mg tablets. Mycophenolate mofetil for injection (as hydrochloride) is supplied as a 500 mg vial for reconstitution.[12] Similar to other discussed immunosuppressants, the IV formulation is only reserved for patients who cannot tolerate PO intake and should only be used intermittently. A loading dose of mycophenolate is usually not indicated, and the recommended initial doses in adults (PO or IV) are 1 g BID (kidney or liver transplant) or 1 to 1.5 g BID (heart transplant).[12] The enteric-coated sodium formulation is typically not the first-line formulation for newly transplanted patients, and the typical dosing is 720 mg BID (comparable, but not bioequivalent, to 1 g BID mycophenolate mofetil).[12,13] Dose adjustments of mycophenolate based on renal or hepatic function are usually not necessary unless renal function is significantly deteriorated (ie, glomerular filtration <25 mL/min/1.73 m^2 in which case a maximum daily dose of 2 g is suggested), but temporarily withholding the drug may be considered in patients developing severe neutropenia.[12,13] Similar to tacrolimus, mycophenolate is not likely removed by hemodialysis based on its physiochemical properties. Mycophenolate is primarily metabolized by UDP-glucuronosyltransferase (UGT) enzymes and transported by hepatic multidrug-resistant transporter 2 proteins (MRP2) and organic anion transporting peptides

(OATP)[62,64]; thus, molecular drug interactions with xenobiotics that affect these metabolic and transport pathways may be possible. Although mycophenolate exhibits wide intraindividual and interindividual variability in its pharmacokinetic parameters, TDM is not commonly practiced and remains a topic of debate.[64,67]

KEY PARAMETERS: Mycophenolate[12,13,62-66]

Therapeutic concentration[a]	30-60 mg·hr/L based on plasma exposure values. Various LSSs for estimating AUC have been proposed.[64,68]
F	70%-90% (depending on the formulation and time post-transplant)
V	Average 3.6 L/kg (mofetil), 54-112 L (enteric-coated sodium)
Cl	Highly variable based on specific transplant population[64,66,69-71]
$t_{1/2}$[b]	8-18 hr
fu (fraction unbound in plasma, binding primarily to albumin)	0.01-0.03

[a]Target exposure ranges may vary with the organ(s) transplanted and transplant center–specific immunosuppression protocols.
[b]Large variability is potentially secondary to the propensity for mycophenolate to undergo enterohepatic recirculation. The half-life is also dependent on the formulation.

THERAPEUTIC AND TOXIC CONCENTRATIONS

The therapeutic exposure range (30-60 mg·hr/L) of mycophenolate has only been established in adult kidney transplant patients but is widely applied to other indications.[64,67] However, routine TDM of mycophenolate in solid organ transplant patients remains controversial.[64,67] Currently, most of the data favor the use of mycophenolate AUC (estimated by LSSs) over trough concentration data for mycophenolate TDM, because the latter does not correlate well with drug exposure in a variety of transplant types.[64,67] Although various LSSs have been proposed to estimate mycophenolate exposure in solid organ transplant patients (the majority of the data have been reported in kidney transplants), these predictive equations should be used only in similar patient populations for which the equations were originally developed/validated.[64,68] In contrast to cyclosporine, tacrolimus, and sirolimus, routine mycophenolate TDM is usually not instituted in most transplant centers. However, LSS-estimated mycophenolate exposure may be used in select kidney transplant recipients with unexplained organ rejection or adverse drug effect to guide dose adjustments to tailor to the empiric therapeutic target (30-60 mg·hr/L).

ADVERSE EFFECTS

Mycophenolate is associated with a wide range of adverse effects.[12,13,19,65] The most common dose-related effects are gastrointestinal pain, nausea, vomiting, diarrhea, abnormal liver function tests, and elevated serum creatinine. Less frequently, neutropenia, which is more likely to occur within the first 18 months after engraftment, can be associated with mycophenolate use.[65] The gastrointestinal side effects may be alleviated by administering with food, dividing the total daily dose into more frequent intervals, or administering a proton-pump inhibitor. Alternatively, patients who do not tolerate mycophenolate mofetil may be switched to the enteric-coated formulation. With respect to neutropenia, frequent monitoring (complete blood count and absolute neutrophil count) during the first post-transplant year after initiation of mycophenolate should be instituted. In the event of suspected mycophenolate-induced neutropenia, the dose of mycophenolate may require reduction until other causes of neutropenia (eg, cytomegalovirus infection, other drugs such as cotrimoxazole or valganciclovir) can be ruled out.[12]

BIOAVAILABILITY (F)

The PO bioavailability of mycophenolate, which is dependent on formulation and time post-transplant, is relatively high compared to that of cyclosporine and tacrolimus.[12,13] Mycophenolate mofetil reaches t_{max} at approximately 1 to 1.8 hours, relatively faster than the enteric-coated formulation (t_{max}, 1.5-2.5 hours), when compared at steady-state conditions.[12] The bioavailability of mycophenolate mofetil is also higher (ie, >90%) than the enteric-coated formulation (~70%), and the prodrug (mofetil salt) requires bioactivation in the vasculature in a reaction that is rapid and complete.[12,62,70] Because the overall exposure of mycophenolate can increase in relation to post-transplant time,[69] dose reduction may be needed to attain the same exposure. The presence of food does not affect the overall exposure of mycophenolate but has been documented to decrease the maximum concentration by up to 40%.[12] To minimize the variability in absorption, mycophenolate (both formulations) should be taken consistently with or without food. In the presence of gastrointestinal upset, clinicians usually recommend ingesting mycophenolate with small amounts of food.

VOLUME OF DISTRIBUTION (V)[12,63,64,66,69]

The volume of distribution of mycophenolate (3.6-4 L/kg for mycophenolate mofetil and 54-112 L for enteric-coated mycophenolate sodium) depends on the formulation.[12] Mycophenolate is primarily distributed in plasma and extensively bound to albumin. The free fraction of mycophenolate is approximately 1% to 3% under normal conditions.

CLEARANCE (Cl)

Mycophenolate mofetil is an inactive prodrug that requires bioactivation (by hydrolysis) to generate the active mycophenolic acid.[12,63,64,69] Mycophenolate is extensively metabolized in the liver by UGT enzymes, primarily UGT1A9 and UGT2B7, in the formation of inactive and active glucuronide metabolites, respectively.[12,63,64,69] The inactive glucuronide constitutes the major, whereas the acyl-glucuronide is the minor metabolite. Both glucuronide metabolites undergo enterohepatic recirculation in a reaction catalyzed by MRP2 and OATP transporters. The enterohepatic recirculation results in the formation of secondary "peaks" observed in the blood concentration-time curves of mycophenolate.[62,64,69] The clearance of mycophenolate is highly variable and can be affected by various patient factors.[66,69,71] Because mycophenolate is a substrate of various phase II enzymes and transporters, its clearance can be altered by drug interactions mediated by modulators of these enzyme and transporter systems. However, in contrast to cyclosporine, tacrolimus, and sirolimus (where the enzymes and transporters of interest are CYP3A4/5 and P-glycoprotein), less data are available documenting the effects of UGT or MRP2/OATP interaction on the clinical pharmacokinetics of mycophenolate.[69]

HALF-LIFE ($t_{1/2}$)

The elimination half-life of mycophenolate is approximately 8 to 18 hours.[12] As indicated in Clearance section, the half-life of mycophenolate may be prolonged if it is administered with an inhibitor (of UGT enzymes or MRP2/OATP transporters) and vice versa for a coadministered inducer.

TIME TO SAMPLE

The utility of TDM for mycophenolate is still subject to debate.[64,67] With respect to the method of monitoring, the majority of the literature favors the use of mycophenolate AUC, estimated with LSSs (usually three to four sampling points in the initial 4-6 hours period after dose), over trough concentration data. This is because poor correlations between trough concentration and mycophenolate exposure have been documented in most transplant populations.[64,67] Various LSSs have been proposed to estimate mycophenolate exposure in solid organ transplant patients, and the majority of the data have been reported in kidney transplant recipients.[64,68] Population pharmacokinetic-based algorithms (ie, Bayesian approaches) are also available, but these methods usually require more sophisticated software programs that may not be practical in the clinical setting.[64,66] The LSS-associated equations should be used only *in similar patient populations for which the equations were originally developed/validated*; therefore, equations developed for mycophenolate mofetil cannot be used for the enteric-coated formulation (and vice versa).

CLINICAL PHARMACOGENOMICS OF MYCOPHENOLATE

Currently (June 2022), there are insufficient data to support a pharmacogenomics-guided dosing for mycophenolate[67] (see Pharmacogenomic Applications).

Question #16 *C.J. (50 years old, 70 kg) just received a cadaveric kidney transplant (panel reactive antibody 5%), and the transplant team wants to start her on mycophenolate, tacrolimus, and valganciclovir (cytomegalovirus mismatch). She was not prescribed a regular maintenance steroids regimen because of the low immunologic risk. She has a history of hypertension and takes amlodipine 5 mg PO daily.*

All of her blood work is within normal limits. Her current GFR is 15 mL/min. The site protocol also starts the patient on cotrimoxazole 3 times weekly as antibacterial prophylaxis and pantoprazole 40 mg PO daily as gastrointestinal prophylaxis. On what dose of mycophenolate would you start C.J.? Is genetic testing/dosing warranted in this setting?

A loading dose of mycophenolate is typically not administered. Because C.J. is able to tolerate PO intake of medications, the conventional starting dose (not based on weight) for C.J. would be mycophenolate mofetil 1 g PO BID. Currently, there is insufficient evidence to recommend routine TDM of mycophenolate, unless there are specific reasons that the team suspects which can alter the pharmacokinetics of mycophenolate (eg, decreased absorption or altered elimination) or there are occurrences of unexplained organ rejection/adverse events. If TDM is warranted, an LSS-based predictive equation to estimate the exposure of mycophenolate can be used. Trough concentrations are usually not the reliable surrogate markers for exposure. Likewise, currently, there is insufficient evidence to support pharmacogenomics-guided dosing of mycophenolate.

Question #17   *It has been 1 month post-transplant and C.J.'s renal function has deteriorated to approximately 10 mL/min. Her serum creatinine has been trending up slightly over 2 weeks. Her current immunosuppressants are mycophenolate mofetil 1 g PO BID and tacrolimus 2.5 mg PO BID (trough concentration within target). Her blood pressure is adequately controlled on amlodipine. She is seronegative with respect to cytomegalovirus and BK virus. Her clinical blood work is within normal limits. She has not experienced any adverse effects from drugs. The team suspects acute graft rejection and has ordered a renal ultrasound to be followed by renal biopsy. Is it appropriate to monitor mycophenolate exposure in this setting? How would you adjust the dose?*

It may be appropriate to monitor mycophenolate exposure in the setting where no other causes can explain the patient's acute rejection episode. The best approach to determine mycophenolate exposure is to estimate AUC using LSS equations.[64] However, the LSS-associated equations should be used only in similar patient populations for which the equations were originally developed/validated.[64] A suitable LSS equation available in the literature describing the use of mycophenolate in a similar population (coadministered with tacrolimus in the absence of steroids) uses three sampling time points[72]:

$$\text{Mycophenolate exposure} = 9.328 + 1.311(C_{1hr}) + 1.455(C_{2hr}) + 2.901(C_{4hr}) \quad \textbf{(Eq. 13.9)}$$

In order to use this equation to estimate C.J.'s mycophenolate exposure, serum mycophenolate concentrations would have to be obtained relatively precisely at 1, 2, and 4 hours after the ingestion of dose.

Question #18   *The laboratory reports the following mycophenolate concentrations: timing of dose (9 A.M.), 4 mg/L (1 hour postdose), 1.5 mg/L (2 hours postdose), and 1 mg/L (4 hours postdose). Calculate C.J.'s mycophenolate exposure based on this information.*

Mycophenolate exposure = 9.328 + 1.311 (4 mg/L) + 1.455 (1.5 mg/L) + 2.901 (1 mg/L)

$$= {\sim}20\ mg{\cdot}hr/L$$

Because the therapeutic target of mycophenolate AUC in kidney transplant is usually 30 to 60 mg·hr/L, one can adjust the mycophenolate dose using Equation 13.7, assuming there is a proportional dose-exposure relationship:

$$\text{Desired dose} = \frac{\text{Exposure desired}}{\text{Exposure current}} \times \text{Current dose}$$

$$= \frac{30\ mg{\cdot}hr/L}{20\ mg{\cdot}hr/L} \times 2\ g/d$$

$$= 3\ g/d\ \text{or}\ 1.5\ g\ q12h$$

Question #19   *C.J.'s kidney rejection episode was reversed with steroid pulse, and her renal function has gradually normalized (GFR of 50 mL/min) at 2 months post-transplant. Her current immunosuppressants are mycophenolate mofetil 1.5 g PO BID and tacrolimus 3 mg PO BID (trough concentrations within target). Her blood pressure is adequately controlled (130/80 mm Hg) on amlodipine 10 mg PO daily. She is still on valganciclovir 900 mg PO daily and cotrimoxazole DS tablet 3 times weekly. Her clinic blood work is within normal limits, but she complains of stomach cramps and occasional diarrhea for the past 1 month (timing associated with increase in mycophenolate dose), which became more intensified/intolerable in the past week. The symptoms are more intense after the ingestion of her BID medication regimens. How would you manage this complaint?*

A thorough history of C.J.'s stomach ailments should be taken. If other differential causes (eg, gastric ulceration, infection) are ruled out by the transplant team, then a drug-associated adverse effect should be considered. Although all of her current medications can potentially cause these symptoms, stomach cramp and diarrhea are often associated with mycophenolate mofetil. The timing of gastrointestinal upset also corresponds with the increase in mycophenolate dose. She can be tried off mycophenolate mofetil and started on enteric-coated mycophenolate sodium, which has been shown to have reduced gastrointestinal adverse effects. Because the two PO formulations are not bioequivalent, the *closest comparable dose* is 1,080 mg PO BID.

Question #20 *A year after C.J.'s transplant, her renal function has remained stable (GFR of 60 mL/min). Her current immunosuppression regimen includes enteric-coated mycophenolate sodium 1,080 mg PO BID, tacrolimus 3.5 mg PO BID (trough concentrations within target), and prednisone 5 mg PO BID. Her cotrimoxazole had been taken off 2 weeks ago because of a significant drop in white blood cell count. Her valganciclovir was stopped 3 months ago because of several, consecutive seronegative cytomegalovirus readings in the blood. Her blood pressure is well controlled with amlodipine. Her current clinic blood work still reveals a depressed white blood cell and neutrophil count. She is afebrile and otherwise asymptomatic. Virology indicates no detectable amounts of BK or cytomegalovirus in the blood. How would you advise the team?*

Neutropenia commonly occurs within the first 1.5 years post-transplant and may be because of a host of reasons. In the setting where the differential causes have been ruled out (eg, virus-associated neutropenia), drug causes should be considered. Because the team had already stopped cotrimoxazole (the first agent likely to be discontinued in the setting of neutropenia), the possibility of over immunosuppression from her other drugs should be considered. In this scenario, the next mostly likely target for drug-induced neutropenia would be mycophenolate, because mycophenolate exposure values are known to increase over post-transplant time. The patient's mycophenolate dose can be dropped by 25% to 50%. An LSS-guided TDM (using an equation developed with the enteric-coated formulation) can be considered in this scenario. The patient's clinical status (eg, complete white blood cell count and renal function) should be monitored closely.

Pharmacogenomic Applications

Cyclosporine, tacrolimus, and sirolimus are primarily metabolized by hepatic/gut CYP3A4/5 and also act as substrates for the P-glycoprotein efflux pumps. Mycophenolate is a substrate of UGT enzymes and MRP2/OATP transporters. Genetic polymorphisms of these enzymes and transporters that result in functional phenotypic alterations can theoretically affect the clearance of these agents. However, currently (as of June 2022), clinical guidelines from the CPIC, which provides peer-reviewed practice recommendations (https://www.pharmgkb.org/page/cpic), are not available for cyclosporine, sirolimus, and mycophenolate. Overall, the absence of clear links between known genetic polymorphisms and clinical outcomes means that genomic-guided dosing for these agents cannot yet be recommended.

On the other hand, a CPIC guideline is available for tacrolimus in the context of CYP3A5 polymorphism.[47] Specifically, patients carrying the CYP3A5*3/*6/*7 alleles (the most common mutations for this gene) exhibit reduced catalytic activity toward tacrolimus compared to the wild type (CYP3A5*1). It has been recommended that three different phenotypic categories can be assigned to subjects based on their genotype: Wild-type homozygous individuals would be classified as "extensive metabolizer," those carrying a wild-type and a mutant allele classified as "intermediate metabolizer," and patients with two mutant alleles classified as "poor metabolizer."[47] A higher tacrolimus dose is recommended (ie, 1.5-2 times the labeled dose) for both extensive and intermediate metabolizers, whereas the original labeled doses are suggested for the poor metabolizers. Although this approach has proven to attain therapeutic tacrolimus concentrations more efficiently, these pharmacogenomic dosing strategies have yet been associated with improved tacrolimus pharmacodynamics (ie, reduced toxicity and graft loss), as evident by the findings of a recent meta-analysis.[48] The most current CPIC guidelines do not recommend the routine testing of CYP3A5 for individuals being prescribed tacrolimus, and standard TDM is still recommended, irrespective of the availability of the CYP3A5 genomic data. However, if CYP3A5 genetic information are already available, then clinicians can provide tacrolimus dose adjustments according to the guidelines, in conjunction with TDM.[47]

ACKNOWLEDGMENT

The important work of David J. Quan on a previous version of this chapter is acknowledged. The current chapter is an update and revision of the previous versions.

REFERENCES

1. Product Monograph. Neoral and Sandimmune IV [Product Monograph]. 2020 [updated January 9, 2015 (Novartis Version: July 14, 2020)]. https://www.novartis.ca/sites/www.novartis.ca/files/neoral_patient_e.pdf

2. Lexicomp Clinical Drug Information. *Cyclosporine (Systemic) [Internet]*. Wolters Kluwer; 2022. Accessed June 9, 2022. https://online.lexi.com/lco/action/login

3. Jennings DLJ, Solid HJ. Solid organ transplantation. In: Dipiro JT, Yee GC, Posey LM, Haines ST, Nolin TD, Ellingrod VL, eds. *Pharmacotherapy: A Pathophysiologic Approach*. 11th ed. McGraw Hill; 2020:1-53.

4. Krensky AM, Azzi JR, Hafler DA. Immunosuppressants and tolerogens. In: Brunton LL, Hilal-Dandan R, Knollmann BC, eds. *Goodman & Gilman's: The Pharmacological Basis of Therapeutics*. 13th ed. McGraw Hill; 2017:e1-33.

5. Ekberg H, Tedesco-Silva H, Demirbas A, et al; ELITE-Symphony Study. Reduced exposure to calcineurin inhibitors in renal transplantation. *N Engl J Med*. 2007;357(25):2562-2575.

6. AHFS Drug Information. *CycloSPORINE (Adult and Pediatric) [Internet]*. American Society of Health-System Pharmacists; 2022. Accessed June 9, 2022. https://online.lexi.com/lco/action/login

7. Wahlberg J, Wilczek HE, Fauchald P, et al. Consistent absorption of cyclosporine from a microemulsion formulation assessed in stable renal transplant recipients over a one-year study period. *Transplantation*. 1995;60(7):648-652.

8. Lexicomp Clinical Drug Information. *Tacrolimus (Systemic) [Internet]*; 2022. Accessed June 9, 2022. https://online.lexi.com/lco/action/login

9. AHFS Drug Information. *Tacrolimus (Adult and Pediatric) [Internet]*. American Society of Health-System Pharmacists; 2022. Accessed June 9, 2022. https://online.lexi.com/lco/action/login

10. Lexicomp Clinical Drug Information. *Sirolimus (Conventional) [Internet]*; 2022. Accessed June 9, 2022. https://online.lexi.com/lco/action/login

11. AHFS Drug Information. *Sirolimus (Adult and Pediatric) [Internet]*. American Society of Health-System Pharmacists; 2022. Accessed June 9, 2022. https://online.lexi.com/lco/action/login

12. Lexicomp Clinical Drug Information. *Mycophenolate [Internet]*. 2022. Accessed June 9, 2022. Available from: https://online.lexi.com/lco/action/login

13. AHFS Drug Information. *Mycophenolate (Adult and Pediatric) [Internet]*. American Society of Health-System Pharmacists; 2022. Accessed June 9, 2022. https://online.lexi.com/lco/action/login

14. D'Alessandro C, Benedetti A, Di Paolo A, Giannese D, Cupisti A. Interactions between food and drugs, and nutritional status in renal patients: a narrative review. *Nutrients*. 2022;14(1);212.

15. Bailey DG, Malcolm J, Arnold O, Spence JD. Grapefruit juice-drug interactions. *Br J Clin Pharmacol*. 1998;46(2):101-110.

16. Yee GC, Stanley DL, Pessa LJ, et al. Effect of grapefruit juice on blood cyclosporin concentration. *Lancet*. 1995;345(8955):955-956.

17. Oellerich M, Armstrong VW, Kahan B, et al. Lake Louise Consensus Conference on cyclosporin monitoring in organ transplantation: report of the consensus panel. *Ther Drug Monit*. 1995;17(6):642-654.

18. Johnston A, Holt DW. Therapeutic drug monitoring of immunosuppressant drugs. *Br J Clin Pharmacol*. 1999;47(4):339-350.

19. BC Transplant. *Medication Guidelines for Solid Organ Transplants*; 2021 June 9. 2022:1-119. http://www.transplant.bc.ca/Documents/Health%20Professionals/Clinical%20guidelines/Clinical%20Guidelines%20for%20Transplant%20Medications.pdf

20. Kahan BD, Welsh M, Schoenberg L, et al. Variable oral absorption of cyclosporine. A biopharmaceutical risk factor for chronic renal allograft rejection. *Transplantation*. 1996;62(5):599-606.

21. Lindholm A, Kahan BD. Influence of cyclosporine pharmacokinetics, trough concentrations, and AUC monitoring on outcome after kidney transplantation. *Clin Pharmacol Ther*. 1993;54(2):205-218.

22. Atkinson K, Biggs JC, Britton K, et al. Oral administration of cyclosporin A for recipients of allogeneic marrow transplants: implications of clinical gut dysfunction. *Br J Haematol*. 1984;56(2):223-231.

23. Lindholm A, Henricsson S, Lind M, Dahlqvist R. Intraindividual variability in the relative systemic availability of cyclosporin after oral dosing. *Eur J Clin Pharmacol*. 1988;34(5):461-464.

24. Gupta SK, Bakran A, Johnson RW, Rowland M. Pharmacokinetics of cyclosporin: influence of rate-duration profile of an intravenous infusion in renal transplant patients. *Br J Clin Pharmacol*. 1989;27(3):353-357.

25. Ptachcinski RJ, Venkataramanan R, Rosenthal JT, Burckart GJ, Taylor RJ, Hakala TR. Cyclosporine kinetics in renal transplantation. *Clin Pharmacol Ther*. 1985;38(3):296-300.

26. Nashan B, Cole E, Levy G, Thervet E. Clinical validation studies of Neoral C(2) monitoring: a review. *Transplantation*. 2002;73(9 suppl):S3-S11.

27. Koristkova B, Grundmann M, Brozmanova H, Perinova I, Safarcik K. Validation of sparse sampling strategies to estimate cyclosporine A area under the concentration-time curve using either a specific radioimmunoassay or high-performance liquid chromatography method. *Ther Drug Monit*. 2010;32(5):586-593.

28. Rousseau A, Leger F, Le Meur Y, et al. Population pharmacokinetic modeling of oral cyclosporin using NONMEM: comparison of absorption pharmacokinetic models and design of a Bayesian estimator. *Ther Drug Monit*. 2004;26(1):23-30.

29. Rodriguez-Antona C, Savieo JL, Lauschke VM, et al. PharmVar GeneFocus: CYP3A5. *Clin Pharmacol Ther*. 2022;112(6):1159-1171.

30. Hesselink DA, van Schaik RH, van der Heiden IP, et al. Genetic polymorphisms of the CYP3A4, CYP3A5, and MDR-1 genes and pharmacokinetics of the calcineurin inhibitors cyclosporine and tacrolimus. *Clin Pharmacol Ther*. 2003;74(3):245-254.

31. Bouamar R, Hesselink DA, van Schaik RH, et al. Polymorphisms in CYP3A5, CYP3A4, and ABCB1 are not associated with cyclosporine pharmacokinetics nor with cyclosporine clinical end points after renal transplantation. *Ther Drug Monit*. 2011;33(2):178-184.

32. von Ahsen N, Richter M, Grupp C, Ringe B, Oellerich M, Armstrong VW. No influence of the MDR-1 C3435T polymorphism or a CYP3A4 promoter polymorphism (CYP3A4-V allele) on dose-adjusted cyclosporin A trough concentrations or rejection incidence in stable renal transplant recipients. *Clin Chem*. 2001;47(6):1048-1052.

33. Hesselink DA, van Gelder T, van Schaik RH, et al. Population pharmacokinetics of cyclosporine in kidney and heart transplant recipients and the influence of ethnicity and genetic polymorphisms in the MDR-1, CYP3A4, and CYP3A5 genes. *Clin Pharmacol Ther*. 2004;76(6):545-556.

34. Qiu XY, Jiao Z, Zhang M, et al. Association of MDR1, CYP3A4*18B, and CYP3A5*3 polymorphisms with cyclosporine pharmacokinetics in Chinese renal transplant recipients. *Eur J Clin Pharmacol*. 2008;64(11):1069-1084.

35. Zhao Y, Song M, Guan D, et al. Genetic polymorphisms of CYP3A5 genes and concentration of the cyclosporine and tacrolimus. *Transplant Proc.* 2005;37(1):178-181.

36. Chu XM, Hao HP, Wang GJ, Guo LQ, Min PQ. Influence of CYP3A5 genetic polymorphism on cyclosporine A metabolism and elimination in Chinese renal transplant recipients. *Acta Pharmacol Sin.* 2006;27(11):1504-1508.

37. Staatz CE, Goodman LK, Tett SE. Effect of CYP3A and ABCB1 single nucleotide polymorphisms on the pharmacokinetics and pharmacodynamics of calcineurin inhibitors: part I. *Clin Pharmacokinet.* 2010;49(3):141-175.

38. Brunet M, van Gelder T, Asberg A, et al. Therapeutic drug monitoring of tacrolimus-personalized therapy: second consensus report. *Ther Drug Monit.* 2019;41(3):261-307.

39. Staatz CE, Tett SE. Clinical pharmacokinetics and pharmacodynamics of tacrolimus in solid organ transplantation. *Clin Pharmacokinet.* 2004;43(10):623-653.

40. Kershner RP, Fitzsimmons WE. Relationship of FK506 whole blood concentrations and efficacy and toxicity after liver and kidney transplantation. *Transplantation.* 1996;62(7):920-926.

41. Venkataramanan R, Swaminathan A, Prasad T, et al. Clinical pharmacokinetics of tacrolimus. *Clin Pharmacokinet.* 1995;29(6):404-430.

42. Tuteja S, Alloway RR, Johnson JA, Gaber AO. The effect of gut metabolism on tacrolimus bioavailability in renal transplant recipients. *Transplantation.* 2001;71(9):1303-1307.

43. Mancinelli LM, Frassetto L, Floren LC, et al. The pharmacokinetics and metabolic disposition of tacrolimus: a comparison across ethnic groups. *Clin Pharmacol Ther.* 2001;69(1):24-31.

44. Kimikawa M, Kamoya K, Toma H, Teraoka S. Effective oral administration of tacrolimus in renal transplant recipients. *Clin Transplant.* 2001;15(5):324-329.

45. Plosker GL, Foster RH. Tacrolimus: a further update of its pharmacology and therapeutic use in the management of organ transplantation. *Drugs.* 2000;59(2):323-389.

46. Gallant J, Wichart J, Kiang TKL. Predictability of capillary blood spot toward venous whole blood sampling for therapeutic drug monitoring of tacrolimus in solid organ transplant recipients. *Eur J Drug Metab Pharmacokinet.* 2019;44(6):729-741.

47. Birdwell KA, Decker B, Barbarino JM, et al. Clinical Pharmacogenetics Implementation Consortium (CPIC) guidelines for CYP3A5 genotype and tacrolimus dosing. *Clin Pharmacol Ther.* 2015;98(1):19-24.

48. Yang H, Sun Y, Yu X, et al. Clinical impact of the adaptation of initial tacrolimus dosing to the CYP3A5 genotype after kidney transplantation: systematic review and meta-analysis of randomized controlled trials. *Clin Pharmacokinet.* 2021;60(7):877-885.

49. Venkataramanan R, Jain A, Cadoff E, et al. Pharmacokinetics of FK 506: preclinical and clinical studies. *Transplant Proc.* 1990;22(1):52-56.

50. Kishino S, Takekuma Y, Sugawara M, et al. Influence of continuous venovenous haemodiafiltration on the pharmacokinetics of tacrolimus in liver transplant recipients with small-for-size grafts. *Clin Transplant.* 2003;17(5):412-416.

51. Tedesco-Silva H, Del Carmen Rial M, Cruz Santiago J, Mazzali M, Pacheco-Silva A, Torres R. Optimizing the clinical utility of sirolimus-based immunosuppression for kidney transplantation. *Clin Transplant.* 2019;33(2):e13464.

52. Shaw LM, Kaplan B, Brayman KL. Advances in therapeutic drug monitoring for immunosuppressants: a review of sirolimus. Introduction and overview. *Clin Ther.* 2000;22(suppl B):B1-13.

53. Kahan BD, Napoli KL, Kelly PA, et al. Therapeutic drug monitoring of sirolimus: correlations with efficacy and toxicity. *Clin Transplant.* 2000;14(2):97-109.

54. McTaggart RA, Gottlieb D, Brooks J, et al. Sirolimus prolongs recovery from delayed graft function after cadaveric renal transplantation. *Am J Transplant.* 2003;3(4):416-423.

55. van den Akker JM, Wetzels JF, Hoitsma AJ. Proteinuria following conversion from azathioprine to sirolimus in renal transplant recipients. *Kidney Int.* 2006;70(7):1355-1357.

56. Zimmerman JJ, Kahan BD. Pharmacokinetics of sirolimus in stable renal transplant patients after multiple oral dose administration. *J Clin Pharmacol.* 1997;37(5):405-415.

57. Le Meur Y, Djebli N, Szelag JC, et al. CYP3A5*3 influences sirolimus oral clearance in de novo and stable renal transplant recipients. *Clin Pharmacol Ther.* 2006;80(1):51-60.

58. Anglicheau D, Le Corre D, Lechaton S, et al. Consequences of genetic polymorphisms for siroli-mus requirements after renal transplant in patients on primary sirolimus therapy. *Am J Transplant.* 2005;5(3):595-603.

59. Woillard JB, Kamar N, Coste S, Rostaing L, Marquet P, Picard N. Effect of CYP3A4*22, POR*28, and PPARA rs4253728 on sirolimus in vitro metabolism and trough concentrations in kidney transplant recipients. *Clin Chem.* 2013;59(12):1761-1769.

60. Sam WJ, Chamberlain CE, Lee SJ, et al. Associations of ABCB1 3435C>T and IL-10-1082G>A poly-morphisms with long-term sirolimus dose requirements in renal transplant patients. *Transplantation.* 2011;92(12):1342-1347.

61. Kaplan B, Meier-Kriesche HU, Napoli KL, Kahan BD. The effects of relative timing of sirolimus and cyclosporine microemulsion formulation coadministration on the pharmacokinetics of each agent. *Clin Pharmacol Ther.* 1998;63(1):48-53.

62. Staatz CE, Tett SE. Pharmacology and toxicology of mycophenolate in organ transplant recipients: an update. *Arch Toxicol.* 2014;88(7):1351-1389.

63. Staatz CE, Tett SE. Clinical pharmacokinetics and pharmacodynamics of mycophenolate in solid or-gan transplant recipients. *Clin Pharmacokinet.* 2007;46(1):13-58.

64. Kiang TK, Ensom MHH. Therapeutic drug monitoring of mycophenolate in adult solid organ trans-plant patients: an update. *Expert Opin Drug Metab Toxicol.* 2016;12(5):545-553.

65. Kiang TKL, Ensom MHH. Exposure-toxicity relationships of mycophenolic acid in adult kidney transplant patients. *Clin Pharmacokinet.* 2019;58(12):1533-1552.

66. Kiang TKL, Ensom MHH. Population pharmacokinetics of mycophenolic acid: an update. *Clin Phar-macokinet.* 2018;57(5):547-558.

67. Bergan S, Brunet M, Hesselink DA, et al. Personalized therapy for mycophenolate: consensus report by the international association of therapeutic drug monitoring and clinical toxicology. *Ther Drug Monit.* 2021;43(2):150-200.

68. Sobiak J, Resztak M. A systematic review of multiple linear regression-based limited sampling strat-egies for mycophenolic acid area under the concentration-time curve estimation. *Eur J Drug Metab Pharmacokinet.* 2021;46(6):721-742.

69. Rong Y, Patel V, Kiang TKL. Recent lessons learned from population pharmacokinetic studies of my-cophenolic acid: physiological, genomic, and drug interactions leading to the prediction of drug ef-fects. *Expert Opin Drug Metab Toxicol.* 2021;17(12):1369-1406.

70. Rong Y, Mayo P, Ensom MHH, Kiang TKL. Population pharmacokinetics of mycophenolic acid co-administered with tacrolimus in corticosteroid-free adult kidney transplant patients. *Clin Pharma-cokinet.* 2019;58(11):1483-1495.

71. Rong Y, Jun H, Kiang TKL. Population pharmacokinetics of mycophenolic acid in paediatric patients. *Br J Clin Pharmacol.* 2021;87(4):1730-1757.

72. Poulin E, Greanya ED, Partovi N, Shapiro RJ, Al-Khatib M, Ensom MHH. Development and valida-tion of limited sampling strategies for tacrolimus and mycophenolate in steroid-free renal transplant regimens. *Ther Drug Monit.* 2011;33(1):50-55.

14

PHENYTOIN

Viet-Huong Nguyen and Sunita Dergalust

8. Describe the elements of capacity-limited metabolism (K_m and V_m) and how K_m and V_m relate to clearance.
9. Describe or demonstrate the relationship between a change in the phenytoin maintenance dose and the new $C_{ss\,ave}$ when:
   a. $C_{ss\,ave}$ is below K_m.
   b. $C_{ss\,ave}$ is the same as K_m.
   c. $C_{ss\,ave}$ is much greater than K_m.
   d. The maintenance dose is greater than V_m.
10. Explain or use examples to demonstrate why the concept of $t_{1/2}$ for phenytoin has little to no usefulness in the clinical setting.
11. Do the following if a dosing history is given:
   a. Predict the time expected to achieve 90% of steady state ($t90\%$).
   b. Determine whether or not a measured plasma concentration is likely to represent steady state ($90\%\ t$).
   c. List the conditions necessary for the $t90\%$ and $90\%\ t$ equations to be employed and the potential errors that can be encountered when using the two equations.
   d. Calculate the time required for a phenytoin concentration to decline from an initial concentration to a defined second concentration, assuming no drug input.
12. Identify, given a patient's phenytoin dosing regimen, based on the product being administered, route of administration, and time of the phenytoin plasma sample, whether or not it would be appropriate to consider the steady-state phenytoin concentration as a $C_{ss\,ave}$ and, if not, how to approximate the $C_{ss\,ave}$.
13. Do the following if a patient history with one $C_{ss\,ave}$ phenytoin level is given:
   a. Use a reasonable assumed K_m to calculate a revised V_m.
   b. Use the revised V_m and assumed K_m to calculate either a new $C_{ss\,ave}$ from a selected dosing regimen or a new dosing regimen from the selected $C_{ss\,ave}$.
14. Determine whether phenytoin is a possible candidate for a patient, given a patient's HLA-B15:02 genotype, and explain how initial maintenance doses might be adjusted, given the CYP2C9 genotype.
15. Explain why, in some patients, the phenytoin concentration remains stable and does not decline significantly for several days following the discontinuation of oral phenytoin.
16. Use the "orbit graph" (see Figure 14.2) to determine the most probable V_m and K_m and then determine a new dosing regimen to achieve a desired $C_{ss\,ave}$, given a patient history with one $C_{ss\,ave}$.
17. Calculate and estimate graphically (see Figure 14.3) the unique K_m and V_m values that are consistent with the data provided, given a patient history with two different phenytoin maintenance doses and corresponding $C_{ss\,aves}$.
18. Do the following if an initial phenytoin concentration and a second "non–steady-state" phenytoin concentration are given:
   a. Use the mass balance technique to estimate a revised estimate of V_m.
   b. Use the revised V_m to design a new dosing regimen to achieve a desired $C_{ss\,ave}$.

   c. Describe the rules or conditions necessary to improve the accuracy of the mass balance technique when applied to phenytoin.
19. Recognize the altered binding condition and calculate the corresponding normal binding concentrations, given a patient with hypoalbuminemia and either normal renal function or receiving dialysis, and then:
   a. Determine whether dosing adjustments would be appropriate.
   b. Revise the V_m (one $C_{ss\,ave}$) or K_m and V_m (two dosing regimens with $C_{ss\,ave}$).
   c. Revise the dosing regimen (incremental loading and maintenance doses) to achieve a desired normal binding concentration.
   d. Calculate the $C_{ss\,ave}$ that would be assayed given the altered binding condition.
   e. Calculate the "therapeutic range" of the altered binding condition that would correspond to the normal binding concentrations of 10 to 20 mg/L.
20. Explain, using the criteria outlined in Dialysis of Drugs: Estimating Drug Dialyzability in Chapter "Drug Dosing in Kidney Disease and Dialysis," why dialysis is not likely to remove significant amounts of phenytoin.
21. Calculate the amount of phenytoin removed by chronic renal replacement therapy (CRRT), given the target unbound phenytoin concentration and the effluent flow rate for a patient receiving CRRT.

Phenytoin is primarily used as an anticonvulsant in the treatment of epilepsy and status epilepticus. It has been used in the past for the treatment of cardiac arrhythmias, but that indication is now obsolete.[1] Phenytoin is available in the acid or sodium salt form and as the phosphate ester prodrug (fosphenytoin) of phenytoin. Phenytoin sodium is available as both an injection solution and an extended-release capsule formulation. Phenytoin in the acid form is available as either an immediate-release suspension or an immediate-release chewable tablet. Fosphenytoin is available only as an injectable dosage form.

   Phenytoin is usually administered orally in single or divided doses of 200 to 400 mg/d. When a rapid therapeutic effect is required, such as for emergent treatment of status epilepticus, a loading dose of 15 to 20 mg/kg can be administered by oral or intravenous (IV) routes.[2,3] Although phenytoin for injection can be administered intramuscularly (IM), this route should be avoided because of slow and erratic absorption. Fosphenytoin is dosed as milligrams of phenytoin equivalents (P.E.) of phenytoin sodium injection and is usually administered by the IV route but can be administered by the IM route. Absorption of fosphenytoin by the IM route is more rapid than the oral route but slower than the IV route of phenytoin administration.[4]

   Individualizing the dose of phenytoin is complicated by two major problems. First, binding of phenytoin to plasma proteins is decreased in patients with renal failure or hypoalbuminemia, and in certain cases, phenytoin can be displaced by other drugs. Second, the metabolic capacity of phenytoin is limited; therefore, changes in the maintenance dose result in disproportionate changes in steady-state plasma concentrations.

The capacity-limited metabolism of phenytoin also eliminates the clinical usefulness of half-life ($t_{1/2}$) as a pharmacokinetic parameter and makes estimates of the time required to achieve steady state difficult. Although phenytoin is still commonly used, the difficulty with the capacity-limited metabolism, multiple drug-drug interactions, as well as the long-term side-effect profile has limited its use in epilepsy to a second- or third-line agent.[5]

KEY PARAMETERS: Phenytoin

Therapeutic plasma concentration	10-20 mg/L
F[a]	1
S[b]	0.92, 1
V	0.65 L/kg
Cl	
V_m[c]	7 mg/kg/d
K_m[d]	4 mg/L
$t_{1/2}$[e]	Concentration dependent
fu (fraction unbound in plasma)	0.1

[a]Oral bioavailability is generally assumed to be 1 (100% absorbed). However, bioavailability is difficult to estimate, and different drug products are not considered to be interchangeable or therapeutically equivalent.
[b]For phenytoin sodium capsules and phenytoin sodium injectable preparations (phenytoin and fosphenytoin), salt factor (S) = 0.92; for the acid phenytoin suspension and acid phenytoin chewable tablet, S = 1.
[c]Adult value, V_m values are >7 mg/kg/d and age dependent for children.
[d]Adult value, K_m values are variable for children.
[e]For time required to achieve steady state (see Half-Life $t_{1/2}$).

THERAPEUTIC AND TOXIC PLASMA CONCENTRATIONS

Phenytoin plasma concentrations of 10 to 20 mg/L are generally accepted as therapeutic.[6-11] Plasma concentrations in the range of 5 to 10 mg/L can be therapeutic for some patients, but concentrations less than 5 mg/L are not likely to be effective.[12] In emergent situations, such as in status epilepticus, levels greater than 20 mg/L during the acute period may be targeted.[13]

A number of long-term phenytoin side effects, such as gingival hyperplasia, folate deficiency, peripheral neuropathy, osteoporosis, hirsutism, and coarsening of facial features, do not appear to be easily related to plasma phenytoin concentrations.[14] Subacutely, idiosyncratic hematologic and hepatic toxicity can occur within days to weeks of phenytoin initiation and are not correlated with plasma phenytoin concentrations. Phenytoin is also highly associated with hypersensitivity syndromes that can range from mild rashes to life-threatening reactions, including drug reaction with eosinophilia and systemic symptoms (DRESS), Stevens-Johnson syndrome (SJS), or toxic epidermal necrolysis (TEN).[14,15] Substantial evidence suggests that patients with the HLA-B15:02 genotype have a higher risk of developing SJS or TEN such that the Clinical Pharmacogenetics Implementation Consortium (CPIC) has issued guidelines that recommend using an anticonvulsant other than phenytoin in patients with this genotype unless the benefits of treating the underlying disease clearly outweigh the risk.[16]

In contrast, central nervous system (CNS) side effects do correlate to some degree with plasma concentration. Far-lateral nystagmus (ocular tremor on far-lateral gaze) usually occurs in patients with plasma phenytoin concentrations greater than 20 mg/L. The concentration range associated with this effect, however, is broad, with some patients showing symptoms at concentrations of 15 mg/L and others having no nystagmus at concentrations greater than 30 mg/L. Although far-lateral nystagmus is often used to monitor phenytoin therapy, it is seldom considered a true drug side effect or toxicity and is not a reason to reduce the phenytoin dose. As an example, if a patient has always presented with far-lateral nystagmus but is no longer exhibiting nystagmus, it is an indication that the phenytoin concentration is probably lower than on previous visits. Other CNS symptoms such as ataxia and diminished mental capacity are frequently observed in patients with concentrations exceeding 30 and 40 mg/L, respectively.[7]

Precautions should be taken when phenytoin for injection is administered by the IV route due to the increased incidence of hypotension, cardiac dysrhythmias, extravasation, and purple glove syndrome, a syndrome of progressive distal limb edema, discoloration, and pain that, in severe cases, can lead to skin necrosis and limb ischemia.[17,18] Phenytoin cardiotoxicity is believed to be increased because the propylene glycol diluent has cardiac depressant properties.[7] Fosphenytoin is more soluble than phenytoin for injection and does not contain propylene glycol as a diluent. However, fosphenytoin does have similar effects on the myocardium and cardiovascular system (bradycardia and hypotension), although to a lesser extent. Clinicians should be aware that the maximum recommended rate of IV administration is 50 mg/min for phenytoin for injection and 150 mg/min for fosphenytoin, and slower rates of infusion (one-half to one-third of the maximum rate) are often used, especially in the older adults and when larger loading doses are administered.[13,17]

Alterations in Plasma Protein Binding

The usual phenytoin therapeutic range of 10 to 20 mg/L represents the total plasma drug concentration that consists of unbound (or free) drug concentration plus the phenytoin that is bound to plasma albumin. The usual fu or free fraction of phenytoin is 0.1. Therefore, approximately 90% of phenytoin in the plasma is bound to serum albumin; about 10% is unbound and free to equilibrate with the tissues where the pharmacologic effects and metabolism occur. It is important to keep in mind that although most of the phenytoin in plasma is bound to plasma albumin, most of the phenytoin is not in plasma. The vascular space represents only a small fraction of the total volume of distribution for phenytoin. Of the total amount of drug in the body, only 5% is within the vascular space because most of the phenytoin is actually in the tissue compartments. Therefore, any phenytoin displaced off the plasma albumin, whereas a large percentage of the drug in plasma, is a small percentage of phenytoin in the tissue. The displaced phenytoin will reequilibrate with the tissue, resulting in a large decrease in the total plasma concentration but very little change in the unbound or free plasma phenytoin concentration in the total body and very little change in the pharmacologic effect. Following reequilibration of the displaced phenytoin, the unbound plasma phenytoin concentration will remain relatively unchanged. The total plasma phenytoin concentration will be decreased because the bound concentration has decreased. As a result, the total level will appear to be low relative to its potential for pharmacologic effect (therapeutic and/or toxic).

There are two approaches one can use to interpret phenytoin levels when protein binding is significantly altered. The first is to adjust all the parameters (ie, therapeutic range, volume of distribution, and K_m) to those that would be observed in the presence of altered plasma binding. The second is to convert the measured or observed plasma concentration with low binding into that which would be observed under normal binding conditions ($C_{Normal Binding}$). In this instance, the parameters (ie, therapeutic range, volume of distribution, and K_m) associated with normal plasma protein binding would also be used in any calculations. Although either of these approaches is acceptable, the latter approach is most used commonly in clinical practice, and thus this approach is used throughout this chapter when alterations in plasma binding are encountered.

The three factors that are known to significantly alter the plasma protein binding of phenytoin are hypoalbuminemia, renal failure, and displacement by other drugs.

Hypoalbuminemia. In patients with low serum albumin, Equation 14.1 can be used to determine the plasma concentration that would have been observed with a normal plasma protein concentration.

$$C_{Normal Binding} = \frac{C'}{(1-fu)\left[\dfrac{P'}{P_{NL}}\right] + fu} \quad \text{(Eq. 14.1)}$$

C' is the observed plasma concentration reported by the laboratory; fu is the normal free fraction of drug (phenytoin fu = 0.1)[19-22]; P' is the patient's serum albumin in units of g/dL; P_{NL} is the normal serum albumin (4.4 g/dL); and $C_{Normal Binding}$ is the plasma drug concentration that would have been observed if the patient's serum albumin concentration had been normal. Placing the corresponding values for fu and a normal serum albumin results in Equation 14.2.

$$\text{Phenytoin concentration normal plasma binding} = \frac{\text{Patient's phenytoin concentration with altered plasma binding}}{\left[0.9 \times \dfrac{\text{Patient's serum albumin}}{4.4\,\text{g/dL}}\right] + 0.1} \quad \text{(Eq. 14.2)}$$

This equation is most useful when a patient has a low serum albumin concentration but does not have significantly diminished renal function and is not taking other drugs known to displace phenytoin. In clinical practice, if one is willing to assume that 0.9 is approximately 1 and 0.1 is approximately 0, the adjustment factor is simply the patient's albumin divided by the normal albumin. This simplification should not be used if the patient's albumin is less than 2 g/dL because it suggests that, at the unbound phenytoin, the concentration would be zero if there were no albumin, and this, of course, is not true.

Renal Failure. In patients with end-stage renal disease, the free fraction of phenytoin increases from 0.1 to 0.2 to 0.35.[19,23-26] Some of this change in plasma binding is because of the decrease in serum albumin concentration associated with end-stage renal disease, and some of the binding changes are because of a change in the binding affinity of phenytoin to serum albumin. When the creatinine clearance is greater than 25 mL/min, the change in the binding affinity appears to be minimal, no adjustment for renal function needs to be made, and Equation 14.2 should be used. However, if the creatinine clearance is less than 10 mL/min and the patient is undergoing hemodialysis treatments, binding changes can be significant.[27]

In the latter circumstance, Equation 14.2 can be altered to accommodate changes in both the serum albumin concentration and the affinity of phenytoin for serum albumin. Hence, Equation 14.3 is given as follows:

$$\frac{\text{Phenytoin concentration}}{\text{normal plasma Binding}} = \frac{\text{Dialysis Patient's phenytoin concentration with altered plasma binding}}{\left[(0.9)(0.48) \times \dfrac{\text{Patient's serum albumin}}{4.4\,\text{g/dL}} + 0.1\right]} \qquad \text{(Eq. 14.3)}$$

These equations should only be used in patients with end-stage renal disease receiving hemodialysis treatments because the factor that represents the decreased affinity for phenytoin binding to serum albumin (0.48) was derived from this type of patient. Note that, in Equation 14.3, fu is again assumed to be 0.1 [ie, 0.9 = (1 − fu)] because the phenytoin concentration normal plasma binding ($C_{\text{Normal Binding}}$) calculated by Equation 14.3 is correct for both serum albumin and renal dysfunction. In addition, it should be recognized that Equations 14.2 and 14.3 are only approximate estimates of normal plasma-binding phenytoin concentrations and that there can be considerable variance among individual patients. The accuracy of Equations 14.2 and 14.3 has been studied, and variances have been identified. This is especially true in critically ill patients.[28,29] Regardless of what equation is used to adjust for altered binding, the general concept that phenytoin binding needs to be considered when evaluating phenytoin concentration is important to remember when using phenytoin concentrations to adjust a patient's dosing regimen. In patients with diminished renal function who are not undergoing intermittent hemodialysis, binding affinity is unpredictably altered when the creatinine clearance is between 10 and 25 mL/min. The plasma concentration of drugs cannot be interpreted accurately for this group of patients using Equation 14.3.[27]

When discussing alterations in plasma binding with a nonpharmacist clinician, it is often useful to consider what would be the target phenytoin concentration in a patient with decreased plasma binding. That is, what is the lower and upper concentration in your patient with altered binding that would be equivalent to the usual range of 10 to 20 mg/L when binding is normal. These values can be calculated by rearranging Equations 14.2 and 14.3.

For patients with hypoalbuminemia and a creatinine clearance greater than 25 mL/min, the equivalent lower and upper end of the concentration range would be as follows:

Patient's therapeutic range with
low albumin that would be equal to 10 mg/L =

$$10 \text{ mg/L} \times \left[\left(0.9 \times \frac{\text{Patient's serum albumin}}{4.4 \text{ g/dL}} \right) + 0.1 \right] \quad \text{(Eq. 14.4)}$$

Patient's therapeutic range with
low albumin that would be equal to 20 mg/L =

$$20 \text{ mg/L} \times \left[\left(0.9 \times \frac{\text{Patient's serum albumin}}{4.4 \text{ g/dL}} \right) + 0.1 \right] \quad \text{(Eq. 14.5)}$$

For patients with hypoalbuminemia who are receiving dialysis, the equivalent lower and upper end of the concentration range would be as follows:

Patient's therapeutic range with
low albumin and on dialysis that would be equal to 10 mg/L =

$$10 \text{ mg/L} \times \left[\left(0.9 \times 0.48 \times \frac{\text{Patient's serum albumin}}{4.4 \text{ g/dL}} \right) + 0.1 \right] \quad \text{(Eq. 14.6)}$$

Patient's therapeutic range with
low albumin and on dialysis that would be equal to 20 mg/L =

$$20 \text{ mg/L} \times \left[\left(0.9 \times 0.48 \times \frac{\text{Patient's serum albumin}}{4.4 \text{ g/dL}} \right) + 0.1 \right] \quad \text{(Eq. 14.7)}$$

Drug Displacement. Drugs can also displace phenytoin from plasma protein–binding sites. As explained in desired plasma concentration (C) in Chapter "Pharmacokinetic Processes and Parameters," it is usually difficult to estimate the extent of drug displacement from protein-binding sites because the concentration of the displacing agent is seldom known. One exception to this rule is the situation in which serum concentrations of both valproic acid and phenytoin are being monitored. When the serum valproic acid concentration is less than 20 mg/L, the displacement of phenytoin appears to be minimal, and adjustment of the phenytoin concentration is probably not warranted. When the valproic acid concentration increases, phenytoin displacement from plasma protein–binding sites increases. At valproic acid concentrations of approximately 70 mg/L, phenytoin serum concentrations decrease by 40% (see Equation 14.8 and Chapter "Valproic Acid").[22,30,31]

In a study by Kerrick et al.,[32] an equation was developed to help correct or adjust for the displacement of phenytoin by valproic acid. Equation 14.8 is a modification of their original equation:

$$\text{Phenytoin concentration normal plasma binding} = \frac{\left[0.095 + (0.001)(\text{Valproic acid concentration})\right](\text{Phenytoin concentration})}{0.1}$$

(Eq. 14.8)

where the Phenytoin Concentration Normal Plasma Binding is the concentration that would have been reported if there had been no displacement by valproic acid (ie, fu = 0.1). The valproic acid and phenytoin concentrations are the concentrations that are reported by the laboratory. Note, however, that Equation 14.8 has the requirement that the two drug concentrations be measured (obtained) at the same time. In addition, there should not be any other factors present that would alter plasma binding (eg, hypoalbuminemia, renal failure, other displacing drugs).

BIOAVAILABILITY (F)

Phenytoin bioavailability is difficult to estimate but is generally greater than 0.8 for most currently available products. However, bioavailability varies with the various dosage forms and different manufacturers' products, and for the purposes of this chapter, phenytoin is assumed to be completely absorbed ($F = 1.0$).[10,33-37] The different dosage forms and manufacturers' products are not considered to be equivalent. Although most data suggest that generic phenytoin products are safe and effective and can be interchangeable, in practice, it is usually recommended that changing manufacturer or dosage form be avoided when possible to rule out the possibility that small differences in absorption might result in a therapeutic failure or toxicity.[38] It is the author's recommendation that if a change in the manufacturer is necessary, it would be best to make the change at a time when the patient's daily routine is normal (eg, not at the start of school, vacations, new job) because changes in the daily routine are more likely to result in nonadherence, making it more uncertain as to whether a change is clinical status is the result of differences in absorption or adherence. In addition, different dosage forms of phenytoin contain different salt forms of phenytoin. The capsule and injectable preparations consist of the sodium salt ($S = 0.92$) of phenytoin, whereas the chewable tablet and suspension contain the free acid form ($S = 1.0$) of phenytoin. There is an approximately 8% increase in drug content with the free acid form over the sodium salt form, and dosage adjustments may be needed when switching from one formulation to another. Although the fosphenytoin injectable product has a salt factor other than 0.92, the content of the fosphenytoin vial is labeled as mg of P.E. or "phenytoin equivalent"; therefore, a salt factor (S) of 0.92 should be used in calculations with this product.

The rate of phenytoin absorption following oral administration is slow because of the limited aqueous solubility of phenytoin. This is true, regardless of whether the immediate-release or extended-release oral products are used.[34] Serum concentrations of phenytoin extended-release products usually peak 3 to 12 hours after oral administration when given as the usual daily maintenance doses.[34]

Because phenytoin is absorbed slowly, the bioavailability could be less than 100% in patients with short gastrointestinal (GI) transit times.[39] Phenytoin concentrations are significantly decreased in patients receiving liquid dietary supplements (nasogastric feedings) and neonates.[40-42] Presumably, rapid GI motility decreases the apparent bioavailability of phenytoin, although the specific mechanism has not been identified. In some patients receiving nasogastric feedings, phenytoin doses of up to 1,200 mg/d were required to achieve therapeutic concentrations. Discontinuation of the enteral feedings resulted in a significant increase in the phenytoin plasma concentrations. It is recommended that patients receiving nasogastric feedings be closely monitored because concentrations within the usual therapeutic range are difficult to achieve and maintain. Similar potential problems may occur when phenytoin is administered concomitantly with antacids.[40,43]

The bioavailability of phenytoin is difficult to evaluate because of the drug's capacity-limited metabolism.[44] The slow absorption of phenytoin also tends to diminish the change in concentration following an oral dose. In most patients receiving oral phenytoin, the change in concentration (ΔC) will be about half that observed when giving the drug by the IV route. The slow rate of absorption also results in delayed peak concentrations that occur between 3 and 12 hours after administration of normal maintenance doses. When loading doses of 1 g are administered orally as the extended absorption (ie, extended-release) product, serum concentrations usually peak in about 24 hours, and if the dose is increased to 1,600 mg, the peak may be delayed by as much as 30 hours.[45,46] The time required to achieve the peak concentration can be decreased if a phenytoin "prompt absorption" (immediate-release) product is administered.[34] Fosphenytoin can be administered orally, and absorption appears to be relatively rapid and complete with peak concentrations at about 1 hour if conditions are optimal, for example, an empty stomach, no delay in gastric emptying.[47] However, the time to peak is still delayed compared to the IV route, and the IV route is preferred when rapid achievement of therapeutic concentrations is required.

Although the absorption of phenytoin is almost certainly a complex process, one approach the author has used is to assume an absorption rate of approximately 50 mg/hr for the extended absorption product Dilantin capsules. This absorption rate is consistent with the observations stated earlier and is sometimes useful when estimating a time when the peak concentration will occur following oral administration. In addition, although it is common practice to divide 15 to 20 mg/kg loading doses into 5 mg/kg increments administered every 2 hours, there are no studies documenting that this procedure is optimal in terms of the dose size or interval between doses.

VOLUME OF DISTRIBUTION (V)

The volume of distribution for phenytoin in patients with normal renal function and with normal serum albumin concentrations is approximately 0.65 L/kg.[19,48,49] Although the apparent volume of distribution for phenytoin is increased in patients with diminished plasma binding, the loading dose should not be changed because the increase in the volume of distribution resulting from changes in plasma binding is accompanied by an equal and opposite decrease in the desired total phenytoin plasma concentration. Also, as previously stated, the amount of phenytoin in the plasma represents only a small fraction of the total amount of phenytoin in the body. The approach taken in this chapter is to correct any measured concentrations altered by binding to the concentration that would be observed under normal plasma-binding conditions. Under these conditions, a "normal binding" volume of distribution of 0.65 L/kg, which represents normal plasma binding (fu = 0.1), should be used in all computations.

In patients with obesity, the volume of distribution for phenytoin is a complex relationship between plasma protein binding, lipid solubility, and tissue perfusion. Equation 14.9 is based on a study by Abernathy and Greenblatt.[50]

For patients with obesity:

$$V_{\text{Phenytoin in } L} = 0.65 \text{L}/\text{kg}\left[\text{IBW} + 1.3\,(\text{TBW} - \text{IBW})\right] \qquad \text{(Eq. 14.9)}$$

where TBW is the patient's total body weight in kilogram and IBW is the patient's ideal body weight in kilogram.

$$\begin{array}{l}\text{Ideal body weight} \\ \text{for males in kg}\end{array} = 50 + (2.3)(\text{Height in inches} > 60) \qquad \text{(Eq. 14.10)}$$

$$\begin{array}{l}\text{Ideal body weight} \\ \text{for females in kg}\end{array} = 45 + (2.3)(\text{Height in inches} > 60) \qquad \text{(Eq. 14.11)}$$

CAPACITY-LIMITED METABOLISM

For most drugs, the rate of metabolism (and/or excretion) is proportional to the plasma concentration. *Clearance* is defined as the volume of plasma that is completely cleared of drug per unit of time (see Clearance [Cl] in Chapter "Pharmacokinetic Processes and Parameters"). For first-order drugs, clearance can be viewed as a fixed proportionality constant that makes the steady-state plasma concentration equal to the rate of drug administration (R_A), as illustrated by Equation 14.12:

$$R_A = (\text{Cl})(C_{\text{ss ave}}) \qquad \text{(Eq. 14.12)}$$

R_A is $(S)(F)(\text{Dose}/\tau)$. This view of first-order pharmacokinetics, however, does not apply to phenytoin because the clearance of phenytoin decreases as $C_{ss\ ave}$ increases.

The clearance of phenytoin from plasma occurs primarily by metabolism, and the rate of phenytoin metabolism approaches its maximum at therapeutic concentrations. Thus, the metabolism of phenytoin is described as being capacity limited.[7,49,51-54] Capacity-limited metabolism results in clearance values that decrease with increasing plasma concentrations. Therefore, when the maintenance dose is increased, the plasma concentration rises disproportionately (Figure 14.1).[51,55-60] This disproportionate rise in the steady-state plasma level makes dosage adjustment difficult.

The model that appears to fit the metabolic pattern for phenytoin elimination is the one originally proposed by Michaelis and Menten. The velocity (V) or rate at which an enzyme system can metabolize a substrate (S) can be described by the following equation:

$$V = \frac{(V_m)(S)}{K_m + S}$$
(Eq. 14.13)

where V_m is the maximum metabolic capacity or maximum rate of metabolism, and K_m is the substrate concentration at which V will be one-half of V_m. When the average steady-state phenytoin concentration ($C_{ss\ ave}$) is substituted for the substrate

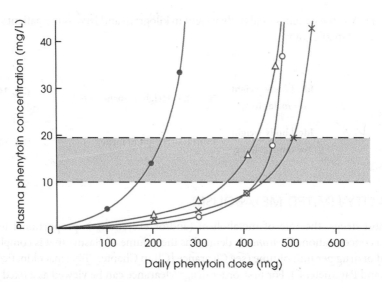

FIGURE 14.1   Changes in steady-state phenytoin plasma concentrations with maintenance dose. Note that for each patient, the plasma phenytoin concentration at steady state increases disproportionately with an increase in the rate of administration, especially as the dose approaches V_m. The patients in the figure represent the following V_m and K_m values: *filled circle*, 300 mg/d, 7 mg/L; *open triangle*, 500 mg/d, 4 mg/L; *open circle*, 500 mg/d, 2 mg/L; and *cross*, 600 mg/d, 4 mg/L. Also note that for patients with a low K_m value, the range of doses that result in a $C_{ss\ ave}$ between 10 and 20 mg/L is very narrow.

concentration (S) and the daily dose or administration rate of phenytoin [R_A or $(S)(F)$ (Dose/τ)] for V,[56,58-60] Equation 14.13 can be rewritten as:

$$(S)(F)(\text{Dose}/\tau) = \frac{(V_m)(C_{ss\,ave})}{K_m + C_{ss\,ave}} \qquad \text{(Eq. 14.14)}$$

In Equation 14.14, the "clearance" that makes $(S)(F)(\text{Dose}/\tau)$ equal to $C_{ss\,ave}$ is a value that will change as the $C_{ss\,ave}$ changes. As a result, there will be a disproportionate change in the $C_{ss\,ave}$ resulting from a change in the administration rate.

$$(S)(F)(\text{Dose}/\tau) = \frac{(V_m)}{K_m + C_{ss\,ave}}(C_{ss\,ave})$$

Equation 14.14 can also be rearranged as follows:

$$C_{ss\,ave} = \frac{(K_m)\left[(S)(F)(\text{Dose}/\tau)\right]}{V_m - \left[(S)(F)(\text{Dose}/\tau)\right]} \qquad \text{(Eq. 14.15)}$$

In accordance with the original definition of V_m and K_m for Equations 14.13 through 14.15, V_m is the maximum rate of metabolism (metabolic capacity), and K_m is the plasma concentration at which the rate of metabolism is one-half the maximum. The units for V_m and K_m are usually mg/d and mg/L, respectively.

Equation 14.15 illustrates the sensitive and disproportionate relationship between the rate of phenytoin administration and $C_{ss\,ave}$ when the rate of administration approaches V_m, the maximum metabolic capacity. If the maintenance dose was equal to V_m, then $V_m - (S)(F)(\text{Dose}/\tau)$ would be 0, and $C_{ss\,ave}$ would be infinity:

$$C_{ss\,ave} = \frac{(K_m)\left[(S)(F)(\text{Dose}/\tau)\right]}{V_m - \left[(S)(F)(\text{Dose}/\tau)\right]}$$

$$= \frac{(K_m)\left[(S)(F)(\text{Dose}/\tau)\right]}{0}$$

$$= [\infty]$$

If $(S)(F)(\text{Dose}/\tau)$ is greater than V_m, $C_{ss\,ave}$ will be a negative number, indicating that steady state can never be achieved. Equation 14.15 is, therefore, invalid as a predictor of $C_{ss\,ave}$ when $(S)(F)(\text{Dose}/\tau)$ is equal to or exceeds V_m.

As can be seen from Equation 14.15, the relationship between steady-state phenytoin concentrations and the maintenance dose can be extremely sensitive. Understanding and being able to use pharmacokinetic parameters for phenytoin help clinicians make initial dose adjustments and use clinical guidelines more effectively. For example, the following dose increments have been suggested using phenytoin concentrations as a guide: increasing the daily dose by 100 mg/d when $C_{ss\,ave}$ concentrations are less than 7 mg/L; by 50 mg/d when $C_{ss\,ave}$ concentrations are 7 to less than

12 mg/L; and a maximum increase of 30 mg/d when $C_{ss\,ave}$ concentrations are greater than 12 mg/L.[61] Although these suggestions are consistent with the usual pharmacokinetic parameters, any increase in dose should be considered carefully in the context of patient adherence and any potential alterations in plasma binding. One should also keep in mind that adding 100 mg/d to patients with a $C_{ss\,ave}$ of 6 mg/L taking 200 mg/d will probably result in a more dramatic rise in the new steady-state phenytoin concentration than for patients with a $C_{ss\,ave}$ of 6 mg/L taking 400 mg/d.

Another factor that can influence phenytoin metabolism and, therefore, the maintenance dose is genetic disposition. The majority of patients (~90%) are genetically classified as normal/extensive metabolizers of phenytoin. Approximately 10% of patients have a CYP2C9 heterozygous variant and are classified as intermediate metabolizers, and about 1% have a homozygous CYP2C9 variant and are classified as poor metabolizers. While phenytoin and fosphenytoin loading doses do not need to be adjusted based on genotype, starting maintenance doses should be adjusted according to genotype. The CPIC guidelines recommend that intermediate and poor metabolizers have their starting maintenance dose reduced by 25% and 50%, respectively.[16,62] Normal/extensive metabolizers do not require adjustments to the starting maintenance dose. In all patients, subsequent doses should be adjusted according to the patient's response to drugs, side effects, and therapeutic drug monitoring. Knowing that genetic disposition is helpful as a starting point, but careful monitoring of phenytoin concentrations over the first few weeks is important because, with this nonlinear drug, small differences in maintenance doses/metabolism can result in significant differences in steady-state phenytoin concentrations.

Because phenytoin can be very sensitive to any change in either the bioavailability or metabolism, relatively minor drug-drug interactions can have significant effects on the steady-state phenytoin concentrations. There are a large number of drugs known to alter the pharmacokinetics of phenytoin (see Table 14.1), but the ability to predict from patient to patient the extent of the interaction is limited. It would be expected, however, that the higher the phenytoin concentration, the more likely that the drug-drug interaction will be significant (see Equation 14.15). Also, although not discussed here, phenytoin can alter the pharmacokinetics of other drugs, most commonly by enzyme induction and as a result of a decrease in efficacy, for example, statins and oral contraceptives.[63,64]

K_m values are usually between 1 and 20 mg/L.[55,57-59,101] V_m appears to be between 5 and 15 mg/kg/d in most patients.[55,58,59] The relationship between K_m and V_m is not clear, but if one of these parameters is low, the other is frequently low as well.[55,56,59] The average values for K_m and V_m are difficult to establish. It is the author's opinion that approximately 4 mg/L for K_m and 7 mg/kg/d for V_m are reasonable initial estimates for the average adult patient. While it is true that the older adults are more likely to have decreased serum albumin and may be more sensitive to side effects, in general, the older adults do not appear to have significantly altered phenytoin pharmacokinetic parameters and the abovementioned V_m and K_m values can be used for this population.[102]

TABLE 14.1 Drugs That Alter Phenytoin Pharmacokinetics[a]

DRUG	EFFECT ON PHENYTOIN CONCENTRATION	MECHANISM
Amiodarone[65,66]	Increase	Inhibition of metabolism
Antacids[b,67-69]	Decrease	Decreased absorption
Carbamazepine[70,71]	Increase or decrease	Induction of metabolism
Chloramphenicol[72,73]	Increase	Inhibition of metabolism
Cimetidine[74,75]	Increase	Inhibition of metabolism
Ciprofloxacin[76,77]	Decrease	Induction of metabolism
Cisplatinum[78]	Decrease	Decreased absorption[c]
Disulfiram[79,80]	Increase	Inhibition of metabolism
Efavirenz[81]	Increase	Inhibition of metabolism
Fluconazole[82]	Increase	Inhibition of metabolism
Fluoxetine[83]	Increase	Inhibition of metabolism
Folic acid[84-86]	Decrease	Induction of metabolism
Isoniazid[87-89]	Increase	Inhibition of metabolism (most significant in phenotypically slow acetylators)
Phenobarbital[d,90,91]	Increase or decrease	Inhibition or induction of metabolism
Rifampin[92]	Decrease	Induction of metabolism
Salicylates[e,93]	Decrease	Plasma protein displacement
Sertraline[94]	Increase	Inhibition of metabolism
Sulfonamides[95,96]	Increase	Inhibition of metabolism and plasma protein displacement
Ticlopidine[97,98]	Increase	Inhibition of metabolism
Trimethoprim[99]	Increase	Inhibition of metabolism
Valproic acid[f,30-32]	Decrease	Plasma protein displacement
Voriconazole[100]	Increase	Inhibition of metabolism

[a]The drugs listed are examples of those that influence phenytoin.
[b]A decrease in absorption is not consistently observed. Both drugs should not be administered at the same time; antacid and phenytoin doses should be taken at least 2 hours apart whenever possible.
[c]There are a number of chemotherapy drugs that appear to alter either phenytoin absorption or metabolism.
[d]The direction of change (if any) for the phenytoin concentration depends on which phenobarbital effect is predominant (ie, induction or inhibition of metabolism).
[e]Plasma protein displacement results in a decrease in the reported total phenytoin concentration but has little effect on the unbound phenytoin concentration or therapeutic effect. Note that high salicylate concentrations, that is, >50 mg/L, are required for displacement and single-daily doses of 80-325 mg should not result in altered binding of phenytoin.
[f]Valproic acid displaces phenytoin from its plasma protein binding. Valproic acid may also inhibit phenytoin metabolism, although this is unclear.

For pediatric patients, the V_m value is usually larger than 7 mg/kg/d. V_m values are approximately 10 to 13 mg/kg/d for children aged 6 months to 6 years and 8 to 10 mg/kg/d for children aged 7 to 16 years.[103-105] K_m values for children vary considerably in the literature; some authors have suggested values of 2 to 3 mg/L,[104,106] whereas others have suggested that a K_m value of 6 to 8 mg/L is more appropriate.[103,107] An average K_m value of 7 mg/L, although uncertain, is not an unreasonable estimate for children between 6 months and 16 years of age. While most standard pediatric references suggest starting with maintenance doses of approximately 5 mg/kg/d, most children will ultimately require maintenance doses of 7 to 10 mg/kg/d. In addition, doses are almost always divided, either every 12 hours or, in some cases, every 8 hours. The divided dose schedule is in part because of the higher V_m and more rapid metabolism, and in addition, many pediatric patients can only take either the suspension or the chewable tablets, and both of these products are immediate release and not intended for once-daily dosing.

CONCENTRATION-DEPENDENT CLEARANCE

The relationship between phenytoin clearance and phenytoin plasma concentration ($C_{ss\,ave}$) can be seen by studying Equation 14.14 and comparing it to the equivalent first-order equation. In the following first-order equation, clearance (Cl) is a constant value with the units of volume/time and can be thought of as the proportionality constant that makes the $C_{ss\,ave}$ equal to $(S)(F)(Dose/\tau)$.

$$(S)(F)(Dose/\tau) = (Cl)(C_{ss\,ave}) \qquad \textbf{(Eq. 14.16)}$$

If we replace Cl in the equation for a first-order drug with the term $(V_m)/(K_m + C_{ss\,ave})$, we again have Equation 14.14 as:

$$(S)(F)(Dose/\tau) = \frac{(V_m)(C_{ss\,ave})}{K_m + C_{ss\,ave}}$$

where the clearance of phenytoin is as follows:

$$Cl_{Phenytoin} = \frac{V_m}{K_m + C} \qquad \textbf{(Eq. 14.17)}$$

Note, in Equation 14.17, that the $C_{ss\,ave}$ has been replaced by C to represent any phenytoin concentration. If C is very small compared to K_m, clearance will be a relatively constant value (V_m/K_m), and the metabolism will appear to follow first-order pharmacokinetics. Most drugs that are metabolized appear to fall into this category (ie, the concentrations used therapeutically are well below the value of K_m). However, if the drug concentration approaches or exceeds K_m, clearance will decrease, and the metabolism will no longer appear to follow a first-order process. As clearance decreases with increasing phenytoin concentration, the velocity or metabolic rate will increase, but not in proportion to the increase in plasma concentration (see Figure 14.1). Because K_m values for phenytoin are generally below the usual therapeutic range, nearly all patients will display capacity-limited metabolism for phenytoin. For example, phenytoin K_m value for adults is approximately 4 mg/L compared to the therapeutic range of phenytoin, which is 10 to 20 mg/L.

Alterations in plasma binding will also alter the apparent K_m value. This is because K_m values are reported as total phenytoin concentration, and it is only the unbound concentration that can cross cell membranes and be available for metabolism. Again, as previously discussed, changes in plasma binding have a profound effect on the total phenytoin concentration, but not on the unbound phenytoin concentration. The general approach taken in this chapter is to adjust the measured concentration to that which would be observed under normal plasma-binding conditions and to use pharmacokinetic parameters (V, K_m, and C or $C_{ss\ ave}$), which are based on normal plasma binding.

CONCENTRATION-DEPENDENT HALF-LIFE

The usual reported half-life ($t_{1/2}$) for phenytoin is approximately 22 hours[52]; however, the $t_{1/2}$ is not a constant value because the clearance of phenytoin changes with the plasma concentration. If Equation 14.17 (the clearance equation for phenytoin):

$$Cl_{Phenytoin} = \frac{V_m}{K_m + C}$$

is substituted into the usual equation for half-life:

$$t_{1/2} = \frac{(0.693)(V)}{Cl} \qquad \text{(Eq. 14.18)}$$

then, the half-life of phenytoin can be derived:

$$t_{1/2\ Phenytoin} = \frac{(0.693)(V)}{V_m}(K_m + C) \qquad \text{(Eq. 14.19)}$$

Based on Equation 14.19, it can be predicted that the half-life of phenytoin will increase as the plasma concentration increases, an observation that has been confirmed.[53] The value and applicability of this observation are very limited, however.

Limited Utility of Half-Life

The clinical usefulness of the phenytoin half-life is limited because the time required to achieve steady state can be much longer than the usual 3 to 4 times the apparent half-life. Likewise, the time required for a plasma concentration to decay following discontinuation of the maintenance dose will be less than predicted by the apparent half-life. The problems associated with capacity-limited metabolism can best be explained by first examining the relationship between the rate of drug administration and elimination for a first-order drug. For a first-order drug, when the rate of administration (R_A) exceeds the rate of drug elimination from the body (R_E), the amount of drug in the body increases and the drug accumulates. If the rate of elimination exceeds the rate of drug administration, the amount of drug in the body will decrease.

$$R_A - R_E = \frac{\Delta \text{ Amount of drug in body}}{t} \qquad \text{(Eq. 14.20)}$$

The rate of drug elimination for a first-order drug is the product of clearance (Cl) and plasma concentration (C). When the pharmacokinetic parameter, clearance, and plasma concentration are substituted into Equation 14.20, the change in the amount of drug in the body per unit of time (Δ Amount of Drug in Body/t) is small when the product of Cl times C approaches the rate of drug administration. This proportional relationship between C and the rate of elimination is the key to the usefulness of $t_{1/2}$. Inspecting Equation 14.21:

$$R_A - (Cl)(C) = \frac{\Delta \text{Amount of drug in body}}{t} \qquad \text{(Eq. 14.21)}$$

it can be seen that when C is 50% of $C_{ss\ ave}$, Δ Amount of Drug in Body/t is 50% of R_A; when C is 90% of $C_{ss\ ave}$, Δ Amount of Drug in Body/t is 10% of R_A. This relationship means that when Δ Amount of Drug in Body/t is small (ie, very slow rate of accumulation) for a first-order drug, then C must be close to $C_{ss\ ave}$.

For capacity-limited drugs, however, clearance [$V_m/(K_m + C)$] is not a constant factor. This expression for clearance is inserted into Equation 14.21 to form Equation 14.22.

$$R_A - \frac{(V_m)}{(K_m + C)}(C) = \frac{\Delta \text{ Amount of drug in body}}{t} \qquad \text{(Eq. 14.22)}$$

As C exceeds K_m, the rate of drug elimination approaches V_m, which is a fixed value (see Capacity-Limited Metabolism). In such cases, it may be possible to have a rate of elimination that is very close to the rate of drug administration, resulting in a slow yet very prolonged accumulation process.

When R_A is equal to or greater than V_m, accumulation would continue forever or at least until the patient develops toxicity symptoms and phenytoin is withheld. Capacity-limited accumulation problems are most dramatic when the plasma concentration greatly exceeds the K_m value. In clinical practice, this means when either the K_m value is low or there is a clinical need to achieve high phenytoin concentrations, accumulation will be slow, and the time required to achieve steady state will be prolonged.

As an example, consider a patient with a V_m of 300 mg/d, a K_m of 4 mg/L, and an R_A of 300 mg/d of phenytoin. Under these conditions, in which the rate of phenytoin administration is equal to V_m, the phenytoin concentrations will continue to increase indefinitely. At a phenytoin concentration of 36 mg/L, the rate of elimination should be 270 mg or 90% of the administration rate, and the accumulation is only 10% of the maintenance dose.

$$R_A - \frac{(V_m)}{(K_m + C)}(C) = \frac{\Delta \text{Amount of drug in body}}{t}$$

$$300 \text{ mg/d} - \frac{(300 \text{ mg/d})}{(4 \text{ mg/L} + 36 \text{ mg/L})}(36 \text{ mg/L}) = \frac{\Delta \text{Amount of drug in body}}{t}$$

$$300 \text{ mg/d} - 270 \text{ mg/d} = 30 \text{ mg/d}$$

If this was a first-order drug, the concentration of 36 mg/L would be 90% of $C_{ss\,ave}$, and there would be very little additional accumulation to the final $C_{ss\,ave}$ of 40 mg/L. However, this is not a first-order drug, and in the example given, although R_E is 90% of R_A, at a C of 36 mg/L, the final theoretical $C_{ss\,ave}$ would be infinity because R_A is equal to V_m.

Again, the key point with phenytoin accumulation is that in a patient with relatively stable concentrations over several days or even weeks, it can be assumed that the rate of elimination is close to the rate of administration, but unlike with first-order drugs, the phenytoin concentrations may or may not be at or near steady state.

Time to Reach Steady State

The time required to achieve 90% of steady state can be calculated as follows[108]:

$$t90\% = \frac{(K_m)(V)}{\left[V_m - (S)(F)(\text{Dose/day})\right]^2}\left[(2.3\,V_m) - (0.9)(S)(F)(\text{Dose/day})\right] \quad \textbf{(Eq. 14.23)}$$

The $t90\%$ is the time required for a patient to achieve 90% of the steady-state plasma concentration on a dosing regimen, given K_m, V, and V_m. The units are mg/L for K_m, L for V, and mg/d for V_m and dose.

Equation 14.23 assumes that the initial plasma concentration is zero. If the initial plasma concentration is between zero and the steady-state concentration, 90% of steady state will be achieved sooner than predicted by Equation 14.23. Nevertheless, it is still reasonable to use Equation 14.23 to predict the time to achieve steady-state concentrations, even when the initial plasma concentration is greater than zero but still relatively low. When therapy with phenytoin is initiated, at first, the drug accumulates rapidly over a short time period so that initial plasma concentrations do not, in most cases, significantly reduce the time required to achieve 90% of steady state. Equation 14.23 should not be used, however, when the initial plasma concentration is greater than the desired steady-state concentration. Because very small differences in V_m or K_m or V can result in significant differences in time to $t90\%$, perhaps the most valuable use of Equation 14.23 is to remind us that accumulation can be slow but prolonged and that the time required to achieve steady state can be very long, especially when steady-state concentrations are high relative to K_m.

When Does a Phenytoin Concentration Represent a Steady-State Value?

When a phenytoin plasma concentration is measured, there is frequently a question as to whether the concentration is likely to represent a steady-state level. This question can be answered using Equation 14.24:

$$90\%t = \frac{\left[115 + (35)(C)\right]\left[C\right]}{(S)(F)(\text{Dose/day})}$$
(Eq. 14.24)

where C is in mg/L, and the Dose/day is in mg/d. This equation is for adults, and the Dose/day should be normalized for a 70-kg patient. The 90% t value, which is calculated by this equation, represents the minimum amount of time the patient must have been receiving the maintenance regimen before it can be assumed that the measured C is at steady state. Equation 14.24 is relatively conservative in that in its derivation, a K_m value of 2 mg/L has been assumed; therefore, the 90% t value is longer than what would be required if the K_m value was actually greater than 2 mg/L. Therefore, steady state may already have been achieved in a patient who has been receiving the maintenance regimen for a shorter period than calculated in Equation 14.24. Also, note that C in Equation 14.24 must reflect normal plasma protein binding.

Rate of Decline: Phenytoin Levels

The decline of phenytoin concentration after discontinuation of therapy can be described by Equation 14.25:

$$t = \frac{\left[K_m\left(\ln\frac{C_1}{C_2}\right) + (C_1 - C_2)\right]}{\dfrac{V_m}{V}}$$
(Eq. 14.25)

where C_1 is the initial plasma concentration, and C_2 is the plasma concentration at the end of the time interval t. When both C_1 and C_2 are much greater than K_m, the rate of metabolism will approach V_m; therefore, the time required to decline from C_1 to C_2 is primarily controlled by the maximum rate of metabolism (V_m) and the apparent volume of distribution (V).

This equation can be used to estimate the V_m value in a patient who has either intentionally or accidentally received excessive phenytoin doses. In this instance, a decline in the phenytoin concentration can be observed over several days. Care should be taken, however, to ensure that no further drug is being administered to the patient. One must also consider that absorption of phenytoin may continue for several days after an acute overdose or following discontinuation of an oral maintenance regimen.[46,109] Given that the usual V_m is about 7 mg/kg/d for patients who have normal/extensive metabolism and V is approximately 0.65 L/kg, the maximum expected decrease in a phenytoin concentration in adults would be approximately 10 mg/L/d.

$$\frac{V_m}{V} = \frac{7\,mg/kg/d}{0.65\,L/kg} \approx 10\,mg/L/d$$

Again, this assumes the average value for V_m and V, no additional absorption of phenytoin, and that the beginning (C_1) and ending (C_2) phenytoin concentrations both are well above the patient's K_m.

There are data to suggest that phenytoin toxic patients with either intermediate or poor metabolism that activated charcoal will increase the rate of phenytoin decline.[110] While the decline in phenytoin concentration was accelerated when activated charcoal was administered, some of the effects may have been because of the sorbitol, administered with the activated charcoal, acting as a laxative and eliminating phenytoin that remained in the GI tract. Regardless of a patient's genetic status or whether activated charcoal is to be used, some type of bowel prep should be considered in patients with significant phenytoin toxicity to make sure that no phenytoin remains in the GI tract following withholding the daily oral maintenance dose.

TIME TO SAMPLE

Depending on the disease state being treated and the clinical condition of the patient, the time of sampling for phenytoin can vary greatly. In patients requiring rapid achievement and maintenance of therapeutic phenytoin concentrations, it is usually wise to monitor phenytoin concentrations within 2 to 3 days of initiating therapy. This is to ensure that the patient's metabolism is not remarkably different from that which would be predicted by average literature-derived pharmacokinetic parameters. A second phenytoin concentration would normally be obtained in another 3 to 5 days; subsequent doses of phenytoin can then be adjusted. If the plasma phenytoin concentrations have not changed over a 3- to 5-day period, the monitoring interval can usually be increased to once weekly in the acute clinical setting. In stable patients requiring long-term therapy, phenytoin plasma concentrations should be monitored until the patient's seizure disorder is stabilized and a steady state with phenytoin has been achieved.[11,111]

The time required to achieve steady state with phenytoin can be prolonged and monitoring before steady state is achieved can avoid sustained periods of low or high phenytoin concentrations. Nevertheless, these early phenytoin concentrations must be used cautiously in the design of new dosing regimens. Once the patient is stable, the phenytoin plasma concentration at this point (ie, the individual therapeutic concentration) should be determined, preferably by measuring steady-state concentrations on at least two separate occasions. Knowledge of the individual therapeutic concentration for a patient is useful when a patient experiences a change in clinical status and can aid in a clinician's assessment of the need for and magnitude of dose adjustments. Routine monitoring of plasma phenytoin levels in stable patients is not necessary unless there are changes in patient status (eg, worsening of seizure frequency, acute illness). Nevertheless, many clinicians still prefer to monitor phenytoin levels at 12 to 24-month intervals in stable patients.[112]

In patients receiving oral phenytoin extended-release dosage forms, especially in divided daily doses, the time of sampling within the dosing interval is not critical because the slow absorption of phenytoin minimizes the fluctuations between peak and trough concentrations. Trough concentrations are generally recommended for routine monitoring. In patients who are receiving phenytoin doses IV, trough concentrations can be adjusted by Equation 14.26 to calculate the average plasma concentration of phenytoin.

$$C_{ss\,ave} = [C_{ss\,min}] + \left[(0.5)\frac{(S)(F)(Dose)}{V}\right]$$ **(Eq. 14.26)**

Following IV administration, sampling within the first 1 to 2 hours after the end of the infusion should be avoided to ensure complete distribution (see Volume of Distribution: Two-Compartment Models in Chapter "Pharmacokinetic Processes and Parameters"). In addition, if fosphenytoin is administered, there may be an assay cross-reactivity between fosphenytoin, which is an inactive prodrug, and the hydrolyzed phenytoin, which is the active drug.[10]

In patients receiving phenytoin orally as an extended-release dosage form, the average concentration can be approximated by multiplying the change in concentration anticipated with the IV dose by 0.25. This 0.25 factor assumes that the fluctuation in plasma concentrations following oral administration is approximately half of that which would be expected if the drug were administered IV. It also assumes that the average concentration lies approximately halfway between the peak and trough concentrations.

$$C_{ss\,ave} = [C_{ss\,min}] + \left[(0.25)\frac{(S)(F)(Dose)}{V}\right]$$ **(Eq. 14.27)**

Use of Equation 14.27 is most appropriate when patients are receiving single-daily doses of greater than 5 mg/kg and when the phenytoin trough concentration is less than 5 mg/L. In patients with phenytoin concentrations greater than 5 mg/L or in those receiving their phenytoin in divided daily doses, use of Equation 14.27 is less critical because the $C_{ss\,peak}$ and C_{ss} trough are both relatively close to $C_{ss\,ave}$.

Question #1 *Calculate the phenytoin loading dose required to achieve a plasma concentration of 20 mg/L in B.F., a 70-kg man. Describe how this loading dose should be administered by the oral and IV routes.*

Equation 14.28 can be used to estimate the loading dose that will produce a plasma concentration of 20 mg/L. If the volume of distribution for phenytoin is assumed to be 0.65 L/kg (see Key Parameters, this chapter), the volume of distribution for B.F. would be 45.5 L (70 kg × 0.65 L/kg). In this case, we are assuming that B.F. has not been receiving phenytoin and, therefore, the $C_{observed}$ or the phenytoin concentration that is present is zero. The salt factor (S) is 0.92 for the oral capsules and injectable phenytoin dosage forms (phenytoin for injection and fosphenytoin), and the bioavailability is 100% (F = 1.0).

$$Loading\,dose = \frac{(V)(C_{desired} - C_{observed})}{(S)(F)}$$ **(Eq. 14.28)**

$$\text{Loading dose} = \frac{(45.5 \text{ L})(20 \text{ mg/L} - 0 \text{ mg/L})}{(0.92)(1)}$$
$$= 989 \text{ mg}$$

This loading dose of 989 mg is reasonably close to the usual, recommended loading dose of 1,000 mg or 15 mg/kg. In certain emergent situations such as in status epilepticus, a plasma concentration of greater than 20 mg/L may be desired, and loading doses for these patients may range from 15 to 20 mg/kg.

If a loading dose is administered IV as phenytoin for injection, it should be administered slowly to minimize the risk of extravasation and cardiovascular toxicities associated with IV infusion and the propylene glycol diluent.[6] A maximum rate of 50 mg/min should be used until the entire loading dose is administered or toxicities are encountered.[6] An administration rate of 50 mg/min for the 1,000-mg dose would mean that the total dose could be administered over 20 minutes. However, because of the potential for cardiovascular side effects, most clinicians administer 1,000-mg loading doses with close monitoring over 45 minutes to 1 hour (ie, about 15-25 mg/min). Also, note that this infusion rate is not size adjusted, and children require much slower infusion rates but are generally given the loading dose at a maximum infusion rate of approximately 1 mg/kg/min but preferably over about the same time as an adult (ie, 45 minutes to 1 hour). If the dose were to be given as fosphenytoin, the total dose would be the same with a maximum infusion rate of 150 mg/min. If possible, fosphenytoin would be given at a slower rate (eg, 75 mg/min) with similar cardiovascular monitoring.

If the 1,000-mg loading dose is to be given orally, a 400-mg dose followed by two 300-mg doses ($\approx$5 mg/kg) at 2-hour intervals is recommended so that the entire loading dose is administered over 4 hours. The oral loading dose is divided into three separate doses to decrease the possibility of nausea and vomiting, which may be associated with a single large dose, and to decrease the time to peak concentration.[45,46] When the loading dose is administered orally, slow absorption causes the peak concentration to be delayed and lower than the expected 20 mg/L, even if an immediate-release product is used.[37,45,46] Following oral administration of the extended-release capsules, the peak concentration is usually about one-half of the value calculated by the IV bolus dose model as predicted by the following equation:

$$\Delta C = (0.5)\frac{(S)(F)(\text{Dose})}{V} \qquad \text{(Eq. 14.29)}$$

This equation is based on the slow absorption associated with the phenytoin extended-release oral products, and the fluctuation in plasma concentration will probably be more than predicted by Equation 14.29 with the immediate-release products.[37] Although the peak concentration is very likely to be less than 20 mg/L following oral administration, it is uncommon to give larger oral doses to compensate for the delay in absorption. Oral absorption is relatively unpredictable, and increasing the oral dose is not likely to reliably correct the problem. If it were imperative, from a clinical standpoint, to achieve a phenytoin level of 20 mg/L or greater, it would be best to give phenytoin by the IV route.

Question #2   *S.B. is a 37-year-old, 70-kg man with a seizure disorder that has only partially been controlled with 300 mg/d of phenytoin oral capsules. His plasma phenytoin concentration has been measured twice over the past year and was 8 mg/L both times. Calculate a maintenance dose to achieve a new steady-state concentration of 15 mg/L.*

To establish the new daily dose, it is necessary to assume a value of V_m or K_m for S.B. The usual approach is to rearrange Equation 14.14:

$$(S)(F)(\text{Dose}/\tau) = \frac{(V_m)(C_{ss\ ave})}{K_m + C_{ss\ ave}}$$

and solve for V_m:

$$V_m = \frac{(S)(F)(\text{Dose}/\tau)(K_m + C_{ss\ ave})}{(C_{ss\ ave})} \qquad \text{(Eq. 14.30)}$$

If K_m is assumed to be 4 mg/L, S to be 0.92 (phenytoin capsules are the sodium salt), and F to be 1.0, then V_m would be 414 mg/d of phenytoin acid.

$$V_m = \frac{(0.92)(1)(300\ \text{mg/d})(4\ \text{mg/L} + 8\ \text{mg/L})}{(8\ \text{mg/L})}$$

$$V_m = \frac{414\ \text{mg}}{\text{Day of phenytoin acid}}$$

To calculate the dose required to achieve a steady-state concentration of 15 mg/L, Equation 14.14:

$$(S)(F)(\text{Dose}/\tau) = \frac{(V_m)(C_{ss\ ave})}{K_m + C_{ss\ ave}}$$

can be rearranged as follows:

$$\text{Dose} = \frac{(V_m)(C_{ssave})(\tau)}{(K_m + C_{ssave})(S)(F)} \qquad \text{(Eq. 14.31)}$$

Using the assumed K_m of 4 mg/L and the calculated V_m of 414 mg/d of phenytoin acid, the daily dose required to achieve a steady-state concentration of 15 mg/L would be:

$$\text{Dose} = \frac{(414\ \text{mg/d})(15\ \text{mg/L})(1\ \text{d})}{(4\ \text{mg/L} + 15\ \text{mg/L})(0.92)(1)}$$

$$= 355\ \text{mg of phenytoin sodium}$$

This 18% dosage adjustment should result in a nearly 100% increase in the steady-state plasma level if the assumed K_m of 4 mg/L is correct. A daily dose of 355 mg would be difficult to administer; therefore, this initial dosing estimate would probably be rounded off to 350 mg/d, and doses of 300 and 400 mg could be prescribed for alternate days. To aid with adherence, it is a common practice to prescribe the 300-mg dose (odd number of capsules) on the odd days of the month and 400 mg (even number of capsules) on the even days of the month. For those months with 31 days, most clinicians tell the patient to simply take the odd number of capsules 2 days in a row.

An alternative approach is illustrated in Figure 14.2. This method allows one to estimate the most probable combination of K_m and V_m values for a patient, given the current dosing regimen and measured average steady-state phenytoin concentration.

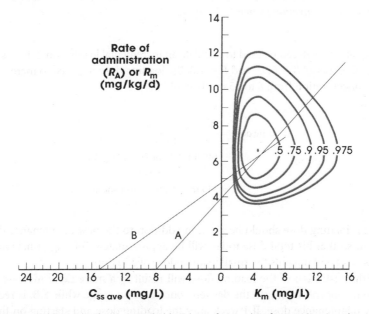

FIGURE 14.2   Orbit graph. The most probable values of V_m and K_m for a patient may be estimated using a single steady-state phenytoin concentration and a known dosing regimen. The eccentric circles or "orbits" represent the fraction of the sample patient population whose K_m and V_m values are within that orbit. (1) Plot the daily dose of phenytoin acid (mg/kg/d) on the vertical line (rate of administration [R_A]). (2) Plot the steady-state concentration ($C_{ss\ ave}$) on the horizontal line. (3) Draw a straight line connecting $C_{ss\ ave}$ and daily dose through the orbits (line A). (4) The coordinates of the midpoint of the line crossing the innermost orbit through which line A passes are the most probable values for the patient's V_m and K_m. (5) To calculate a new maintenance dose, draw a line from the point determined in step 4 to the new desired $C_{ss\ ave}$ (line B). The point at which line B crosses the vertical line (rate of administration [R_A]) is the new maintenance dose (mg/kg/d) of phenytoin acid. Line A represents a C_{ss} of 8 mg/L on 3.94 mg/kg/d or 276 mg/d of phenytoin acid (0.92 × 300 mg/d of sodium phenytoin) for a 70-kg person. The new steady-state concentration was 15 mg/L. From reference,[104] the original figure is modified so that R_A, R_E, and V_m are in mg/kg/d of phenytoin acid. (Reprinted with permission from Burton ME. *Applied Pharmacokinetics: Principles of Therapeutic Drug Monitoring*. 4th ed. Lippincott Williams & Wilkins; 2006.)

If the steps outlined in Figure 14.2 are followed, a K_m value of 5 mg/L and a V_m value of 6.4 mg/kg/d (448 mg/d for this 70-kg patient) can be determined. When these values are used in Equation 14.31 (or when Figure 14.2 is used), a new dose of approximately 365 mg/d is calculated. This method of using the "orbit graph" is perhaps slightly superior to the first in which a K_m value of 4 mg/L was assumed. This is because the "orbit" method attempts to define the most likely set or combination of K_m and V_m values for the patient, given the dosing history and measured phenytoin concentration.

Figure 14.2 can only be used for adult patients, and the phenytoin concentrations used in plotting lines A and B must represent normal plasma protein–binding conditions. Figure 14.2 also requires that the phenytoin concentration be an average steady-state value.

Question #3 *Calculate a loading dose that would rapidly increase S.B.'s plasma phenytoin concentration from 8 to 15 mg/L.*

Equation 14.28 can be used to calculate an incremental loading dose. If V is 45.5 L (70 kg × 0.65 L/kg), $S = 0.92$, and $F = 1.0$, the loading dose required to increase S.B.'s plasma concentration from 8 to 15 mg/L would be:

$$\text{Loading dose} = \frac{(V)(C_{desired} - C_{observed})}{(S)(F)}$$

$$= \frac{(45.5 \text{ L})(15 \text{ mg/L} - 8 \text{ mg/L})}{(0.92)(1)}$$

$$= 346 \text{ mg of phenytoin sodium}$$

This loading dose should be given in addition to the new maintenance dose of 350 mg/d so that his total dose today will be approximately 700 mg (a new maintenance dose of 350 mg plus the small loading dose of 350 mg).

Administration of the loading dose will result in a more rapid increase in the phenytoin concentration into the desired concentration range while S.B. is receiving the new maintenance dose. If 1 week after the loading dose and starting on the new maintenance dose the plasma concentration is less than 10 mg/L, it would suggest that the maintenance dose should again be adjusted. If a loading dose is not given and, at the end of 1 week, the plasma concentration is less than 10 mg/L, it would be difficult to determine why the level was low. One possibility would be that the phenytoin level has not yet reached steady state, and further accumulation on the new regimen would result in levels near our target of 15 mg/L. A second possibility is that our estimates are incorrect, and steady state has been achieved at a lower-than-expected concentration. In this case, an adjustment in the maintenance dose would be appropriate. Administration of the small or incremental loading dose limits the time when the patient has a low phenytoin level and decreases the risk of a seizure. In addition, it helps us to determine in a relatively short time (1-2 weeks) whether we have selected a reasonable maintenance dose for S.B. that, with time, may require at most only minor adjustments as true steady state is achieved.

> **Question #4** *L.C., a 40-year-old, 80-kg man who has been receiving 300 mg/d of phenytoin sodium for the past 3 weeks (21 days), has a phenytoin level of 14 mg/L. Is this reported level likely to represent a steady-state concentration?*

If phenytoin was eliminated according to first-order pharmacokinetics, 21 days would have been more than enough time for steady state to have been achieved based on a half-life of 15 to 24 hours.

Phenytoin, however, exhibits capacity-limited metabolism; therefore, the time required to achieve steady state is frequently much longer than one would estimate using first-order pharmacokinetic principles. Equation 14.24 should be used to calculate the minimum number of days phenytoin must be administered before it can be reasonably assumed that the measured concentration represents a steady-state level. First, the daily dose of phenytoin should be normalized to 262.5 mg for a 70-kg individual using a ratio of 300 mg/80 kg in proportion to $\times$ mg/70 kg:

$$\left[\frac{300\,mg}{80\,kg} \right] [70\,kg] = 262.5\,mg$$

When this value is placed into Equation 14.24 along with an assumed F of 1 and an S of 0.92, the 90% t value can be calculated.

$$\begin{aligned} 90\%\, t &= \frac{[115 + (35)(C)][C]}{(S)(F)(\text{Dose/day})} \\ &= \frac{[115 + (35)(14)][14]}{(0.92)(1)(262.5)} \\ &= 35\ \text{days} \end{aligned}$$

The calculated 90% t value of 35 days is longer than the actual duration of therapy (21 days), suggesting that steady state may not yet have been achieved. If an additional loading dose was administered within the first 21 days of therapy, or if the K_m value is larger than expected, then the plasma level obtained at 21 days may actually represent a steady-state concentration. Owing to this uncertainty, additional phenytoin plasma concentrations should be monitored to detect possible accumulation of phenytoin into a potentially toxic concentration range. Although the phenytoin concentration may not yet be at steady state, it is unlikely that the phenytoin concentrations will change rapidly, even if it is not yet at steady state. Therefore, some time (eg, 2 weeks or so) could be allowed before additional levels are obtained. In addition, the patient should be educated about the potential side effects so that if they do occur, their healthcare provider can be contacted.

> **Question #5**   *A.P., a 52-year-old, 60-kg woman, received a 1,000-mg IV loading dose of phenytoin followed by a daily maintenance regimen of 300 mg. Eight days following the initial loading dose, A.P.'s plasma phenytoin level was 11 mg/L. Should her dose be adjusted at this time to achieve the desired phenytoin concentration of 10 to 20 mg/L?*

According to Equation 14.32, the 1,000-mg loading dose administered to A.P. should have resulted in an initial concentration of 23.5 mg/L:

$$C_0 = \frac{(S)(F)(\text{Loading dose})}{V} \qquad \text{(Eq. 14.32)}$$

$$= \frac{(0.92)(1)(1,000\,\text{mg})}{(0.65\,\text{L/kg})(60\,\text{kg})}$$

$$= \frac{920\,\text{mg}}{39\,\text{L}}$$

$$= 23.5\,\text{mg/L}$$

Therefore, the plasma concentration of 11 mg/L 8 days later has declined significantly, and given the nonlinearity of phenytoin, it is unlikely to represent steady state. The concentration of 11 mg/L will probably continue to decline if the maintenance regimen remains at 300 mg/d.

The first step in calculating the new maintenance dose would be to estimate the rate at which the body had been eliminating phenytoin as it declined from the initial concentration of 23.5 mg/L to the observed concentration of 11 mg/L. The amount eliminated per unit of time can be calculated using Equation 14.33, which considers the rate of phenytoin administration $(S)(F)(\text{Dose}/\tau)$ and the net change in the amount of phenytoin in the body $[(C_2 - C_1)(V)/t]$.

$$\frac{\text{Amount eliminated}}{t} = (S)(F)(\text{Dose}/\tau) - \left[\frac{(C_2 - C_1)(V)}{t}\right] \qquad \text{(Eq. 14.33)}$$

In this equation, C_1 is the initial phenytoin concentration, which is either predicted or measured, and C_2 is the second phenytoin concentration; t is the time interval between C_1 and C_2. It should be pointed out that both C_1 and C_2 phenytoin concentrations should represent the same plasma protein–binding circumstances as V in Equation 14.32 (ie, 0.65 L/kg). As suggested earlier, the author recommends calculating a plasma concentration that represents normal binding conditions rather than correcting the volume of distribution for the altered plasma binding. Assuming the phenytoin levels represent normal plasma binding, the elimination rate for phenytoin during this 8-day interval would be 337 mg/d of phenytoin acid, which corresponds to approximately 366 mg/d of phenytoin sodium.

$$\frac{\text{Amount eliminated}}{t} = (S)(F)(\text{Dose}/\tau) - \left[\frac{(C_2 - C_1)(V)}{t}\right]$$

$$= [(0.92)(1)(300\text{mg}/\text{d})] - \left[\frac{(11\,\text{mg}/\text{L} - 23.5\,\text{mg}/\text{L})(39\,\text{L})}{8\,\text{days}}\right]$$

$$= 276\ \text{mg}/\text{d} - [-61\ \text{mg}/\text{d}]$$

$$= 276\ \text{mg}/\text{d} + 61\ \text{mg}/\text{d}$$

$$= \frac{337\ \text{mg}}{\text{day of phenytoin acid}}$$

or

$$= 366\ \text{mg}/\text{d of sodium phenytoin}\left(\frac{337\,\text{mg}/\text{d}}{0.92}\right)$$

This elimination rate represents an average of A.P.'s actual elimination rate (>366 mg/d when her phenytoin concentration was 23 mg/L and <366 mg/d when her phenytoin concentration was 11 mg/L). Therefore, a dose of approximately 360 mg/d should maintain an average phenytoin concentration somewhere between 23 and 11 mg/L.

Question #6 *T.L., a 70-kg patient, initially received a phenytoin loading dose to achieve a concentration of 20 mg/L and then received the usual maintenance dose of 300 mg/d of phenytoin oral capsules. Ten days later, he had CNS symptoms that were consistent with phenytoin toxicity. A level was drawn and reported as 26 mg/L. What would be a new maintenance dose that would eventually achieve a $C_{ss\ ave}$ of approximately 15 mg/L?*

This problem is similar to the previous example. First, using a volume of distribution of 45.5 L (0.65 L/kg × 70 kg) and Equation 14.33, we can calculate the average rate of phenytoin elimination as the level rose from 20 to 26 mg/L over the 10 days of treatment.

$$\frac{\text{Amount eliminated}}{t} = (S)(F)(\text{Dose}/\tau) - \left[\frac{(C_2 - C_1)(V)}{t}\right]$$

$$= [(0.92)(1)(300\,\text{mg}/\text{d})] - \left[\frac{(26\ \text{mg}/\text{L} - 20\ \text{mg}/\text{L})(45.5\,\text{L})}{10\ \text{day}}\right]$$

$$= 276\ \text{mg}/\text{d} - [27.3\,\text{mg}/\text{d}]$$

$$= 248.7\ \text{mg}/\text{d of phenytoin acid}$$

If, as in the previous example, we administered 248.7 mg/day of phenytoin acid, the final steady-state level would probably be about 23 mg/L or halfway between the initial concentration of 20 mg/L and the level at 10 days of 26 mg/L. In this case, the desired steady-state phenytoin concentration is not between C_1 and C_2; thus, additional steps are required to estimate the new maintenance dose that will achieve a $C_{ss\,ave}$ between 10 and 20 mg/L. Using the amount eliminated per unit of time and the average of C_1 and C_2 in the following equation, we can approximate the patient's V_m.

$$V_m = \frac{\left[\dfrac{\text{Amount eliminated}}{t}\right]\left[K_m + \left(\dfrac{C_1 + C_2}{2}\right)\right]}{\left(\dfrac{C_1 + C_2}{2}\right)} \qquad \text{(Eq. 14.34)}$$

Assuming a K_m value of 4 mg/L, a V_m of 292 mg/d of acid phenytoin is calculated.

$$V_m = \frac{[248.7\,\text{mg/d}]\left[4\,\text{mg/L} + \left(\dfrac{20\,\text{mg/L} + 26\,\text{mg/L}}{2}\right)\right]}{\left(\dfrac{20\,\text{mg/L} + 26\,\text{mg/L}}{2}\right)}$$

$$= \frac{[248.7\,\text{mg/d}][27\,\text{mg/L}]}{(23\,\text{mg/L})}$$

$$= 292\,\text{mg/d}$$

This new V_m of 292 mg/d of acid phenytoin and the assumed K_m value of 4 mg/L would then be used in Equation 14.31 to calculate the new phenytoin maintenance dose of 250 mg/d of phenytoin administered as the sodium salt.

$$\text{Dose} = \frac{(V_m)(C_{ss\,ave})(\tau)}{(K_m + C_{ss\,ave})(S)(F)}$$

$$= \frac{(292\,\text{mg/d})(15\,\text{mg/L})(1\,\text{day})}{(4\,\text{mg/L} + 15\,\text{mg/L})(0.92)(1)}$$

$$= 250\,\text{mg of phenytoin sodium}$$

This approach is more uncertain than the example in Question 5 for several reasons. In both cases, we had to assume a volume of distribution and there is likely to be some assay error in the reported drug concentrations. However, in this second case, we assumed a value for K_m and, more importantly, we are extrapolating to a new concentration that is outside the concentration range we used to estimate the rate of phenytoin elimination. Given the nonlinear metabolism of phenytoin, any errors are compounded in the extrapolation to a new steady-state concentration range.

In addition, if the following three rules are not met, Equations 14.33 and 14.34 are less likely to accurately predict the patient's rate of metabolism, V_m, and any subsequent maintenance dose adjustments.

1. The time between C_1 and C_2 should be 3 days or more.
2. C_2 should be $\leq 2 \times C_1$ if the plasma concentrations are rising. C_2 should be $\geq 1/2$ of C_1 if the plasma concentrations are declining.
3. The phenytoin dose, dosage form, and route of administration should be consistent.

If any of the these rules is broken, Equations 14.33 and 14.34 do not necessarily become invalid, but their accuracy is less than the usual uncertainties associated with phenytoin dose adjustments.

Question #7 *If T.L.'s phenytoin dose was held, what would be the expected time required for T.L. to have his phenytoin level decline to approximately 15 mg/L?*

If T.L.'s dose is held, the decay time can be calculated using Equation 14.25.

$$t = \frac{\left[K_m \left(\ln \frac{C_1}{C_2} \right) \right] + (C_1 - C_2)}{\dfrac{V_m}{V}}$$

If we substitute our literature estimates of 45.5 L for volume of distribution (0.65 L/kg $\times$ 70 kg), 4 mg/L for K_m, and our patient-specific estimate of V_m, the time required to decline to 15 mg/L would be 2 days.

$$t = \frac{\left[K_m \left(\ln \frac{C_1}{C_2} \right) \right] + (C_1 - C_2)}{\dfrac{V_m}{V}}$$

$$t = \frac{\left[4\,\text{mg/L} \left(\ln \frac{26\,\text{mg/L}}{15\,\text{mg/L}} \right) \right] + (26\,\text{mg/L} - 15\,\text{mg/L})}{\dfrac{292\,\text{mg/d}}{45.5\,\text{L}}}$$

$$t = \frac{[4\,\text{mg/L}\,(0.55)] + (11\,\text{mg/L})}{6.4\,\text{mg/L/d}}$$

$$= 2\,\text{days}$$

Note that because both C_1 and C_2 are well above our estimate of K_m (4 mg/L), we could have estimated the daily drop in phenytoin concentration by V_m/V because, at these concentrations, the rate of metabolism is relatively fixed at a value approaching V_m. Therefore, this simple method would suggest that the phenytoin concentration should decrease by approximately 6.4 mg/L in 1 day (292 mg/d/45.5 L). Therefore, in 2 days, the phenytoin concentration would fall by 12.8 mg/L, a value close to our desired decline of 11 mg/L (ie, 26-15 mg/L). In either case, it is important that, for our estimates to be reasonably correct, the patient does not continue to receive (or absorb from previously administered oral doses) additional phenytoin. In any case, the patient should be monitored closely. If after only 1 day the symptoms of phenytoin toxicity have cleared, it might be appropriate to initiate the new maintenance dose at that time (to avoid the risk of seizures). If after holding the dose for 2 days the symptoms are still present, it would be appropriate to obtain another phenytoin level to confirm that the levels are declining as we expected. In addition, if the patient was at "high seizure risk" and the toxicity symptoms were not considered serious, many clinicians might elect to simply reduce the maintenance dose and allow the levels to decline slowly.

Question #8 *R.M., a 32-year-old, 80-kg nonobese man, had been taking 300 mg/d of acid phenytoin; however, his dose was increased to 350 mg/d of acid phenytoin, because his seizures were poorly controlled and because his plasma concentration was only 8 mg/L. Now he complains of minor CNS side effects, and his reported plasma phenytoin concentration is 20 mg/L. Renal and hepatic function are normal. Assume that both of the reported plasma concentrations represent steady-state levels and that R.M. has complied with the prescribed dosing regimens. Calculate R.M.'s apparent V_m and K_m and a new daily dose of phenytoin that will result in a steady-state level of approximately 15 mg/L.*

The relationship between daily dose and C_{ss} can be made linear by plotting daily dose (R_A) versus daily dose divided by $C_{ss\ ave}$ (clearance) for at least two steady-state plasma levels. The graph for R.M. is plotted in Figure 14.3, in which the rate-in intercept (390 mg/d) is V_m and the slope of the line (-2.5 mg/L) is the negative value of K_m.

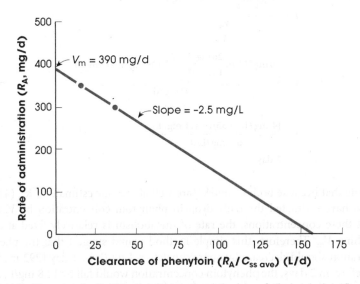

FIGURE 14.3 The rate of administration (R_A) or the daily dose of phenytoin (mg/d) versus the clearance of phenytoin ($R_A/C_{ss\ ave}$, L/d) is plotted for two or more different daily doses of phenytoin. A straight line of the best fit is drawn through the points plotted. The intercept on the rate of administration axis is V_m (mg/d), and the slope of the line is the negative value of K_m.

Using these values, the daily dose of phenytoin that will achieve a steady-state level of 15 mg/L can be calculated using Equation 14.31.

$$\text{Dose} = \frac{(V_m)(C_{ss\,ave})(\tau)}{(K_m + C_{ss\,ave})(S)(F)}$$
$$= \frac{(390\ \text{mg/d})(15\ \text{mg/L})(1\,\text{d})}{(2.5\ \text{mg/L} + 15\ \text{mg/L})(1)(1)}$$
$$= 334\ \text{mg}$$

The most convenient dose for a calculated value of 334 mg/d, administered as acid phenytoin, would be 325 mg/d, which could be administered as the suspension. The suspension is available as 125 mg/5 mL (25 mg/mL) and, therefore, the volume to administer would be 13 mL. The suspension should be shaken vigorously and measured accurately to ensure that the proper dose is delivered. In addition, the suspension is not recommended to be given on a once-daily basis, and the dose should be divided into at least a twice-daily regimen (ie, 162.5 mg or 6.5 mL twice daily).

If, for the convenience of once-daily dosing, the acid phenytoin dose was to be converted to a sodium phenytoin extended-release product, the following equation could be used to calculate an equivalent dose (also see Bioavailability [F]: Chemical Form [S] in Chapter "Pharmacokinetic Processes and Parameters"):

$$\frac{\text{Dose of new}}{\text{dosage form}} = \frac{\begin{array}{c}\text{Amount of drug absorbed}\\ \text{from current dosage form}\end{array}}{(S)(F)\text{ of new dosage form}} \qquad \textbf{(Eq. 14.35)}$$

$$\text{Slope} = \frac{R_{A1} - R_{A2}}{\left(\dfrac{R_{A1}}{C_{ss\,ave_1}}\right) - \left(\dfrac{R_{A2}}{C_{ss\,ave_2}}\right)}$$

Assuming S to be 0.92 and F to be 1 for phenytoin sodium, the equivalent dose would be 363 mg.

$$\frac{\text{Dose of new}}{\text{dosage form}} = \frac{334\ \text{mg}}{(0.92)(1)\text{ of new dosage form}}$$
$$= 363\ \text{mg of phenytoin sodium}$$

This dose might be rounded off to 350 mg/d (300 mg alternating with 400 mg given as 100-mg capsules), or 360 mg/d given as three of the 100-mg capsules and two of the 30-mg capsules.

If it were decided to round off the dose to the average dose of 350 mg/d, the expected $C_{ss\,ave}$ can be calculated using Equation 14.15:

$$C_{ss\,ave} = \frac{(K_m)[(S)(F)(Dose/\tau)]}{V_m - [(S)(F)(Dose/\tau)]}$$

Using the patient-specific K_m value of 2.5 mg/L and V_m of 390 mg/d of acid phenytoin for R.M. obtained from the graph in Figure 14.3, we calculate a $C_{ss\,ave}$ on 350 mg/d of phenytoin sodium of 11.8 mg/L.

$$C_{ss\,ave} = \frac{(2.5\,mg/L)[(0.92)(1)(350\,mg/1\,day)]}{390\,mg/d - [(0.92)(1)(350\,mg/1\,day)]}$$
$$= 11.8\,mg/L$$

Assuming the concentration of 11.8 mg/L is satisfactory, the patient could be converted from the current acid phenytoin to phenytoin sodium extended-release capsules. It is important to remember that phenytoin products are not equivalent, and if a change in the dosage form is to be considered, a careful discussion with both the patient and the patient's provider should take place before any changes are made. It is also recommended that follow-up of phenytoin levels be obtained to ensure that the conversion from one dosage form to another results in the expected outcome.

An alternate approach to plotting the data for R.M. would be to calculate the negative value of K_m using Equation 14.36:

$$-K_m = \frac{R_1 - R_2}{\left(\dfrac{R_1}{C_{ss_1}}\right) - \left(\dfrac{R_2}{C_{ss_2}}\right)} \qquad \text{(Eq. 14.36)}$$

where R_1 and R_2 represent the first and second maintenance doses, respectively. C_{ss_1} and C_{ss_2} represent the steady-state concentrations produced by these doses. Again, assuming S and F to be 1.0, a value of -2.5 mg/L is calculated.

$$-K_m = \frac{R_1 - R_2}{\left(\dfrac{R_1}{C_{ss_1}}\right) - \left(\dfrac{R_2}{C_{ss_2}}\right)}$$
$$= \frac{300\,mg/d - 350\,mg/d}{\left(\dfrac{300\,mg/d}{8\,mg/L}\right) - \left(\dfrac{350\,mg/d}{20\,mg/L}\right)}$$
$$= \frac{-50\,mg/d}{(37.5\,L/d) - (17.5\,L/d)}$$
$$= -2.5\,mg/L$$

The value of 2.5 mg/L can then be used in Equation 14.30 with either of the maintenance doses and the corresponding steady-state levels to calculate V_m:

$$V_m = \frac{(S)(F)(\text{Dose}/\tau)(K_m + C_{ss\ ave})}{(C_{ss\ ave})}$$

$$= \frac{(1)(1)(300\ \text{mg/d})(2.5\ \text{mg/L} + 8\ \text{mg/L})}{(8\ \text{mg/L})}$$

$$= 393.75\ \text{mg/d} \approx 390\ \text{mg/d}$$

With only two data points, the calculated and graphically determined values for K_m and V_m should be exactly the same. Small differences sometimes occur, however, because of differences in mechanical drawing skills or rounding off errors in the calculation.

Question #9   *How long will it take for R.M.'s phenytoin concentration of 20 mg/L to decline to 15 mg/L?*

As with Question 7, the important clinical decision is whether to hold the dose and allow the phenytoin levels to decline as rapidly as possible or to start a new lower dosing regimen and let the phenytoin concentrations decline slowly with time. The decision would be based on a balance between the severity of the phenytoin side effects and R.M.'s seizure risk. The phenytoin half-life will be of no value in predicting the time required for the plasma concentration to decay because the apparent half-life will change as the plasma concentration changes.

The time required for the phenytoin plasma concentration to fall from an initial concentration (C_1) to a lower concentration (C_2), if we hold the dose, can be calculated using Equation 14.25.

$$t = \frac{\left[K_m\left(\ln\dfrac{C_1}{C_2}\right)\right] + (C_1 - C_2)}{\dfrac{V_m}{V}}$$

For R.M., who has a volume of distribution of 52 L (0.65 L/kg × 80 kg), a V_m of 390 mg/d, and a K_m of 2.5 mg/L, the time required for the initial plasma concentration of 20 mg/L to decline to 15 mg/L will be about 0.76 days:

$$t = \frac{\left[K_m\left(\ln\dfrac{C_1}{C_2}\right)\right] + (C_1 - C_2)}{\dfrac{V_m}{V}}$$

$$= \frac{\left[2.5\,\text{mg/L}\left(\ln\dfrac{20\,\text{mg/L}}{15\,\text{mg/L}}\right)\right] + (20\,\text{mg/L} - 15\,\text{mg/L})}{\dfrac{390\ \text{mg/d}}{52\ \text{L}}}$$

$$= 0.76\ \text{days}$$

This rate of decline assumes that phenytoin will not continue to be absorbed from the GI tract for a significant period following the discontinuation of the drug. In the author's experience, however, the initial rate of decline for 1 to 3 days is often less than expected because of prolonged absorption.[46,109]

Question #10   *E. W., a 56-year-old, 60-kg woman, has chronic renal failure and a seizure disorder. She undergoes hemodialysis treatments 3 times a week, has a serum albumin of 3.3 g/dL, and takes 300 mg/d of phenytoin oral capsules. Her reported steady-state plasma phenytoin concentration is 5 mg/L. What would be her phenytoin concentration if she had a normal serum albumin concentration and normal renal function? Should her daily phenytoin dose be increased?*

It is critical to carefully evaluate measured phenytoin plasma concentrations in uremic patients because plasma protein binding is altered in these individuals. In patients with normal renal function, about 90% of the measured plasma phenytoin concentration is bound to albumin and 10% is free (fu normal binding = 0.1).[19-21,27] Because binding affinity and albumin concentrations are decreased in uremic patients, the fraction of the total phenytoin concentration that is unbound or free in patients with very poor renal function increases from 0.1 to a range of 0.2 to 0.35[19,23,27] (see also Figures 1.3 through 1.5, and Desired Plasma Concentration in Chapter "Pharmacokinetic Processes and Parameters").

Because the fraction free (fu) for phenytoin is increased in uremic individuals, lower plasma concentrations will produce pharmacologic effects that are equivalent to those produced by higher levels in nonuremic individuals. E.W.'s case can be used as an illustration.

Using E.W.'s serum albumin of 3.3 g/dL and her phenytoin concentration of 5 mg/L (Dialysis Patient's Phenytoin Concentration with Altered Plasma Binding) in Equation 14.3, a phenytoin concentration of 11.9 mg/L is calculated.

$$\frac{\text{Phenytoin concentration}}{\text{normal plasma binding}} = \frac{\text{Dialysis patient's phenytoin concentration with altered plasma binding}}{\left[(0.9)(0.48)\left(\dfrac{\text{Patient's serum albumin}}{4.4 \text{ g/dL}}\right) + 0.1\right]}$$

$$= \frac{5 \text{ mg/L}}{\left[(0.9)(0.48)\left(\dfrac{3.3 \text{ g/dL}}{4.4 \text{ g/dL}}\right) + 0.1\right]}$$

$$= \frac{5 \text{ mg/L}}{0.42}$$

$$= 11.9 \text{ mg/L} \approx 12 \text{ mg/L}$$

Therefore, E.W.'s measured plasma phenytoin concentration of 5 mg/L with altered binding is comparable to a concentration of 12 mg/L in a patient with normal plasma binding. That is, we would expect the reported concentration of 5 mg/L to have the same unbound or free phenytoin concentration as a concentration of 12 mg/L, which represents normal plasma binding. The usually accepted therapeutic range for phenytoin in patients with normal binding is 10 to 20 mg/L, and E.W.'s adjusted or normal binding concentration of 12 mg/L would be expected to correspond to the low end of this range. If E.W.'s seizure disorder is well controlled, no adjustment in the maintenance dose is necessary, even though the reported concentration of 5 mg/L appears to be well below the usual "therapeutic range." However, if seizures are poorly controlled and phenytoin doses must be adjusted, the comparable plasma concentration for a patient with normal plasma binding (12 mg/L) should be used in all calculations because the values for phenytoin parameters reported in the literature were determined in patients with normal plasma protein binding.

Question #11 *Is it necessary to make dose adjustments or to administer a phenytoin replacement dose following dialysis?*

Using the principles outlined in Estimating Drug Dialyzability under Dialysis of Drugs in Chapter "Drug Dosing in Kidney Disease and Dialysis," it can be seen that the unbound volume of distribution is very large.

$$\text{Unbound volume of distribution} = \frac{V}{fu} \qquad \text{(Eq. 14.37)}$$

$$= \frac{0.65 \, \text{L/kg}}{0.1}$$

$$= 6.5 \, \text{L/kg}$$

Given that the unbound volume of distribution is 6.5 L/kg or 390 L (6.5 L/kg × 60 kg), a very small percentage of the total body phenytoin would be removed during hemodialysis. In addition, there are studies supporting this prediction.[23,24,113] It is also known that dialysis does not change the protein-binding characteristics of the uremic patient.[23,24,113] Therefore, doses should not be adjusted for E.W. based on dialysis. Even though the binding has been decreased, it is important to remember that the unbound concentration for the uremic patient is not affected by the decreased albumin, nor the decreased affinity of phenytoin for albumin. In acute renal failure, changes in plasma protein binding occur within a few days after the development of acute renal failure.[114] Conversely, there is some evidence that following a renal transplant, the plasma protein binding of phenytoin increases rapidly over the first 2 to 4 postoperative days and is almost normal 2 weeks after a successful transplant.[25]

Question #12 *Mr. T.B. is an 80-kg man in the intensive care unit receiving chronic renal replacement therapy (CRRT). His serum albumin is 4.2, and his serum creatinine is 3.8. His CRRT effluent flow is 2 L/hr (1 L/hr of ultrafiltration and 1 L/hr of dialysate). The patient is receiving phenytoin for a seizure disorder. At the start of CRRT, his phenytoin level was 9.8 mg/L. In addition to T.B.'s phenytoin maintenance dose, should he receive an additional CRRT phenytoin replacement dose?*

The answer is possibly. Unlike hemodialysis and plasmapheresis, CRRT does remove some phenytoin. Data suggest that the concentration of phenytoin in the CRRT effluent is approximately equal to the unbound phenytoin concentration in plasma.[115] The amount removed by CRRT would depend on the target unbound phenytoin concentration and the CRRT effluent flow rate. Guideline recommended CRRT effluent flow rates for acute kidney injury range from 20 to 25 mL/kg/hr and is continuous until the CRRT is discontinued.[116] In most cases, CRRT is a temporary procedure and is seldom continued for more than a few days to a week.

In order to calculate T.B.'s phenytoin removal by CRRT, we first need to estimate his unbound phenytoin concentration. We could use the reported phenytoin level of 9.8 mg/L and then one of the equations to correct the reported value to a normal binding value (eg, Equations 14.2 and 14.3). The difficulty is that if T.B.'s renal dysfunction is recent Equation 14.3 for patients on dialysis may not be appropriate, and in addition, as previously stated, estimating corrected phenytoin concentrations in critical care patients is difficult. A simpler approach might be to consider that an unbound concentration of 1 to 2 mg/L is associated with normal binding concentrations of 10 to 20 mg/L. Using the middle of the usual targeted unbound concentration of 1.5, we could use Equation 14.38 to calculate a daily phenytoin CRRT replacement dose.

$$\text{Amount of phenytoin removed by CRRT} = (C_{UNBOUND})(\text{Effluent flow L/hr})(\text{Number of hours})$$

$$\text{(Eq. 14.38)}$$

Substituting 1.5 mg/L for the $C_{UNBOUND}$, 2 L/hr for the effluent flow, and 24 hours for the number of hours in a day, the amount removed per day would be 72 mg.

$$\text{Amount of phenytoin removed by CRRT} = (1.5\text{mg/L})\ (2\ \text{L/hr})\ (24\ \text{hr})$$

$$= 72\ \text{mg/d}$$

Although 72 mg is not a large amount, it could be significant if CRRT is to be continued for several days. Because the duration of CRRT is uncertain, it would be logical to add approximately 70 mg to T.B.'s daily maintenance dose and to adjust the CRRT replacement dose if the effluent flow rate is changed or to discontinue the replacement dose if CRRT is discontinued.

Question #13   *I.A. is a 52-year-old, 77-kg man with chronic renal failure who is receiving hemodialysis 3 times a week. Because of a seizure disorder, he has been receiving 300 mg of extended-release phenytoin sodium each evening for the past year. He has had three seizures over the past year and one in the past month. His phenytoin concentration has been reported to be 3 mg/L on several occasions. His serum albumin is 2.7 g/dL, and his SCr fluctuates between 3 and 5 mg/dL. Should I.A. have his phenytoin dose increased? What would you recommend?*

Although a Cl_{Cr} of more than 10 mL/min can be calculated using the creatinine clearance equations, it would not be appropriate to use these equations. When a patient is receiving any type of dialysis, the creatinine clearance equations are invalid (see Creatinine Clearance [Cl_{Cr}] in Chapter "Drug Dosing in Kidney Disease and Dialysis"). Therefore, to calculate I.A.'s phenytoin concentration that represents normal plasma, we should use Equation 14.3 as he is a dialysis patient.

$$\frac{\text{Phenytoin concentration}}{\text{normal plasma binding}} = \frac{\text{Dialysis patient's phenytoin concentration with altered plasma binding}}{\left[(0.9)(0.48)\left(\dfrac{\text{Patient's serum albumin}}{4.4\,\text{g/dL}}\right)\right] + 0.1}$$

$$= \frac{3\,\text{mg/L}}{\left[(0.9)(0.48)\left(\dfrac{2.7\,\text{g/dL}}{4.4\,\text{g/dL}}\right)\right] + 0.1}$$

$$= \frac{3\,\text{mg/L}}{[0.265] + 0.1}$$

$$= \frac{3\,\text{mg/L}}{0.365}$$

$$= 8.2\,\text{mg/L or} \approx 8\,\text{mg/L}$$

The normal plasma-binding concentration of 8 mg/L is below the usual target concentration range of 10 to 20 mg/L, and he is experiencing breakthrough seizures. Assuming I.A. should have his concentration increased to prevent further seizures, we will need to calculate his V_m using an assumed average value of 4 mg/L for K_m and the normal plasma-binding concentration of 8 mg/L in Equation 14.30 to calculate V_m:

$$V_m = \frac{(S)(F)(\text{Dose}/\tau)(K_m + C_{ss\,ave})}{(C_{ss\,ave})}$$

$$V_m = \frac{(0.92)(1)(300\,\text{mg/d})(4\,\text{mg/L} + 8\,\text{mg/L})}{(8\,\text{mg/L})}$$

$$= 414\,\text{mg/d}$$

Note again in this equation that the Phenytoin Concentration Normal Plasma Binding of 8 mg/L is used and not the observed value of 3 mg/L, which represents altered binding.

This revised V_m estimate of 414 mg/d of acid phenytoin, along with our assumed K_m, can then be used in Equation 14.31 to calculate a new maintenance dose of 355 mg/d of phenytoin sodium to achieve a target level of 15 mg/L.

$$\text{Dose} = \frac{(V_m)(C_{ss\,ave})(\tau)}{(K_m + C_{ss\,ave})(S)(F)}$$

$$\text{Dose} = \frac{(414\,\text{mg/d})(15\,\text{mg/L})(1\,\text{d})}{(4\,\text{mg/L} + 15\,\text{mg/L})(0.92)(1)}$$

$$= 355\,\text{mg}$$

If the patient is started on this new regimen of 350 mg/d of phenytoin sodium (probably as 300 mg on odd days and 400 mg on even days), it will require some time to accumulate to the new steady-state concentration. To avoid the prolonged period of accumulation toward the new steady state, a small loading dose could be administered. This incremental loading dose can be calculated using Equation 14.28.

$$\text{Loading dose} = \frac{(V)(C_{desired} - C_{observed})}{(S)(F)}$$

Again the normal binding concentration of 8 mg/L will be used for $C_{observed}$, and the V represents the usual value of 0.65 L/kg or 50 L for this 77-kg nonobese patient (0.65 L/kg × 77 kg).

$$\text{Loading dose} = \frac{(50\,\text{L})(15\,\text{mg/L} - 8\,\text{mg/L})}{(0.92)(1)}$$
$$= 380 \text{ mg or about 400 mg}$$

This small loading dose of 400 mg of phenytoin sodium, if given orally, may not increase I.A.'s phenytoin level to 15 mg/L, but should increase it to above 10 mg/L and shorten the time required for I.A. to achieve his new steady-state concentration on 350 mg/d. Remember that I.A. should receive both his loading dose and his new maintenance dose so that today he will receive a total of about 700 or 800 mg, probably as 300 or 400 mg increments separated by at least 2 hours.

Question #14 *What would you expect the measured or observed phenytoin concentration to be in I.A. when he achieves the new steady-state concentration?*

The value reported by the laboratory can be calculated by placing the targeted normal plasma-binding concentration of 15 mg/L in Equation 14.3 and solving for the Patient's Phenytoin Concentration with Altered Plasma Binding.

$$\frac{\text{Phenytoin concentration}}{\text{normal plasma binding}} = \frac{\text{Dialysis patient's phenytoin concentration with altered plasma binding}}{\left[(0.9)(0.48)\left(\dfrac{\text{Patient's serum albumin}}{4.4\,\text{g/dL}}\right) + 0.1\right]}$$

$$15\,\text{mg/L} = \frac{\text{Dialysis patient's phenytoin concentration with altered plasma binding}}{\left[(0.9)(0.48)\left(\dfrac{2.7\,\text{g/dL}}{4.4\,\text{g/dL}}\right) + 0.1\right]}$$

$$15\,\text{mg/L} = \frac{\text{Dialysis patient's phenytoin concentration with altered plasma binding}}{0.365}$$

$$(15\,\text{mg/L})(0.365) = \text{Dialysis patient's phenytoin concentration with altered plasma binding}$$

$$5.5\,\text{mg/L} = \text{Dialysis patient's phenytoin concentration with altered plasma binding}$$

This phenytoin concentration of 5.5 mg/L for I.A. would be expected to have the same unbound or free phenytoin concentration as a level of 15 mg/L in a patient with normal binding.

It might also be reasonable to provide the clinicians caring for I.A. with a "therapeutic range" that they could use to compare to the assayed or reported phenytoin concentration. Equations 14.6 and 14.7 could be used to calculate a "therapeutic range" for I.A. that is approximately 3.5 to 7 mg/L.

Using Equation 14.6:

$$\text{Patient's therapeutic range with low albumin and on dialysis that would be equal to 10 mg/L} =$$

$$10\,\text{mg/L} \times \left[\left(0.9 \times 0.48 \times \frac{\text{Patient's serum albumin}}{4.4\,\text{g/dL}} \right) + 0.1 \right]$$

$$\text{Patient's therapeutic range with low albumin and on dialysis that would be equal to 10 mg/L} =$$

$$10\,\text{mg/L} \times \left[\left(0.9 \times 0.48 \times \frac{2.7\,\text{g/dL}}{4.4\,\text{g/dL}} \right) + 0.1 \right]$$

$$\text{Patient's therapeutic range with low albumin and on dialysis that would be equal to 10 mg/L} =$$

$$10\,\text{mg/L} \times [0.365]$$

$$\text{Patient's therapeutic range with low albumin and on dialysis that would be equal to 10 mg/L} = 3.65\,\text{mg/L}$$

and using Equation 14.7:

$$\text{Patient's therapeutic range with low albumin and on dialysis that would be equal to 20 mg/L} =$$

$$20\,\text{mg/L} \times \left[\left(0.9 \times 0.48 \frac{\text{Patient's serum albumin}}{4.4\,\text{g/dL}} \right) + 0.1 \right]$$

$$\text{Patient's therapeutic range with low albumin and on dialysis that would be equal to 20 mg/L} =$$

$$20\,\text{mg/L} \times \left[\left(0.9 \times 0.48 \times \frac{2.7\,\text{g/dL}}{4.4\,\text{g/dL}} \right) + 0.1 \right]$$

$$\text{Patient's therapeutic range with low albumin and on dialysis that would be equal to 20 mg/L} =$$

$$20\,\text{mg/L} \times [0.365]$$

$$\text{Patient's therapeutic range with low albumin and on dialysis that would be equal to 20 mg/L} = 7.3\,\text{mg/L}$$

Question #15 *Because phenytoin is bound to plasma protein to a significant extent, will a substantial amount of drug be lost during plasmapheresis or plasma exchange?*

Although 90% of the phenytoin in the serum is bound to albumin, the vascular space represents only a small fraction of the total volume of distribution for phenytoin. Of the total amount of drug in the body, only 5% is within the vascular space. Because most of the phenytoin is actually in the tissue compartments, plasmapheresis or plasma volume exchange should not result in a significant loss of phenytoin from the body. Most studies indicate that somewhere between 5% and 10% of phenytoin is lost from the body during plasmapheresis.[117] Of course, if the procedure was to be repeated many times, the cumulative effect could result in a significant amount of drug loss and the requirement of a replacement dose.

Question #16   *S.T. is a 47-year-old, 60-kg man with glomerular nephritis. His creatinine clearance is reasonably good, but he has a serum albumin concentration of 2.0 g/dL. S.T. is receiving 300 mg/d of phenytoin oral capsules and has a steady-state phenytoin concentration of 6 mg/L. What would his phenytoin concentration be if his serum albumin was normal?*

The fraction of a drug concentration that is bound to plasma proteins is a function of the drug's affinity for the binding sites on the plasma protein and the number of binding sites available. The number of binding sites is proportional to the amount or concentration of plasma protein to which the drug is bound. Phenytoin is an acidic drug and appears to be bound primarily to albumin.[20] The relationship between a phenytoin concentration that is observed (Patient's Phenytoin Concentration with Altered Plasma Binding) when a patient has a low serum albumin relative to the phenytoin concentration that would be observed if the serum albumin were normal is described by Equation 14.2 (also see Desired Plasma Concentration in Chapter "Pharmacokinetic Processes and Parameters").

$$\frac{\text{Phenytoin concentration}}{\text{normal plasma binding}} = \frac{\text{Patient's phenytoin concentration with altered plasma binding}}{\left[0.9 \times \dfrac{\text{Patient's serum albumin}}{4.4 \text{ g/dL}} \right] + 0.1}$$

The plasma phenytoin concentration that corresponds to a concentration that would be observed if S.T.'s albumin concentration was normal is calculated as follows:

$$\frac{\text{Phenytoin concentration}}{\text{normal plasma binding}} = \frac{6 \text{ mg/L}}{\left[0.9 \times \dfrac{2.0 \text{ g/dL}}{4.4 \text{ g/dL}} \right] + 0.1}$$

$$= \frac{6 \text{ mg/L}}{0.509}$$

$$= 11.8 \text{ mg/L}$$

The Phenytoin Concentration Normal Plasma Binding value of 11.8 mg/L should be used when comparing S.T.'s phenytoin concentration to the usual therapeutic range of 10 to 20 mg/L or in any of our calculations.

Question #17 *A.R., a 66-year-old, 60-kg man, was admitted to the hospital because of poor seizure control. He had been receiving 350 mg/d of phenytoin acid as an outpatient. On admission, he had a phenytoin plasma concentration of 3 mg/L. Nonadherence was suspected, and a dose of 350 mg/d as sodium phenytoin was ordered. Five days after administration, a second phenytoin level was reported as 18 mg/L. Has steady state been achieved? Is it reasonable to assume that A.R.'s V_m is close to the average values reported in the literature (ie, 7 mg/kg/d)?*

The usual guideline of three to four half-lives as the time required to achieve steady state does not hold true for phenytoin because its metabolism is capacity limited. The rate of phenytoin accumulation is the difference between the rate of metabolism and the rate of administration. Unlike drugs following first-order elimination, the rate of elimination is not proportional to the plasma concentration. Therefore, the time required to reach steady state can be prolonged. This will be especially true when the plasma concentrations are much greater than K_m. After the daily dose of 350 mg for this 60-kg patient is corrected to 408.3 mg/d for a 70-kg patient:

$$\left[\frac{350\,\text{mg}}{60\,\text{kg}}\right][70\,\text{kg}] = 408.3\,\text{mg}$$

Equation 14.24 can be used to calculate a 90% t value of 35.7 days.

$$90\%t = \frac{[115 + (35)(C)][C]}{(S)(F)(\text{Dose/day})}$$
$$= \frac{[115 + (35)(18)][18]}{(0.92)(1)(408.3)}$$
$$= 35.7\,\text{days}$$

A.R. has been receiving this maintenance regimen for only 5 days; therefore, the plasma concentration of 18 mg/L is very unlikely to represent a steady-state condition. Equation 14.33 can be used to estimate the amount of drug eliminated per day.

$$\frac{\text{Amount eliminated}}{t} = (S)(F)(\text{Dose}/\tau) - \left[\frac{(C_2 - C_1)(V)}{t}\right]$$
$$= [(0.92)(1)(350\,\text{mg/d})] - \left[\frac{(18\,\text{mg/L} - 3\,\text{mg/L})(0.65\,\text{L/kg} \times 60\,\text{kg})}{5\,\text{days}}\right]$$
$$= 322\,\text{mg/d} - \left[\frac{(15\,\text{mg/L})(39\,\text{L})}{5\,\text{days}}\right]$$
$$= 322\,\text{mg/d} - [117\,\text{mg/d}]$$
$$= 205\,\text{mg/d}$$

If a K_m of 4 mg/L is assumed, a V_m of about 283 mg/d or 4.7 mg/kg/d is calculated for A.R. using Equation 14.34.

$$V_m = \frac{\left[\dfrac{\text{Amount eliminated}}{t}\right]\left[K_m + \left(\dfrac{C_1 + C_2}{2}\right)\right]}{\left(\dfrac{C_1 + C_2}{2}\right)}$$

$$= \frac{\left[\dfrac{205\,\text{mg}}{1\,\text{day}}\right]\left[4\,\text{mg/L} + \left(\dfrac{3\,\text{mg/L} + 18\,\text{mg/L}}{2}\right)\right]}{\left(\dfrac{3\,\text{mg/L} + 18\,\text{mg/L}}{2}\right)}$$

$$= \frac{\left[\dfrac{205\,\text{mg}}{1\,\text{day}}\right]\left[4\,\text{mg/L} + 10.5\,\text{mg/L}\right]}{\left(10.5\,\text{mg/L}\right)}$$

$$= 283\,\text{mg / d}$$

or

$$= \frac{283\,\text{mg/d}}{60\,\text{kg}} = 4.7\,\text{mg/kg/d}$$

This V_m value of approximately 4.7 mg/kg/d is less than the average value of 7 mg/kg/d but is not unreasonable, and it can be used as a first approximation of a new maintenance dose. Note that even though C_2 was not $\leq 2 \times C_1$, the mass balance approach can be used as an initial adjustment, and the estimate of 4.7 mg/kg/d is probably a better guess than the literature average of 7 mg/kg/d for A.R.'s V_m.

Question #18   *Why does changing from oral to IM phenytoin for injection result in a sudden and dramatic decrease in phenytoin levels? Is there a difference between phenytoin for injection and fosphenytoin?*

Phenytoin is a relatively insoluble compound that crystallizes within the muscle following IM administration.[118] The phenytoin crystals are slowly absorbed, and the absorption rate is decreased initially. The subsequent decline in the plasma concentration of phenytoin will be more than proportional to the reduction in absorption from the IM injection because phenytoin metabolism is capacity limited. In one study,[107] a change from oral to IM administration resulted in an initial 40% to 60% decrease in the phenytoin plasma level, whereas the metabolite elimination decreased by only 16% to 20%. Therefore, the IM route of administration for phenytoin should be avoided.

Fosphenytoin for injection is a more soluble ester of phenytoin and has a much more reliable and rapid absorption pattern when administered by the IM route than phenytoin for injection. When administered by the IM route, the majority of patients achieve plasma concentrations in the therapeutic range within 30 minutes.[119] Whereas IM fosphenytoin is more rapidly absorbed than oral phenytoin, most clinicians prefer the IV route when rapid attainment of therapeutic concentrations is required, regardless of whether phenytoin for injection or fosphenytoin is used.

Question #19   *What effect does phenobarbital have on steady-state phenytoin concentrations? What other drugs might interact with phenytoin?*

Clinically, the addition of phenobarbital does not change steady-state phenytoin concentrations, although there are effects of phenobarbital on phenytoin kinetics.[91] Phenobarbital may induce the metabolism of phenytoin and thereby increase the metabolic capacity of phenytoin (ie, increase V_m). If V_m is increased, phenytoin clearance will increase, and the phenytoin concentration will decrease. However, competition between phenobarbital and phenytoin for the same metabolic enzymes could have the effect of increasing K_m. If K_m is increased, phenytoin clearance will decrease, and the phenytoin concentration will increase; therefore, there may be no consistent effect on the phenytoin concentration (see Equation 14.15).

$$C_{ss\,ave} = \frac{(K_m)[(S)(F)(Dose/\tau)]}{V_m - [(S)(F)(Dose/\tau)]}$$

Similar problems exist in evaluating the mechanism for the increased phenytoin concentrations associated with drugs, such as isoniazid, chloramphenicol, and cimetidine. In the case of isoniazid, animal data suggest that there is noncompetitive inhibition of metabolic enzymes that reduces V_m.[89] The interaction appears to be more significant in patients who are phenotypically slow acetylators of isoniazid.[89]

Valproic acid, phenylbutazone, and salicylates reportedly displace phenytoin from albumin.[32,93,120] This protein displacement would decrease the total phenytoin concentration, but not the free or unbound concentration. Assuming no change in metabolism, the result of the altered binding would be a decreased bound concentration, no change in the free concentration, an increased free fraction, and a decrease in the total concentration, which would be associated with a corresponding and equally offsetting decreased therapeutic range. While monitoring of unbound phenytoin concentrations would seem to be the most logical approach, it is still an uncommon practice.[121]

The number of drugs reported to interact with phenytoin is large (see Table 14.1). Many of the drugs are easily recognized because they are commonly reported to either increase (eg, carbamazepine) or decrease (eg, amiodarone) the metabolism of other drugs. Phenytoin is a more complex issue because due to capacity-limited metabolism, even small changes in either absorption (F) or metabolism (V_m or K_m) can result in significant changes in the final steady-state concentration of phenytoin. The potential for even small changes in metabolism to result in substantial changes in the steady-state concentration makes it difficult to predict which drugs will result in clinically significant drug-drug interaction with phenytoin (see Table 14.1).

Question #20   *Ms. A.C. is a 48-year-old Asian woman who was admitted to the emergency department for an acute seizure. She weighs 55 kg. In reviewing A.C.'s medical record, you note that her recent lab results indicated a normal serum albumin and creatinine. In addition, she has had genetic screening and is HLA-B15:02* *negative and is classified as an intermediate metabolizer for CYP2C9. What would you recommend for her phenytoin loading and maintenance dose?*

Because Ms. A.C. is HLA-B15:02 negative, phenytoin is not contraindicated, and if it is decided that it is appropriate, she can be given phenytoin. The phenytoin loading dose is a function of the target concentration and the volume of distribution, and V is not altered by genetics. Therefore, she can receive a standard 15 mg/kg or about 800 mg (15 mg/kg × 55 kg = 825 mg) loading dose. If the loading dose is administered IV as either sodium phenytoin for injection or fosphenytoin, the initial phenytoin concentration should be approximately 17 mg/L as calculated by Equation 14.32 ($S = 0.92$, $F = 1$, loading dose = 800 mg, and $V = 42$ L or 0.65 L/kg × 55 kg).

$$C_0 = \frac{(S)(F)(\text{Loading dose})}{V}$$
$$= \frac{(0.92)(1)(800\,\text{mg})}{42\,\text{L}}$$
$$= 17\,\text{mg/L}$$

Most patients are started on a phenytoin daily maintenance dose of 300 mg (~5 mg/kg/d). Because Ms. A.C. has been identified as an intermediate CYP2C9 metabolizer, her maintenance dose should be reduced by 25%, suggesting a maintenance dose of 225 mg/d. Because this specific dose would be difficult to prescribe, given the dosage forms available, and because we do not know with any certainty that her final maintenance dose will be 225 mg, A.C. should probably be started on 200 mg/d of extended-release sodium phenytoin. As with all patients starting phenytoin, she will require relatively frequent plasma monitoring over the next few days to weeks. A.C. should probably have an initial level within 3 days to ensure that our initial dose is approximately correct. If our initial dose was much higher or lower than the dose that will maintain a therapeutic phenytoin concentration, it would be important to identify early that her phenytoin levels were declining or rising rapidly. Assuming her phenytoin level at 2 or 3 days is near our predicted 17 mg/L, the next sample should be in about a week. Then, depending on whether the phenytoin levels appear to be relatively stable, less frequent monitoring would be required. If the phenytoin concentrations are changing significantly, then more frequent monitoring with dose adjustments may be necessary (see Time to Sample and Questions #5 and #6).

REFERENCES

1. Bigger JT Jr, Schmidt DH, Kutt H. Relationship between the plasma level of diphenylhydantoin sodium and its cardiac antiarrhythmic effects. *Circulation*. 1968;38:363-374.

2. Glauser T, Shinnar S, Gloss D, et al. Evidence-based guideline: treatment of convulsive status epilepticus in children and adults: report of the Guideline Committee of the American Epilepsy Society. *Epilepsy Curr*. 2016;16(1):48-61.

3. Brophy GM, Bell R, Claasen J, et al; Neurocritical Care Society Status Epilepticus Guideline Writing Committee. Guidelines for the evaluation and management of status epilepticus. *Neurocrit Care*. 2012;17(1):3-23.

4. Pyror FM, Gidal B, Ramsay RE, DeToledo J, Morgan RO. Fosphenytoin: pharmacokinetics and tolerance of intramuscular loading doses. *Epilepsia*. 2001;42(2):245-250.

5.   National Institute for Clinical Excellence. *Clinical Guideline.* April 27, 2022:65. Accessed June 1, 2022. https://www.nice.org.uk/guidance/ng217/resources/epilepsies-in-children-young-people-and-adults-pdf-66143780239813

6.   Louis S, Kutt H, McDowell F. The cardiocirculatory changes caused by intravenous Dilantin and its solvent. *Am Heart J.* 1967;74:523-529.

7.   Kutt H, Winters W, Kokenge R, Mcdowell F. Diphenylhydantoin metabolism, blood levels and toxicity. *Arch Neurol.* 1964;11:642-648.

8.   Lund L. Effects of phenytoin in patients with epilepsy in relation to its concentration in plasma. In: David DS, Prichard NBC, eds. *Biological Effects of Drugs in Relation to Their Concentration in Plasma.* University Park Press; 1972:227.

9.   Abou-Khalil BW. Antiepileptic Drugs. *Continuum (Minneap Minn).* 2016;22:132-156.

10. Kugler AR, Annesley TM, Nordblom GD, Koup JR, Olson SC. Cross-reactivity of fosphenytoin in two human plasma phenytoin immunoassays. *Clin Chem.* 1998;44:1474-1480.

11. Yukawa E. Optimization of antiepileptic drug therapy. The importance of serum drug concentration monitoring. *Clin Pharmacokinet.* 1996;31:120-130.

12. Lascelles PT, Kocen RS, Reynolds EH. The distribution of plasma phenytoin levels in epileptic patients. *J Neurol Neurosurg Psychiatry.* 1970;33:501-505.

13. Cloyd JC, Gumnit RJ, McLain W Jr. Status epilepticus: the role of intravenous phenytoin. *JAMA.* 1980;244:1479-1481.

14. Powers NG, Carson SH. Idiosyncratic reactions to phenytoin. *Clin Pediatr (Phila).* 1986;26(3):120-124.

15. Zacarra G, Franciotta D, Perucca E. Idiosyncratic adverse reactions to antiepileptic drugs. *Epilepsia.* 2007;48(7):1223-1244.

16. Karnes JH, Rettie AE, Smogyi AA, et al. Clinical pharmacogenetics implementation consortium guidelines for CYP2C9 and HLA-B genotypes and phenytoin dosing: 2020 update. *Clin Phamacol Ther.* 2021;109(2):302-309.

17. Craig S. Phenytoin poisoning. *Neurocrit Care.* 2005;3:161-170.

18. O'Brien TJ, Cascino D, So EL, Hanna DR. Incidence and clinical consequences of the purple glove syndrome in patients receiving intravenous phenytoin. *Neurology.* 1998;51:1034-1039.

19. Odar-Cederlof I, Borgå O. Kinetics of diphenylhydantoin in uremic patients: consequence of decreased protein binding. *Eur J Clin Pharmacol.* 1974;7:31-37.

20. Koch-Weser J, Sellers EM. Binding of drugs to serum albumin. *N Engl J Med.* 1976;294:311-316.

21. Lund L, Berlin A, Lunde KM. Plasma protein binding of diphenylhydantoin in patients with epilepsy. Agreement between the unbound fraction in plasma and the concentration in the cerebrospinal fluid. *Clin Pharmacol Ther.* 1972;13:196-200.

22. Joerger M, Huitema AD, Boogerd W, van der Sande JJ, Schellens JH, Beijnen JH. Interactions of serum albumin, valproic acid and carbamazepine with the pharmacokinetics of phenytoin in cancer patients. *Basic Clin Pharmacol Toxicol.* 2006;96:133-140.

23. Adler DS, Martin E, Gambertoglio JG, Tozer TN, Spire JP. Hemodialysis of phenytoin in a uremic patient. *Clin Pharmacol Ther.* 1975;18:65-69.

24. Reidenberg MM, Odar-Cedelöf L, von Bahr C, Borgå O, Sjöqvist F. Protein binding of diphenylhydantoin and desmethylimipramine in plasma from patients with poor renal function. *N Engl J Med.* 1971;285:264-267.

25. Odar-Cederlof I. Plasma protein binding of phenytoin and warfarin in patients undergoing renal transplantation. *Clin Pharmacokinet.* 1977;2:147-153.

26. Reidenberg MM. The binding of drugs to plasma proteins and the interpretation of measurements of plasma concentrations of drugs in patients with poor renal function. *Am J Med.* 1977;62:466-470.

27. Liponi DF, Winter ME, Tozer TN. Renal function and therapeutic concentrations of phenytoin. *Neurology.* 1984;34:395-397.

28. Kiang, TK, Ensom MH. A comprehensive review on the predictive performance of the Sheiner-Tozer derivative equations for the correction of phenytoin concentrations. *Ann Pharmacother.* 2016;50(4):311-325.

29. Sadeghi K, Hadi F, Ahmadi A, et al. Total phenytoin concentration is not well correlated with active free drug in critically-ill head trauma patients. *J Res Pharm Pract.* 2013;2(3):105-109.

30. Mattson RH, Cramer JA, Williamson PD, Novelly RA. Valproic acid in epilepsy: clinical and pharma-cological effects. *Ann Neurol.* 1978;3:20-25.

31. Monks A, Richens A. Effect of single dose of sodium valproate on serum phenytoin levels and protein binding in epileptic patients. *Clin Pharmacol Ther.* 1980;27:89-95.

32. Kerrick JM, Wolff DL, Graves NM. Predicting unbound phenytoin concentrations in patients receiv-ing valproic acid: a comparison of two prediction methods. *Ann Pharmacother.* 1995;29:470-474.

33. Jusko WJ, Koup JR, Alvan G. Nonlinear assessment of phenytoin bioavailability. *J Pharmacokinet Bio-pharm.* 1976;4:327-336.

34. Gugler R, Manion CV, Azarnoff DL. Phenytoin: pharmacokinetics and bioavailability. *Clin Pharmacol Ther.* 1976;19:135-142.

35. Wilder BJ, Leppik I, Hietpas TJ, Cloyd JC, Randinitis EJ, Cook J. Effect of food on absorption of Dilan-tin Kapseals and Mylan extended phenytoin sodium capsules. *Neurology.* 2001;57(4):582-589.

36. Rosenbaum DH, Rowan AJ, Tuchman L, French JA. Comparative bioavailability of generic phenytoin and Dilantin. *Epilepsia.* 1994;35:656-660.

37. Goff DA, Spunt AL, Jung D, Bellur SN, Fischer JH. Absorption characteristics of three phenytoin so-dium products after administration of oral loading doses. *Clin Pharm.* 1984;3:634-638.

38. Jankovic SM, Ignjatovic Ristic D. Is bioavailability altered in generic vs brand anticonvulsants? *Expert Opin Drug Metab Toxicol.* 2015;11(3):329-332.

39. Cacek AT. Review of alterations in oral phenytoin bioavailability associated with formulation, antac-ids, and food. *Ther Drug Monit.* 1986;8:166-171.

40. Bauer LA. Interference of oral phenytoin absorption by continuous nasogastric feedings. *Neurology.* 1982;32:570-572.

41. Faraji B, Yu PP. Serum phenytoin levels of patients on gastrostomy tube feeding. *J Neurosci Nurs.* 1998;30:55-59.

42. Doak KK, Haas CE, Dunnigan KJ, et al. Bioavailability of phenytoin acid and phenytoin sodium with enteral feedings. *Pharmacotherapy.* 1998;18:637-645.

43. Carter BL, Garnett WR, Pellock JM, Stratton MA, Howell JR. Effect of antacids on phenytoin bioavail-ability. *Ther Drug Monit.* 1981;3(4):333-340.

44. Neuvonen PJ. Bioavailability of phenytoin: clinical pharmacokinetic and therapeutic implications. *Clin Pharmacokinet.* 1979;4:91-103.

45. Wilder BJ, Serrano EE, Ramsay RE. Plasma diphenylhydantoin levels after loading and maintenance doses. *Clin Pharmacol Ther.* 1973;14:797-801.

46. Jung D, Powell JR, Walson P, Perrier D. Effect of dose on phenytoin absorption. *Clin Pharmacol Ther.* 1980;28:479-485.

47. Kaucher KA, Acquisto NM, Rao GG, et al. Relative bioavailability of orally administered fosphenytoin sodium injection compared with phenytoin sodium injection in healthy volunteers. *Pharmacotherapy.* 2015;35(5):482-488.

48. Havidberg E, Dam M. Clinical pharmacokinetics of anticonvulsants. *Clin Pharmacokinet.* 1976;1:161-188.

49. Glazko AJ, Chang T, Baukema J, Dill WA, Goulet JR, Buchanan RA. Metabolic disposition of di-phenylhydantoin in normal human subjects following intravenous administration. *Clin Pharmacol Ther.* 1969;10:498-504.

50. Abernathy DR, Greenblatt DJ. Phenytoin disposition in obesity. determination of loading dose. *Arch Neurol.* 1985;42:468-471.

51. Bochner F, Hooper WD, Tyrer JH, Eadie MJ. Effects of dosage increments on blood phenytoin concen-trations. *J Neurol Neurosurg Psychiatry.* 1972;35:873-876.

52. Arnold K, Gerber N. The rate of decline of diphenylhydantoin in human plasma. *Clin Pharmacol Ther.* 1970;11:121-134.

53. Houghton GW, Richens A. Rate of elimination of tracer doses of phenytoin at different steady-state serum phenytoin concentrations in epileptic patients. *Br J Clin Pharmacol.* 1974;1:155-161.

54. Lund L, Alvan G, Berlin A, Alexanderson B. Pharmacokinetics of single and multiple doses of phenyt-oin in man. *Eur J Clin Pharmacol.* 1974;7:81-86.

55. Mawer GE, Mullen PW, Rodgers M, Robins AJ, Lucas SB. Phenytoin dose adjustments in epileptic patients. *Br J Clin Pharmacol.* 1974;1:163-168.

56. Lambie DG, Johnson RH, Nanda RN, Shakir RA. Therapeutic and pharmacokinetic effects of increasing phenytoin in chronic epileptics on multiple drug therapy. *Lancet.* 1976;2:386-389.

57. Richens A. A study of the pharmacokinetics of phenytoin (diphenylhydantoin) in epileptic patients, and the development of a nomogram for making dose increments. *Epilepsia.* 1975;16:627-646.

58. Ludden TM, Allen JP, Valutsky WA, et al. Individualization of phenytoin dosage regimens. *Clin Pharmacol Ther.* 1977;21:287-293.

59. Martin E, Tozer TN, Sheiner LB, Riegelman S. The clinical pharmacokinetics of phenytoin. *J Pharmacokinet Biopharm.* 1977;5:579-596.

60. Mullen PW. Optimal phenytoin therapy: a new technique for individualizing dosage. *Clin Pharmacol Ther.* 1978;23:228-232.

61. Privitera MD. Clinical rules for phenytoin dosing. *Ann Pharmacother.* 1993;27:1169-1173.

62. Franco V, Perucca E. CYP2C0 polymorphisms and phenytoin metabolism: implications for adverse effects. *Expert Opin Drug Metab Toxicol.* 2015;11(8):1269-1279.

63. Khandwala HM. Lipid lowering inefficiency of high-dose statin therapy due to concurrent use of phenytoin. *South Med J.* 2006;99:1385-1387.

64. Thomas SV. Management of epilepsy and pregnancy. *J Postgrad Med.* 2006;52:57-64.

65. Nolan PE Jr, Marcus FI, Hoyer GL, Bliss M, Gear K. Pharmacokinetic interaction between intravenous phenytoin and amiodarone in healthy volunteers. *Clin Pharmacol Ther.* 1989;46:43-50.

66. Shackleford EJ, Watson FT. Amiodarone—phenytoin interaction. *Drug Intell Clin Pharm.* 1987;21:921.

67. Garrett WR, Carter BL, Pellock JM. Bioavailability of phenytoin administered with antacids. *Ther Drug Monit.* 1979;1:435-437.

68. O'Brien WM, Orme ML, Breckenridge AM. Failure of antacids to alter the pharmacokinetics of phenytoin. *Br J Clin Pharmacol.* 1978;6:276-277.

69. Smart HL, Somerville KW, Williams J, Richens A, Langman MJ. The effects of sucralfate upon phenytoin absorption in man. *Br J Clin Pharmacol.* 1985;20:238-240.

70. Hansen JM, Siersbaek-Nielsen K, Skovsted L. Carbamazepine-induced acceleration of diphenylhydantoin and warfarin metabolism in man. *Clin Pharmacol Ther.* 1971;12:539-543.

71. Brown TR, Szabo GK, Evans JE, Evans BA, Greenblatt DJ, Mikati MA. Carbamazepine increases phenytoin serum concentrations and reduces phenytoin clearance. *Neurology.* 1988;38:1146-1150.

72. Harper JM, Yost RL, Stewart RB, Ciezkowski J. Phenytoin–chloramphenicol interaction: a retrospective study. *Drug Intell Clin Pharm.* 1979;13:425-429.

73. Rose JQ, Choi HK, Schentag JJ, et al. Intoxication caused by interaction of chloramphenicol and phenytoin. *JAMA.* 1977;237:2630-2631.

74. Phillips P, Hansky J. Phenytoin toxicity secondary to cimetidine administration. *Med J Aust.* 1984;141:602.

75. Bartle WR, Walker SE, Shapero T. Dose-dependent effect of cimetidine on phenytoin kinetics. *Clin Pharmacol Ther.* 1983;33:649-655.

76. Pollak PT, Slayter KL. Hazards of doubling phenytoin dose in the face of an unrecognized interaction with ciprofloxacin. *Ann Pharmacother.* 1997;31:61-64.

77. Dillard ML, Fink RM, Parkerson R. Ciprofloxacin-phenytoin interaction. *Ann Pharmacother.* 1992;26:263.

78. Sylvester RK, Lewis FB, Caldwell KC, Lobell M, Perri R, Sawchuk RA. Impaired phenytoin bioavailability secondary to cisplatinum, vinblastine and bleomycin. *Ther Drug Monit.* 1984;6:302-305.

79. Olesen OV. Disulfiram (Antabuse) as inhibitor of phenytoin metabolism. *Acta Pharmacol Toxicol (Copenh).* 1966;24:317-322.

80. Brown CG, Kaminsky MJ, Feroli ER Jr, Gurley HT. Delirium with phenytoin and disulfiram administration. *Ann Emerg Med.* 1983;12:310-313.

81. Robertson SM, Penzak SR, Lane J, Pau AK, Mican JM. A potentially significant interaction between efavirenz and phenytoin: a case report and review of the literature. *Clin Infect Dis.* 2005;41:e15-e18.

82. Blum RA, Wilton JH, Hilloigoss DM, et al. Effect of fluconazole on the disposition of phenytoin. *Clin Pharmacol Ther.* 1991;49:420-425.

83. Jalil P. Toxic reaction following the combined administration of fluoxetine and phenytoin: two case reports. *J Neurol Neurosurg Psychiatry.* 1992;55:412-413.

84. Lewis DP, Van Dyke DC, Willhite LA, Stumbo PJ, Berg MJ. Phenytoin-folic acid interaction. *Ann Pharmacother.* 1995;29:726-735.

85. Seligmann H, Potasman I, Weller B, Schwartz M, Prokocimer M. Phenytoin-folic acid interactions: a lesson to be learned. *Clin Neuropharmacol.* 1999;22:268-272.

86. Berg MJ, Stumbo PJ, Chenard CA, Fincham RW, Schneider PJ, Schottelius DD. Folic acid improves phenytoin pharmacokinetics. *J Am Diet Assoc.* 1995;95:352-356.

87. Miller RR, Porter J, Greenblatt DJ. Clinical importance of the interaction of phenytoin and isoniazid: a report from the Boston Collaborative Drug Surveillance Program. *Chest.* 1979;75:356-358.

88. Brennan RW, Dehejia H, Kutt H, Verebely K, McDowell F. Diphenylhydantoin intoxication attendant to slow inactivation of isoniazid. *Neurology.* 1970;20:687-693.

89. Kutt H, Winters W, McDowell FH. Depression of parahydroxylation of diphenylhydantoin by antituberculosis chemotherapy. *Neurology.* 1966;16:594-602.

90. Kutt H, Haynes J, Verebely K, McDowell F. The effect of phenobarbital on plasma diphenylhydantoin level and metabolism in man and in rat liver microsomes. *Neurology.* 1969;19:611-616.

91. Morselli PL, Rizzo M, Garaltini S, et al. Interaction between phenobarbital and diphenylhydantoin in animals and in epileptic patients. *Ann N Y Acad Sci.* 1971;179:88-107.

92. Kay L, Kampmann JP, Svendsen TL, et al. Influence of rifampicin and isoniazid on the kinetics of phenytoin. *Br J Clin Pharmacol.* 1985;20:323-326.

93. Odar-Cederlöf I, Borga O. Impaired plasma protein binding of phenytoin in uremia and displacement effect of salicylic acid. *Clin Pharmacol Ther.* 1976;20:36-47.

94. Haselberger MB, Freedman LS, Tolbert S. Elevated serum phenytoin concentrations associated with coadministration of sertraline. *J Clin Psychopharmacol.* 1997;17:107-109.

95. Lumholtz B, Siersbaek-Nielsen K, Skovsted L, et al. Sulfamethizole-induced inhibition of diphenylhydantoin, tolbutamide and warfarin metabolism. *Clin Pharmacol Ther.* 1975;17:731-734.

96. Lunde PK, Rane A, Yaffe SJ, Lund L, Sjöqvist F. Plasma protein binding of diphenylhydantoin in man. Interaction with other drugs and the effect of temperature and plasma dilution. *Clin Pharmacol Ther.* 1970;11:846-855.

97. Privitera M, Welty TE. Acute phenytoin toxicity followed by seizure breakthrough from a ticlopidine-phenytoin interaction. *Arch Neurol.* 1996;53:1191-1192.

98. Donahue S, Flockhart, DA, Abernethy, DR. Ticlopidine inhibits phenytoin clearance. *Clin Pharmacol Therap.* 1999;66:563-568.

99. Hansen JM, Kampmann JP, Siersbaek-Nielsen K, et al. The effect of different sulfonamides on phenytoin metabolism in man. *Acta Med Scand Suppl.* 1979;624:106-110.

100. Purkins L, Wood N, Ghahramani P, Love ER, Eve MD, Fielding A. Coadministration of voriconazole and phenytoin: pharmacokinetic interaction, safety, and toleration. *Br J Clin Pharmacol.* 2003;56:37-44.

101. Atkinson AJ Jr, Shaw JM. Pharmacokinetic study of a patient with diphenylhydantoin toxicity. *Clin Pharmacol Ther.* 1973;14:521-528.

102. Ahn JE, Cloyd JC, Brundage RC, et al. Phenytoin half-life and clearance during maintenance therapy in adults and elderly patients with epilepsy. *Neurology.* 2008;71:38-43.

103. Bauer LA, Blouin RA. Phenytoin Michaelis-Menten pharmacokinetics in Caucasian pediatric patients. *Clin Pharmacokinet.* 1983;8:545-549.

104. Grasela TH, Sheiner LB, Rambeck B, et al. Steady-state pharmacokinetics of phenytoin from routinely collected patient data. *Clin Pharmacokinet.* 1983;8:355-364.

105. Dodson WE. Nonlinear kinetics of phenytoin in children. *Neurology.* 1982;32:42-48.

106. Chiba K, Ishizaki T, Miura H, Minagawa K. Michaelis-Menten pharmacokinetics of diphenylhydantoin and application in the pediatric age patient. *J Pediatr.* 1980;96:479-484.

107. Wilder BJ, Serrano EE, Ramsey E, Buchanan RA. A method for shifting from oral to intramuscular diphenylhydantoin administration. *Clin Pharmacol Ther.* 1974;16:507-513.

108. Tozer TN, Winter ME. Phenytoin. In: Burton ME, Evans WE, Shaw LM, et al, eds. *Applied Pharmacokinetics: Principles of Therapeutic Drug Monitoring*. 4th ed. Lippincott Williams and Wilkins; 2006.

109. Wilder BJ, Buchanan RA, Serrano EE. Correlation of acute diphenylhydantoin intoxication with plasma levels and metabolite excretion. *Neurology*. 1973;23:1329-1332.

110. Chan BS, Sellors K, Chiew AL, Buckley NA. Use of multi-dose activated charcoal in phenytoin toxicity secondary to genetic polymorphism. *Clin Toxicol (Phila)*. 2015;53(2):131-133.

111. Warner A, Privitera M, Bates D. Standards of laboratory practice: antiepileptic drug monitoring. National Academy of Clinical Biochemistry. *Clin Chem*. 1998;44:1085-1095.

112. Patsalos PN, Berry DJ, Bourgeois BFD, et al. Antiepileptic drugs—best practice guidelines for therapeutic drug monitoring: a position paper by the subcommission on therapeutic drug monitoring, ILAE Commission on Therapeutic Strategies. *Epilepsia*. 2008;49(7):1239-1276.

113. Martin E, Gambertoglio JG, Adler DS, Tozer TN, Roman LA, Grausz H. Removal of phenytoin by hemodialysis in uremic patients. *JAMA*. 1977;238:1750-1753.

114. Andreasen F, Jakobsen P. Determination of furosemide in blood plasma and its binding to proteins in normal plasma and in plasma from patients with acute renal failure. *Acta Pharmacol Toxicol (Copenh)*. 1974;35:49-57.

115. Oltrogge KM, Peppard WJ, Saleh M, Regner KR, Herrmann DJ. Phenytoin removal by continuous venovenous hemofiltraton. *Ann Pharmacother*. 2013;47(9):1218-1222.

116. KDIGO Worgroup. KDIGO clinical practice guidelines for acute kidney injury. *Kidney Int Suppl*. 2012;2(6):1-141.

117. Silberstein LE, Shaw LM. Effect of plasma exchange on phenytoin plasma concentration. *Ther Drug Monit*. 1986;8:172-176

118. Wilensky AJ, Lowden JA. Inadequate serum levels after intramuscular administration of diphenylhydantoin. *Neurology*. 1973;23:318-324.

119. Uthman BM, Wilder BJ, Ramsay RE. Intramuscular use of fosphenytoin: an overview. *Neurology*. 1996;46(6 suppl 1):S24-S28.

120. Richens A, Dunlop A. Serum-phenytoin levels in the management of epilepsy. *Lancet*. 1975;2:247-248.

121. Dasgupta A. Usefulness of monitoring free (unbound) concentrations of therapeutic drugs in patient management. *Clin Chim Acta*. 2007;377:1-13.

15

VALPROIC ACID

Irving Steinberg and Autumn Walkerly

Learning Objectives

By the end of the valproic acid chapter, the learner shall be able to:

1. Assess bioavailability factors and differences in absorption rates of various dosage forms of valproic acid (VPA) and the impact on therapeutic choices and dosing strategies.
2. Describe the therapeutic concentration range of VPA and the specific target concentrations for each clinical indication.
3. Comprehend all clinical and pharmacokinetic (PK) aspects of the saturable protein binding of VPA, execute proper interpretation of serum concentrations in the context of changes in protein binding and drug clearance, and calculate a free VPA level, given a total drug level and albumin concentration or binding displacing drug.
4. Understand the volume of distribution range in various populations and factors that impact these values, and calculate the serum concentration resulting from a loading dose.
5. Elucidate the varied metabolic pathways of VPA, the patient-drug interaction (and relevant mechanism), pharmacogenetic factors that influence its clearance, and active/toxic metabolite production. Describe typical clearance rates and elimination half-life values in various patient groups.
6. Calculate the clearance of VPA given a steady-state level, or using two levels within a dosage interval, and construct a dosage regimen to meet therapeutic levels and pharmacologic success.
7. Describe the impact of the presence of an interacting drug or changes in protein binding on clearance.
8. Detail the concentration- or dose-related adverse effects of VPA.
9. Utilize population PK models to calculate parameter estimates and initial and revised VPA dosage regimens.

Valproic acid (VPA), a simple branch-chain aliphatic acid, is among the most versatile central nervous system active drugs in the pharmacopeia and whose clinical uses and dosing strategies continue to be explored and refined.[1] It remains a drug of choice for various idiopathic generalized and focal epileptic disorders (classic and atypical absence, tonic-clonic, atonic and myoclonic seizures, Dravet syndrome, juvenile myoclonic epilepsy, focal onset seizures, post-traumatic epilepsy),[2,3] as well as an approved use in bipolar disorder (BPD)[4] and migraine prophylaxis.[5] VPA has also been investigated for use in the treatment of brain cancer (eg, glioma),[6] delirium,[7] acute migraine,[8] post-traumatic brain injury epilepsy, anxiety, and irritability.[9,10] The unique nature of VPA and the clinical need for therapeutic drug monitoring are highlighted by the following:

a. Concentration-dependent protein binding within the therapeutic range and dose-dependent pharmacokinetic (PK) parameters[11,12]
b. Large variability in concentration-dose ratio that depends on numerous demographic and clinical factors[13,14]
c. Multitude of metabolic pathways with primary phase 1 and phase 2 reactions whose balance is age dependent and genetically determined[15,16]
d. Significant adverse effects that are concentration or dose dependent[17]

Drug interactions are numerous and mostly feature inhibiting the clearance of other hepatically eliminated drugs via cytochrome (CYP) P450 and glucuronidation mechanisms. Likewise, other interacting medicines and genetic polymorphisms may interfere with the clearance of VPA and increase its adverse event risk profile.

MECHANISM OF ACTION

Enhanced inhibitory neurotransmission by γ-amino butyric acid (GABA) and VPA is done via increased synthesis, decreased degradation and turnover,[18] and inhibition of succinate semialdehyde dehydrogenase, along with inhibition of GABA transaminase at higher concentrations.[19] In addition, antiseizure effects derive from the blockade of voltage-gated sodium, potassium, and calcium channels.[3] Likely, the effects on serotonergic and dopaminergic receptor transmission modulate the benefits seen in migraine prophylaxis and the treatment of BPD, anxiety, and other psychiatric and mood disorders. The histone deacetylase inhibition observed with VPA is responsible for apoptotic and antitumor gene upregulation, consistent with the encouraging experimental and clinical data seen with this drug against certain forms of cancer.[6,20] Other pharmacologic mechanisms for anti-inflammatory, neuroprotective, and renal protective effects with additional clinical indications are actively studied.[21]

DOSAGE FORMS AND ABSORPTION

VPA is absorbed through the small intestine, and delayed- and extended-release forms are designed to extend the dosage interval and bypass the stomach to reduce dyspepsia. The liquid and tablet forms have a more than 10-fold higher absorption rate constant than the extended-release forms and peak at 1 to 3 hours after ingestion.[22] The delayed-release divalproex sodium (which combines equal amounts of

VPA and sodium valproate) has a lag time (T^{lag}) of 2 hours and then releases quickly for small intestinal absorption at a rapid rate much like the liquid-filled capsule. The extended-release form of divalproex slowly absorbs with a time to peak of 8 to 16 hours ($ka = 0.2$) and provides for efficient 24-hour dosing in adolescents and adults. Beyond the available liquid ($ka = 4$), tablet ($ka = 4$), and capsule ($ka = 4$) where three to four daily doses are needed to sustain adequate trough levels, the oversized sprinkle capsule ($ka = 1.2$, $T^{lag} = 1$ hour) provides sufficiently slow release to allow twice-daily dosing. Complete bioavailability is evident for all the dosage forms, except the extended release where 80% to 90% of bioavailability is seen.[22] Coingested food moderately lengthens the T_{max} for the sprinkle capsule and can double it for the delayed-release tablet. Rectal administration of the syrup or suppositories can provide an alternative route to obtain therapeutic plasma levels.[23] Valpromide is a carboxamide derivative of VPA, available in Italy and France, with no efficacy advantages but a heightened concern when combined with carbamazepine (CBZ), as this form of VPA has 100 times higher potency of inhibiting epoxide hydrolase metabolism of CBZ.[24]

Male and female adults differ in disposition for sustained-release valproate, as the higher concentration-to-dose ratio was observed in adult females than in males.[13] This is likely less to do with differences in intrinsic hepatic clearance than the amount of enterohepatic recirculation, which is twice as high in females than males. This manifests in a larger area under the curve (AUC) for an equivalent dose and a significant "second peak" in females.[25]

PROTEIN BINDING

Although proportional serum protein binding is present for the great majority of drugs that bind primarily to albumin, VPA exhibits saturable binding within the therapeutic concentration range, because the molar concentration of VPA approaches and exceeds that of its binding protein, albumin.[11,12,14,26] When evaluated after intravenous (IV) dosing and normal albumin levels, the unbound fraction for VPA was variable with the total serum concentration, demonstrating saturable binding to albumin, as has been consistently reported. Binding percentages ranging from 5% to 19%[27] and 3.9% to 20.6%[28] have been reported in children when normal albumin-binding capacity and affinity are present; the latter over a 6-fold range of total VPA concentrations.[28] Large variability in the unbound VPA fraction is also found in intensive care unit (ICU) patients, in whom the free VPA concentration cannot be reliably predicted by the total drug concentration.[29]

Nonlinear approaches to model protein binding based on a maximum binding site concentration and dissociation constant show VPA binding in children ranging from 8.5% at total concentrations of 50 mg/L, 11% at 75 mg/L, 15% at 100 mg/L, and 27.2% at 150 mg/L.[30] Likewise, older patients showed an unbound fraction of 10%, 13%, and 17.4% at VPA daily doses of 500, 1,000, and 1,500 mg, respectively.[12] In vitro studies show the increase in unbound fraction with lower human serum albumin concentrations, with a 3-fold increase observed when the albumin concentration was varied from 4 to 2 g/dL.[31] Brain-to-plasma concentration ratios follow similarly to the free fraction of VPA, and the variability is similar to that of the 4-fold range of serum protein binding of VPA in humans.[32] There are linear and nonlinear equations to estimate the unbound fraction or free concentration of VPA, taking into account hypoalbuminemia, age, concentration dependency, or displacement interactions,[11,14,28,30] but none thus far accounts for them together in one multivariate expression. A pediatric population PK model of VPA clearance based on size and maturation jointly with a model for bound and free VPA concentrations has been produced.[33]

Binding of VPA is also subject to displacement interactions and, as expected, is decreased when hypoalbuminemia exists. Maximum binding capacity is lower at the extremes of age in infants and older adults, with lower albumin levels more typical in these age groups.[34,35] The older adults also can have reduced affinity for binding,[36] likely due to higher serum free fatty acid concentrations and correlations of free fatty acid content and unbound fraction of VPA are seen in diabetes.[37] Therefore, unbound concentrations will be higher for a given total concentration in the older adults than in younger adults and children. The unbound fraction of VPA increases in late pregnancy, patients with renal disease, chronic liver disease, nephrotic syndrome, protein-losing enteropathy, traumatic brain injury, critical illness, and other conditions associated with low albumin concentrations.

Displacement interactions of VPA also occur with endogenous free fatty acid excess or exogenous administration of fatty acids–containing products (eg, propofol),[38] salicylates, highly bound nonsteroidal anti-inflammatory drugs such as ibuprofen and naproxen,[39,40] and with uremic compounds disrupting albumin binding in patients with renal failure.[41] Significant renal impairment can more than double the free fraction to 20%.[42] Aspirin and other salicylates create an increased toxicity risk as they can additionally impair mitochondrial β-oxidation (and the intrinsic clearance) of VPA, while increasing the unbound fraction, leading to elevation of the receptor-available VPA.[43] Risperidone may displace protein binding, leading to increase in valproate-induced encephalopathy.[44] Highly protein-bound drugs with weaker affinity will be displaced by VPA, leading to changes in PK, pharmacodynamics (PD), and serum level interpretation for drugs such as warfarin, oral (PO) sulfonylurea agents, CBZ, the active monohydroxy metabolite of oxcarbazepine, and phenytoin (PHT).[45] Equations to determine the degree of displacement of other narrow therapeutic index agents by VPA can be clinically utilized to "correct" for the protein-binding disturbance and assist blood level interpretation.[46,47]

Within numerous population PK modeling studies of VPA, surrogates to saturable protein binding are found in the form of clearance estimates taken as an additive or power function of daily VPA dose; the latter with a model exponent less than 1.[48-52] As the dose increases, total clearance for this low extraction ratio drug will increase by virtue of declining albumin binding,[48] and the rise in VPA C_{ss} will be less than proportional to the increase in daily dose (see later in this chapter). Validation of such models has shown greater predictive success compared to those not taking account of this relationship.[53,54]

VOLUME OF DISTRIBUTION

Although lipid soluble by chemistry, V is restricted to 0.1 to 0.4 L/kg owing to the high plasma protein binding of 90% to 95% and a pK_a of 4.8, with the drug being mostly ionized at blood pH. The mean V approximates 0.2 L/kg[11,27] in adults and is higher with decreased protein binding.[14,27,51] When standardized to body weight, VPA V is higher in infants and young children because of lower protein binding, reduced albumin content, and altered body composition compared to adolescents and young adults.[55] The relatively lower V for VPA compared with other antiseizure medications (ASMs) results in serum concentrations that exceed those in tissues by 8- to 9-fold.[56]

Higher VPA doses would be expected to increase the unbound fraction for peak plasma levels and thereby increase the distribution volume as more drug exits the intravascular space. This is supported by data showing higher distribution volume (and disproportionately higher peak-free concentrations) after a 30 mg/kg IV loading dose of VPA compared with a 20 mg/kg dose.[57] Total concentrations after the 30 mg/kg dose were, however, only 20% higher during the first 60 minutes postinfusion despite a 50% higher dose. This is meaningful in the context of the recommendations for the management of status epilepticus during the second phase of therapy that call for loading doses as high as 40 mg/kg (maximum 3,000 mg) as a single dose.[58] Response in status epilepticus with postbolus total concentrations of 103 to 135 mg/L was more prompt than delayed response seen with levels of 85 to 102 mg/L.[59] This is likely owing to the higher delivery of free drug to the brain and cerebrospinal fluid.[32]

METABOLISM, CLEARANCE, AND PHARMACOGENETICS

Three main routes of metabolism produce about 10 to 20 metabolites for VPA,[16] some purported to have central nervous system (CNS) activity during long-term therapy. Glucuronidation to VPA glucuronide is responsible for 40% to 50% of the disposition of VPA, predominantly using UGT1A3 and UGT2B7. Mitochondrial β-oxidation accounts for 30% to 40%, and from the cytochrome P450 system (mainly CYP2C9), a more minor 10% produces hydroxylated metabolites and unsaturated moieties.[16] Children have more accentuated CYP2C9 activity compared to adults and utilize this pathway more, with a longer time to full maturation of some glucuronidation enzymes.[60] This is one reason why the production of 4-ene VPA via this pathway, and its potential to cause fatal hepatotoxicity, is more selected toward younger children, with additional risks including mitochondrial diseases, inborn errors of metabolism, and/or polytherapy with enzyme-inducing ASMs.[61] Moreover, the therapeutic use of carnitine, in those at greater risk for hyperammonemia and drug-induced liver injury, in part prevents the incorporation of the toxic 4-ene VPA into mitochondria, where 2,4-diene-VPA-CoA can be produced, itself a hepatotoxin.[62]

Selected polymorphisms in UDP-glucuronosyltransferase (UGT) and CYP2C9 can reduce VPA clearance via these pathways,[16] resulting in higher dose-normalized VPA concentrations. Loss-of-function alleles CYP2C9*2 and CYP2C9*3 significantly diminish VPA clearance via this pathway and are particularly impactful in children and certain ethnic groups. Studies show a nearly double the frequency of the A1075C allele in Asian patients (11.7%) compared to Caucasians (6.5%), with this variant found to be more prevalent in children of Chinese descent.[63] Even when carrying wild-type CYP2C9*1/*1, there can be transient reductions of VPA metabolism based on a low level of gene expression, as CYP2C9 expression (as measured by CYP2C9 mRNA levels) is downregulated in children with epilepsy after seizures compared to healthy adults.[64,65] Discordance between phenotypic expression and genotype observed with VPA ("phenoconversion") can be influenced by interacting drugs, hormonal balance, nutrition, and disease activity.[65] Dose guidance using CYP2C9 genotype and phenotypic expression in children more precisely predicted VPA dose, achieved therapeutic range serum concentrations, and reduced hyperammonemia and other metabolic adverse effects.[60,65] The same impact of CYP2C9 polymorphisms was not seen in adults, where no differences in concentration-dose ratio were observed between patients with wild-type and poor metabolism alleles.[13,65] Other pharmacogenetic influences include select polymorphisms of CYP2A6 and CYP2B6, and UGT2B7 and UGT1A4 can result in higher plasma VPA levels,[66] whereas altered alleles of CYP2C19, UGT1A6, and UGT1A3 result in higher VPA dose requirements to reach target plasma concentrations.[67] Increases in *ABCB1* gene expression and P-glycoprotein (P-gp) activity may additionally account for VPA clearance changes, and the addition of genotyping may further refine population models for VPA and interacting drugs.[68]

Relatively reduced drug metabolic activity is observed in the older adults, with the concentration-dose ratio of VPA higher than in young adults.[12,13,35] Decreased intrinsic clearance coupled with lower protein binding will often manifest as total drug concentrations being similar to younger adults but with higher free concentrations and clinical effects. Furthermore, the greater likelihood of polytherapy and interacting medications in this age group makes the older adults of specific concern for VPA toxicity, with needs for closer clinical and therapeutic drug monitoring. Similar considerations are present for patients with hepatic and renal impairment with reduced clearance and altered protein binding.

Given the concentration-dependent protein binding and low extraction ratio (ie, rate limitation is with intrinsic clearance), total VPA clearance increases with increasing unbound fraction and concentration-dose ratios will decrease, as seen with the addition of ibuprofen[69]:

$$Cl_{hepatic} = fu \times Cl_{intrinsic}$$

$$C_{ss} = (Dose)(F)/Cl_{hepatic}$$

Therefore, as the fraction unbound increases with higher doses and total concentrations, so too will the total clearance, and total steady-state concentration will increase less than proportionately with increases in dose.

Since mathematically:

$$C_{unbound} = fu \times C_{total}$$

The C_{total} decrease and fraction unbound increase will eventually offset each other at steady state, leaving a relatively stable unbound VPA concentration. Total levels must be interpreted carefully with a recognition that the relationship between free levels and total levels changes when protein binding changes and that any factor altering intrinsic clearance will alter the accumulation of free VPA concentrations.

Clearances of VPA on monotherapy are within typical ranges of 12 to 25 mL/hr/kg in children and 6 to 12 mL/kg/hr in adults, with elimination half-lives ranging from 6 to 12 hours and 8 to 20 hours, respectively. The half-life may be shorter when protein binding is lower, depending on whether expansion of V offsets the increase in total Cl. Larger clearance and shorter half-life are expected when enzyme-inducing comedications are prescribed. Increased intrinsic clearance of VPA is also recognized in traumatic brain injury.[70] Within the numerous population PK models developed for VPA, the factors most often found to influence clearance include age, weight, VPA dose, and interacting medications; for V, they include age, weight, and dose.[71] Addition of genotype, when tested, may add to the precision of proposed models for VPA clearance.

INTERACTIONS

Comprehensive review of all VPA PK drug interactions is beyond the scope of this chapter, and thorough reviews are available.[45,72,73] Select examples are discussed later and provided in the cases at the end of this chapter.

Most interactions involving VPA are PK based. VPA is an inhibitor of the enzymes CYP2C9, epoxide-hydroxylase, and UGT, thereby slowing the metabolism of ASMs such as PHT, phenobarbital (PB), clobazam, CBZ (to its 10-11 epoxide), and lamotrigine to varying degrees.[72] At high serum concentrations, VPA may decrease its own intrinsic clearance,[12] further complicating its kinetics and level interpretation. Enzyme-inducing ASMs (eg, PB, PHT, CBZ) and non-ASMs (eg, rifampin) can accelerate VPA metabolism to varying degrees and motivate an increase in VPA doses necessary to sustain therapeutic levels. Therefore, the nature of the complex induction and inhibition of the ASMs involved in polytherapy with VPA commands attention to measuring serum levels of all interacting, narrow therapeutic index ASMs during therapy, even when the dose is adjusted for a single agent within the regimen. Moreover, VPA upregulates gene expression and activity of P-gp in a concentration-dependent manner[74] and can thereby negatively affect the activity of substrates. such as direct-acting thrombin inhibitors (DOACs). Caution must be addressed when a combination of VPA with DOACs is administered, with the increased risk of bleeding[75] or thrombosis and death[76] having been reported compared to combinations with ASMs that have no effects on P-gp.[76]

Potent inhibitors of VPA P450 enzyme metabolism, such as isoniazid, selective serotonin reuptake inhibitors (SSRIs) (eg, fluoxetine, paroxetine),[77] and imidazoles (eg, voriconazole), can increase serum levels and AUC of VPA and enhance its toxicity profile.[73] When combined, competitive inhibition by VPA of UGT2B7-mediated glucuronidation of lamotrigine can double the latter's elimination half-life, increase its levels 2- to 3-fold,[78] and potentiate its toxicity, including the risk of Stevens-Johnson syndrome and toxic epidermal necrolysis. This can be furthered by specific polymorphisms in UGT2B7 and UGT1A4 in the presence of higher VPA concentrations.[79] Therefore, slow titration with small incremental doses of lamotrigine is necessary, especially when added to VPA.[80] In parallel, specific polymorphisms in UTG2B7 may also heighten VPA serum concentrations and are amplified by concomitant lamotrigine competition for glucuronidation, enhancing VPA toxicity risk.[81] In contrast, there is an enhanced clearance of monohydroxy-oxcarbazepine (MHD, the active metabolite of oxcarbazepine) in a Chinese patient sample, with a 46% increase in MHD clearance incorporated into the proposed population PK model.[82] In addition, VPA decreases the median concentration-dose ratio of norclozapine (the major active clozapine metabolite) and the norclozapine-to-clozapine ratio, both by 44%.[83] The mechanism is suggested to be through induction of UGT2B10 activity.[84] However, significant gender differences in the magnitude of the norclozapine metabolite formation have been observed.[85]

VPA can show different interactions within the same class of medications. For instance, VPA raises the AUC of injectable paliperidone by 50%, yet has a mostly neutral effect on risperidone levels, and lowers the concentration-dose ratio of olanzapine, potentially resulting in breakthrough psychiatric symptoms.[77,86-88] A 26.4% increase in olanzapine clearance was described in a population PK model where sex and concurrent use VPA were the influential covariates.[89] Inhibition of CYP2C9 and CYP3A4 by VPA leads to increased CNS side effects of amitriptyline, with the mean concentration-dose ratio for amitriptyline 67% higher than for those patients not concomitantly taking VPA and a 228% higher value for the active nortriptyline metabolite.[90]

Important functional and PK interactions involve females of childbearing age. Attempts to mitigate the well-established teratogenic effects of VPA in early-stage pregnancy embody pregnancy avoidance via contraception, choosing other ASMs that can provide similar clinical response to patient, or using the lowest possible effective dose within provider-patient shared informed decision.[91] Withdrawal of VPA in an attempt to avoid pregnancy complications engenders its own risk of increased breakthrough seizure activity,[92] so this must be performed carefully and with appropriate replacement therapy.

Among ASM monotherapies, VPA had the largest differential effect on hormonal contraception versus nonhormonal contraception. When VPA was combined with hormonal contraception, 32% of patients had an increase in seizures compared with none on nonhormonal methods.[93] Notably, VPA has significantly lower serum levels when women take active combined PO contraceptives as compared to inactive pills, with a 21% and 45% increase in total and intrinsic VPA clearance, respectively, likely due to induction of glucuronosyltransferase by ethinylestradiol.[94] Understanding among clinicians of these drug interactions is lacking and adds to the potential risks of combined PO contraceptive and VPA use[95] and the need for pharmacist input.

DOSING AND THERAPEUTIC DRUG MONITORING

Doses of VPA vary somewhat by the indication. Low doses of 500 to 1,500 mg/d in adolescents and adults may be sufficient for prophylaxis of migraine headaches,[96] with low therapeutic levels also providing adjunctive benefit to alcohol withdrawal treatment[97] and in the primary management of juvenile myoclonic epilepsy.[98] Higher doses with blood level monitoring may be necessary for other seizure types, particularly of focal origin, and also where enzyme-inducing comedications are in use. VPA dose ranges of 10 to 30 mg/kg/d for adults and 15 to 60 mg/kg/d in pediatric patients are most common for the drug's indications. As a guideline-based choice for second-line treatment for status epilepticus, IV loading doses range up to 40 mg/kg, with an adult maximum of 3 g in a single dose.[58] Children studied under this treatment protocol given 40 mg/kg infused over 10 minutes had a range of serum concentrations at 20 to 240 minutes postdose of 126 to 223 mg/L for total drug and a corresponding 31 to 114 mg/L for free drug, with nonlinear concentration-dependent binding exhibited (fu = 17%-51%).[99] An institutional review of adults given loading doses higher than 30 mg/kg of VPA showed no added effect of aborting status epilepticus, but large variability in trough levels of total VPA were measured (10-110 mg/L), with significant overlap between responders and nonresponders. Optimum target levels, taking protein binding into account, for this indication are needed, and the concentration-related risk of hyperammonemia with IV VPA must be regarded.[100]

The generally accepted therapeutic range for epilepsy is 50 to 100 mg/L,[101] with some patients requiring higher levels if only partial response is obtained within the stated range. Further validation of the therapeutic range has been documented in a population PK/PD evaluation with probit analysis for the concentrations associated with diminished seizure activity in patients on monotherapy and polytherapy. Highest probability of antiseizure response to VPA was in the 50 to 70 mg/L range,[51] so it is sensible that the lower end of the therapeutic range should be the first target to evaluate efficacy in individuals. In bipolar mania, VPA levels of 50 to 125 mg/L have established efficacy.[102] In addition, some children may tolerate levels up to 120 mg/L without additional concentration-related adverse effects.[103]

There are a number of adverse effects of VPA that are dose or concentration related.[104] Hyperammonemia, via depletion of L-carnitine in the urea cycle, and associated encephalopathy have been related to VPA dose, treatment duration, and serum concentrations,[105] free levels in particular,[106] though not in all cases as other comorbid factors with VPA use exist.[107] This CNS adverse effect is particularly concerning for confusion with, or adding to, the CNS conditions that VPA is used to treat. Topiramate increases the risk of VPA-induced encephalopathy, though VPA may lower topiramate concentrations by 10% to 15%.[108]

Thrombocytopenia and other blood dyscrasias for many drugs are idiosyncratic and irrespective of concentration exposure. This is not the case for VPA, where platelet counts may decrease to less than 100,000/μL when VPA concentrations exceed 100 mg/L for females and 130 mg/L for males,[68] and is seen comparatively more in patients with diabetes with status epilepticus receiving VPA, presumably due to glycosylation of albumin disrupting VPA binding.[109] Free concentrations of VPA may be more defining of the risk of this adverse effect, with a negative correlation of platelet count with the free level and 3-fold higher average trough-free concentrations in those with platelet counts cutoff of 150 and 100 K.[110] Separate equations and probability curves for predicted platelet counts in males and females were posited based on baseline platelet count and free VPA concentrations, with the free VPA concentration best discriminating risk of a platelet count of 100 K or less of 16.65 mg/L[110] Dangerously low platelet counts are rarely observed if this cell line is solely involved, clotting is not usually compromised, and recovery to normal platelet counts occurs with either temporarily suspending VPA or reducing VPA dosage and concentration. The more rare occurring neutropenia can also be dose related.[111]

KEY PARAMETERS: Valproic Acid

Therapeutic plasma concentration	50-100 mg/L (up to 125 mg/L for BPD/mania)
	100-130 mg/L postdose for status epilepticus
	Unbound concentration: 2.5-12.5 mg/L
F	
Extended-release tablets	0.8-0.9
All other forms	1.0
S	1.0
$V_d{}^a$	0.2 (range: 0.1-0.4) L/kg
$Cl^{b,c}$ (mL/kg/hr)	
Children	10-25
Adults	6-12
$t_{1/2}$ (hr)	
Children	6-12
Adults	10-20
fu^d (fraction unbound in plasma)	0.1-0.5, typical value = 0.1

[a] Volume of distribution may be increased in infants, older adults, liver and renal disease, hypoalbuminemia, or with displacers of VPA binding.

[b] Clearance is decreased in the older adults, neonates and infants, functional liver disease, drugs that impair intrinsic clearance, or compete for glucuronidation; the presence of poor function allelic polymorphisms of CYP2C9 or UGT.

[c] Clearance may be increased in patients receiving co-therapy with enzyme-inducing antiepileptic agents or other drugs that induce P450 or glucuronidation, or in patients with polymorphisms imparting higher-than-normal metabolic enzymatic function. Free drug clearance may be decreased at higher VPA concentrations. Higher clearance is seen in patients with traumatic brain injury in the absence of liver impairment.

[d] Protein binding is concentration dependent within the therapeutic range; the fraction unbound increases with higher VPA levels and with drugs and free fatty acids that displace VPA from albumin-binding sites. Protein binding will be lower in disease states where poor synthesis (liver disease, malnutrition, older adults, critical illness) or increased losses (nephrotic syndrome, other renal diseases, protein-losing enteropathy, critical illness) of albumin exist.

Quality-of-life measures in patients with epilepsy can be affected by the disease itself, comorbidities, and comedications. Although VPA affects psychomotor functions and mental acuity less than some other antiepileptic drugs, overall quality-of-life measures are observed to be inversely proportional to serum VPA levels.[112]

Along with the indirect relationship of VPA fatal hepatotoxicity to concentration (via toxic metabolite formation/accumulation) described earlier, γ-glutamyltransferase (GGT) elevations, an indicator of hepatobiliary disease, have been correlated with VPA concentrations.[113] Other serious abdominal adverse effects such as VPA-induced pancreatitis are not concentration or dose related.[114] Weight gain, low thyroid levels, and tremors have been linked to some extent with dose exposure or serum VPA levels.[115,116] Weight gain has also been related to specific CYP2C19 and UGT1A6 genetic polymorphisms.[117] The incidence of major congenital malformations increases exponentially with advancing maternally administered VPA doses,[118] with each type of anomaly demonstrating an individual dose-toxicity relationship.[119]

VPA levels are best obtained at steady state for patients on maintenance therapy for epilepsy, to ensure compliance and correlation with clinical benefit and avoid potential concentration-related toxicities. This is less necessary with use in migraine headaches, as low doses are usually sufficient for prophylaxis and are useful for bipolar mania treatment, especially if therapeutic endpoints are not met. Repeat measurements of VPA levels should be done when toxicity occurs, when the dose is changed, when anticipated PK drug interactions exist, and when efficacy is lost. Levels may also be obtained upon admission to the hospital for recurrence or breakthrough seizures and after loading doses are given to ensure achievement of the target concentration. Predose levels taken with rapidly absorbed syrup, tablet, and IV preparations will likely overestimate the actual clearance when calculated as Dose $\times$ F/C_{ss}, as the steady-state trough level will generally be lower than the average C_{pss}, especially those with faster clearances such as children or those taking metabolism-inducing drugs. The C_{ss} is better represented with trough level sampling for extended- and delayed-release preparations. For practical purposes, if trough concentrations are monitored consistently in the individual patient, the concentration-dose ratio is a useful surrogate to clearance and can be compared on different doses, and the relationship between serum concentration and effectiveness can then be accurately evaluated.

Unbound drug concentration measurement of VPA, using ultrafiltration methods, may be needed when correlation to effect or toxicity is elusive, or if liver or renal disease, traumatic brain injury, hypoalbuminemia, or protein-binding displacement is present, and especially if a combination of binding-altering factors exists.[120] The free level can then be used to more precisely assess efficacy and toxicity end points than total concentrations, particularly with dose alterations. Unbound concentrations may be elevated, whereas total VPA serum concentrations remain within the therapeutic range, leading to potential toxicity. An observational study of patients who had both total and unbound VPA concentrations drawn found 5% of patients had an elevated total VPA concentration compared to 37% of those same patients with elevated unbound VPA concentrations (Figure 15.1).[121]

Question #1   *B.I. is a 46-year-old, 82-kg male admitted to the neurointensive care unit after having serial tonic-clonic seizures emanating from a newly diagnosed glioblastoma. Repeated bolus doses of levetiracetam were not successful in suppressing the seizure activity, and it is decided to administer IV VPA. He has normal liver enzymes and function tests, and his albumin is 4.2 g/dL. A 1,500 mg loading dose given over 30 minutes is prescribed, with a 30-minute postinfusion serum level to be obtained. What peak concentration might be expected?*

Because the typical half-life of valproate in adults ranges between 10 and 20 hours, no significant drug loss would occur between the time to load dose and the time to peak concentration. Therefore, the peak concentration can be estimated using the single-dose bolus model (Equation 15.1), assuming the average V for an adult is 0.2 L/kg.

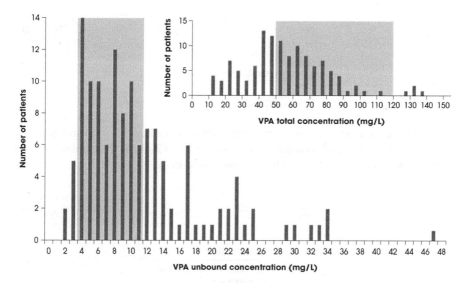

FIGURE 15.1 Total and unbound VPA matched concentration measurements ($n = 273$) in 132 patients. Free levels were measured due to renal insufficiency in 34% and hypoalbuminemia in 27%. The reference range depicted by gray shading was 50 to 120 mg/L for total concentration (inset graph) and 4 to 12 for free concentration. Only 5% of the measured total VPA concentrations were above the reference range, whereas the unbound VPA concentrations were elevated above the reference range in 37% of patients.[121]

$$V = 0.2 \text{ L/kg } (82 \text{ kg})$$
$$= 16.4 \text{ L}$$

$$C_{peak} = \frac{(S)(F)(Dose)}{V} \qquad \text{(Eq. 15.1)}$$

$$= \frac{(1)(1)(1,500 \text{ mg})}{16.4 \text{ L}}$$
$$= 91.5 \text{ mg/L}$$

Question #2 *What is an appropriate maintenance dose to be administered by continuous IV infusion to achieve an average steady-state concentration of 70 mg/L? If the drug is administered through a nasogastric (NG) tube, what would be an appropriate dosing regimen?*

Using the population Cl = 10 mL/hr/kg, the maintenance dose to achieve the average steady-state concentration of 70 mg/L can be calculated using the continuous infusion model.

$$\text{Cl} = 10 \text{ mL/hr/kg } (82 \text{ kg})(1 \text{ L/1,000 mL})$$
$$= 0.82 \text{ L/hr}$$

$$\text{Dose}/\tau = \frac{(C_{ss\,ave}\ [\text{mg/L}])(Cl\ [\text{L/hr}])}{(S)(F)} \qquad \textbf{(Eq. 15.2)}$$

$$= \frac{(70\ \text{mg/L})(0.82\ \text{L/hr})}{(1)(1)}$$

$$= 57.4\ \text{mg/hr}$$

This can also be given by syrup if the gastrointestinal tract is used and access is gained (eg, NG tube). Based on the population values of Cl and V, the elimination rate constant (K) and half-life ($t_{1/2}$) can be calculated as follows:

$$K = \frac{Cl}{V} \qquad \textbf{(Eq. 15.3)}$$

$$= \frac{0.82\ \text{L/hr}}{16.4\ \text{L}}$$

$$= 0.05\ \text{hr}^{-1}$$

$$t_{1/2} = \frac{0.693}{K} \qquad \textbf{(Eq. 15.4)}$$

$$= \frac{0.693}{0.05\ \text{hr}^{-1}}$$

$$= 13.9\ \text{hr}$$

In order to minimize peak-to-trough fluctuation in plasma concentrations, the dosing interval for a rapid-release product should be much less than the half-life. Using an interval of every 6 hours, the dose can be calculated using Equation 15.2 as follows:

$$= \frac{(70\ \text{mg/L})(0.82\ \text{L/hr})(6\ \text{hr})}{(1)(1)}$$

$$= 344\ \text{mg} \approx 350\ \text{mg}$$

Question #3 *B.I. was receiving an emergent computed tomography scan immediately after receiving his IV load of VPA. Instead of the planned postbolus level, a serum level is obtained 8 hours after completed infusion and measures 55 mg/L. What maintenance dose would be recommended to maintain an average steady-state concentration of 70 mg/L? What are the estimated steady-state C_{max} and C_{min} concentrations on this prescribed dose?*

The estimated peak and the 8-hour postinfusion measured concentrations can be used to determine the revised VPA clearance.

$$K = \frac{\ln\left(\dfrac{C_1}{C_2}\right)}{\Delta t} \qquad \text{(Eq. 15.5)}$$

$$= \frac{\ln\left(\dfrac{91.5 \text{ mg/L}}{55 \text{ mg/L}}\right)}{7 \text{ hr}}$$

$$= 0.073 \text{ hr}^{-1}$$

$$t_{\frac{1}{2}} = \frac{0.693}{K}$$

$$= \frac{0.693}{0.073 \text{ hr}^{-1}}$$

$$= 9.5 \text{ hr}$$

The revised Cl can be calculated using the population V and revised K.

$$\text{Cl} = (K)(V)$$

$$= (0.073 \text{ hr}^{-1})(16.4 \text{ L})$$

$$= 1.2 \text{ L/hr}$$

The revised dose can then be calculated using Equation 15.2 to achieve the desired average steady-state concentration of 70 mg/L.

$$= \frac{(70 \text{ mg/L})(1.2 \text{ L/hr})(6 \text{ hr})}{(1)(1)}$$

$$= 504 \text{ mg} \approx 500 \text{ mg IV or syrup q6h}$$

We can use the parameters determined here to calculate the steady-state peak and trough (predose) concentrations of the 500 mg IV every 6-hour regimen using the steady-state bolus Equation 15.6. Because $t_{\frac{1}{2}}$ is 9.5 hours, we consider the drug lost and gained during the short infusion negligible.

The steady-state C_{max} can also be calculated using Equation 15.6.

$$C_{ss\,max} = \frac{\dfrac{(S)(F)(\text{Dose})}{V}}{1 - e^{-(K)(\tau)}} \qquad \text{(Eq. 15.6)}$$

$$= \frac{\dfrac{(1)(1)(500 \text{ mg})}{16.4}}{1 - e^{-(0.073)(6)}}$$

$$= 85.96 \text{ mg/L} \approx 86 \text{ mg/L}$$

The steady-state C_{min} can then be calculated using the C_{max} and revised K with Equation 15.7 as follows:

$$C_{ss\,min} = (C_{ss\,max})e^{-(K)(\tau)} \qquad \text{(Eq. 15.7)}$$

$$= (86 \text{ mg/L})\, e^{-(0.073 \text{ hr}^{-1})(6 \text{ hr})}$$

$$= 55.5 \text{ mg/L}$$

Question #4   *B.I. has his seizures controlled while in the ICU on a dose of VPA of 500 mg every 8 hours, but spikes a fever and has an elevated neutrophil count. He has a history of documented urinary tract infections with an extended-spectrum β-lactamase producing Escherichia coli and is placed on meropenem 1,000 mg every 8 hours on suspicion of recurrence. Two days later, he has a breakthrough tonic-clonic seizure, and a STAT mid-interval VPA level comes back at 25 mg/L. All of the doses are checked, and another serum sample is sent for verification, and it results as 19 mg/L. A 1,000 mg loading dose is given, and the maintenance dose is increased to 750 mg every 8 hours. The next morning, B.I. has another brief breakthrough seizure, and the VPA level sent is 25 mg/L. Rapid calculation demonstrates a clearance value that is not physiologically plausible. What accounts for the repeated low levels?*

A major pathway of VPA metabolism is via glucuronidation, and deglucuronidation by hydrolysis may contribute active drug back into the circulation. The carbapenem antibiotics (eg, imipenem, doripenem, meropenem) all feature inhibition of the VPA glucuronidase enzyme acylpeptide hydrolase, located in the cytosol of the liver and kidney, which blocks the deglucuronidation of VPA and enhances the urinary elimination of VPA glucuronide.[122,123] This increases the apparent clearance dramatically, and VPA levels fall more than 50%, even with increased dosing,[123,124] hence precipitating seizures in those vulnerable to breakthrough. Even increases in dose may not sustain a therapeutic level or outcome, and other antimicrobials, susceptibility permitting, or additional antiepileptic drugs may be required. Despite the relatively short half-lives of the carbapenems, the effect on blocking deglucuronidation lasts for several days, and levels may take a week or more to return to pre-carbapenem values. Meropenem and ertapenem show greater decreases in VPA levels in patients than with imipenem. Care must be taken to recognize the interaction and prevent seizure activity appropriately[125] and to reduce the dose of VPA back to the baseline VPA doses that had been significantly raised in an attempt to obtain therapeutic concentrations, because once the interaction reverses, the VPA levels may rise dramatically to levels promoting toxicity. Perhaps, more concerning is the convenience of the use of parenteral ertapenem to treat various community infections in the nonhospital setting, thereby increasing the risk of breakthrough seizure activity in a less monitored location. This interaction has been exploited in the management of VPA overdoses by administering a carbapenem as an antidote.[126]

Question #5   *B.I.'s seizures are eventually controlled on a regimen of Depakote delayed-release tablets of 500 mg PO every 8 hours, while he receives chemotherapy and radiation for his brain tumor. He has maintained a VPA trough level of 50 mg/L. He is diagnosed with depression, and fluoxetine is added to his regimen. He is seen in the clinic a month later, and it is noted that his nutrition is poor and he has lost 7 kg. His depression is slightly improved, but a noticeable tremor in his right hand is present, and he is sleepy during the day. His labs show that his albumin is low at 2.8 g/dL, his ammonia level has risen to 98 μmol/L, and his follow-up trough VPA level is now 70 mg/L. What assessment can be made regarding any changes in the PK of VPA and associated toxicity findings? Should a change in VPA dose be recommended?*

B.I.'s VPA revised Cl can be calculated from the trough level. Because the time to maximum concentrations (T_{max}) with the delayed-release tablets is approximately 8 hours, the fluctuation between peak and trough concentrations with every 8-hour dosing is minimal, and, therefore, the trough concentration can be considered an average steady state. The revised Cl can then be calculated using Equation 15.8.

$$\text{Cl (L/hr)} = \frac{(S)(F)(\text{Dose})}{C_{ss\,ave}\,(\tau)} \qquad \textbf{(Eq. 15.8)}$$

$$= \frac{(1)(1)(500\text{ mg})}{(50\text{ mg/L})\,(8\text{ hr})}$$
$$= 1.25\text{ L/hr or } 16.67\text{ mL/hr/kg}$$

After adding fluoxetine, we have

$$= \frac{(1)(1)(500\text{ mg})}{(70\text{ mg/L})(8\text{ hr})}$$
$$= 0.89\text{ L/hr}$$

With the 40% increase in steady-state blood level to 70 mg/L, B.I.'s VPA clearance is reduced to 0.893 L/hr, or 11.90 mL/hr/kg, a decrease of 28.6%. Fluoxetine can moderately inhibit CYP2C9 metabolism, an important pathway in the metabolism of VPA, thus limiting its intrinsic clearance. [29,48,49,45,72,73,77]

However, the total concentration measured is not outside the therapeutic range, or consistent with levels of dose-related toxicities, though individual sensitivities should be clinically considered.

Concentration-dependent protein binding is evident within the therapeutic range, and considering that hypoalbuminemia is present in B.I., an assessment of the free concentration given reduced binding capacity may be useful in sorting out these apparent concentration-related toxicities. There are a number of equations and graphic relationships that illustrate the nonlinearity of the relationship between free and total (free + bound) concentrations. A simple linearized version of this nonlinear relationship is the following: fraction unbound (fu) = 0.0015 C_p total. [127]

$$\text{Fraction unbound (fu)} = 0.0015\ C_p\ \text{total} \qquad \textbf{(Eq. 15.9)}$$

$$\text{For B.I., fu} = 0.0015\ (70)$$
$$= 0.105\text{ or } 10.5\%$$

The free concentration can be calculated from the total (measured) concentration and the estimated fraction unbound (fu) as follows:

$$\text{Free concentration} = \text{Total concentration (fu)} \qquad \textbf{(Eq. 15.10)}$$

$$= 70 \text{ mg/L } (0.105)$$
$$= 7.35 \text{ mg/L}$$

The therapeutic range of free VPA is 2.5 to 10.0 for epilepsy and 2.5 to 12.5 mg/L for bipolar mania (based on normal fu of 0.05–0.1).

With B.I.'s hypoalbuminemia, the free fraction is increased when the binding capacity (ie, albumin concentration) diminishes. For total VPA concentrations greater than 75 mg/L, an accurate corrected level can be calculated as % free $= 130.2 \times e^{(-0.72 \times ALB)}$, where ALB is the albumin concentration in g/dL.[30] The fu for B.I. at an albumin concentration of 2.8 g/dL is estimated to be 17.34%, and therefore, the free concentration $= 0.1734 \times 70 \text{ mg/L} = 12.14 \text{ mg/L}$, which exceeds the therapeutic range for free drug in epilepsy and can explain the adverse effects seen in this patient.

These equations provide calculated free levels that are different, with the Hermida method being recognized to be inaccurate at total serum levels over 75 mg/L.[120] A 20% reduction in dose will decrease the free concentration closer to 10 mg/L, with a total level $= 10 \text{ mg/L}/0.1734 = 57.3 \text{ mg/L}$ at the current albumin concentration.

Question #6 *B.I. is receiving treatment for his brain tumor and has a break-through seizure during a clinic visit despite adequate VPA serum concentrations. PHT is added at a dose of 400 mg/d, and B.I.'s seizures are controlled. The PHT steady-state concentration is 6.6 mg/L, and the physician is contemplating increasing the PHT dose to achieve the therapeutic range of 10 to 20 mg/L. B.I. still has an albumin concentration of 2.8 g/dL. Should the PHT dose be increased?*

A calculation of the free fraction of PHT can be made using an equation derived from the literature[46]:

$$\text{Phenytoin fu} = 0.1 + [0.0151 \times (4.08 - ALB)] + (0.0525 \times VPA) + (0.0385 \times CBZ) \qquad \textbf{(Eq. 15.12)}$$

where ALB is the albumin concentration in g/dL, VPA and CBZ are 1 if the patient is on those comedications (which raise the free fraction of PHT by 52.5% and 38.5%, respectively), otherwise it is zero. 0.1 is the normal free fraction of PHT.

Therefore, for B.I.:

$$\text{Phenytoin fu} = 0.1 + [0.0151 \times (4.08 - ALB)] + (0.0525 \times VPA) + (0.0385 \times CBZ) = 0.1718 \text{ (or 17.2\%)}$$

$$\text{Phenytoin free concentration} = fu \times C_{ss} = 0.1718 \times 6.6 \text{ mg/L} = 1.14 \text{ mg/L}$$

The estimated free PHT concentration would be in the stated therapeutic range for unbound PHT concentrations of 1 to 2 mg/L.

Alternatively, the corrected total PHT concentration can be calculated as follows:

$$C_{ss\ corrected} = C_{ss\ measured} \left(\frac{fu\ calculated}{fu\ normal} \right) \quad \text{(Eq. 15.13)}$$

$$= 6.6\ mg/L \left(\frac{0.1718}{0.1} \right)$$

$$= 11.4\ mg/L$$

Therefore, B.I. should not require a dose change, given the free PHT level estimate and corrected total PHT level are within their respective therapeutic ranges, and B.I. is sustaining good antiseizure response from the combination.

Question #7 *M.Z. is an 11-year-old, 42-kg prepubescent female with a history of focal convulsive epilepsy that is incompletely controlled by high therapeutic doses of CBZ, and VPA will be added. To accommodate her school schedule, she is prescribed 500 mg of Depakote to be taken at 0800 and 2,000 daily (23.8 mg/kg/d). What would be her estimated average steady-state serum level?*

Concomitant use of other antiepileptic agents is known to increase the metabolic clearance of VPA. CBZ induces CYP3A4 metabolism of VPA, which requires increased doses of VPA to maintain therapeutic concentrations. In addition, as stated previously, VPA exhibits dose-dependent changes in clearance as a function of saturable protein binding. Several population PK models have been published that relate dose-dependent changes in VPA clearance as a surrogate to saturable protein binding, as well as incorporating adjustments for common drug interactions. One such model developed from a pediatric population is represented in Equation 15.14.

$$Cl\ (L/hr) = 0.012\ (\text{weight in kg})^{0.715} \times Dose\ (mg/kg/d)^{0.306} \times (1 + 0.359 \times CBZ) \quad \text{(Eq. 15.14)}$$

where CBZ is 1 if comedicated with CBZ, otherwise it is 0 (indicating an increase in VPA clearance by 35.9% when CBZ is present).[49]

$$= 0.012 \times (42\ kg)^{0.715} \times (23.8\ mg/kg/d)^{0.306} \times (1 + 0.359 \times 1)$$

$$= 0.012 \times 14.475 \times 2.638 \times 1.359$$

$$= 0.6226\ L/hr$$

$$= 14.83\ mL/hr/kg$$

The average steady-state concentration can be calculated using Equation 15.15 as follows:

$$C_{ss\ ave} = \frac{(S)(F)(\text{Dose})}{(Cl)(\tau)} \quad \text{(Eq. 15.15)}$$

$$= \frac{(1)(1)(500 \text{ mg})}{(0.62 \text{ L/hr})(12 \text{ hr})}$$

$$= 67 \text{ mg/L}$$

A model constructed and tested in adults from the same investigators[48] has a similar structure, including clearance induction terms for PHT and PB:

$$Cl (L/hr) = 0.004 (wt \text{ in } kg) \times Dose (mg/kg/d)^{0.304} \times (1 + (0.363 \times CBZ))$$
$$\times (1 + (0.541 \times PHT)) \times (1 + (0.397 \times PB))$$

Other mathematical expressions encompassing the same and other covariates in ethnically and pharmacogenetically diverse populations have been published, with lower and higher magnitudes of the effect of comedications on clearance.[50-52,128-130] Conversely, the statistical magnitude of VPA effect on the clearance of other ASMs and non-ASMs has been captured in population PK models of those agents.[85,86,128,131,132]

REFERENCES

1.   Tomson T, Battino D, Perucca E. Valproic acid after five decades of use in epilepsy: time to reconsider the indications of a time-honoured drug. *Lancet Neurol.* 2016;15(2):210-218.

2.   Guerrini R. Valproate as a mainstay of therapy for pediatric epilepsy. *Paediatr Drugs.* 2006;8(2):113-129.

3.   Rahman M, Nguyen H. *Valproic Acid.* StatPearls; 2022.

4.   Yee CS, Vazquez GH, Hawken ER, Biorac A, Tondo L, Baldessarini RJ. Long-term treatment of bipolar disorder with valproate: updated systematic review and meta-analyses. *Harv Rev Psychiatry.* 2021;29(3):188-195.

5.   Rollo E, Romozzi M, Vollono C, Calabresi P, Geppetti P, Iannone LF. Antiseizure medications for the prophylaxis of migraine during the anti-CGRP drugs era. *Curr Neuropharmacol.* 2022.

6.   Han W, Guan W. Valproic acid: a promising therapeutic agent in glioma treatment. *Front Oncol.* 2021;11:687362.

7.   Swayngim R, Preslaski C, Dawson J. Use of valproic acid for the management of delirium and agitation in the intensive care unit. *J Pharm Pract.* 2022:8971900221128636.

8.   Dogruyol S, Gur STA, Akbas I, et al. Intravenous ibuprofen versus sodium valproate in acute migraine attacks in the emergency department: a randomized clinical trial. *Am J Emerg Med.* 2022;55:126-132.

9.   Chen A, Sharoha N. Valproate efficacy for agitation management in a patient with paroxysmal sympathetic hyperactivity due to traumatic brain injury. *Prim Care Companion CNS Disord.* 2021;23(5):20cr02892.

10. Beresford T, Ronan PJ, Hipp D, et al. A double-blind placebo-controlled, randomized trial of divalproex sodium for posttraumatic irritability greater than 1 year after mild to moderate traumatic brain injury. *J Neuropsychiatry Clin Neurosci.* 2022;34(3):224-232.

11. Panomvana Na Ayudhya D, Suwanmanee J, Visudtibhan A. Pharmacokinetic parameters of total and unbound valproic acid and their relationships to seizure control in epileptic children. *Am J Ther.* 2006;13(3):211-217.

12. Felix S, Sproule BA, Hardy BG, Naranjo CA. Dose-related pharmacokinetics and pharmacodynamics of valproate in the elderly. *J Clin Psychopharmacol.* 2003;23(5):471-478.

13. Smith RL, Haslemo T, Refsum H, Molden E. Impact of age, gender and CYP2C9/2C19 genotypes on dose-adjusted steady-state serum concentrations of valproic acid-a large-scale study based on naturalistic therapeutic drug monitoring data. *Eur J Clin Pharmacol.* 2016;72(9):1099-1104.

14. Cloyd JC, Fischer JH, Kriel RL, Kraus DM. Valproic acid pharmacokinetics in children. IV. Effects of age and antiepileptic drugs on protein binding and intrinsic clearance. *Clin Pharmacol Ther.* 1993;53(1):22-29.

15. Xu S, Chen Y, Zhao M, Guo Y, Wang Z, Zhao L. Population pharmacokinetics of valproic acid in epileptic children: effects of clinical and genetic factors. *Eur J Pharm Sci.* 2018;122:170-178.

16. Ghodke-Puranik Y, Thorn CF, Lamba JK, et al. Valproic acid pathway: pharmacokinetics and pharmacodynamics. *Pharmacogenet Genomics.* 2013;23(4):236-241.

17. Vakrinou A, Murphy E, Sisodiya SM, Vivekananda U, Balestrini S. Risk factors and outcome of hyperammonaemia in people with epilepsy. *J Neurol.* 2022;269(12):6395-6405.

18. Schmidt D, Schachter SC. Drug treatment of epilepsy in adults. *BMJ.* 2014;348:g254.

19. Hakami T. Neuropharmacology of antiseizure drugs. *Neuropsychopharmacol Rep.* 2021;41(3):336-351.

20. Salminen JK, Tammela TL, Auvinen A, Murtola TJ. Antiepileptic drugs with histone deacetylase inhibition activity and prostate cancer risk: a population-based case-control study. *Cancer Causes Control.* 2016;27(5):637-645.

21. Singh D, Gupta S, Verma I, Morsy MA, Nair AB, Ahmed AF. Hidden pharmacological activities of valproic acid: a new insight. *Biomed Pharmacother.* 2021;142:112021.

22. Dutta S, Reed RC. Distinct absorption characteristics of oral formulations of valproic acid/divalproex available in the United States. *Epilepsy Res.* 2007;73(3):275-283.

23. DiScala SL, Tran NN, Silverman MA. Valproic acid suppositories for management of seizures for geriatric patients. *Consult Pharm.* 2016;31(6):313-319.

24. Delage C, Palayer M, Etain B, et al. Valproate, divalproex, valpromide: are the differences in indications justified? *Biomed Pharmacother.* 2023;158:114051.

25. Ibarra M, Vazquez M, Fagiolino P, Derendorf H. Sex related differences on valproic acid pharmacokinetics after oral single dose. *J Pharmacokinet Pharmacodyn.* 2013;40(4):479-486.

26. Charlier B, Coglianese A, De Rosa F, et al. The effect of plasma protein binding on the therapeutic monitoring of antiseizure medications. *Pharmaceutics.* 2021;13(8):1208.

27. Cloyd JC, Dutta S, Cao G, Walch JK, Collins SD, Granneman GR; Depacon Study Group. Valproate unbound fraction and distribution volume following rapid infusions in patients with epilepsy. *Epilepsy Res.* 2003;53(1-2):19-27.

28. Otten N, Hall K, Irvine-Meek J, Leroux M, Budnik D, Seshia S. Free valproic acid: steady-state pharmacokinetics in patients with intractable epilepsy. *Can J Neurol Sci.* 1984;11(4):457-460.

29. Riker RR, Gagnon DJ, Hatton C, et al. Valproate protein binding is highly variable in ICU patients and not predicted by total serum concentrations: a case series and literature review. *Pharmacotherapy.* 2017;37(4):500-508.

30. Ueshima S, Aiba T, Makita T, et al. Characterization of non-linear relationship between total and unbound serum concentrations of valproic acid in epileptic children. *J Clin Pharm Ther.* 2008;33(1):31-38.

31. Bailey DN, Briggs JR. The binding of selected therapeutic drugs to human serum alpha-1 acid glycoprotein and to human serum albumin in vitro. *Ther Drug Monit.* 2004;26(1):40-43.

32. Shen DD, Ojemann GA, Rapport RL, Dills RL, Friel PN, Levy RH. Low and variable presence of valproic acid in human brain. *Neurology.* 1992;42(3 Pt 1):582-585.

33. Gu X, Zhu M, Sheng C, et al. Population pharmacokinetics of unbound valproic acid in pediatric epilepsy patients in China: a protein binding model. *Eur J Clin Pharmacol.* 2021;77(7):999-1009.

34. Ueshima S, Aiba T, Ishikawa N, et al. Poor applicability of estimation method for adults to calculate unbound serum concentrations of valproic acid in epileptic neonates and infants. *J Clin Pharm Ther.* 2009;34(4):415-422.

35. Lampon N, Tutor JC. Apparent clearance of valproic acid in elderly epileptic patients: estimation of the confounding effect of albumin concentration. *Ups J Med Sci.* 2012;117(1):41-46.

36. Butler JM, Begg EJ. Free drug metabolic clearance in elderly people. *Clin Pharmacokinet.* 2008; 47(5):297-321.

37. Gatti G, Crema F, Attardo-Parrinello G, Fratino P, Aguzzi F, Perucca E. Serum protein binding of phenytoin and valproic acid in insulin-dependent diabetes mellitus. *Ther Drug Monit.* 1987;9(4):389-391.

38. Hatton C, Riker RR, Gagnon DJ, May T, Seder DB, Fraser GL. Free serum valproate concentration more reliable than total concentration in critically ill patients. *Resuscitation.* 2016;105:e15-e16.

39. Christensen H, Baker M, Tucker GT, Rostami-Hodjegan A. Prediction of plasma protein binding displacement and its implications for quantitative assessment of metabolic drug-drug interactions from in vitro data. *J Pharm Sci.* 2006;95(12):2778-2787.

40. Lana F, Marti-Bonany J, de Leon J. Ibuprofen may increase pharmacological action of valproate by displacing it from plasma proteins: a case report. *Am J Psychiatry.* 2016;173(9):941-942.

41. Dasgupta A, Jacques M, Malhotra D. Diminished protein binding capacity of uremic sera for valproate following hemodialysis: role of free fatty acids and uremic compounds. *Am J Nephrol.* 1996;16(4):327-333.

42. Gugler R, Mueller G. Plasma protein binding of valproic acid in healthy subjects and in patients with renal disease. *Br J Clin Pharmacol.* 1978;5(5):441-446.

43. Sandson NB, Marcucci C, Bourke DL, Smith-Lamacchia R. An interaction between aspirin and valproate: the relevance of plasma protein displacement drug-drug interactions. *Am J Psychiatry.* 2006;163(11):1891-1896.

44. Rodrigues-Silva N, Venancio A, Bouça J. Risperidone, a risk factor for valproate-induced encephalopathy? *Gen Hosp Psychiatry.* 2013;35(4):452.e5-452.e6.

45. Zaccara G, Perucca E. Interactions between antiepileptic drugs, and between antiepileptic drugs and other drugs. *Epileptic Disord.* 2014;16(4):409-431.

46. Joerger M, Huitema AD, Boogerd W, van der Sande JJ, Schellens JH, Beijnen JH. Interactions of serum albumin, valproic acid and carbamazepine with the pharmacokinetics of phenytoin in cancer patients. *Basic Clin Pharmacol Toxicol.* 2006;99(2):133-140.

47. Ratnaraj N, Hjelm M. Prediction of free levels of phenytoin and carbamazepine in patients comedicated with valproic acid. *Ther Drug Monit.* 1995;17(4):327-332.

48. Blanco-Serrano B, Otero MJ, Santos-Buelga D, Garcia-Sanchez MJ, Serrano J, Dominguez-Gil A. Population estimation of valproic acid clearance in adult patients using routine clinical pharmacokinetic data. *Biopharm Drug Dispos.* 1999;20(5):233-240.

49. Serrano BB, Garcia Sanchez MJ, Otero MJ, Buelga DS, Serrano J, Dominguez-Gil A. Valproate population pharmacokinetics in children. *J Clin Pharm Ther.* 1999;24(1):73-80.

50. Lin WW, Jiao Z, Wang CL, et al. Population pharmacokinetics of valproic acid in adult Chinese epileptic patients and its application in an individualized dosage regimen. *Ther Drug Monit.* 2015;37(1):76-83.

51. Nakashima H, Oniki K, Nishimura M, et al. Determination of the optimal concentration of valproic acid in patients with epilepsy: a population pharmacokinetic-pharmacodynamic analysis. *PLoS One.* 2015;10(10):e0141266.

52. Methaneethorn J. Population pharmacokinetics of valproic acid in patients with mania: implication for individualized dosing regimens. *Clin Ther.* 2017;39(6):1171-1181.

53. Methaneethorn J, Leelakanok N. Predictive ability of published population pharmacokinetic models of valproic acid in Thai manic patients. *J Clin Pharm Ther.* 2021;46(1):198-207.

54. Zang YN, Guo W, Dong F, Li AN, de Leon J, Ruan CJ. Published population pharmacokinetic models of valproic acid in adult patients: a systematic review and external validation in a Chinese sample of inpatients with bipolar disorder. *Expert Rev Clin Pharmacol.* 2022;15(5):621-635.

55. Chiba K, Suganuma T, Ishizaki T, et al. Comparison of steady-state pharmacokinetics of valproic acid in children between monotherapy and multiple antiepileptic drug treatment. *J Pediatr.* 1985;106(4):653-658.

56. Ogungbenro K, Aarons L; CRESim & Epi-CRESim Project Groups. A physiologically based pharmacokinetic model for valproic acid in adults and children. *Eur J Pharm Sci.* 2014;63:45-52.

57. Limdi NA, Knowlton RK, Cofield SS, et al. Safety of rapid intravenous loading of valproate. *Epilepsia.* 2007;48(3):478-483.

58. Glauser T, Shinnar S, Gloss D, et al. Evidence-based guideline: treatment of convulsive status epilepticus in children and adults: report of the Guideline Committee of the American Epilepsy Society. *Epilepsy Curr.* 2016;16(1):48-61.

59. Uberall MA, Trollmann R, Wunsiedler U, Wenzel D. Intravenous valproate in pediatric epilepsy patients with refractory status epilepticus. *Neurology.* 2000;54(11):2188-2189.

60. Budi T, Toth K, Nagy A, et al. Clinical significance of CYP2C9-status guided valproic acid therapy in children. *Epilepsia*. 2015;56(6):849-855.

61. Star K, Edwards IR, Choonara I. Valproic acid and fatalities in children: a review of individual case safety reports in VigiBase. *PLoS One*. 2014;9(10):e108970.

62. Lheureux PE, Hantson P. Carnitine in the treatment of valproic acid-induced toxicity. *Clin Toxicol (Phila)*. 2009;47(2):101-111.

63. Fang H, Wang X, Hou K, et al. The association of adjusted plasma valproic acid concentration with CYP2C9 gene polymorphism in patients with epilepsy: a systematic review and meta-analysis. *Ann Transl Med*. 2021;9(10):846.

64. Toth K, Budi T, Kiss A, et al. Phenoconversion of CYP2C9 in epilepsy limits the predictive value of CYP2C9 genotype in optimizing valproate therapy. *Per Med*. 2015;12(3):199-207.

65. Monostory K, Nagy A, Toth K, et al. Relevance of CYP2C9 function in valproate therapy. *Curr Neuropharmacol*. 2019;17(1):99-106.

66. Du Z, Jiao Y, Shi L. Association of UGT2B7 and UGT1A4 polymorphisms with serum concentration of antiepileptic drugs in children. *Med Sci Monit*. 2016;22:4107-4113.

67. Zhu MM, Li HL, Shi LH, Chen XP, Luo J, Zhang ZL. The pharmacogenomics of valproic acid. *J Hum Genet*. 2017;62(12):1009-1014.

68. Shen X, Chen X, Lu J, et al. Pharmacogenetics-based population pharmacokinetic analysis and dose optimization of valproic acid in Chinese southern children with epilepsy: effect of ABCB1 gene polymorphism. *Front Pharmacol*. 2022;13:1037239.

69. Gao P, Wang J, Zhang L, et al. The impact of ibuprofen on valproic acid plasma concentration in pediatric patients. *Xenobiotica*. 2022;52(6):535-540.

70. Anderson GD, Temkin NR, Awan AB, Winn HR. Effect of time, injury, age and ethanol on interpatient variability in valproic acid pharmacokinetics after traumatic brain injury. *Clin Pharmacokinet*. 2007;46(4):307-318.

71. Methaneethorn J. A systematic review of population pharmacokinetics of valproic acid. *Br J Clin Pharmacol*. 2018;84(5):816-834.

72. Patsalos PN. Drug interactions with the newer antiepileptic drugs (AEDs)—Part 1: pharmacokinetic and pharmacodynamic interactions between AEDs. *Clin Pharmacokinet*. 2013;52(11):927-966.

73. Patsalos PN. Drug interactions with the newer antiepileptic drugs (AEDs)—Part 2: pharmacokinetic and pharmacodynamic interactions between AEDs and drugs used to treat non-epilepsy disorders. *Clin Pharmacokinet*. 2013;52(12):1045-1061.

74. Grewal GK, Kukal S, Kanojia N, Madan K, Saso L, Kukreti R. In vitro assessment of the effect of antiepileptic drugs on expression and function of ABC transporters and their interactions with ABCC2. *Molecules*. 2017;22(10):1484.

75. Stollberger C, Finsterer J. Interactions between non-vitamin K oral anticoagulants and antiepileptic drugs. *Epilepsy Res*. 2016;126:98-101.

76. Ip BY, Ko H, Wong GL, et al. Thromboembolic risks with concurrent direct oral anticoagulants and antiseizure medications: a population-based analysis. *CNS Drugs*. 2022;36(12):1313-1324.

77. Spina E, Pisani F, de Leon J. Clinically significant pharmacokinetic drug interactions of antiepileptic drugs with new antidepressants and new antipsychotics. *Pharmacol Res*. 2016;106:72-86.

78. Lalic M, Cvejic J, Popovic J, et al. Lamotrigine and valproate pharmacokinetics interactions in epileptic patients. *Eur J Drug Metab Pharmacokinet*. 2009;34(2):93-99.

79. Liu L, Zhao L, Wang Q, Qiu F, Wu X, Ma Y. Influence of valproic acid concentration and polymorphism of UGT1A4*3, UGT2B7 -161C > T and UGT2B7*2 on serum concentration of lamotrigine in Chinese epileptic children. *Eur J Clin Pharmacol*. 2015;71(11):1341-1347.

80. Nakamura T, Tomita M, Hirota S, Matsunaga T, Uchimura N. Impact of selected initial titration schedules on safety and long-term effectiveness of lamotrigine for the treatment of mood disorders. *J Clin Psychopharmacol*. 2022;42(4):350-356.

81. Wang Q, Zhao L, Liang M, et al. Effects of UGT2B7 genetic polymorphisms on serum concentrations of valproic acid in Chinese children with epilepsy comedicated with lamotrigine. *Ther Drug Monit*. 2016;38(3):343-349.

82. Yang Q, Hu Y, Zhang X, Zhang X, Dai H, Li X. Population pharmacokinetics of oxcarbazepine 10-monohydroxy derivative in Chinese adult epileptic patients. *Eur J Hosp Pharm*. 2022;30(e1):e90-e96.

83. Hommers L, Scharl M, Hefner G, et al. Comedication of valproic acid is associated with increased metabolism of clozapine. *J Clin Psychopharmacol*. 2018;38(3):188-192.

84. Sanguesa E, Cirujeda C, Concha J, Padilla PP, Garcia CB, Ribate MP. Pharmacokinetic interactions between clozapine and valproic acid in patients with treatment-resistant schizophrenia: does UGT polymorphism affect these drug interactions? *Chem Biol Interact*. 2022;364:110042.

85. Marazziti D, Palego L, Betti L, et al. Effect of valproate and antidepressant drugs on clozapine metabolism in patients with psychotic mood disorders. *Ther Drug Monit*. 2018;40(4):443-451.

86. Habibi M, Hart F, Bainbridge J. The impact of psychoactive drugs on seizures and antiepileptic drugs. *Curr Neurol Neurosci Rep*. 2016;16(8):71.

87. Deng SH, Wang ZZ, Lu HY, et al. A retrospective analysis of steady-state olanzapine concentrations in Chinese patients using therapeutic drug monitoring: effects of valproate and other factors. *Ther Drug Monit*. 2020;42(4):636-642.

88. Ding J, Zhang Y, Zhang Y, et al. Effects of age, sex, and comedication on the plasma concentrations of olanzapine in Chinese patients with schizophrenia based on therapeutic drug monitoring data. *J Clin Psychopharmacol*. 2022;42(6):552-559.

89. Xiao T, Hu JQ, Liu SJ, et al. Population pharmacokinetics and dosing optimization of olanzapine in Chinese paediatric patients: based on the impact of sex and concomitant valproate on clearance. *J Clin Pharm Ther*. 2022;47(11):1811-1819.

90. Unterecker S, Burger R, Hohage A, Deckert J, Pfuhlmann B. Interaction of valproic acid and amitriptyline: analysis of therapeutic drug monitoring data under naturalistic conditions. *J Clin Psychopharmacol*. 2013;33(4):561-564.

91. Nucera B, Brigo F, Trinka E, Kalss G. Treatment and care of women with epilepsy before, during, and after pregnancy: a practical guide. *Ther Adv Neurol Disord*. 2022;15:17562864221101687.

92. Tomson T, Battino D, Bonizzoni E, et al; EURAP Study Group. Withdrawal of valproic acid treatment during pregnancy and seizure outcome: observations from EURAP. *Epilepsia*. 2016;57(8):e173-e177.

93. Herzog AG, Mandle HB, Cahill KE, Fowler KM, Hauser WA. Differential impact of contraceptive methods on seizures varies by antiepileptic drug category: findings of the epilepsy birth control registry. *Epilepsy Behav*. 2016;60:112-117.

94. Galimberti CA, Mazzucchelli I, Arbasino C, Canevini MP, Fattore C, Perucca E. Increased apparent oral clearance of valproic acid during intake of combined contraceptive steroids in women with epilepsy. *Epilepsia*. 2006;47(9):1569-1572.

95. Suto HS, Braga GC, Scarpellini GR, et al. Neurologist knowledge about interactions between antiepileptic drugs and contraceptive methods. *Int J Gynaecol Obstet*. 2016;134(3):264-267.

96. Kinze S, Clauss M, Reuter U, et al. Valproic acid is effective in migraine prophylaxis at low serum levels: a prospective open-label study. *Headache*. 2001;41(8):774-778.

97. De Iuliis V, Gelormini R, Flacco M, et al. Comparison of serum total valproic acid levels and %CDT values in chronic alcohol addictive patients in an Italian clinic: a retrospective study. *Drugs Real World Outcomes*. 2016;3(1):7-12.

98. Hernandez-Vanegas LE, Jara-Prado A, Ochoa A, et al. High-dose versus low-dose valproate for the treatment of juvenile myoclonic epilepsy: going from low to high. *Epilepsy Behav*. 2016;61:34-40.

99. Sathe AG, Mishra U, Ivaturi V, et al. Early exposure of fosphenytoin, levetiracetam, and valproic acid after High-dose intravenous administration in young children with benzodiazepine-refractory status epilepticus. *J Clin Pharmacol*. 2021;61(6):763-768.

100. Lind J, Nordlund P. Intravenous use of valproic acid in status epilepticus is associated with high risk of hyperammonemia. *Seizure*. 2019;69:20-24.

101. Abou-Khalil BW. Update on antiseizure medications 2022. *Continuum (Minneap Minn)*. 2022;28(2):500-535.

102. Bowden CL, Janicak PG, Orsulak P, et al. Relation of serum valproate concentration to response in mania. *Am J Psychiatry*. 1996;153(6):765-770.

103. Young MR, Bisaccia EK, Romantseva L, Hovey SW. Valproic acid serum concentration and incidence of toxicity in pediatric patients. *J Child Neurol.* 2022;37(6):461-470.

104. Nanau RM, Neuman MG. Adverse drug reactions induced by valproic acid. *Clin Biochem.* 2013;46(15):1323-1338.

105. Hosseini H, Shafie M, Shakiba A, et al. Valproic acid-induced hyperammonemia in neuropsychiatric disorders: a 2-year clinical survey. *Psychopharmacology (Berl).* 2023;240(1):149-156.

106. Itoh H, Suzuki Y, Fujisaki K, Sato Y, Takeyama M. Correlation between plasma ammonia level and serum trough concentration of free valproic acid in patients with epilepsy. *Biol Pharm Bull.* 2012;35(6):971-974.

107. Chopra A, Kolla BP, Mansukhani MP, Netzel P, Frye MA. Valproate-induced hyperammonemic encephalopathy: an update on risk factors, clinical correlates and management. *Gen Hosp Psychiatry.* 2012;34(3):290-298.

108. Blackford MG, Do ST, Enlow TC, Reed MD. Valproic acid and topiramate induced hyperammonemic encephalopathy in a patient with normal serum carnitine. *J Pediatr Pharmacol Ther.* 2013;18(2):128-136.

109. Muller A, von Hofen-Hohloch J, Awissus C, Przybilla J, Mrestani A, Classen J. Does diabetes mellitus affect the safety profile of valproic acid for the treatment of status epilepticus? A retrospective cohort study. *Neurol Res Pract.* 2022;4(1):52.

110. Nasreddine W, Atweh SF, Beydoun AA, Dirani M, Nawfal O, Beydoun A. Predicting the occurrence of thrombocytopenia from free valproate levels: a prospective study. *Seizure.* 2022;94:33-38.

111. Stoner SC, Deal E, Lurk JT. Delayed-onset neutropenia with divalproex sodium. *Ann Pharmacother.* 2008;42(10):1507-1510.

112. Jakovljevic MB, Jankovic SM, Jankovic SV, Todorovic N. Inverse correlation of valproic acid serum concentrations and quality of life in adolescents with epilepsy. *Epilepsy Res.* 2008;80(2-3):180-183.

113. Ogusu N, Saruwatari J, Nakashima H, et al. Impact of the superoxide dismutase 2 Val16Ala polymorphism on the relationship between valproic acid exposure and elevation of gamma-glutamyltransferase in patients with epilepsy: a population pharmacokinetic-pharmacodynamic analysis. *PLoS One.* 2014;9(11):e111066.

114. Pawlowska-Kamieniak A, Krawiec P, Pac-Kozuchowska E. Acute pancreatitis as a complication of antiepileptic treatment: case series and review of the literature. *Pediatr Rep.* 2021;13(1):98-103.

115. Kim SH, Chung HR, Kim SH, et al. Subclinical hypothyroidism during valproic acid therapy in children and adolescents with epilepsy. *Neuropediatrics.* 2012;43(3):135-139.

116. Hamed SA, Abdellah MM. The relationship between valproate induced tremors and circulating neurotransmitters: a preliminary study. *Int J Neurosci.* 2017;127(3):236-242.

117. Mani B, Nair PP, Sekhar A, Kamalanathan S, Narayan SK, Kesavan R. CYP2C19 & UGT1A6 genetic polymorphisms and the impact on valproic acid-induced weight gain in people with epilepsy: prospective genetic association study. *Epilepsy Res.* 2021;177:106786.

118. Tomson T, Battino D, Perucca E. Teratogenicity of antiepileptic drugs. *Curr Opin Neurol.* 2019;32(2):246-252.

119. Vajda FJE, O'Brien TJ, Graham JE, Hitchcock AA, Lander CM, Eadie MJ. Valproate-associated foetal malformations—rates of occurrence, risks in attempted avoidance. *Acta Neurol Scand.* 2019;139(1):42-48.

120. Lin K, Cao VFS, Au C, Dahri K. Clinical pharmacokinetic monitoring of free valproic acid levels: a systematic review. *Clin Pharmacokinet.* 2022;61(10):1345-1363.

121. Wallenburg E, Klok B, de Jong K, et al. Monitoring protein-unbound valproic acid serum concentrations in clinical practice. *Ther Drug Monit.* 2017;39(3):269-272.

122. Suzuki E, Nakai D, Ikenaga H, et al. In vivo inhibition of acylpeptide hydrolase by carbapenem antibiotics causes the decrease of plasma concentration of valproic acid in dogs. *Xenobiotica.* 2016;46(2):126-131.

123. Wu CC, Pai TY, Hsiao FY, Shen LJ, Wu FL. The effect of different carbapenem antibiotics (ertapenem, imipenem/cilastatin, and meropenem) on serum valproic acid concentrations. *Ther Drug Monit.* 2016;38(5):587-592.

124. Park MK, Lim KS, Kim TE, et al. Reduced valproic acid serum concentrations due to drug interactions with carbapenem antibiotics: overview of 6 cases. *Ther Drug Monit.* 2012;34(5):599-603.

125. Fratoni AJ, Colmerauer JL, Linder KE, Nicolau DP, Kuti JL. A retrospective case series of concomitant carbapenem and valproic acid Use: are best practice advisories working? *J Pharm Pract.* 2023;36(3):537-541.

126. Cunningham D, Clark K, Lord K. Treatment of valproic acid overdose with meropenem in an epileptic patient. *Am J Emerg Med.* 2022;53:284.e1-284.e3.

127. Hermida J, Tutor JC. A theoretical method for normalizing total serum valproic acid concentration in hypoalbuminemic patients. *J Pharmacol Sci.* 2005;97(4):489-493.

128. Correa T, Rodriguez I, Romano S. Population pharmacokinetics of valproate in Mexican children with epilepsy. *Biopharm Drug Dispos.* 2008;29(9):511-520.

129. EL Desoky ES, Fuseau E, EL Din Amry S, Cosson V. Pharmacokinetic modelling of valproic acid from routine clinical data in Egyptian epileptic patients. *Eur J Clin Pharmacol.* 2004;59(11):783-790.

130. Ding J, Wang Y, Lin W, et al. A population pharmacokinetic model of valproic acid in pediatric patients with epilepsy: a non-linear pharmacokinetic model based on protein-binding saturation. *Clin Pharmacokinet.* 2015;54(3):305-317.

131. Arzimanoglou A, Ferreira JA, Satlin A, et al. Safety and pharmacokinetic profile of rufinamide in pediatric patients aged less than 4 years with Lennox-Gastaut syndrome: an interim analysis from a multicenter, randomized, active-controlled, open-label study. *Eur J Paediatr Neurol.* 2016;20(3):393-402.

132. Vucicevic K, Jovanovic M, Golubovic B, et al. Nonlinear mixed effects modelling approach in investigating phenobarbital pharmacokinetic interactions in epileptic patients. *Eur J Clin Pharmacol.* 2015;71(2):183-190.

16

VANCOMYCIN

Timothy J. Bensman and Emi Minejima

Learning Objectives

By the end of the vancomycin chapter, the learner should be able to:

1. Describe the relationship between plasma vancomycin concentration and its bactericidal and postantibiotic effects.
2. Describe the rationale for monitoring AUC_{24hr} to maximize the efficacy and safety of vancomycin.
3. Devise a plasma sampling strategy to obtain an accurate estimate of the individual's AUC_{24hr}.
4. Devise dosing schemes for patients on standard hemodialysis, high-flux hemodialysis, continuous ambulatory peritoneal dialysis (CAPD), and continuous renal replacement therapy (CRRT).
5. Describe the effect of obesity on the pharmacokinetic parameters for vancomycin.
6. Describe appropriate monitoring parameters to minimize dose-related adverse effects

Vancomycin is a glycopeptide antibiotic with a gram-positive spectrum of activity that is effective in the treatment of infections involving methicillin-resistant *Staphylococcus aureus* (MRSA). It is also an alternative to penicillin in patients who have a history of serious penicillin allergy.[1-6] Vancomycin is bactericidal for most gram-positive organisms, except against enterococci, and it is synergistic with gentamicin against most strains of *S. aureus*, streptococci, and enterococci.[5,7] There has been a resurgence in the use of vancomycin because of the increased prevalence of MRSA.

Vancomycin is poorly absorbed orally and has been used to treat gastrointestinal overgrowths of gram-positive bacteria. When used to treat systemic infections, vancomycin must be given by the intravenous route or intraperitoneally for those patients receiving continuous ambulatory peritoneal dialysis (CAPD). The usual adult dose, in patients with normal renal function, is 1 g (10-15 mg/kg) administered intravenously over 60 minutes every 8 to 12 hours.[4-6] Vancomycin is eliminated by renal excretion and requires dosage adjustment, particularly in the older patients and in patients with diminished renal function.

Vancomycin use is associated with several dose-related adverse effects, including a pseudoallergic reaction, nephrotoxicity, and ototoxicity. The pseudoallergic reaction (Red man syndrome) is characterized by flushing around the head and neck region and pruritis and is mediated by histamine release. The reaction can be mitigated by administering by a slower infusion rate and/or adding an antihistamine. Therapeutic drug monitoring is employed to reduce the risk for the development of nephrotoxicity and ototoxicity. The ideal vancomycin dosing regimen is one that results in trough concentrations that are in the range of 5 to 15 and peak concentrations less than 50 mg/L.[1,2,5,6,8-15] Patients most likely to benefit from vancomycin plasma concentration monitoring are those at highest risk for therapeutic failure or potential drug toxicity. These include pediatrics patients, patients with burn, and patients with cystic fibrosis owing to high clearances and short half-lives. In addition, it is important to monitor plasma vancomycin concentrations in patients with poor renal function who are receiving empiric dosages, because they are at greater risk of toxicity.

THERAPEUTIC AND TOXIC PLASMA CONCENTRATIONS

Efficacy

The efficacy of vancomycin therapy has been associated with attainment of target steady-state trough concentrations, although accumulating clinical evidence indicates a stronger association with achievement of a 24-hour area under the curve/minimum inhibitory concentration (AUC_{24hr}/MIC) of greater than 400.[16,17] The Clinical Laboratory Standards Institute susceptibility breakpoint for vancomycin is 2 μg/mL for S. aureus and typically ranges from 0.5 to 2 μg/mL.[18] It has been demonstrated that serum unbound trough concentrations 5 times the MIC are optimal for bacterial eradication and clinical success.[15] Considering plasma protein binding of 50%, the target trough concentrations for efficacy range from 5 to 20 mg/L (0.5-2 μg/mL times 5 divided by 50%). High-dose regimens achieving 10 to 20 μg/mL are favored in patients with endocarditis, nosocomial infections, pneumonia, and other systemic infections who are at greater risk of therapeutic failure.[8,10,11,15,19-21] However, the high-dose regimens need to be evaluated in the context of the patient's risk for nephrotoxicity (see Safety).

A growing body of evidence supports the AUC_{24hr}/MIC ratio of 400 as the clinically relevant therapeutic target, where AUC_{24hr} is expressed as mg·hr/L and MIC is expressed as mg/L.[14,15,22,23] The rationale for targeting an AUC_{24hr}/MIC for vancomycin is based on the pharmacodynamic properties of concentration-independent killing and a modest dose–dependent postantibiotic effect of 0.5 to 3 hours.[5,24] Alternative antibiotic agents should be considered in patients with infections involving MRSA strains with MIC 2 μg/mL or higher because of the inability to achieve an AUC_{24hr}/MIC of greater than 400 without significantly increasing the risk for the development of nephrotoxicity.[25]

Safety

A relatively high incidence of adverse effects was initially associated with vancomycin. However, it is believed that some of these adverse reactions were caused by impurities in the original products; the current formulations are more pure.[1] Phlebitis and a histamine reaction that presents as flushing, tachycardia, and hypotension are known side effects associated with vancomycin therapy. To minimize the histamine response, vancomycin should be infused slowly over 60 to 120 minutes, and/or premedication with an antihistamine should be considered.[26,27] In addition, vancomycin therapy is associated with dose-related nephrotoxicity and ototoxicity. As a single agent, vancomycin is associated with a low incidence of nephrotoxicity (5%); however, when it is combined with aminoglycoside antibiotics, the incidence may be as high as 30%.[28] Higher rates of nephrotoxicity (11-20%) have been observed when trough vancomycin concentrations of 15 to 20 mg/L are targeted[18,22,26] and more so (30-45%) when high-dose therapy is maintained for 2 weeks or longer.[15,29,30] Best available evidence suggests vancomycin AUC_{24hr} values (assuming an MIC of 1 mg/L) should be maintained 600 mg·h/L or less to minimize the likelihood of nephrotoxicity.[31] In terms of ototoxicity, peak concentrations greater than 50 mg/L have been associated with hearing loss; with the majority of cases reported at concentration greater than 80 mg/L.[1,3,28]

KEY PARAMETERS: Vancomycin

	ADULT	PEDIATRIC
Therapeutic plasma concentration[a]		
Peak	<40-50 mg/L	<40-50
Trough	5-15 mg/L	5-15
F (oral)	<5%	<5%
V^b	$V = 0.72$ L/kg if Cl_{Cr} is ≥60 mL/min $V = 0.9$ L/kg if Cl_{Cr} is <60 mL/min	V (L) = 0.636 × Wt
Cl^c	Cl (mL/min) = (Cl_{Cr} × 0.689) + 3.66	Cl (L/hr) = 0.248 × $Wt^{0.75}$ × (0.48/$SCr)^{0.361}$ × (ln(age)/7.8)$^{0.995}$
$t_{\frac{1}{2}}$	6-7 hr	2-4 hr
fu^d (fraction unbound in plasma)	0.45-0.7	0.61-0.95

[a]A total drug peak concentration of approximately 30 mg/L is a reasonable target; however, to ensure efficacy, trough concentrations should be maintained at or above 5 mg/L.
[b]Actual body weight (ABW).
[c]ABW and age in days.
[d]The fraction unbound in plasma may be as high as 0.8 to 0.9 in patients with end-stage renal disease.

With respect to determining patient-specific dosages, a variety of methods have been developed and proposed to estimate the pharmacokinetic (PK) parameters.[32-34] Although most of the methods yield reasonable estimates of plasma vancomycin concentrations from a given dosage, the parameters used are based on population averages with sufficient variability such that therapeutic drug monitoring is still necessary when indicated.

BIOAVAILABILITY (F)

Vancomycin is poorly absorbed following oral administration (ie, <5%); as a result, parenteral or intraperitoneal administration is necessary for the treatment of systemic infections. Vancomycin's limited oral bioavailability has been used advantageously to treat enterocolitis.[1,4-6]

VOLUME OF DISTRIBUTION (V)

The volume of distribution for vancomycin ranges between 0.5 and 1 L/kg.[32,35,36] In clinical practice, an average value of 0.7 L/kg is often used; however, the method described by Matzke et al for estimating V for vancomycin in adults (ie, those older than 18 years) splits population estimates by creatinine clearance (Cl_{Cr}) and has the highest precision and least bias.[34,37] In Pediatrics, weight has been shown to influence volume of distribution.[38]

Adults:

$$V = 0.72 \text{ L/kg if } Cl_{Cr} \text{ is } \geq 60 \text{ mL/min} \qquad \text{(Eq. 16.1)}$$

$$V = 0.9 \text{ L/kg if } Cl_{Cr} \text{ is } <60 \text{ mL/min} \qquad \text{(Eq. 16.2)}$$

Pediatrics:

$$V \text{ (L)} = 0.636 \times \text{Weight} \qquad \text{(Eq. 16.3)}$$

A two- or three-compartment model best describes the distribution of vancomycin. The complexity of this model can be problematic when peak plasma samples are obtained during the distribution phase. In clinical practice, a one-compartment model is frequently used.[13,32,39] Vancomycin has moderate plasma protein binding. The fraction unbound (fu) in plasma is approximately 0.6, with a reported range of 0.45 to 0.70.[35,40-42] Data in patients with end-stage renal disease suggest that the fu in plasma may be as high as 0.8 to 0.9.[43,44]

CLEARANCE (Cl)

Vancomycin is eliminated primarily by the renal route; approximately 5% of the dose is metabolized.[35,45] The clearance of vancomycin is highly correlated with creatinine clearance[32,36,39]:

$$Cl_{Cr} \text{ for males (mL/min)} = \frac{(140 - \text{Age in years})(\text{Weight in kg})}{(72)(SCr_{ss})} \qquad \textbf{(Eq. 16.4)}$$

$$Cl_{Cr} \text{ for females (mL/min)} = (0.85)\frac{(140 - \text{Age in years})(\text{Weight in kg})}{(72)(SCr_{ss})} \quad \textbf{(Eq. 16.5)}$$

For issues that should be considered when estimating creatinine clearance, see Chapter "Drug Dosing in Kidney Disease and Dialysis."

Vancomycin clearance in adults:

$$Cl \text{ (mL/min)} = (Cl_{Cr} \times 0.689) + 3.66 \qquad \textbf{(Eq. 16.6)}$$

Vancomycin clearance in pediatrics:

$$Cl \text{ (L/hr)} = 0.248 \times Wt^{0.75} \times (0.48/SCr)^{0.361} \times (\ln (\text{Age in days})/7.8)^{0.995} \qquad \textbf{(Eq. 16.7)}$$

Very little vancomycin is cleared by standard hemodialysis or peritoneal dialysis.[10,46,47] In patients undergoing CAPD, the small but continuous drug loss caused by peritoneal dialysis exchanges is significant. The usual approach is to replace vancomycin with intermittent intravenous injections on a somewhat more frequent basis than is usually done for patients with end-stage renal disease (in some cases, as often as every 3-5 days), or to instill vancomycin directly into the peritoneal space to treat peritonitis and achieve systemic concentrations of vancomycin.[48,49] Some caution should be used in evaluating plasma concentrations in patients with end-stage renal disease. Some immunoassays that use polyclonal antibodies overestimate actual vancomycin concentrations owing to an accumulation of pseudometabolites (crystalline degradation products) that cross-react with the assay.[49,50] In patients undergoing high-flux or high-efficiency hemodialysis, a significant amount of vancomycin can be removed. Early studies estimated that as much as 30% of vancomycin was removed during high-flux hemodialysis; recent reports indicate that only 17% of vancomycin is removed during these procedures. Early investigators did not recognize that a redistribution of vancomycin occurs after the completion of dialysis.[51,52] Owing to wide interpatient variability, monitoring plasma vancomycin concentrations to determine individual dosing requirements is often required.

HALF-LIFE ($t_{1/2}$)

The usual serum half-life of vancomycin in adults is 6 to 7 hours; in patients with end-stage renal disease, the half-life may approach 7 days.[10,32,35,44] This wide range in the serum half-life partially explains the variability in the dose and dosing intervals used for vancomycin. Adult patients with normal renal function may receive the drug every 8 to 12 hours, whereas those with end-stage renal disease may receive a dose once a week.[10,46]

NOMOGRAMS

Dosing nomograms for vancomycin are available.[10,53] However, an understanding of the desired therapeutic range and the PK parameters of vancomycin provides the clinician more flexibility to tailor doses and dosing intervals that meet the specific needs of the patient. For example, using PK parameters allows targeting plasma vancomycin AUC_{24hr}/MIC, which is particularly advantageous when treating infections with vancomycin-intermediate–sensitive bacteria.

TIME TO SAMPLE

Steady-state trough concentration monitoring is currently the standard of care[25]; however, given the discordance between trough levels and AUC_{24hr}, it is advisable to measure both peak and trough concentrations to more accurately estimate the AUC_{24hr}.[54] Measurement of both peak and trough concentrations may also be helpful in patients in whom the PK parameters may be difficult to estimate with confidence (eg, very overweight or underweight patients).

If only a steady-state trough concentration is available, peak concentrations can be estimated with reasonable accuracy based on the dose administered, an estimate of the volume of distribution, and a measured trough concentration. This is especially true in patients with diminished renal function and a long vancomycin half-life.

If the trough concentration is known, the peak concentration ($C_{ss\ max}$) can be approximated using Equation 16.8.

$$C_{ssmax} = [C_{ssmin}] + \left[\frac{(S)(F)(Dose)}{V} \right]$$ (Eq. 16.8)

The $(S)(F)(Dose)/V$ represents the change in concentration (ΔC) following a dose.

As described in Part I (see Chapter "Selecting the Appropriate Equation and Interpretation of Measured Drug Concentrations"), the use of this equation requires that several conditions be met, including:

1. Steady state has been achieved.
2. The measured plasma concentration is a trough concentration.
3. The bolus dose is an acceptable model.

In the clinical setting, trough concentrations are often obtained slightly before the true trough. Because vancomycin has a relatively long half-life, most plasma concentrations obtained within 1 hour of the true trough can be assumed to have met condition 2.

Because vancomycin follows a multicompartmental model, it is difficult to avoid the distribution phase when obtaining peak plasma concentrations.[55] If a one-compartment model is to be applied, samples should be obtained at least 1 or possibly 2 hours after the end of the infusion period. It is difficult to evaluate the appropriateness of a dosing regimen that is based on plasma samples obtained before steady state. Additional plasma concentrations are required to more accurately estimate a patient's apparent clearance and half-life and to ensure that any dosing adjustments based on a non–steady-state trough concentration achieve the targeted steady-state concentrations.

Question #1   *B.C., a 65-year-old, 45-kg man with a serum creatinine concentration of 2.2 mg/dL, is being treated for a presumed hospital-acquired MRSA infection. Design a dosing regimen that will produce peak concentrations less than 50 mg/L and trough concentrations of 5 to 15 mg/L.*

The first step in calculating an appropriate dosing regimen for B.C. is to estimate his PK parameters (ie, clearance, volume of distribution, elimination rate constant, and half-life).

B.C.'s creatinine clearance is estimated to be approximately 21.3 mL/min, as shown using Equation 16.4:

$$\text{Cl}_{Cr} \text{ for males (mL/min)} = \frac{(140 - \text{Age in years})(\text{Weight in kg})}{(72) \times (\text{SCr}_{ss})}$$

$$= \frac{(140 - 65)(45 \text{ kg})}{72(2.2 \text{ mg/dL})}$$

$$= 21.3 \text{ mL/min}$$

Using Equation 16.6, the corresponding vancomycin clearance for B.C. is 1.1 L/hr.

$$\text{Cl (mL/min)} = (\text{Cl}_{Cr} \times 0.689) + 3.66$$
$$= 21.3 \text{ mL/min} (0.689) + 3.66$$
$$= 18.3 \text{ mL/min}$$

or

$$= 18.3 \text{ mL/min} \times \frac{60 \text{ min/hr}}{1,000 \text{ mL/L}}$$

$$= 1.1 \text{ L/hr}$$

The volume of distribution for B.C. can be calculated using Equation 16.2 (see Key Parameters, this chapter). According to the following calculations, B.C.'s expected volume of distribution would be 40.5 L.

$$V(L) = 0.9 \text{ L/kg } (45 \text{ kg}) = 40.5 \text{ L}$$

The calculated vancomycin clearance of 1.1 L/hr and the volume of distribution of 40.5 L can then be used to estimate the elimination rate constant of 0.027 hr^{-1} using Equation 16.9.

$$K = \frac{Cl}{V} \qquad \text{(Eq. 16.9)}$$

$$= \frac{1.1 \text{ L/hr}}{40.5 \text{ L}}$$

$$= 0.027 \text{ hr}^{-1}$$

and the corresponding vancomycin half-life can be calculated using Equation 16.10:

$$t_{\frac{1}{2}} = \frac{(0.693)(V)}{Cl} \qquad \text{(Eq. 16.10)}$$

$$= \frac{(0.693)(V)}{Cl}$$

$$= \frac{(0.693)(40.5 \text{ L})}{1.1 \text{ L/hr}}$$

$$= 25.5 \text{ hr}$$

Using Equation 16.11, with the patient's weight, and the volume of distribution of 40.5 L that we calculated, and substituting the usual maintenance dose as 15 mg/kg for the dose, it can be seen that the initial plasma concentration should be approximately 17 mg/L.

$$C_0 = \frac{(S)(F)(\text{Loading dose})}{V} \qquad \text{(Eq. 16.11)}$$

$$C_0 = \frac{(1)(1)(15 \text{ mg/kg} \times 45 \text{ kg})}{40.5}$$

$$= 16.7 \text{ mg/L}$$

This value is below the usual targeted peak concentration of about 30 mg/L. The initial dose (ie, loading dose) can be calculated using the assumed volume of distribution of 40.5 L using Equation 16.12. The salt form and bioavailability are assumed to be

1.0 when vancomycin is administered intravenously. Using an initial target of 30 mg/L, the loading dose would be approximately 1,250 mg.

$$\text{Loading dose} = \frac{(V)(C)}{(S)(F)} \qquad \text{(Eq. 16.12)}$$

$$= \frac{(40.5)(30 \text{ mg/L})}{(1)(1)}$$
$$= 1,215 \text{ mg} \approx 1,250 \text{ mg}$$

There are no known renal or ototoxicities associated with elevated vancomycin levels that occur during the distribution phase. However, to minimize the cardiovascular effects associated with rapid administration, the initial and subsequent doses should be administered over approximately 60 minutes. In addition, if peak concentrations are measured, samples should be drawn at least 1 to 2 hours after completion of the infusion period to avoid the distribution phase (if using a one-compartment model as demonstrated here).

The maintenance dose can be calculated by a number of methods. One approach might be to first approximate the hourly infusion rate required to maintain the desired average concentration. Then, the hourly infusion rate can be multiplied by an appropriate dosing interval to calculate a reasonable dose to be given on an intermittent basis. For example, if an average concentration of 20 mg/L is selected (approximately halfway between the desired peak concentration of $\approx$30 mg/L and trough concentration of $\approx$10 mg/L), the hourly administration rate would be 22 mg/hr (Equation 16.13).

$$\text{Maintenance dose} = \frac{(Cl)(C_{ss \text{ ave}})(\tau)}{(S)(F)} \qquad \text{(Eq. 16.13)}$$

$$= \frac{(1.1 \text{ L/hr})(20 \text{ mg/L})(1 \text{hr})}{(1)(1)}$$
$$= 22 \text{ mg/hr}$$

Although a number of dosing intervals could be selected, 24 hours is reasonable because it is a convenient interval and approximates B.C.'s half-life for vancomycin of 25.5 hours. A dosing interval of approximately 1 half-life should result in peak concentrations of 30 mg/L and trough concentrations that are within the 5 to 15 mg/L range, in this case. If an interval of 24 hours is selected, the dose would be approximately 500 mg.

$$\text{Maintenance dose} = \frac{(1.1 \text{ L/hr})(20 \text{ mg/L})(24 \text{ hr})}{(1)(1)}$$
$$= 528 \text{ mg} \approx 500 \text{ mg}$$

This method assumes that the average concentration is halfway between the peak and trough. As mentioned in Part I (see Chapter "Selecting the Appropriate Equation and Interpretation of Measured Drug Concentrations"), this is approximately correct as long as the dosing interval is less than or approximately equal to the drug's half-life. When dosing intervals greatly exceed the half-life, the true average concentration is much lower than halfway between the peak and trough levels.

A second approach that can be used to calculate the maintenance dose is to select a desired peak and trough concentration that is consistent with the therapeutic range and B.C.'s vancomycin half-life. For example, if steady-state peak concentrations of 30 mg/L are desired, it would take approximately two half-lives for that peak level to fall to 7.5 mg/L (a level of 30 mg/L declines to 15 mg/L in one half-life and to 7.5 mg/L in another half-life). Because the vancomycin half-life in B.C. is approximately 1 day, the dosing interval would be 48 hours. The dose to be administered every 48 hours can be calculated using Equation 16.14.

$$\text{Dose} = \frac{(V)(C_{ss\,max} - C_{ss\,min})}{(S)(F)} \qquad \textbf{(Eq. 16.14)}$$

$$= \frac{(40.5 \text{ L})(30 \text{ mg/L} - 7.5 \text{ mg/L})}{(1)(1)}$$

$$= 911 \text{ mg} \approx 900 \text{ mg}$$

The peak and trough concentrations that are expected using this dosing regimen can be calculated using Equations 16.15 and 16.17, respectively.

$$C_{ss\,max} = \frac{\dfrac{(S)(F)(\text{Dose})}{V}}{1 - e^{-K\tau}} \qquad \textbf{(Eq. 16.15)}$$

$$= \frac{\dfrac{(1)(1)(900 \text{ mg})}{40.5 \text{ L}}}{(1 - e^{-(0.027 \text{ hr}^{-1})(48\,\text{hr})})}$$

$$= 30.6 \text{ mg/L}$$

Note that although 30.6 mg/L is an acceptable peak, the actual clinical peak would normally be obtained approximately 1 hour after the end of a 1-hour infusion, or 2 hours after this calculated peak concentration, and would be about 29 mg/L, as calculated by Equation 16.16.

$$C_2 = C_1(e^{-Kt}) \qquad \textbf{(Eq. 16.16)}$$

$$= 30.6 \text{ mg/L} \, (e^{-(0.027 \text{ hr}^{-1})(2\,\text{hr})})$$

$$= 29 \text{ mg/L}$$

The calculated trough concentration would be about 8 mg/L (Equations 16.17 and 16.18).

$$C_{ss\,min} = \frac{\frac{(S)(F)(Dose)}{V}}{1 - e^{-K\tau}}(e^{-K\tau}) \qquad \text{(Eq. 16.17)}$$

$$C_{ss\,min} = C_{ss\,max} \times (e^{-K\tau}) \qquad \text{(Eq. 16.18)}$$

$$= 30.6 \text{ mg/L } (e^{-(0.027\,hr^{-1})\,(48\,hr)})$$
$$= 8.4 \text{ mg/L}$$

This process of checking the expected peak and trough concentrations is most appropriate when the dose or the dosing interval has been changed from a calculated value (eg, twice the half-life) to a practical value (eg, 8, 12, 18, 24, 36, or 48 hours). If different plasma vancomycin concentrations are desired, Equations 16.15 and 16.17 can be used to target specific vancomycin concentrations by adjusting the dose and/or the dosing interval. For example, a dosage regimen of 1,000 mg every 48 hours would result in calculated peak and trough concentrations of 34 and 9.3 mg/L, respectively. Alternatively, 800 mg every 36 hours would result in an expected peak concentration of 31.7 mg/L and a trough concentration of 12.0 mg/L, at steady state.

A third alternative is to rearrange Equation 16.17:

$$C_{ss\,min} = \frac{\frac{(S)(F)(Dose)}{V}}{1 - e^{-K\tau}}(e^{-K\tau})$$

such that the dose can be calculated.

$$Dose = \frac{(C_{ss\,min})(V)(1 - e^{-K\tau})}{(S)(F)(e^{-K\tau})} \qquad \text{(Eq. 16.19)}$$

Note that it is the $C_{ss\,min}$ or trough concentration that is used to solve for dose. Making the appropriate substitutions for the parameters indicated in Equation 16.19 and choosing a target trough concentration of 10 mg/L and a dosing interval of 24 hours, a dose of approximately $369 \approx 400$ mg is calculated.

$$Dose = \frac{(Trough)(1 - e^{-K\tau}(V))}{e^{-K\tau}}$$
$$= \frac{(10 \text{ mg/L})(1 - e^{-(0.027\,hr^{-1})(24\,hr)})(40.5 \text{ L})}{e^{-(0.027\,hr^{-1})(24\,hr)}}$$
$$= 369 \text{ mg} \approx 400 \text{ mg}$$

Alternatively, doses could have been calculated for dosing intervals of 36 or 48 hours if those intervals were deemed to be appropriate.

Question #2   *E.K., is a 60-year-old, 5-foot 1-inch, 50-kg woman with a serum creatinine of 1.0 mg/dL, has been empirically started on 750 mg of vancomycin every 12 hours (infused over 1 hour) for the treatment of a hospital-acquired staphylococcal infection. What are the expected peak and trough vancomycin concentrations for E.K.?*

To calculate the peak and trough concentrations, E.K.'s clearance, volume of distribution, and elimination rate constant (or half-life) need to be estimated.

E.K.'s creatinine clearance can be calculated using Equation 16.5, and Equation 16.6 can be used to calculate her vancomycin clearance of 2.2 L/hr, as shown in the following:

$$\text{Cl}_{Cr} \text{ for females (mL/min)} = (0.85)\frac{(140 - \text{Age in years})(\text{Weight in kg})}{(72)(\text{SCr}_{ss})}$$

$$= (0.85)\frac{(140 - 60)(50 \text{ kg})}{(72)(1.0 \text{ mg/dL})}$$

$$= 47.2 \text{ mL/min}$$

Using Equation 16.6 to calculate vancomycin clearance:

$$\text{Cl (mL/min)} = (\text{Cl}_{Cr} \times 0.689) + 3.66$$

$$= 47.2 \text{ mL/min } (0.689) + 3.66$$

$$= 36.2 \text{ mL/min}$$

or

$$= 36.2 \text{ mL/min} \times \frac{60 \text{ min/hr}}{1,000 \text{ mL/L}}$$

$$= 2.2 \text{ L/hr}$$

Using Equation 16.2, the expected volume of distribution for E.K. is 45 L.

$$V(L) = 0.9 \text{ L/kg (50 kg)}$$

$$= 45 \text{ L}$$

Equation 16.9 can now be used to calculate E.K.'s elimination rate constant and Equation 16.10 to calculate the corresponding half-life.

$$K = \frac{\text{Cl}}{V}$$

$$= \frac{2.2 \text{ L/hr}}{45 \text{ L}}$$

$$= 0.049 \text{ hr}^{-1}$$

and the corresponding vancomycin half-life can be calculated as follows:

$$t_{1/2} = \frac{(0.693)(V)}{Cl}$$

$$= \frac{(0.693)(V)}{Cl}$$

$$= \frac{(0.693)(45\ L)}{2.2\ L/hr}$$

$$= 14.2\ hr$$

Equations 16.15 and 16.17 can be used to calculate the expected peak and trough concentrations for E.K.

$$C_{ss\ max} = \frac{\dfrac{(S)(F)(Dose)}{V}}{1 - e^{-K\tau}}$$

$$= \frac{\dfrac{(1)(1)(750\ mg)}{45\ L}}{(1 - e^{-(0.049\ hr^{-1})(12)})}$$

$$= 37.6\ mg/L$$

To calculate the clinical peak concentration, which is usually sampled 2 hours after the start of a vancomycin infusion (1 hour after the end of a 1-hour infusion), the $C_{ss\ max}$ could be decayed for 2 hours using Equation 16.16.

$$= 37.6\ mg/L\ (e^{-(0.049\ hr^{-1})(2\ hr)})$$

$$= 34.1\ mg/L$$

$C_{ss\ min}$ can be calculated using Equation 16.17 and the dosing interval of 12 hours.

$$C_{ss\ min} = (C_{ss\ max})(e^{-K\tau})$$

$$= 37.6\ mg/L\ (e^{-(0.049\ hr^{-1})(12\ hr)})$$

$$= 20.9\ mg/L$$

Although the expected peak concentration of approximately 34 mg/L is not above the usually accepted range for peak concentrations, the trough concentration of 20.9 mg/L is above the usual targeted range of 5 to 15 mg/L, which is targeted for efficacy/safety. This suggests that decreasing the dose and/or increasing the dosing interval, as well as monitoring plasma concentrations of vancomycin, would be appropriate.

Question #3   *A culture indicates that the infection is caused by MRSA with an MIC of 1.0 mg/L. A steady-state trough concentration of 25 mg/L was obtained for E.K. Design a dosing regimen that will produce therapeutic vancomycin concentrations and an AUC_{24hr}/MIC of 400 or more for E.K.*

To design such a regimen, E.K.'s PK parameters should first be revised so that they are consistent with the observed trough concentration of 25 mg/L. Some assumptions will have to be made. Because the measured trough concentration is higher than predicted, her half-life is longer than the estimate of 14.2 hours. For E.K., the percentage fluctuation between peak and trough concentrations should be relatively small at steady state because her dosing interval of 12 hours is shorter than her apparent half-life. Therefore, the best approach is to use the literature estimate for volume of distribution and then calculate the corresponding elimination rate constant and clearance values.

If E.K.'s volume of distribution is assumed to be 45 L (see previous calculation using Equation 16.1) and the observed trough concentration of 25 mg/L is used, a peak concentration of approximately 42 mg/L can be calculated by using Equation 16.8, as follows:

$$C_{ss\ max} = [25\ mg/L] + \left[\frac{(1)(1)(750\ mg)}{45.0\ L} \right]$$

$$= 41.7\ mg/L \approx 42\ mg/L$$

Using the observed trough concentration of 25 mg/L and the predicted peak concentration of 42 mg/L, an elimination rate constant (K) can be calculated using Equation 16.20, where C_1 is the peak concentration of 42 mg/L, C_2 is the trough concentration of 25 mg/L, and the interval between those two concentrations, t, is the dosing interval of 12 hours.

$$K = \frac{\ln\left(\dfrac{C_1}{C_2}\right)}{t} \qquad \text{(Eq. 16.20)}$$

$$= \frac{\ln\left(\dfrac{42\ mg/L}{25\ mg/L}\right)}{12\ hr}$$

$$= 0.043\ hr^{-1}$$

This apparent elimination rate constant of 0.043 hr^{-1} corresponds to a half-life of approximately 16 hours (Equation 16.21).

$$t_{\frac{1}{2}} = \frac{0.693}{K} \qquad \text{(Eq. 16.21)}$$

$$= \frac{0.693}{0.052 \ hr^{-1}}$$

$$= 16 \ hr$$

The apparent elimination rate constant of 0.043 hr^{-1} and the assumed volume of distribution of 45 L can be used in Equation 16.22 to calculate E.K.'s vancomycin clearance.

$$Cl = (K)(V) \qquad \text{(Eq. 16.22)}$$

$$= (0.043 \ hr^{-1})(45 \ L)$$

$$= 1.94 \ L/hr$$

Because the revised $t_{1/2} \geq \tau$, we expect $C_{ss \ ave}$ to be halfway between $C_{ss \ max}$ and $C_{ss \ min}$. Therefore, clearance could have been approximated by assuming $C_{ss \ ave}$ is approximately equal to:

$$C_{ss \ ave} = C_{ss \ min} + \left(\frac{1}{2}\right)\frac{(S)(F)(Dose)}{V} \qquad \text{(Eq. 16.23)}$$

and then calculating clearance by using Equation 16.24 (see Chapter "Selecting the Appropriate Equation and Interpretation of Measured Drug Concentrations"):

$$Cl = \frac{(S)(F)(Dose/\tau)}{C_{ss \ ave}} \qquad \text{(Eq. 16.24)}$$

The maintenance dose can then be calculated using Equation 16.17. Because the apparent half-life is approximately 16 hours, the most logical dosing interval and $C_{ss \ min}$ would be 24 hours and 10 to 15 mg/L, respectively.

$$Dose = \frac{(C_{ss \ min})(V)(1 - e^{-K\tau})}{(S)(F)(e^{-K\tau})}$$

$$Dose = \frac{(12.5 \ mg/L)(45 \ L)(1 - e^{-(0.043hr^{-1})(24hr)})}{(1)(1)(e^{-(0.043hr^{-1})(24hr)})}$$

$$= 1,016 \ mg \approx 1,000 \ mg$$

We can round the dose to 1,000 mg every 24 hours, which should result in a steady-state C_{max} concentration of approximately 35 mg/L by using Equation 16.15.

$$C_{ss\,max} = \frac{\dfrac{(S)(F)(\text{Dose})}{V}}{1-e^{-K\tau}}$$

$$= \frac{\dfrac{(1)(1)(1,000\ \text{mg})}{45\ \text{L}}}{(1-e^{-(0.043\,\text{hr}^{-1})(24\,\text{hr})})}$$

$$= 34.5\ \text{mg/L}$$

A trough concentration of approximately 12 mg/L can be calculated using Equation 16.18.

$$C_{ss\,min} = (C_{ss\,max})(e^{-K\tau})$$

$$= (34.5\ \text{mg/L})(e^{-(0.043\ \text{hr}^{-1})(24\ \text{hr})})$$

$$-12.3\ \text{mg/L}$$

This trough concentration of approximately 12 mg/L is within the usual therapeutic range (5-15 mg/L).

The AUC_{24hr}/MIC for this case can be determined by employing Equation 16.25:

$$AUC_{24hr}/MIC = \frac{\text{Dose}_{24hr}\ (\text{mg})}{\text{Cl}\ (\text{L/hr})\times \text{MIC}\ (\text{mg/L})} \qquad \textbf{(Eq. 16.25)}$$

$$= \frac{1,000\ \text{mg}}{(1.94\ \text{L/hr})(1\ \text{mg/L})}$$

$$= 515$$

Hence, the dose of 1,000 mg every 24 hours produces peak and trough vancomycin concentrations within the usual therapeutic range, and also yields a desirable AUC_{24hr}/MIC of greater than 400.

If a peak (1 hours after a 1-hour infusion; 40 mg/L) and trough (25 mg/L) were available, then one could use the peak-trough approach to revise patient-specific parameters and to calculate the dose required to achieve an AUC_{24hr}/MIC of around 400. Assuming that the trough was drawn right before the start of infusion and using Equation 16.20, we have

$$K = \frac{\ln\left(\dfrac{C_1}{C_2}\right)}{t}$$

$$= \frac{\ln\left(\dfrac{40}{25}\right)}{10}$$

$$= 0.047$$

This apparent elimination rate constant of 0.047 hr^{-1} corresponds to a half-life of approximately 15 hours (Equation 16.21).

$$t_{1/2} = \frac{0.693}{K}$$

$$= \frac{0.693}{0.047 \text{ hr}^{-1}}$$

$$= 14.7 \text{ hr} \approx 15 \text{ hr}$$

Because the infusion time (1 hour) is short relative to the half-life (13 hours), the bolus model is appropriate to determine the revised V.

$$V = \frac{\dfrac{\text{Dose}}{C_{\text{ss peak}}}}{1 - e^{-(K)(\tau)}} e^{-(K)(t)}$$

$$= \frac{\dfrac{750 \text{ mg}}{40 \text{ mg/L}}}{1 - e^{-(0.047)(12)}} e^{-(0.047)(2)}$$

$$= 39.6 \text{ L}$$

The revised clearance can be calculated using the revised K and V and Equation 16.22:

$$Cl \text{ (L/hr)} = (K)(V)$$

$$= 0.047 \text{ hr}^{-1} (39.6 \text{ L})$$

$$= 1.86 \text{ L/hr} \approx 1.9 \text{ L/hr}$$

Now, we can calculate a dose to achieve a target AUC_{24hr}/MIC of 400 using Equation 16.25.

$$AUC_{24hr}/MIC = \frac{\text{Dose}_{24hr}}{Cl \times MIC}$$

$$\text{Dose}_{24hr} = AUC_{24hr}/MIC \times Cl \times MIC$$

$$= 400 \times 1.9 \times 1$$

$$= 760 \text{ mg}$$

We can round this dose to 750 mg every 24 hours and check the steady-state $C_{\text{ss max}}$ concentration using Equation 16.15.

$$C_{\text{ss max}} = \frac{\dfrac{(S)(F)(\text{Dose})}{V}}{1 - e^{-K\tau}}$$

$$= \frac{(1)(1)(750 \text{ mg})}{1 - e^{-(0.047 \text{ hr}^{-1})(24 \text{ hr})}}$$

$$= \frac{39.6 \text{ L}}{}$$

$$= 28 \text{ mg/L}$$

A steady-state trough concentration can be calculated using Equation 16.18.

$$C_{ss\,min} = (C_{ss\,max})(e^{-K\tau})$$

$$= (28)(e^{-(0.047 \text{ hr}^{-1})(24 \text{ hr})})$$

$$= 9.1 \text{ mg/L} \approx 9 \text{ mg/L}$$

Here, we see that the target AUC_{24hr}/MIC of greater than 400 is achieved while also maintaining a therapeutic trough concentration. The peak concentration minimizes ototoxicity risks.

It should be noted that without the peak level, we would have to assume the population average for volume of 45 L compared with our revised estimate of 39.6 L. Using the peak-trough approach, a dose reduction of 250 mg was observed.

Bear in mind, generating vancomycin AUC_{24hr} estimates through Bayesian modeling techniques is now a preferred approach recommended by vancomycin therapeutic monitoring guidelines.[31] Advantages of using the Bayesian modeling software over two-level monitoring (peak and trough levels) in clinical practice include the ability to draw vancomycin concentrations before reaching steady state, the flexibility of timing of the levels (can use peak, random, or trough levels), ability to more accurately estimate the AUC with just one level instead of two levels, and the software can be integrated with the hospital's electronic medical record saving the pharmacist time from inputting the information by hand. One of the major limitations currently from integrating a commercially available Bayesian modeling software is the cost associated with the programs. However, there are some free available to the public (eg, ClinCalc; https://clincalc.com/Vancomycin/). Although the Bayesian modeling software may be preferred, if the sampling of vancomycin concentrations are timed and obtained correctly, the median error in AUC estimation using 2-level monitoring is 2% or less.[56]

Providing E.K's patient information, dosing history, and steady-state trough vancomycin concentration as inputs to the vancomycin PK calculator with Bayesian modeling (priors) from ClinCalc, the dosing regimen of 750 mg vancomycin infused over 1 hour administered every 24 hours results in an AUC_{24hr}/MIC of 377 and vancomycin peak and trough concentration of 23.7 and 9.7 mg/L, respectively. This predicted AUC_{24hr}/MIC is below the goal (between 400 and 600). The software proposes a dosing regimen of 1,000 mg vancomycin infused over 1 hour administered every 24 hours, same as ours using first-order PK equations with a measured steady-state trough level. If one entered the entire vancomycin concentration history (ie, both steady-state vancomycin peak and trough concentrations), then the software proposes a dosing regimen of 1,000 mg vancomycin infused over 1 hour administered every 24 hours. Although it should be noted that the dosing regimen of 750 mg vancomycin infused over 1 hour administered every 24 hours is also reasonable as the $AUC_{24hr}/$ MIC of 377 is just below the target of 400. This example illustrates that measuring both peak and trough concentrations provides a more precise means to determine individualized PK parameters (ie, Cl, V) to achieve therapeutic success and minimize toxicities (ie, nephrotoxicity).

Finally, the reader is strongly encouraged to read the excellent commentary in the practice guidelines[31] for greater details on the vancomycin Bayesian modeling approach and its role in clinical practice.

Question #4   *A.C., a 50-year-old, 60-kg woman with end-stage renal disease and a serum creatinine of 9 mg/dL, is undergoing standard intermittent hemodialysis treatments 3 times a week and, currently, has an apparent shunt infection that is to be treated with vancomycin. Calculate an appropriate dose for A.C.*

Vancomycin is extensively cleared by the kidneys; consequently, patients with end-stage renal disease have prolonged half-lives that average 5 to 7 days. This extended half-life is consistent with a residual vancomycin clearance of 3 to 4 mL/70 kg/min (0.18-0.24 L/70 kg/hr) and an average volume of distribution. Depending on A.C.'s residual renal function, the half-life may be shorter or longer than this general range. Note that for dialysis patients, it is not appropriate to use their SCr to estimate creatinine clearance with Equation 16.9 or 16.21 because the SCr is not at steady state. The duration and frequency of A.C.'s hemodialysis is not a factor in vancomycin dosing because the amount of vancomycin cleared during standard hemodialysis is negligible.

The usual approach to the use of vancomycin in patients receiving intermittent hemodialysis is to administer 1 g every 5 days to 2 weeks. Using Equation 16.2 to estimate the volume of distribution gives:

$$V = 0.9 \text{ L/kg if } Cl_{Cr} \text{ is } <60 \text{ mL/min}$$

$$= 0.9 \text{ L/kg (60 kg)}$$

$$= 54 \text{ L}$$

Then, one can see from Equation 16.26 that the first 1-g dose should result in an initial peak concentration of 18.5 mg/L.

$$C_0 = \frac{(S)(F)(\text{Loading dose})}{V} \qquad \textbf{(Eq. 16.26)}$$

$$= \frac{(1)(1)(1,000 \text{ mg})}{54 \text{ L}}$$

$$= 18.5 \text{ mg/L}$$

For a dose of 1 g administered weekly, steady-state peak and trough levels of approximately 38.5 and 20 mg/L, respectively, can be calculated using an average vancomycin clearance of 3.5 mL/min (0.21 L/hr), a volume of distribution of 54 L, and a corresponding elimination rate constant of 0.0039 hr^{-1} (Equations 16.15 and 16.18).

$$C_{ss\,max} = \frac{(S)(F)(Dose)}{1-e^{-K\tau}}$$

$$= \frac{(1)(1)(1,000\ mg)}{\dfrac{54\ L}{1-e^{-(0.0039\ hr^{-1})(24\,hr/d)(7\,days)}}}$$

$$= 38.5\ mg/L$$

$$C_{ss\,min} = (C_{ss\,max})(e^{-K\tau})$$

$$= (38.5)(e^{-(0.0039)(24\,hr/d)(7\ days)})$$

$$= 20\ mg/L$$

If the 1-g dose had been administered every 2 weeks, the expected peak and trough vancomycin concentrations would have been approximately 25 and 7 mg/L, respectively. However, because of the long half-life of vancomycin in renal failure (~1 week) and a usual course of therapy of 2 weeks, steady state would not be achieved. Alternatively, if a dose of 500 mg was given weekly for a prolonged period, the expected steady-state peak and trough concentrations would have been approximately 19 and 10 mg/L, respectively. When the same average dosing rate $[(S)(F)(Dose/\tau)]$ is administered as a smaller dose given more frequently, the steady-state peak concentration is lower and the steady-state trough concentration is higher, but the average steady-state concentration is the same, as demonstrated by Equation 16.27 (also see Interpretation of Plasma Drug Concentrations in Chapter "Selecting the Appropriate Equation and Interpretation of Measured Drug Concentrations").

$$C_{ss\,ave} = \frac{\dfrac{(S)(F)(Dose/\tau)}{V}}{Cl} \qquad \text{(Eq. 16.27)}$$

$$= \frac{(1)(1)(1,000\ mg)\,/\,(14\ days)(24\ hr/d)}{0.21\ L/hr}$$
$$= 14.2\ mg/L$$

versus

$$= \frac{(1)(1)(500\ mg)/(7\ d)(24\ hr/d)}{0.21\ L/hr}$$
$$= 14.2\ mg/L$$

If an extended course of therapy is anticipated, it is probably advisable to obtain vancomycin plasma levels to make certain that A.C.'s actual plasma levels are within an acceptable range. In seriously ill patients, it might be appropriate to obtain an initial vancomycin level 3 to 5 days after the initiation of therapy. The purpose is to ensure that the patient's actual clearance is not unusually large, resulting in vancomycin levels that are below the desired therapeutic range.

If A.C. had been receiving CAPD as her method of dialysis, it is probable that the vancomycin would be administered via her peritoneal dialysis fluid. The usual approach is to place 15 to 30 mg/kg of vancomycin (~1-2 g for A.C.) into an initial dialysate exchange, which should result in approximately 50% of that dose being absorbed during the usual 4- to 6-hour dwell time. Her maintenance dose would then be administered in one of two ways. An additional 15 to 30 mg/kg dose could be administered in single exchanges every 3 to 5 days such that her predose trough vancomycin concentration would be maintained at approximately 10 mg/L. A less common, alternative method for maintenance therapy is to place in each dialysis exchange enough vancomycin to achieve a dialysate concentration of 15 to 20 mg/L (30-40 mg in a 2-L exchange). This technique of placing vancomycin in each exchange results in an average steady-state plasma concentration approximately equal to the concentration of vancomycin in the dialysate fluid, after multiple exchanges (ie, 15-20 mg/L).[42,43]

Question #5 *Suppose A.C. was given an initial 1-g dose and 3 days later, she underwent high-flux hemodialysis for 2 hours. Calculate a replacement dose after the dialysis session.*

Although the amount of vancomycin removed by standard hemodialysis is negligible, high-flux hemodialysis has been reported to remove approximately 17% over 2 hours.[47] Assuming the initial plasma concentration is 18.5 mg/L and using the estimated K of 0.0039 hr^{-1}, as calculated previously for A.C., the predialysis concentration can be determined using Equation 16.16.

$$C_2 = C_1(e^{-Kt})$$

$$= 18.5 \text{ mg/L } (e^{-(0.0039 \text{ hr}^{-1})(72 \text{ hr})})$$

$$= 14 \text{ mg/L}$$

If the plasma concentration declines by approximately 17% because of high-flux hemodialysis, then the postdialysis plasma concentration will be 83% of the predialysis concentration. This ignores any additional elimination from the intrinsic clearance during the 2-hour dialysis period, because it is negligible.

$$C_{\text{post dialysis}} = 14 \text{ mg/L } (0.83)$$

$$= 11.6 \text{ mg/L}$$

If a replacement dose is desired at this point, the dose can be calculated using Equation 16.28.

$$\text{Dose} = \frac{(V)(\Delta C)}{(S)(F)} \qquad \text{(Eq. 16.28)}$$

$$= \frac{(54 \text{ L})(18.5 \text{ mg/L} - 11.6 \text{ mg/L})}{(1)(1)}$$

$$= 373 \text{ mg} \approx 375 \text{ mg}$$

A similar approach can be used in a stepwise manner to determine dosing needs on any particular day and dialysis schedule. The amount of actual drug loss will depend on the intrinsic Cl, V, time of decay (t), duration of hemodialysis, and efficiency of the dialysis treatment.

Question #6   *A.C. became hemodynamically unstable. Therefore, hemodialysis was discontinued, and continuous renal replacement therapy (CRRT) was initiated with an ultrafiltration rate of 1 L/hr. How should the vancomycin dosage be changed?*

In this case, it would be advisable to monitor vancomycin concentrations until the level declines to a point where therapy can be reinstituted (eg, 5-15 mg/L). Recall from Chapter "Drug Dosing in Kidney Disease and Dialysis" that not all CRRT is the same. Here the patient is undergoing Continuous Veno-Venous Hemofiltration (CVVH), given the reported ultrafiltration rate. Since no sieve coefficient is reported, a good approximation is the fraction of unbound drug. Using the population average (fu = 0.6), we can estimate the clearance owing to CRRT as follows:

$$Cl_{CRRT\,max} = (fu)(CRRT \text{ flow rate})$$

$$= (0.6)(1 \text{ L/hr})$$

The total vancomycin clearance would be the sum of the clearance owing to CRRT, and the estimated intrinsic clearance previously estimated as 0.21 L/hr.

$$Cl = Cl_{CRRT} + Cl_{pat}$$

$$= 0.6 \text{ L/hr} + 0.21 \text{ L/hr}$$

$$= 0.81 \text{ L/hr}$$

Now that we have estimated the Cl, using the previously estimated V, we can use Equation 16.9 to calculate the elimination rate constant as 0.015 hr^{-1} and Equation 16.10 to calculate the half-life of 46 hours. Based on this information, we can employ Equations 16.15 and 16.18 to estimate the steady-state peak and trough concentrations, respectively, for a dose of 750 mg every 48 hours.

$$C_{ss\,min} = \frac{\dfrac{(S)(F)(Dose)}{V}}{1 - e^{-K\tau}}$$

$$= \frac{(1)(1)(750 \text{ mg})}{54 \text{ L}}{(1 - e^{-(0.015 \text{ hr}^{-1})(48 \text{ hr})})}$$

$$= 27.1 \text{ mg/L}$$

$$C_{ss \, min} = (C_{ss \, max})(e^{-K\tau})$$

$$= (27.1 \text{ mg/L})(e^{-(0.015 \text{ hr}^{-1}) \, (48 \text{ hr})})$$

$$= 13.2 \text{ mg/L}$$

Question #7 *K.G., a 10-year-old, 45-kg female with a serum creatinine of 0.6 mg/dL, requires vancomycin for an MRSA infection with MIC = 1. Based on this information, estimate K.G.'s vancomycin maintenance regimen to achieve a trough of 10 to 15 mg/L and AUC$_{24hr}$/MIC of greater than 400.*

The V and Cl can be estimated using the pediatric population parameters described in the Key Parameters table and using Equation 16.3.

$$V = 0.636 \times \text{Wt}$$

$$= 28.62 \text{ L}$$

and Equation 16.7

$$Cl = 0.248 \times \text{Wt}^{0.75} \times \left(\frac{0.48}{\text{Scr}} \right)^{0.361} \times (\ln (\text{Age in days})/7.8)^{0.995}$$

Recall from the Key Parameters table that Age should be in days and Weight as actual kg.

$$Cl = 0.248 \times 45^{0.75} \times \left(\frac{0.48}{0.6} \right)^{0.361} \times (\ln (3,650)/7.8)^{0.995}$$

$$= 4.31 \times 0.923 \times 1.05$$

$$= 4.18 \text{ L/hr}$$

To determine the dosing interval, we can calculate the half-life using the above-mentioned parameters with Equation 16.10.

$$t_{\frac{1}{2}} = \frac{(0.693)(V)}{Cl}$$

$$= \frac{(0.693)(28.62 \text{ L})}{(4.18 \text{ L/hr})}$$

$$= 4.7 \text{ hr}$$

Given this half-life, we dose every 6 hours, which is within the recommended one to two half-lives. Now, we are left to determine what dose to administer at each 6-hour interval. Because AUC_{24hr}/MIC of 400 is associated with efficacy and, therefore, the primary target for dosing is calculated using Equation 16.24.

$$\text{Dose}_{24hr} = AUC_{24hr}/\text{MIC} \times \text{Cl} \times \text{MIC}$$

$$= 400 \times 4.18 \times 1$$

$$= 1,672 \text{ mg}$$

We round the daily dose to 1,600 mg for ease of dosing. Based on the half-life of 5 hours, a dosing frequency of every 6 hours is appropriate (eg, 400 mg intravenously every 6 hours). Vancomycin is commonly dosed at every 6 hours in pediatrics owing to the short half-life. Alternatively, because the AUC_{24hr}/MIC is the pharmacodynamic driver, another option is to dose 500 mg every 8 hours. However, higher doses administered less frequently increase the chance for Red man syndrome. Now that we have a proposed plan that hits the AUC goal, let us also ensure that it achieves a safe and effective trough between 10 and 15 mg/L. Before we do that however, we need to calculate the elimination rate constant by rearranging Equation 16.20.

$$K = 0.693/t_{\frac{1}{2}}$$

$$= 0.693/4.7$$

$$= 0.147$$

Now, using Equation 16.17, we can calculate the expected trough level.

$$C_{ss \text{ min}} = \frac{\dfrac{(S)(F)(\text{Dose})}{V}}{1 - e^{-K\tau}} (e^{-K\tau})$$

$$= \frac{\dfrac{(1)(1)(400)}{28.6}}{1 - e^{-(0.147)(6)}} (e^{-(0.147)(6)})$$

$$= 9.9 \text{ mg/L} \approx 10 \text{ mg/L}$$

The trough estimate is both within efficacy and safety parameters. Finally, we should ensure that the estimated peak is also within safety limits for ototoxicity. Following Equation 16.15,

$$C_{ss\,max} = \frac{\dfrac{(S)(F)(Dose)}{V}}{1-e^{-K\tau}}$$

$$= \frac{\dfrac{(1)(1)(400)}{28.6}}{1-e^{-0.147(6)}}$$

$$= 23.9 \text{ mg/L}$$

A peak of 24 mg/L is far below 50 mg/L associated with an increased risk for ototoxicity.

Therefore, 400 mg every 6 hours is an appropriate initial dosing regimen.

Question #8 *C.U. is a 40-year-old, 5-foot 7-inch, 105-kg man with a serum creatinine of 1.2 mg/dL. He has a penicillin allergy history, and, for that reason, vancomycin is being considered for empiric therapy. What size descriptor (eg, ideal body weight [IBW], actual body weight [ABW], adjusted ABW [ABW$_{adj}$]) should the dosing regimen of vancomycin be based on for C.U.?*

The volume of distribution of vancomycin is greater in obese subjects than that in nonobese subjects. The apparent volume of distribution for vancomycin tends to correlate best with actual (total) body weight, although there is a fair degree of variability.[9,32,36,57-59] For clearance, some investigators have reported higher vancomycin clearances in patients with obesity, whereas others have observed that vancomycin clearance is still essentially equivalent to creatinine clearance.[9,32,36,57-59] The use of ABW$_{adj}$ in the Cl$_{Cr}$ equation is recommended for patients with a body mass index (BMI) between 30 and 40 and lean body weight (LBW$_{2005}$) for those with BMI greater than 40 (see Chapter "Drug Dosing in Kidney Disease and Dialysis").[60-62] However, when ABW was used to calculate Cl$_{Cr}$, the Matzke method to estimate vancomycin PK was shown to be the most precise and least biased among seven published methods where 61% (116/189) of subjects were obese.[34] Owing to the wide variability in the PK parameters, monitoring serum vancomycin concentrations in patients with obesity is advisable. To calculate the expected PK parameters for C.U., first estimate the patient's BMI using Equation 16.29

$$BMI \ (kg/m^2) = \frac{Weight \ (kg)}{Height \ in \ m^2} \qquad \textbf{(Eq. 16.29)}$$

$$C.U.'s \ BMI = \frac{105 \ kg}{1.7 \ m^2}$$

$$= 36.3 \ kg/m^2$$

Estimated Cl$_{Cr}$ depends on BMI (see earlier). Because C.U.'s BMI is between 30 and 40, ABW$_{adj}$ will be used in lieu of ABW to estimate Cl$_{Cr}$.

To calculate ABW_{adj} we first need to estimate IBW using Equation 16.30 (male) or Equation 16.31 (female).

> IBW for male: 50 kg + 2.3 kg for each inch over 5 feet   **(Eq. 16.30)**

> IBW for female: 45.5 kg + 2.3 kg for each inch over 5 feet   **(Eq. 16.31)**

Following Equation 16.30,

$$C.U.'s\ IBW = 50\ kg + (2.3\ kg \times 7)$$

$$= 66.1\ kg$$

Next, calculate ABW_{adj} using Equation 16.32.

> ABW_{adj}= IBW + 0.4 (ABW − IBW)   **(Eq. 16.32)**

$$C.U.'s\ ABW_{adj} = 66.1\ kg + 0.4(105\ kg - 66.1\ kg)$$

$$= 81.7\ kg$$

If C.U. had a BMI of 40 or more, then Equation 16.33 (male) or 16.34 (female) for LBW would have been used as calculated by Janmahasatian et al[63] and Cl_{Cr} estimated using this body size descriptor to calculate vancomycin Cl using the Matzke method. This approach is supported by the observation that at extreme, BMI's ABW does not scale proportionally; thus, lower mg/kg doses can be used.[64]

> $LBW_{Male} = (9,270 \times TBW)/(6,680 + 216 \times BMI)$ **(Eq. 16.33)**

> $LBW_{Female} = (9,270 \times TBW)/(8,780 + 244 \times BMI)$ **(Eq. 16.34)**

After calculating ABW_{adj}, creatinine clearance can be obtained using Equation 16.9.

$$Cl_{Cr}\ for\ males = \frac{(140 - Age\ in\ years)(Weight\ in\ kg)}{72 \times SCr_{ss}(mg/dL)}$$

$$= \frac{(140 - 40)(81.7\ kg)}{(72)(1.2\ mg/dL)}$$

$$= 94.6\ mL/min$$

We can then calculate vancomycin clearance using Equation 16.6:

$$Cl \ (mL/min) = (Cl_{Cr} \times 0.689) + 3.66$$

$$= (94.6 \ mL/min \times 0.689) + 3.66$$

$$= 68.8 \ mL/min$$

To convert to L/hr:

$$Cl \left(L/hr\right) = 68.8 \ mL/min \times \left(\frac{60 \ min/hr}{1,000 \ mL/L} \right)$$

$$= 4.1 \ L/hr$$

Recall that vancomycin clearance (Cl) is best estimated using ABW. To adjust Cl estimated by ABW_{adj} ($Cl_{ABW_{adj}}$) to Cl estimated by ABW (Cl_{ABW}), we simply scale by using the ABW to ABW_{adj} ratio as follows:

$$Cl_{ABW} = Cl_{ABW_{adj}} \left(\frac{ABW}{ABW_{adj}} \right)$$

$$= 4.1 \left(\frac{105 \ kg}{81.7 \ kg} \right)$$

$$= 5.3 \ L/hr$$

Equation 16.1 can be used to calculate C.U.'s volume of distribution:

$$V = 0.72 \ L/kg \ if \ Cl_{Cr} \ is > 60 \ mL/min$$

$$= 0.72 \ L/kg \ (105 \ kg)$$

$$= 75.6 \ L$$

and Equation 16.9 can be used with the clearance of 5.3 L/hr and the volume of distribution of 75.6 L to calculate an elimination rate constant of 0.054 hr^{-1}.

$$K = \frac{Cl}{V}$$

$$= \frac{5.3}{75.6}$$

$$= 0.07 \ hr^{-1}$$

Finally, using Equation 16.10, the vancomycin $t_{1/2}$ can be estimated to be 10 hours.

$$t_{\frac{1}{2}} = \frac{0.693}{K}$$

$$= \frac{0.693}{0.07}$$

$$= 9.9 \text{ hr}$$

Given the half-life and the desire to choose a dosing interval that is between one and two half-lives for vancomycin, a logical approach would be to use a convenient dosing interval of 12 hours, an AUC_{24hr}/MIC ratio 400 or higher, and trough concentration between 10 and 15 mg/L. If we assume an $MIC = 1$, use Equation 16.24 to solve for a dose.

$$\text{Dose}_{24hr} = AUC_{24hr}/MIC \times Cl \times MIC$$

$$= 400 \times 5.3 \times 1$$

$$= 2{,}120 \text{ mg}$$

This dose would usually be rounded off to a reasonable amount (closest 250 interval). Based on the half-life of 9.9 hours, a dosing interval of every 12 hours is appropriate (ie, 1,000 mg given every 12 hours). The steady-state trough and peak concentrations on this new dose could be confirmed by using Equations 16.17 and 16.15, respectively.

$$C_{ssmin} = \frac{\dfrac{(S)(F)(\text{Dose})}{V}}{1-e^{-K\tau}}(e^{-K\tau})$$

$$= \frac{\dfrac{(1)(1)(1{,}000)}{75.6}}{1-e^{-(0.07)(12)}}(e^{-(0.07)(12)})$$

$$= 10 \text{ mg/L}$$

$$C_{ss\,peak} = \frac{\dfrac{(S)(F)(\text{Dose})}{V_d}}{1-e^{-K\tau}}$$

$$= \frac{\dfrac{(1)(1)(1{,}000)}{75.6}}{1-e^{-0.07(12)}}$$

$$= 23.3 \text{ mg/L}$$

If an alternative trough is desired (eg, 15 mg/L), the new dose can be calculated by simply using a ratio of the new target concentration to the current concentration. At a dose of 1,000 mg, the vancomycin $C_{ss\,min} = 10$ mg/L and will be labeled as (current trough).

$$\text{New dose} = \text{Current dose}\left(\frac{\text{New trough}}{\text{Current trough}}\right)$$

$$= (1,000 \text{ mg})\left(\frac{15 \text{ mg/L}}{10 \text{ mg/L}}\right)$$

$$= 1,500 \text{ mg } q12h$$

This technique of using a ratio of concentrations to calculate the new dose is appropriate as long as the dosing interval and time of sampling have not changed for a drug that exhibits stable linear PK. Note that any difference between the plasma concentrations calculated by the two methods is because of rounding-off errors and not due to any other assumptions.

Finally, therapeutic monitoring and revision with two-sample measurement approach (peak and trough) is shown to significantly improve target trough concentration attainment in the obese population and is, therefore, strongly advocated for revision of initial dosing regimens.[65]

REFERENCES

1. Alexander MR. A review of vancomycin: after 15 years of use. *Ann Pharmacother*. 1974;8(9):520-525.

2. Kirby WM, Perry DM, Bauer AW. Treatment of staphylococcal septicemia with vancomycin: report of thirty-three cases. *N Eng J Med*. 1960;262:49-55.

3. Banner W Jr, Ray CG. Vancomycin in perspective. *Am J Dis Child*. 1984;138(1):14-16.

4. Cunha BA, Ristuccia AM. Clinical usefulness of vancomycin. *Clin Pharm*. 1983;2(5):417-424.

5. Wilhelm MP. Vancomycin. *Mayo Clin Proc*. 1991;66(11):1165-1170.

6. Lundstrom TS, Sobel JD. Antibiotics for gram-positive bacterial infections. Vancomycin, teicoplanin, quinupristin/dalfopristin, and linezolid. *Infect Dis Clin North Am*. 2000;14(2):463-474.

7. Watanakunakorn C, Tisone JC. Synergism between vancomycin and gentamicin or tobramycin for methicillin-susceptible and methicillin-resistant *Staphylococcus aureus* strains. *Antimicrob Agents Chemother*. 1982;22(5):903-905.

8. Rotschafer JC, Crossley K, Zaske DE, Mead K, Sawchuk RJ, Solem LD. Pharmacokinetics of vancomycin: observations in 28 patients and dosage recommendations. *Antimicrob Agents Chemother*. 1982;22(3):391-394.

9. Blouin RA, Bauer LA, Miller DD, Record KE, Griffen WO. Vancomycin pharmacokinetics in normal and morbidly obese subjects. *Antimicrob Agents Chemother*. 1982;21(4):575-580.

10. Moellering RC Jr, Krogstad DJ, Greenblatt DJ. Vancomycin therapy in patients with impaired renal function: a nomogram for dosage. *Ann Intern Med*. 1981;94(3):343-346.

11. Zimmermann AE, Katona BG, Plaisance KI. Association of vancomycin serum concentrations with outcomes in patients with gram-positive bacteremia. *Pharmacotherapy*. 1995;15(1):85-91.

12. Mulhern JG, Braden GL, O'Shea MH, Madden RL, Lipkowitz GS, Germain MJ. Trough serum vancomycin levels predict the relapse of gram-positive peritonitis in peritoneal dialysis patients. *Am J Kidney Dis*. 1995;25(4):611-615.

13. Welty TE, Copa AK. Impact of vancomycin therapeutic drug monitoring on patient care. *Ann Pharmacother*. 1994;28(12):1335-1339.

14. American Thoracic Society; Infectious Diseases Society of America. Guidelines for the management of adults with hospital-acquired, ventilator-associated, and healthcare-associated pneumonia. *Am J Respir Crit Care Med*. 2005;171(4):388-416.

15. Hidayat LK, Hsu DI, Quist R, Shriner KA, Wong-Beringer A. High-dose vancomycin therapy for methicillin-resistant *Staphylococcus aureus* infections: efficacy and toxicity. *Arch Intern Med*. 2006; 166(19):2138-2144.

16. Men P, Li HB, Zhai SD, Zhao RS. Association between the AUC0-24/MIC ratio of vancomycin and its clinical effectiveness: a systematic review and meta-analysis. *PLoS One*. 2016;11(1):e0146224.

17. Prybylski JP. Vancomycin trough concentration as a predictor of clinical outcomes in patients with *Staphylococcus aureus* bacteremia: a meta-analysis of observational studies. *Pharmacotherapy*. 2015;35(10):889-898.

18. Clinical and Laboratory Standards Institute (CLSI). *Performance Standards for Antimicrobial Susceptibility Testing, 16th Informational Supplement*. Clinical and Laboratory Standards Institute; 2006.

19. Karchmer AW. Staphylococcal endocarditis. Laboratory and clinical basis for antibiotic therapy. *Am J Med*. 1985;78(6b):116-127.

20. Lodise TP, Patel N, Lomaestro BM, Rodvold KA, Drusano GL. Relationship between initial vancomycin concentration-time profile and nephrotoxicity among hospitalized patients. *Clin Infect Dis*. 2009;49(4):507-514.

21. Wong-Beringer A, Joo J, Tse E, Beringer P. Vancomycin-associated nephrotoxicity: a critical appraisal of risk with high-dose therapy. *Int J Antimicrob Agents*. 2011;37(2):95-101.

22. Mohr JF, Murray BE. Point: vancomycin is not obsolete for the treatment of infection caused by methicillin-resistant *Staphylococcus aureus*. *Clin Infect Dis*. 2007;44(12):1536-1542.

23. Moise-Broder PA, Forrest A, Birmingham MC, Schentag JJ. Pharmacodynamics of vancomycin and other antimicrobials in patients with *Staphylococcus aureus* lower respiratory tract infections. *Clin Pharmacokinet*. 2004;43(13):925-942.

24. Aeschlimann JR, Hershberger E, Rybak MJ. Analysis of vancomycin population susceptibility profiles, killing activity, and postantibiotic effect against vancomycin-intermediate *Staphylococcus aureus*. *Antimicrob Agents Chemother*. 1999;43(8):1914-1918.

25. Liu C, Bayer A, Cosgrove SE, et al. Clinical practice guidelines by the infectious diseases society of america for the treatment of methicillin-resistant *Staphylococcus aureus* infections in adults and children: executive summary. *Clin Infect Dis*. 2011;52(3):285-292.

26. Newfield P, Roizen MF. Hazards of rapid administration of vancomycin. *Ann Intern Med*. 1979; 91(4):581.

27. Cook FV, Farrar WE Jr. Vancomycin revisited. *Ann Intern Med*. 1978;88(6):813-818.

28. Farber BF, Moellering RC Jr. Retrospective study of the toxicity of preparations of vancomycin from 1974 to 1981. *Antimicrob Agents Chemother*. 1983;23(1):138-141.

29. Jeffres MN, Isakow W, Doherty JA, Micek ST, Kollef MH. A retrospective analysis of possible renal toxicity associated with vancomycin in patients with health care-associated methicillin-resistant *Staphylococcus aureus* pneumonia. *Clin Ther*. 2007;29(6):1107-1115.

30. Lodise TP, Lomaestro B, Graves J, Drusano GL. Larger vancomycin doses (at least four grams per day) are associated with an increased incidence of nephrotoxicity. *Antimicrob Agents Chemother*. 2008; 52(4):1330-1336.

31. Rybak MJ, Le J, Lodise TP, et al. Therapeutic monitoring of vancomycin for serious methicillin-resistant *staphylococcus aureus* infections: a revised consensus guideline and review by the American Society of Health-system Pharmacists, the Infectious Diseases Society of America, the Pediatric Infectious Diseases Society, and the Society of Infectious Diseases Pharmacists. *Clin Infect Dis*. 2020;71(6): 1361-1364.

32. Rushing TA, Ambrose PJ. Clinical application and evaluation of vancomycin dosing in adults. *J Pharm Technol*. 2001;17(2):33-38.

33. Lee E, Winter ME, Boro MS. Comparing two predictive methods for determining serum vancomycin concentrations at a Veterans Affairs Medical Center. *Am J Health Syst Pharm*. 2006;63(19):1872-1875.

34. Murphy JE, Gillespie DE, Bateman CV. Predictability of vancomycin trough concentrations using seven approaches for estimating pharmacokinetic parameters. *Am J Health Syst Pharm*. 2006; 63(23):2365-2370.

35. Krogstad DJ, Moellering RC Jr, Greenblatt DJ. Single-dose kinetics of intravenous vancomycin. *J Clin Pharmacol*. 1980;20(4 Pt 1):197-201.

36. Ducharme MP, Slaughter RL, Edwards DJ. Vancomycin pharmacokinetics in a patient population: effect of age, gender, and body weight. *Ther Drug Monit*. 1994;16(5):513-518.

37. Matzke GR, McGory RW, Halstenson CE, Keane WF. Pharmacokinetics of vancomycin in patients with various degrees of renal function. *Antimicrob Agents Chemother*. 1984;25(4):433-437.

38. Le J, Bradley JS, Murray W, et al. Improved vancomycin dosing in children using area under the curve exposure. *Pediatr Infect Dis J*. 2013;32(4):e155-e163.

39. Leonard AE, Boro MS. Vancomycin pharmacokinetics in middle-aged and elderly men. *Am J Hosp Pharm*. 1994;51(6):798-800.

40. Ackerman BH, Taylor EH, Olsen KM, Abdel-Malak W, Pappas AA. Vancomycin serum protein binding determination by ultrafiltration. *Drug Intell Clin Pharm*. 1988;22(4):300-303.

41. Rodvold KA, Blum RA, Fischer JH, et al. Vancomycin pharmacokinetics in patients with various degrees of renal function. *Antimicrob Agents Chemother*. 1988;32(6):848-852.

42. Rybak MJ, Albrecht LM, Berman JR, Warbasse LH, Svensson CK. Vancomycin pharmacokinetics in burn patients and intravenous drug abusers. *Antimicrob Agents Chemother*. 1990;34(5):792-795.

43. Bickley SK. Drug dosing during continuous arteriovenous hemofiltration. *Clin Pharm*. 1988;7(3): 198-206.

44. Dupuis RE, Matzke GR, Maddux FW, O ddux MG. Vancomycin disposition during continuous arteriovenous hemofiltration. *Clin Pharm*. 1989;8(5):371-374.

45. Nielsen HE, Hansen HE, Korsager B, Skov PE. Renal excretion of vancomycinin in kidney disease. *Acta Med Scand*. 1975;197(4):261-264.

46. Lindholm DD, Murray JS. Persistence of vancomycin in the blood during renal failure and its treatment by hemodialysis. *N Engl J Med*. 1966;274(19):1047-1051.

47. Ayus JC, Eneas JF, Tong TG, et al. Peritoneal clearance and total body elimination of vancomycin during chronic intermittent peritoneal dialysis. *Clin Nephrol*. 1979;11(3):129-132.

48. Paton TW, Cornish WR, Manuel MA, Hardy BG. Drug therapy in patients undergoing peritoneal dialysis. Clinical pharmacokinetic considerations. *Clin Pharmacokinet*. 1985;10(5):404-425.

49. Morse GD, Farolino DF, Apicella MA, Walshe JJ. Comparative study of intraperitoneal and intravenous vancomycin pharmacokinetics during continuous ambulatory peritoneal dialysis. *Antimicrob Agents Chemother*. 1987;31(2):173-177.

50. Smith PF, Morse GD. Accuracy of measured vancomycin serum concentrations in patients with end-stage renal disease. *Ann Pharmacother*. 1999;33(12):1329-1335.

51. Lanese DM, Alfrey PS, Molitoris BA. Markedly increased clearance of vancomycin during hemodialysis using polysulfone dialyzers. *Kidney Int*. 1989;35(6):1409-1412.

52. Pollard TA, Lampasona V, Akkerman S, et al. Vancomycin redistribution: dosing recommendations following high-flux hemodialysis. *Kidney Int*. 1994;45(1):232-237.

53. Karam CM, McKinnon PS, Neuhauser MM, Rybak MJ. Outcome assessment of minimizing vancomycin monitoring and dosing adjustments. *Pharmacotherapy*. 1999;19(3):257-266.

54. Neely MN, Youn G, Jones B, et al. Are vancomycin trough concentrations adequate for optimal dosing? *Antimicrob Agents Chemother*. 2014;58(1):309-316.

55. Schaad UB, McCracken GH Jr, Nelson JD. Clinical pharmacology and efficacy of vancomycin in pediatric patients. *J Pediatr*. 1980;96(1):119-126.

56. Pai MP, Neely M, Rodvold KA, Lodise TP. Innovative approaches to optimizing the delivery of vancomycin in individual patients. *Adv Drug Deliv Rev*. 2014;77:50-57.

57. Vance-Bryan K, Guay DR, Gilliland SS, Rodvold KA, Rotschafer JC. Effect of obesity on vancomycin pharmacokinetic parameters as determined by using a Bayesian forecasting technique. *Antimicrob Agents Chemother*. 1993;37(3):436-440.

58. Bearden DT, Rodvold KA. Dosage adjustments for antibacterials in obese patients: applying clinical pharmacokinetics. *Clin Pharmacokinet*. 2000;38(5):415-426.

59. Grace E. Altered vancomycin pharmacokinetics in obese and morbidly obese patients: what we have learned over the past 30 years. *J Antimicrob Chemother*. 2012. doi:10.1093/jac/dks066.

60. Winter MA, Guhr KN, Berg GM. Impact of various body weights and serum creatinine concentrations on the bias and accuracy of the Cockcroft-Gault equation. *Pharmacotherapy*. 2012;32(7):604-612.

61. Bouquegneau A, Vidal-Petiot E, Moranne O, et al. Creatinine-based equations for the adjustment of drug dosage in an obese population. *Br J Clin Pharmacol*. 2016;81(2):349-361.

62. Park EJ, Pai MP, Dong T, et al. The influence of body size descriptors on the estimation of kidney function in normal weight, overweight, obese, and morbidly obese adults. *Ann Pharmacother*. 2012;46(3):317-328.

63. Janmahasatian S, Duffull SB, Ash S, Ward LC, Byrne NM, Green B. Quantification of lean bodyweight. *Clin Pharmacokinet*. 2005;44(10):1051-1065.

64. Morrill HJ, Caffrey AR, Noh E, LaPlante KL. Vancomycin dosing considerations in a real-world Cohort of obese and extremely obese patients. *Pharmacotherapy*. 2015;35(9):869-875.

65. Hong J, Krop LC, Johns T, Pai MP. Individualized vancomycin dosing in obese patients: a two-sample measurement approach improves target attainment. *Pharmacotherapy*. 2015;35(5):455-463.

Nomograms for Calculating Body Surface Area

Nomogram for Calculating the Body Surface Area of Children[a]

Height	Surface area	Weight

[a]From the formula of DuBois and DuBois. *Arch Intern Med.* 1916;17:863: $S = W^{0.425} \times H^{0.725} \times 71.84$, or $\log S = 0.425 \log W + 0.725 \log H + 1.8564$, where S is body surface area in cm^2, W is weight in kg, and H is height in cm. (Reprinted with permission from Lontmer C, ed. *Geigy Scientific Tables.* Vol 1., 8th ed. Ciba-Geigy; 1981:226-227.)

Nomogram for Calculating the Body Surface Area of Adults[a]

Height | Surface area | Weight

[a]From the formula of DuBois and DuBois. *Arch Intern Med*. 1916;17:863: $S = W^{0.425} \times H^{0.725} \times 71.84$, or $\log S = 0.425 \log W + 0.725 \log H + 1.8564$, where S is body surface area in cm², W is weight in kg, and H is height in cm. (Reprinted with permission from Lontmer C, ed. *Geigy Scientific Tables*. Vol 1., 8th ed. Ciba-Geigy; 1981:226-227.)

Common Equations Used Throughout the Text

The following is a list of equations that are frequently used in pharmacokinetic calculations. They are grouped together according to specific dosing situations. For a complete discussion, refer to the text and figures cited next to each equation. Although some of the equations may appear complicated, most are simple rearrangements of basic equations that can be broken down into one or more of the following components:

$\dfrac{(S)(F)(\text{Dose})}{V}$	The change in plasma concentration following a dose (ΔC_p)
$\dfrac{(S)(F)(\text{Dose}/t)}{Cl}$	Average steady-state concentration
(e^{-Kt})	Fraction remaining after time of decay (t)
$(1 - e^{-Kt})$	Fraction lost during decay phase *or* fraction of steady state achieved during infusion

SINGLE DOSE (ABSORPTION TIME OR $t_{in} \leq \frac{1}{6}\, t_{\frac{1}{2}}$)

$\text{Loading dose} = \dfrac{(V)(C)}{(S)(F)}$	Part I: Chapter 1: Basic Principles, Equation 1.11; Part I: Chapter 2: Selecting the Appropriate Equation and Interpretation of Measured Drug Concentrations, Figure 2.1
$\begin{aligned}\text{Incremental} \\ \text{loading dose}\end{aligned} = \dfrac{(V)(C_{\text{desired}} - C_{\text{initial}})}{(S)(F)}$	Part I: Chapter 1: Basic Principles, Equation 1.12
$\begin{aligned}C &= \dfrac{(S)(F)(\text{Loading dose})}{(V)} \\ &= (\text{Change in concentration})\end{aligned}$	Part I: Chapter 2: Selecting the Appropriate Equation and Interpretation of Measured Drug Concentrations, Equation 2.1; Figure 2.1

$C_1 = \dfrac{(S)(F)(\text{Loading dose})}{V}(e^{-Kt_1})$ $= \begin{pmatrix} \text{Change in} \\ \text{concentration} \end{pmatrix}\begin{pmatrix} \text{Fraction remaining} \\ \text{after time of decay } t_1 \end{pmatrix}$	Part I: Chapter 2: Selecting the Appropriate Equation and Interpretation of Measured Drug Concentrations, Equation 2.2; Figure 2.1

HALF-LIFE ($t_{\frac{1}{2}}$) AND ELIMINATION RATE CONSTANT (K)

$K = \dfrac{Cl}{V}$	Part I: Chapter 1: Basic Principles, Equation 1.27
$t_{\frac{1}{2}} = \dfrac{(0.693)(V)}{Cl}$	Part I: Chapter 1: Basic Principles, Equation 1.30
$K = \dfrac{0.693}{t_{\frac{1}{2}}}$	Part II: Chapter 12: Precision Oncology: Pharmacokinetics and Genomics to Guide Cancer Therapy, Equation 12.7
$t_{\frac{1}{2}} = \dfrac{0.693}{K}$	Part I: Chapter 1: Basic Principles, Equation 1.29
$K = \dfrac{\ln\left(\dfrac{C_1}{C_2}\right)}{t}$	Part I: Chapter 1: Basic Principles, Equation 1.28

SINGLE DOSE (ABSORPTION OR $t_{in} > \frac{1}{6}\, t_{\frac{1}{2}}$)

$C_2 = \dfrac{(S)(F)(\text{Dose}/t_{in})}{Cl}\left(1 - e^{-Kt_{in}}\right)\left(e^{-Kt_2}\right)$	Part I: Chapter 2: Selecting the Appropriate Equation and Interpretation of Measured Drug Concentrations, Equation 2.6; Figure 2.4

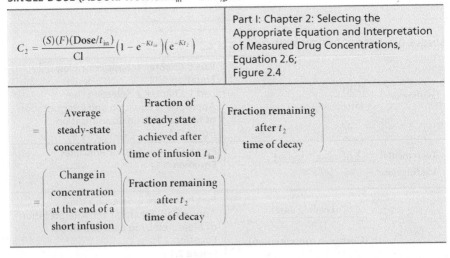

$= \begin{pmatrix} \text{Average} \\ \text{steady-state} \\ \text{concentration} \end{pmatrix}\begin{pmatrix} \text{Fraction of} \\ \text{steady state} \\ \text{achieved after} \\ \text{time of infusion } t_{in} \end{pmatrix}\begin{pmatrix} \text{Fraction remaining} \\ \text{after } t_2 \\ \text{time of decay} \end{pmatrix}$

$= \begin{pmatrix} \text{Change in} \\ \text{concentration} \\ \text{at the end of a} \\ \text{short infusion} \end{pmatrix}\begin{pmatrix} \text{Fraction remaining} \\ \text{after } t_2 \\ \text{time of decay} \end{pmatrix}$

CONTINUOUS INFUSION

AT STEADY STATE

$\text{Maintenance dose} = \dfrac{(\text{Cl})(C_{ss\,ave})(\tau)}{(S)(F)}$	Part I: Chapter 1: Basic Principles, Equation 1.16
$C_{ss\,ave} = \dfrac{(S)(F)(\text{Dose}/\tau)}{\text{Cl}}$ = Average steady-state concentration	Part I: Chapter 1: Basic Principles, Equation 1.33; Part I: Chapter 2: Selecting the Appropriate Equation and Interpretation of Measured Drug Concentrations, Figure 2.2

DECAY FROM STEADY STATE

$C_2 = \dfrac{(S)(F)(\text{Dose}/\tau)}{\text{Cl}}\left(e^{-Kt_2}\right)$ $= \begin{pmatrix} \text{Average} \\ \text{steady-state} \\ \text{concentration} \end{pmatrix}\begin{pmatrix} \text{Fraction remaining} \\ \text{after } t_2 \\ \text{time of decay} \end{pmatrix}$	Part I: Chapter 2: Selecting the Appropriate Equation and Interpretation of Measured Drug Concentrations, Equation 2.4; Figure 2.2

NON–STEADY STATE

$C_1 = \dfrac{(S)(F)(\text{Dose}/\tau)}{\text{Cl}}\left(1 - e^{-Kt_1}\right)$	Part I: Chapter 1: Basic Principles, Equation 1.35; Figure 1.19
$= \begin{pmatrix} \text{Average} \\ \text{steady-state} \\ \text{concentration} \end{pmatrix}\begin{pmatrix} \text{Fraction of} \\ \text{steady state} \\ \text{achieved } t_1 \text{ time} \\ \text{after starting infusion} \end{pmatrix}$	

DECAY FROM NON–STEADY STATE

$C_2 = \dfrac{(S)(F)(\text{Dose}/\tau)}{\text{Cl}}\left(1 - e^{-Kt_1}\right)\left(e^{-Kt_2}\right)$	Part I: Chapter 1: Basic Principles, Equation 1.39; Figure 1.19
$= \begin{pmatrix} \text{Average} \\ \text{steady-state} \\ \text{concentration} \end{pmatrix}\begin{pmatrix} \text{Fraction of} \\ \text{steady state} \\ \text{achieved } t_1 \\ \text{time after} \\ \text{starting infusion} \end{pmatrix}\begin{pmatrix} \text{Fraction} \\ \text{remaining} \\ \text{after } t_2 \\ \text{time of decay} \end{pmatrix}$	

MULTIPLE DOSE
(CONSISTENT τ AND DOSE): STEADY STATE

ABSORPTION OR $t_{in} \leq \frac{1}{6} t_{\frac{1}{2}}$

$$C_{ss_1} = \frac{\dfrac{(S)(F)(Dose)}{V}}{\left(1 - e^{-Kt}\right)}\left(e^{-K\tau_1}\right)$$	Part I: Chapter 1: Basic Principles, Equation 1.46 Part I: Chapter 2: Selecting the Appropriate Equation and Interpretation of Measured Drug Concentrations, Figure 2.6
$$= \frac{\left(\begin{array}{c}\text{Change in}\\\text{concentration}\end{array}\right)\left(\begin{array}{c}\text{Fraction}\\\text{remaining}\\\text{after } t_1\\\text{time of decay}\end{array}\right)}{\left(\begin{array}{c}\text{Fraction lost in}\\\text{dosing interval}\end{array}\right)}$$ $$= \left(\begin{array}{c}\text{Steady-state}\\\text{peak}\\\text{concentration}\end{array}\right)\left(\begin{array}{c}\text{Fraction remaining}\\\text{after } t_1\\\text{time of decay}\end{array}\right)$$	

ABSORPTION OR $t_{in} > \frac{1}{6} t_{\frac{1}{2}}$

$$C_{ss_2} = \frac{\dfrac{(S)(F)(Dose/t_{in})}{Cl}\left(1 - e^{-Kt_{in}}\right)}{1 - e^{-K\tau}}\left(e^{-Kt_2}\right)$$	Part I: Chapter 2: Selecting the Appropriate Equation and Interpretation of Measured Drug Concentrations, Equation 2.10 Part II: Chapter 6: Aminoglycoside Antibiotics, Equation 6.21; Figure 6.2
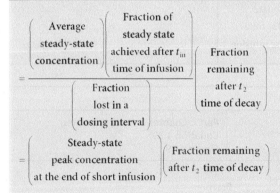	

$$= \left(\begin{array}{c}\text{Steady-state}\\\text{peak concentration}\\\text{at the end of short infusion}\end{array}\right)\left(\begin{array}{c}\text{Fraction remaining}\\\text{after } t_2 \text{ time of decay}\end{array}\right)$$

MULTIPLE DOSE
(CONSISTENT τ AND DOSE): NON–STEADY STATE

ABSORPTION OR $t_{in} \leq \frac{1}{6} t_{\frac{1}{2}}$

$C_{ss_2} = \dfrac{\dfrac{(S)(F)(\text{Dose})}{V}}{1 - e^{-K\tau}}\left(1 - e^{-K(N)\tau}\right)\left(e^{-Kt_2}\right)$	Part I: Chapter 2: Selecting the Appropriate Equation and Interpretation of Measured Drug Concentrations, Equation 2.8
$= \left(\dfrac{\text{Change in concentration}}{\text{Fraction lost in dosing interval}}\right)\left(\begin{array}{c}\text{Fraction of}\\\text{steady state}\\\text{achieved}\\\text{after } N \text{ doses}\end{array}\right)\left(\begin{array}{c}\text{Fraction}\\\text{remaining}\\\text{after } t_2 \text{ time}\\\text{of decay}\end{array}\right)$	
$= \left(\begin{array}{c}\text{Steady-state}\\\text{peak}\\\text{concentration}\end{array}\right)\left(\begin{array}{c}\text{Fraction of}\\\text{steady state}\\\text{achieved}\\\text{after } N \text{ doses}\end{array}\right)\left(\begin{array}{c}\text{Fraction}\\\text{remaining}\\\text{after } t_2 \text{ time}\\\text{of decay}\end{array}\right)$	

MASS BALANCE

$\dfrac{(S)(F)(\text{Dose}/\tau) - \dfrac{(C_2 - C_1)V}{t}}{C_{ave}} = \text{Cl}$	Part I: Chapter 2: Selecting the Appropriate Equation and Interpretation of Measured Drug Concentrations, Equation 2.17

CREATININE CLEARANCE (Cl$_{Cr}$)

$\begin{array}{c}\text{Cl}_{Cr} \text{ for males}\\\text{(mL/min)}\end{array} = \dfrac{(140 - \text{Age})(\text{Weight})}{(72)(\text{SCr}_{ss})}$	Part I: Chapter 3: Drug Dosing in Kidney Disease and Dialysis, Equation 3.4
$\begin{array}{c}\text{Cl}_{Cr} \text{ for females}\\\text{(mL/min)}\end{array} = (0.85)\dfrac{(140 - \text{Age})(\text{Weight})}{(72)(\text{SCr}_{ss})}$	Part I: Chapter 3: Drug Dosing in Kidney Disease and Dialysis, Equation 3.5

where age in years, weight in kg, and SCr$_{ss}$ in mg/dL

$\begin{array}{c}\text{GFR}\\(\text{mL/min}/1.73\,\text{m}^2)\end{array} = \dfrac{(0.41)(\text{Height in cm})}{\text{SCr}_{ss}}$	Part I: Chapter 3: Drug Dosing in Kidney Disease and Dialysis, Equation 3.13

where SCr$_{ss}$ in mg/dL

$\text{BSA in m}^2 = \left(\dfrac{\text{Patient's weight in kg}}{70\,\text{kg}}\right)^{0.7}(1.73\,\text{m}^2)$	Part I: Chapter 1: Basic Principles, Equation 1.17

NONLINEAR EQUATIONS (PHENYTOIN)

$(S)(F)(\text{Dose}/\tau) = \dfrac{(\text{Vm})(C_{ss\,ave})}{\text{Km} + C_{ss\,ave}}$	Part II: Chapter 14: Phenytoin, Equation 14.14
$C_{ss} = \dfrac{(\text{Km})\big[(S)(F)(\text{Dose}/\tau)\big]}{\text{Vm} - \big[(S)(F)(\text{Dose}/\tau)\big]}$	Part II: Chapter 14: Phenytoin, Equation 14.15

TIME REQUIRED TO ACHIEVE 90% OF STEADY STATE (t90%)

$t90\% = \dfrac{(\text{Km})(V)}{\big[\text{Vm} - (S)(F)(\text{Dose/day})\big]^{2}}[(2.3\,\text{Vm})$ $-(0.9)(S)(F)(\text{Dose/day})]$	Part II: Chapter 14: Phenytoin, Equation 14.23

HAS STEADY STATE BEEN ACHIEVED?

$90\%t = \dfrac{\big[115 + (35)(C)\big]\big[C\big]}{(S)(F)(\text{Dose/day})}$	Part II: Chapter 14: Phenytoin, Equation 14.24

Days on current maintenance regimen must exceed 90%*t* value to ensure that steady state has been achieved. Dose is in mg/day normalized to 70 kg.

ADJUSTMENT FOR PLASMA PROTEIN BINDING (PHENYTOIN)

ADJUSTMENT FOR SERUM ALBUMIN IF CL$_{CR}$ > 25 ML/MIN

$\dfrac{\text{Phenytoin concentration}}{\text{normal plasma binding}} = \dfrac{\begin{array}{c}\text{Patient's phenytoin concentration}\\\text{with altered plasma binding}\end{array}}{\left[0.9 \times \dfrac{\text{Patient's serum albumin}}{4.4 \text{ g/dL}}\right] + 0.1}$	Part II: Chapter 14: Phenytoin, Equation 14.2

ADJUSTMENT FOR SERUM ALBUMIN IF PATIENT RECEIVING DIALYSIS

$\dfrac{\text{Phenytoin concentration}}{\text{normal plasma binding}} = \dfrac{\begin{array}{c}\text{Dialysis patient's phenytoin concentration}\\\text{with altered plasma binding}\end{array}}{\left[(0.9)(0.48)\left(\dfrac{\text{Patient's serum albumin}}{4.4 \text{ g/dL}}\right)\right] + 0.1}$	Part II: Chapter 14: Phenytoin, Equation 14.3

Algorithm for Evaluating and Interpreting Plasma Concentrations

Step 1. Initial Data Collection

Before one can interpret the patient's pharmacokinetic parameters or plasma drug concentrations, appropriate information must be collected so that factors that may influence drug absorption and disposition can be considered.

Relevant Physical Data, Medical and Surgical History:

Height, weight, age, sex, race, current diseases, and symptoms.

Relevant Laboratory Data:

Renal Function: SCr, BUN, Cl_{Cr} (Is the collection complete?)

Hepatic Function: Serum albumin, bilirubin, prothrombin time, serum enzymes.

Protein Binding: Plasma protein concentration. Acidic drugs—Albumin. Basic drugs—Globulins. Evaluate displacing factors such as other drugs or presence of uremia

Thyroid Function

Drug Administration History:

Collect dosing data (dose, frequency, and route) for 3-5 half-lives. In acute care settings, consider history before admissions as well as during hospital stay.

It is critical to determine the exact time of administration for those doses taken just before drug level sampling.

Time of Sampling Relative to the Last Dose:

The best time to sample is usually just before the next dose. For drugs with a short half-life, peak and trough levels may be appropriate. Avoid absorption and distribution phase when peak levels are obtained.

(Continued on next page)

Step 2. Evaluation of Reported Plasma Concentrations

Has the patient been receiving constant dosing for >3-4 half-lives before obtaining the plasma sample?

Yes

No

Non-Steady State Plasma Concentration

The plasma concentration must be evaluated by considering the contribution of each dose at the time the plasma sample was obtained. Use Equation 2.2 for each bolus dose or Equation 2.6 for each "short infusion." If several different sustained infusion rates have been used during the accumulation period, Equation 1.35 or 1.39 should be used for each infusion rate.

C Is Greater Than Expected:

See List A.

V may be less than expected.
Sample may have been obtained during distribution phase.

C Is Less Than Expected:

See List B.

V may be greater than expected.
Sample may have been obtained too soon after the dose was administered and absorption was not yet complete.

List A

When drug concentrations are greater than expected, consider:

1. Increased bioavailability. This is only important if the drug's bioavailability is usually low.
2. Nonadherence. Intake is greater than prescribed.
3. Decreased clearance.
4. Increased plasma protein binding. Changes in plasma protein binding will be most important if fu is ≤0.1 and are unlikely to be significant if fu is >0.5. Increased plasma protein binding will also decrease the volume of distribution and clearance of most drugs.

List B

When drug concentrations are less than expected, consider:

1. Decreased bioavailability.
2. Nonadherence. Intake is less than prescribed.
3. Increased clearance.
4. Decreased plasma protein binding. Changes in plasma protein binding will be most important if fu is ≤0.1. It is unlikely to be significant if fu is >0.5. Decreased plasma protein binding will also increase the volume of distribution and the clearance of most drugs.

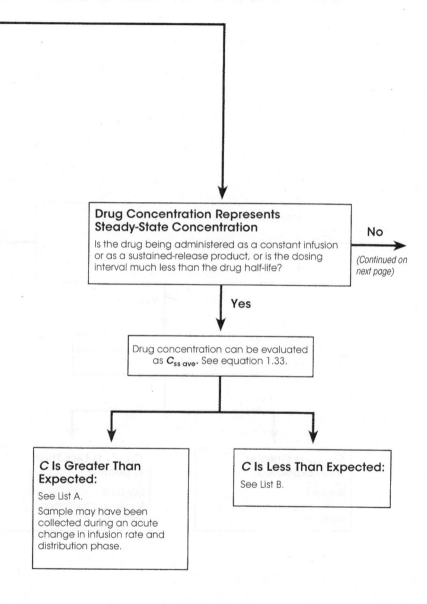

Drug Concentration Represents Steady-State Concentration

Is the drug being administered as a constant infusion or as a sustained-release product, or is the dosing interval much less than the drug half-life?

No

(Continued on next page)

Yes

Drug concentration can be evaluated as $C_{ss\ ave}$. See equation 1.33.

C Is Greater Than Expected:

See List A.

Sample may have been collected during an acute change in infusion rate and distribution phase.

C Is Less Than Expected:

See List B.

Step 2. Evaluation of Reported Plasma Concentrations
(Continued)

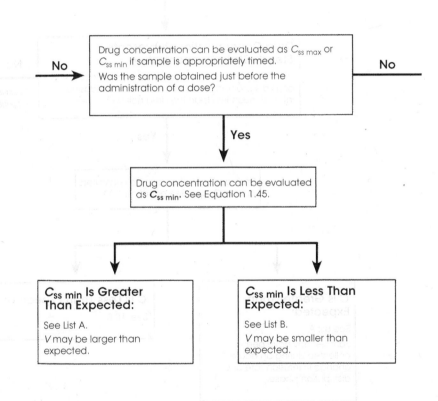

No →

Drug concentration can be evaluated as $C_{ss\,max}$ or $C_{ss\,min}$ if sample is appropriately timed.
Was the sample obtained just before the administration of a dose?

← **No**

Yes

Drug concentration can be evaluated as $C_{ss\,min}$. See Equation 1.45.

$C_{ss\,min}$ Is Greater Than Expected:

See List A.
V may be larger than expected.

$C_{ss\,min}$ Is Less Than Expected:

See List B.
V may be smaller than expected.

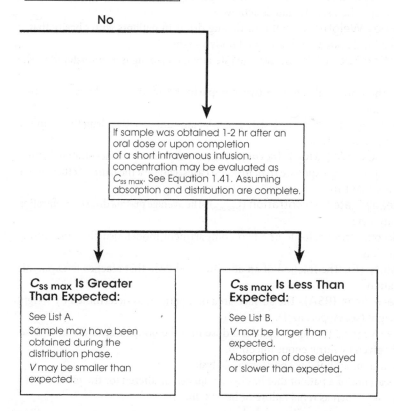

List A

When drug concentrations are greater than expected, consider:

1. Increased bioavailability. This is only important if the drug's bioavailability is usually low.
2. Nonadherence. Intake is greater than prescribed.
3. Decreased clearance.
4. Increased plasma protein binding. Changes in plasma protein binding will be most important if fu is ≤0.1 and are unlikely to be significant if fu is >0.5. Increased plasma protein binding will also decrease the volume of distribution and clearance of most drugs.

List B

When drug concentrations are less than expected, consider:

1. Decreased bioavailability.
2. Nonadherence. Intake is less than prescribed.
3. Increased clearance.
4. Decreased plasma protein binding. Changes in plasma protein binding will be most important if fu is ≤0.1. It is unlikely to be significant if fu is >0.5. Decreased plasma protein binding will also increase the volume of distribution and the clearance of most drugs.

No

If sample was obtained 1-2 hr after an oral dose or upon completion of a short intravenous infusion, concentration may be evaluated as $C_{ss\,max}$. See Equation 1.41. Assuming absorption and distribution are complete.

$C_{ss\,max}$ Is Greater Than Expected:

See List A.

Sample may have been obtained during the distribution phase.

V may be smaller than expected.

$C_{ss\,max}$ Is Less Than Expected:

See List B.

V may be larger than expected.

Absorption of dose delayed or slower than expected.

Appendix 4

Glossary of Terms and Abbreviations

Accumulation Factor: $1/(1 - e^{-K\tau})$ or the degree to which a maintenance dose will accumulate when steady state is achieved.

Adjusted Body Weight: A weight for dosing drugs in patients with obesity that is between ideal body weight and total body weight.

Administration Rate (R_A): The average rate at which a drug is administered to the patient.

Alpha (α): The initial half-life in a two-compartment model, usually representing distribution (see Figure 1.9).

Amount of Drug in the Body (Ab): The total amount of active drug that is in the body at any given time.

Area Under the Curve (AUC_{24}): The concentration area in units of concentration $\times$ time. A measure of drug exposure that, in some cases, can be a measure of efficacy. See Chapters 6 and 16.

Average Steady-State Concentration ($C_{ss\,ave}$): The average plasma drug concentration at steady state.

Beta (β): Second decay half-life in a two-compartment model, usually representing elimination.

Bioavailability (F): The fraction of an administered dose that reaches the systemic circulation.

Body Surface Area (BSA): The surface area of a patient, as determined by weight and height (see Appendix 1).

Bolus Dose: A model for rapid input of a dose into the body or an individual dose, usually given by intravenous injection.

CAPD: Continuous ambulatory peritoneal dialysis.

$Cl_{adjusted}$: Clearance of a patient that has been adjusted or altered for the presence of a disease state such as renal failure or heart failure.

Cl_{CAPD}: Drug clearance by peritoneal dialysis.

Cl_{CRRT}: Drug clearance by CRRT (see CRRT).

Cl_{dial}: Drug clearance by dialysis.

Cl_{pat}: Drug clearance of a patient, usually associated with decreased renal function.

Clearance (Cl_t or Cl): Total body clearance is a measure of how well a patient can metabolize or eliminate drug. It is used to calculate maintenance doses or average steady-state plasma concentrations.

Clearance, Metabolic (Cl_m): A measure of how well the body can metabolize drugs. The major metabolic organ is usually the liver.

Clearance, Renal (Cl_r): A measure of how well the kidneys can excrete unchanged or unmetabolized drug. It is usually assumed to be proportional to creatinine clearance.

C': Plasma concentration measured in the patients with altered plasma protein binding.

C_1: The initial plasma concentration at the beginning of a decay phase, usually following a loading dose.

C_2: The drug concentration at the end of a decay phase.

$C_{desired}$: Plasma concentration desired following an incremental loading dose.

C free: Unbound or free plasma concentration.

C Normal Binding: Plasma concentration that would be observed or measured if a patient's plasma protein binding is normal.

$C_{initial}$: Plasma concentration present in a patient before an incremental loading dose.

$C_{t_{in}}$: Plasma concentration at the end of a short infusion or at the end of absorption.

$C_{ss\,ave}$: Average plasma concentration at steady state.

$C_{ss\,max}$: The maximum or peak concentration at steady state, when a constant dose is administered at a constant dosing interval.

$C_{ss\,min}$: The minimum or trough concentration at steady state, when a constant dose is administered at a constant dosing interval.

Continuous Renal Replacement Therapy: A type of hemodialysis that is continuous versus intermittent.

Creatinine Clearance (Cl_{Cr}): A measure of the kidney's ability to eliminate creatinine from the body. Total renal function is usually assumed to be proportional to creatinine clearance.

CRRT: See Continuous Renal Replacement Therapy.

ΔC: Change in plasma concentration resulting from a single dose.

Dosing Interval (τ): The time interval between doses when a drug is given intermittently.

Dry Weight: Weight of a patient before excessive third-space fluid weight gain.

Dwell Time (T_D): The time between instillation and removal of a peritoneal dialysis exchange volume.

e^{-Kt}: Fraction remaining at the end of a time interval.

$1 - e^{-Kt}$: (a) Fraction lost during a dosing interval at steady state, if $t = \tau$; (b) fraction of steady state achieved during a constant infusion t hours after starting the infusion.

Elimination Rate Constant (K): The fractional rate of drug loss from the body or the fraction of the volume of distribution that is cleared of drug during a time interval.

Elimination Rate (R_E): The amount of drug eliminated from the body during a time interval.

Extraction Ratio: Fraction of drug that is removed from the blood or plasma as it passes through the eliminating organ.

First-Pass: Drug removed from the blood or plasma, following absorption from the gastrointestinal tract, before reaching the systemic circulation.

First-Order Elimination: A process whereby the amount or concentration of drug in the body diminishes logarithmically over time. The rate of elimination is proportional to the drug concentration.

fu: Fraction of total plasma concentration that is free or unbound.

Half-Life ($t_{1/2}$): Time required for the plasma concentration to be reduced to one-half of the original value.

Half-Life, Alpha ($\alpha\ t_{1/2}$): Initial decay half-life, usually representing distribution of drug into the tissue or slowly equilibrating second compartment in a two-compartmental model.

Half-Life, Beta ($\beta\ t_{1/2}$): Second decay half-life, usually representing the elimination half-life. Half-life, β for most drugs can be calculated using the elimination rate constant.

Ideal Body Weight (IBW): Body weight used as an estimate of nonobese weight.

Incremental Loading Dose: An adjusted loading dose required to achieve a desired plasma concentration (C desired) when a preexisting plasma concentration (C observed) is present.

Initial Volume of Distribution (V_i): Initial volume into which the drug rapidly equilibrates following an intravenous bolus dose injection.

Iterative Search: A trial-and-error process to determine patient-specific pharmacokinetic parameters when direct solutions are not possible owing to the nature of the pharmacokinetic model.

$K_{adjusted}$: Elimination rate constant that has been adjusted or altered for the presence of a disease state such as renal failure.

K_{dial}: Elimination rate constant representing both the patient's drug clearance and the drug clearance by dialysis.

Km (Michaelis-Menten Constant): Plasma concentration at which the rate of metabolism is half the maximum rate.

$K_{metabolic}$ (K_m): Elimination rate constant calculated from the metabolic clearance and the volume of distribution (Cl_m/V).

K_{renal} (K_r): Elimination rate constant calculated from the renal clearance and the volume of distribution (Cl_r/V).

Linear Pharmacokinetics: Assumes the elimination rate constant is not affected by plasma drug concentration and that the rate of drug elimination is directly proportional to the concentration of drug in plasma.

ln: Natural logarithm using the base 2.718 rather than 10, which is used for the common logarithm or log.

Loading Dose: Initial total dose required to rapidly achieve a desired plasma concentration.

Maintenance Dose: The dose required to replace the amount of drug lost from the body so that a desired plasma concentration can be maintained.

Mass Balance: The process of comparing drug administration rate (R_A) to the rate of change of drug in the body ((ΔC)(V)/t) in order to estimate drug elimination rate (R_E).

Modified Diet in Renal Disease (MDRD): Equation used for estimating glomerular filtration rate (GFR).

N: The number of doses that have been administered at a fixed-dosing interval.

One-Compartment Model: Assumes that drug distributes rapidly and equally to all areas of the body. Most drugs can be modeled this way if sampling during the initial distribution phase is avoided.

P_{NL} or P': Plasma protein concentration. P_{NL} refers to the normal plasma protein concentration and P' refers to the plasma protein concentration of the specific patient.

Pharmacokinetics: Study of the absorption, distribution, metabolism, and excretion of a drug and its metabolites in the body.

Plasma Concentration (C): Concentration of drug in plasma. Usually refers to the total drug concentration and includes both the bound and unbound or free drug concentration.

Salt Form (S): Fraction of administered salt or ester form of the drug that is the active moiety.

Sensitivity Analysis: The practice of examining the relationship between a change in either clearance or volume of distribution and the corresponding change in the calculated plasma concentration (see Chapter 2: Interpretation of Plasma Drug Concentrations: Sensitivity Analysis).

SCr: Serum creatinine concentration.

Steady State: Steady state is achieved when the rate of drug administration is equal to the rate of drug elimination.

$t_{90\%}$: Time required to achieve 90% of steady state for phenytoin on a fixed-dosing regimen in a patient with known values of V, Vm, and Km.

Tau (τ): See Dosing Interval.

$\tau - t_{in}$: Time from end of infusion to trough concentration when using a short infusion model.

t_d: Time of dialysis for intermittent hemodialysis.

t_{in}: Time required for drug to be infused or absorbed.

Tissue Concentration (C_t): Concentration of drug in the tissue.

Tissue Volume of Distribution (V_t): Apparent volume into which the drug appears to distribute following rapid equilibration with the initial volume of distribution.

Total Body Weight (TBW): Total weight of a patient usually used for patients with obesity.

Two-Compartment Model: Composed of an initial, rapidly equilibrating volume of distribution (V_i) and an apparent second, more slowly equilibrating volume of distribution (V_t).

Unbound V: Volume of distribution based on the free or unbound plasma concentration.

Vm: Maximum rate at which metabolism can occur.

Volume of Distribution (V): The apparent volume required to account for all the drug in the body if it was present throughout the body in the same concentration as in the sample obtained from the plasma.

90%t: Duration of therapy on a fixed-dosing regimen that must be exceeded to assure that a measured phenytoin concentration represents steady state.

Index

Note: Page numbers in italics denote figures; those followed by t denote tables